FROM CELLS TO ORGANS.

FROM CELLS TO ORGANS.

A Histology Textbook and Atlas.

Alfons T.L. Van Lommel, Ph.D.

Leuven Catholic University,
Medical Faculty,
Department of Morphology and Medical Imaging,
Section of Morphology and Molecular Pathology,
Minderbroedersstraat 12, 3000 Leuven, Belgium.

Alfons.vanLommel@uz.kuleuven.ac.be

Springer-Science+Business Media, B.V.

Lommel, Alfons T. L. van
    From cells to organs : a histology textbook and atlas / Alfons T.L. van Lommel.
      p.cm.
    Includes bibliographical references and index.
    ISBN 978-1-4613-5035-4   ISBN 978-1-4615-0353-8 (eBook)
    DOI 10.1007/978-1-4615-0353-8

    1. Histology. 2. Histology--Atlases. I. Title.

QM551 .L74 2002
611'.018--dc21

                                2002034121

I dedicate this book to the memory of my father: KAREL VAN LOMMEL (1928-2000)

ACKNOWLEDGEMENTS.

It was not difficult to start writing this book. It was another matter altogether to bring it to completion. Years ago, in the long bygone days when I was a college student, I used a textbook of animal physiology, written by Knut Schmidt-Nielsen. I still vividly remember my surprise when my eye fell on the first sentence of the introduction (in those days, I actually read textbook introductions). I can still cite the exact sentence from memory: "This book was written in anger and frustration.". I did not understand this at the time. It all looked so very easy! Now I know better, much better. Writing a book is like getting married or having children. You don't know what you have begun, but don't worry: you'll know soon enough. Dickens and Tolstoi were heard to complain, when they were writing what later was to become one of their immortal masterpieces, that they wished they had never begun it. I wouldn't dream of comparing myself with these Olympian gods, but I have felt something very similar. This doesn't mean that I regret having written this book, far from it. It made me think about histology, it taught me histology, and I feel that I know far more about histology now than when I got started.

Writing this book, and preparing its numerous illustrations, took many lonely hours, more, in fact, than I care to recall. But I did not do it entirely by myself. Many people, one way or another, have assisted me. I take this opportunity to express my gratitude to them.

First of all, I have to thank my editors at Kluwer: Mimi Breed, Joanne Tracy, and Arno Flier, who helped me in the complex task of bringing this work before an international public. Their interest and constant encouragement, from the very start, have been an immense stimulus.

You can't write a book like this without illustrations. Histology is a very "visual" science, and pictures say so much more than words. For illustrations you need appropriately processed tissue sections that can be photographed. Making a good job of this calls for the kind of professionalism and dexterity which take years to acquire, and doing this yourself may theoretically be possible, but in practice it is out of the question. That is why I am immensely indebted to my laboratory technicians: Rolande Renwart, Chris Armee, and Martine Verhoeven. I taxed their time, their patience, and their professional skills to the limit, but they did a splendid job, and the quality of the illustrations is entirely their merit, not mine.

Although I can dimly remember the days when it was different, nowadays almost everything that matters is done with computers. So is writing and preparing illustrations, which involves working with specific computer programs: Word, Powerpoint, Imaging, and Photo Editor, to name only the most important. This project was an opportunity to familiarize myself with their subtlest applications. Needless to say, I got hopelessly stuck from time to time. It was my good fortune always to run into someone who had just the right item of knowledge to get me going again. To name but a few: Prof. Jos Mebis, Dr. Filip Rega, Dr. Pieter Leyssen, Mireille Goedhuys, Vanessa Van De Plas, Marcella Bervoets, and Mariette Van Aerschot. For photographic assistance, I thank Andre Vandormael and Michel Rooseleer.

Another of my handicaps is that English is not my mother tongue (which is Dutch, by the way). My book proposal was professionally translated into English by Agius Translating Agency, London. The sample chapters were proofread by Prof. Ed Conway, department of Molecular and Vascular Biology, and Prof. Neil Taylor, department of Human Genetics, both of the KULeuven medical faculty. I found their positive appreciation of the text and its contents most encouraging.

I shall never know who the reviewers are who were approached by Kluwer to evaluate my proposal. Apparently, they reviewed it positively, otherwise I would not now be writing these words. I thank them, whoever they may be, for their constructive evaluation.

I owe a special word of thanks to my colleague Prof. Erik Verbeken. His moral and, on occasion, material support have vitally contributed to the completion of this book, and for this, I continue to be appreciative.

Last but not least I have to thank my parents and my family. Indirectly, they made it possible for me to devote my time to this book, and to acquire the talents necessary for it. My parents gave me every opportunity to study and to pursue an education. I now understand that I would not be what I am and where I am today if they had not kept believing in me, no matter how difficult this may have been sometimes. I also see now that there have been times when I was so occupied with this book that I tended to forget that I still am husband and father. When I ran into problems, I often took them home with me. The rest of the family had no alternative but to endure this and hope for better times. So let me very warmly thank my wife Christl, my son Joris, and my daughter Katrien, for bearing with me all the time I was working on this book, and for still being with me now that it is completed.

TABLE OF CONTENTS.

Abbreviations used in the figure legends: HE: hematoxylin-eosin, a standard combination of stains in routine
light microscopy.
TEM: transmission electron microscopy.
SEM: scanning electron microscopy.

INTRODUCTION.

Histology is the science that investigates the microscopic structure of the body and, from this, attempts to draw inferences regarding its functions. Of course, the body's functions can never be completely understood from this morphological approach alone. Nevertheless, the body's morphology is one of its basic aspects and histology has contributed, and continues to do so to this day, to analyze and understand it. Histology's central dogma is that form is related to function. This principle does not always work equally well. Examples can be found of cells and tissues, the functions of which can hardly be understood from their morphology alone. In general though, this principle has stood the test of time.

The microscopic structure of the body can be studied at three levels: cells, tissues, and organs.
The most fundamental building blocks of the body are the **cells**. The human body contains an impressive number of them. Estimates are in excess of ten thousand billion (something in the order of 10^{13}). Cells are the smallest, least complex entities that show all the characteristics we associate with life, such as metabolism, motility, sensitivity to stimuli, and reproduction. They are the only components of the body that, in theory, are capable of independent life: they can be maintained, for longer or shorter periods of time, in culture. Another indication of the cell's capability of independent life is the existence of unicellular organisms. Cells may be the least complex entities which are capable of independent life, but that doesn't mean that they are simple. In fact, cells are quite complex themselves. They are composed of smaller and simpler (again, this term has to be understood in the relative sense) entities: **organelles**. Organelles are not capable of independent life. They are the organs of the cell, which they maintain. They also enable the cell to carry out functions which do not benefit the cell itself, but which contribute to the well being of the body. This is the essence of multicellular life. There are several kinds of organelles, and cells may possess various selections and combinations of them, depending on their function. This means that many cell types are in existence. They will be discussed in the following pages. Cells combine into structures with a higher level of organization: **tissues**. A tissue is a collection of identical, or at least closely cooperating, cells. Cells have various shapes and may be joined in various ways. This means that several types of tissue exist, from simple to complex ones. Tissues participate in the formation of something more complex still: **organs**. Organs vary regarding the number of tissues they are made of and the complexity of these tissues. In simple organs, only a single tissue may be apparent. Complex organs may contain five or six different tissues.

This, in a few words, is the essence of what will be discussed in the following pages. For better understanding, it may be useful to start with a brief representation of the most fundamental methods used in microscopic investigation.

Only a few lines of what follows, those about pulmonary endocrine cells, are based on my own personal research and observations. The rest has been gathered from the very kind of textbooks I used during my own training as a scientist and a teacher, and from more recent publications of other scientists. At the end of each chapter, a number of references are appended. Most of these are reviews: overviews and summaries of basic research papers, written by an expert in the field. These references are included for a double reason. It is only fair that fellow scientists are given their due credit by citing their publications. Also, by including these references, the reader may be encouraged to check things for him or herself (You don't have to take my word for anything!), thereby adopting the scientific way of doing things.

I. METHODS OF STUDY.

In this chapter, a brief survey will be given of the most common routine methods to study the microscopic structure of cells, tissues, and organs.

I.1. Microscopes.

Cells, the fundamental building blocks of the body, are minute objects: their dimensions are expressed in **micrometers**. One micrometer is 0.001 millimeter. Organelles, the subcomponents of cells, are smaller still: their dimensions are usually expressed in **nanometers**. A nanometer is 0.001 micrometer, or 0.000 001 millimeter. Even in ideal conditions, the human eye cannot make out objects smaller than about 0.15 millimeter, or 150 micrometers. This is the eye's maximal **resolution**. It means that cells are much too small to be seen by naked human eyes. Cells can only be observed with the help of a more powerful lens system: a microscope. Conform to the laws of optics, microscopes form images of small objects, magnified to such an extent that the resolution of the human eye is sufficient to make them out.

The optic microscope or **light microscope** is, at least in its basic form, a fairly simple instrument, everyone with scientific notions is familiar with. It contains glass lenses and uses visible light. The most primitive models were built as long ago as the 17th century. In the course of four centuries, the performance of light microscopes has been pushed to the limits of what is technically possible. Nevertheless, there remains a physical limit to the amount of detail a light microscope can show: light's wavelength. The mean wavelength of visible light is about 0.55 micrometer (550 nanometers). The smallest object which can be made out with a light microscope cannot be much smaller than this. Actually, the size of the smallest object that a good light microscope can show is close to 0.2 micrometer. In other words, the resolution of the light microscope is about 750 (150 / 0.2) times better than that of the naked eye. In the previous alinea, it was mentioned that a microscope produces a magnified image of an object, to enable the eye to make it out. In order for the eye to see an object with a diameter of 0.2 micrometer, magnification must be 750 times, so that its apparent diameter is 0.15 millimeter. Can magnification be increased still further, in order to see still smaller things? Intuitively, one may be inclined to think so, but things are not as simple as that. Technically, it is a piece of cake to magnify more than 750 times. In lecture rooms, microscopic images are projected on a screen, which

amounts to magnifications of thousands or millions of times. Still, objects smaller than 0.2 micrometer will not pop into view. The resolution of the light microscope, or any optic system using visible light, such as a projector, simply does not suffice to produce images of objects that small. Thus, the maximal practical or useful magnification that is attainable with a light microscope is about 750 times. The resolution of a microscope is a measure of the amount of detail it can show. The light microscope has sufficient resolution to observe single cells and the way they are arranged into tissues and organs. It has insufficient resolution to make out the details of the cell's internal structure.

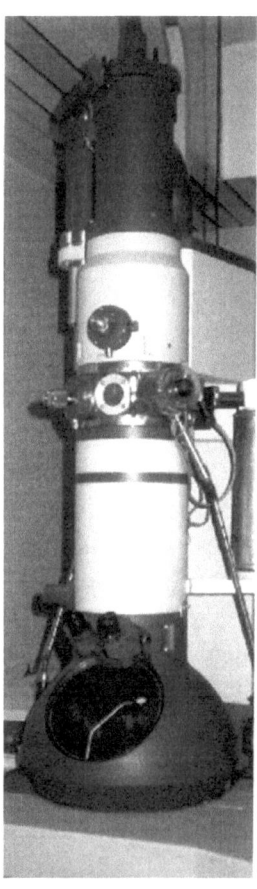

Fig. 1.1. A transmission electron microscope has the shape of a column (c). The radiation source is a filament that is at the upper end of the column. A sample is introduced into the column through an air lock (a). The column houses strong electromagnets that focus the electron beam, produced by the filament. The electron beam strikes a fluorescent screen at the bottom of the column, which can be observed through a pair of binoculars (b).

In the fifties of the 20th century, the **electron microscope** (Fig. 1.1.) came into general use, although its working principle had been discovered some 20

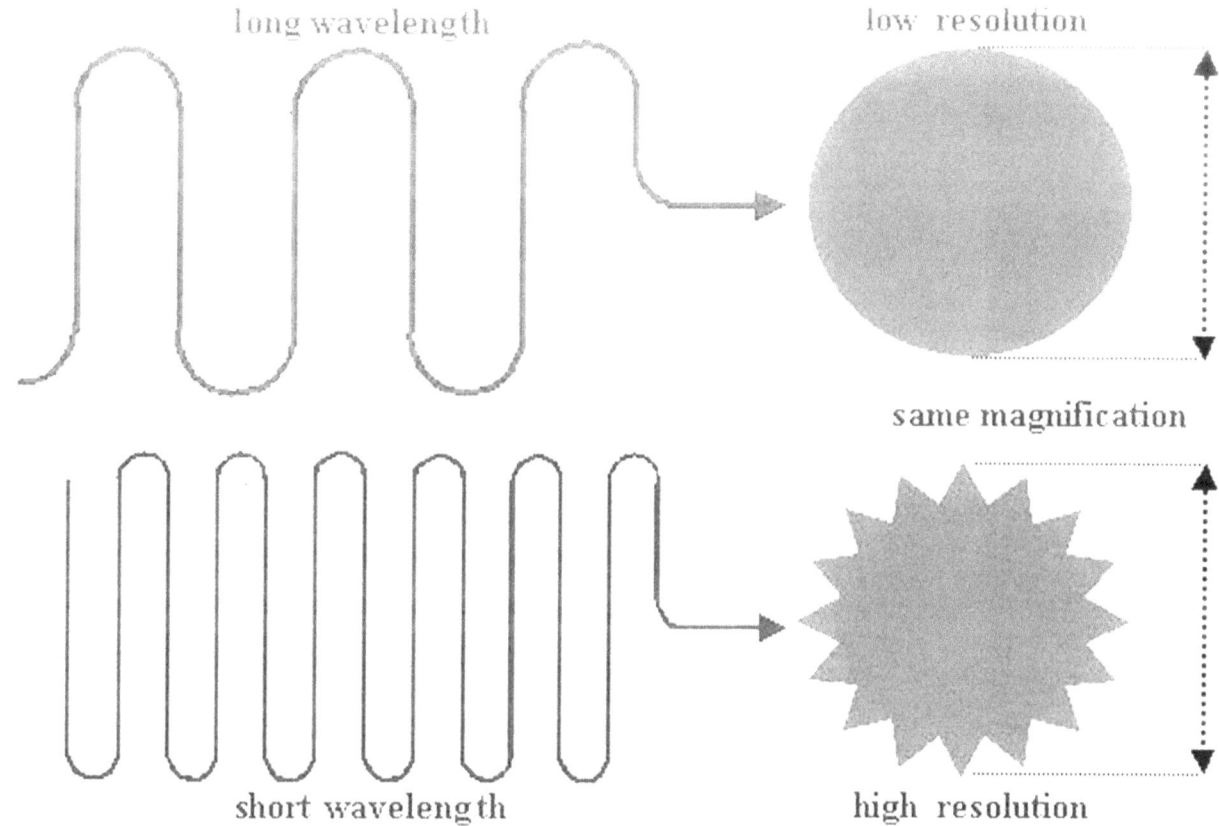

long wavelength

low resolution

same magnification

short wavelength

high resolution

Fig. 1.2. The link between wavelength and resolution. At the same magnification, the use of radiation with a smaller wavelength allows demonstration of smaller details: the resolution of the image increases.

years earlier. This device makes use of electromagnets, which serve as "lenses", focusing a bundle of electrons which, when accelerated under sufficient voltage, behave like electromagnetic radiation. The wavelength of this radiation depends on the acceleration voltage, and can be as small as a fraction of a nanometer. Consequently, the resolution of an electron microscope is at least a thousand times better than that of a light microscope. This allows useful (i.e. showing more detail) magnifications of several ten thousand times. At the resolution made possible by electron microscopy, the ultrastructure of the cell, with its organelles, can be observed. Observation must be indirect, however, since the human eye is insensitive to electrons. After having interacted with the object under observation, the electron beam falls on a fluorescent screen, producing an image. One of several major problems that had to be solved to make electron microscopy feasible was the inability of electron beams to travel through air. The electron beam is handled in an airtight column, in which a high vacuum is maintained.

In conclusion, there is a direct link between the wavelength of the electromagnetic radiation used and the resolution that can be obtained at a certain magnification (Fig. 1.2.). People intuitively think that it is sufficient simply to increase the magnification to see more details. A microscope is indeed a device that produces enlarged, or magnified, images. But magnification is secondary. The primary purpose of a microscope is to allow better resolution. Magnification only makes sense if resolution can be increased proportionally. These points are beautifully illustrated by comparison of a light microscopic and an electron microscopic image of the same type of cell at the same magnification (Figs. 1.3.-4.).

Other types of microscopes exist, which are variations on the two fundamental types, light and electron microscopes.

Fluorescence microscopy is a routinely used variant of light microscopy. Fluorescence is the emission of light of a certain wavelength by an object upon excitation with light of a shorter wavelength (and thus higher energy). A **fluorescence microscope** excites objects to be visualized at a specified shorter wavelength by means of ultraviolet light or a laser,

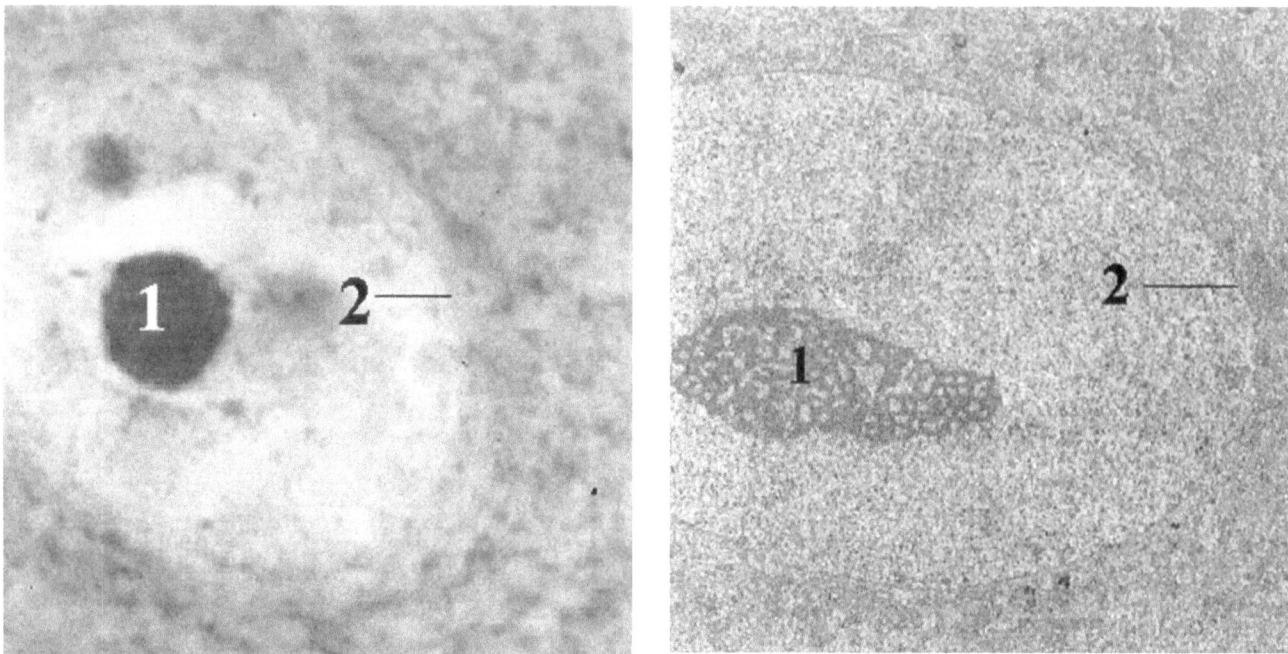

Fig. 1.3. (left) A light microscopic image of a sensory nerve cell's perikaryon, magnified about 8000 times, which is far beyond the useful magnification of the light microscope. Indicative for this is the unsharp, hazy aspect of the picture. Spinal ganglion, rabbit, HE. **Fig. 1.4.** (right) An electron microscopic image of the same cell as in Figure 1.3., also magnified about 8000 times. Although the magnification is the same, the electron microscopic image is far sharper and shows much more detail than the light optic one, i.e. its resolution is far greater. Identical parts are indicated with the same numbers. Figures 1.3. and 1.4. illustrate the link between wavelength and resolution. Spinal ganglion, rabbit, TEM.

inducing emission in the visible part of the spectrum. The emission can be viewed, or, by means of a photodetector, be analyzed quantitatively (intensity) or qualitatively (spectrum). Fluorescence can be natural, but most often an object is made to fluoresce by attaching a fluorescent label to it. The eye is sensitive to fairly low light intensities and to color, making fluorescence microcopy a powerful tool in the detection of various cell and tissue components (I.3.).

The latest novelty concerning light microscopy is the **confocal microscope** (Fig. 1.5.). This is a fluorescence microscope, equipped with a diaphragm, which is placed in a confocal position relative to the objective lens. A commonly encountered problem with fluorescence microscopy is that not all of the emission one obtains is in focus, i.e. originating in the focal plane of the objective lens. The diaphragm used by the confocal microscope is positioned thus that it only allows the focused part of the light beam to enter a photodetector. In this way, only a single focused point is produced, however, not an entire image. To obtain this, a laser beam systematically scans the whole object, and a pattern of points is generated, all of them in focus. These points are stored, in digital form (pixels), on the hard disk of a computer, and used to build up an image. The resulting image, or optic

section, is sharper than one that is obtained with conventional fluorescence microscopy, because the "noise" has been filtered out. The essence of a confocal microscope is that the image formation process is not entirely optical, but involves computer technology. Confocal images cannot be seen by looking into the microscope. They are in the computer's memory, and appear on a monitor. While a conventional fluorescence microscope can only focus on a single plane, and record single images, the computer connected with a confocal microscope can store images obtained at successive levels of the same object. These can be stacked, producing an extended depth of focus image, which is sharp throughout its entire thickness (Figs. 3.6.2., 4.4.15.). Successive optical sections can also be stored individually, allowing three-dimensional reconstruction. When several lasers are used, different emissions can be obtained and recorded, each of them highlighting different parts of the object. Computer technology allows superposition of two or more emissions to obtain a composite image (Fig. 3.6.1.).

The electron microscope comes in several variants as well. The type shown in Fig. 1.1. is a **transmission electron microscope**, which produces images by means of radiation that falls through the object to be

confocal microscopy

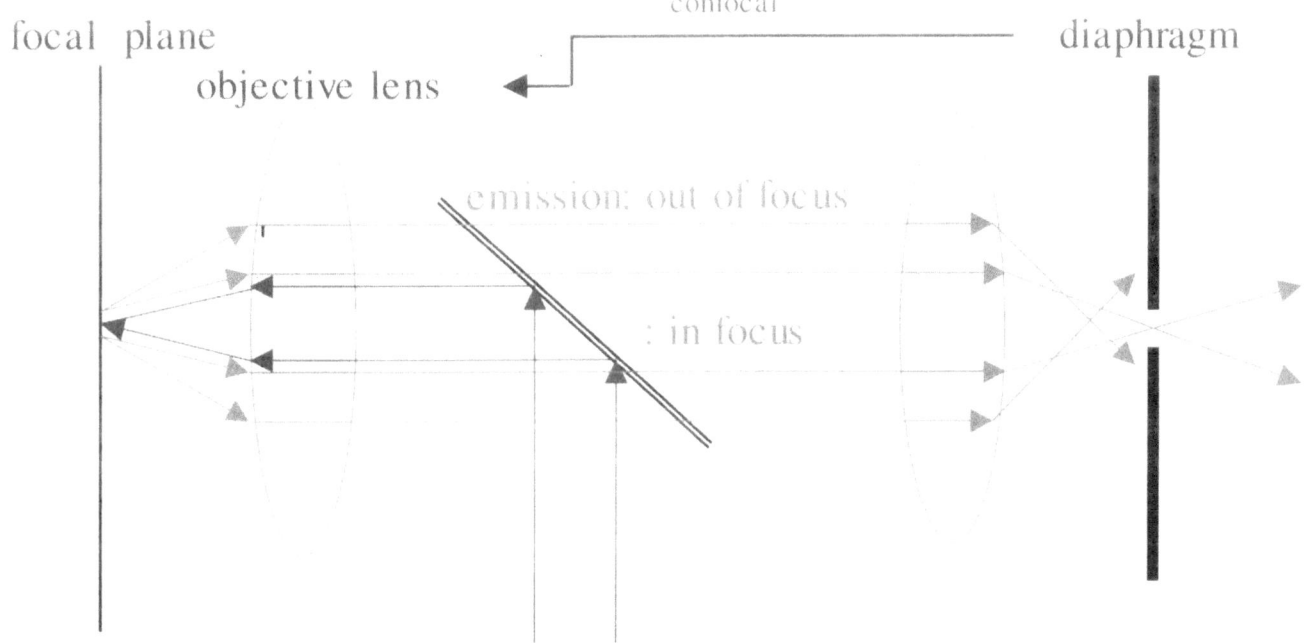

excitation: laser

Fig. 1.5. The principle of confocal microscopy. A tissue slide is scanned by a laser, which excites certain fluorescent substances in the tissue, which produces a characteristic emission. A diaphragm or pinhole, placed confocally relative to the objective lens, only allows passage of emission in focus. Thus, a focused point is obtained. Systematic scanning of a slide results in a series of points or pixels, which are digitally processed and used to construct an image.

observed. Light microscopes are also transmission microscopes. Another type of electron microscope is the **scanning electron microscope**. This type makes use of reflected radiation to obtain images. This allows three-dimensional observation (compare Figs. 3.1.2. and 3.1.3.). Images are observed on a monitor. Preparation of objects for observation with scanning electron microscopy involves coating them with an electron-reflecting heavy metal layer.

I.2. Histologic sections.

The microscopic structure of biological material usually cannot be studied without special preparation. It has to be fixated, embedded, sectioned, mounted, and stained. In this way, histologic sections can be prepared which can be kept permanently.

Biological material is perishable, and the first step in converting it into permanent sections is to fixate it. A

sample is treated with a **fixative**, a chemical solution that irreversibly changes the sample's chemical structure, so that any enzymes it contains are inactivated and that it becomes unfit as a substrate for enzymes and microorganisms. Many kinds of fixatives exist, from simple solutions to quite complicated mixtures. Most often, fixatives are used as watery, buffered solutions. In light microscopy, frequent use is made of **formaldehyde**, or mixtures based on it, such as Bouin's fixative (formaldehyde, acetic acid, and picric acid). In electron microscopy, the most popular fixatives are **glutaraldehyde** and **osmium tetroxide**, most often used in combination. Glutaraldehyde has two aldehyde groups, in contrast to formaldehyde's single one, and is able to form cross-links between proteins, resulting in better fixation. This is important, since electron microscopy allows observation of greater detail. The use of osmium tetroxide results in better preservation of lipids, so that cell membranes show more clearly. Fixative penetrates a biological sample by diffusion, a

5

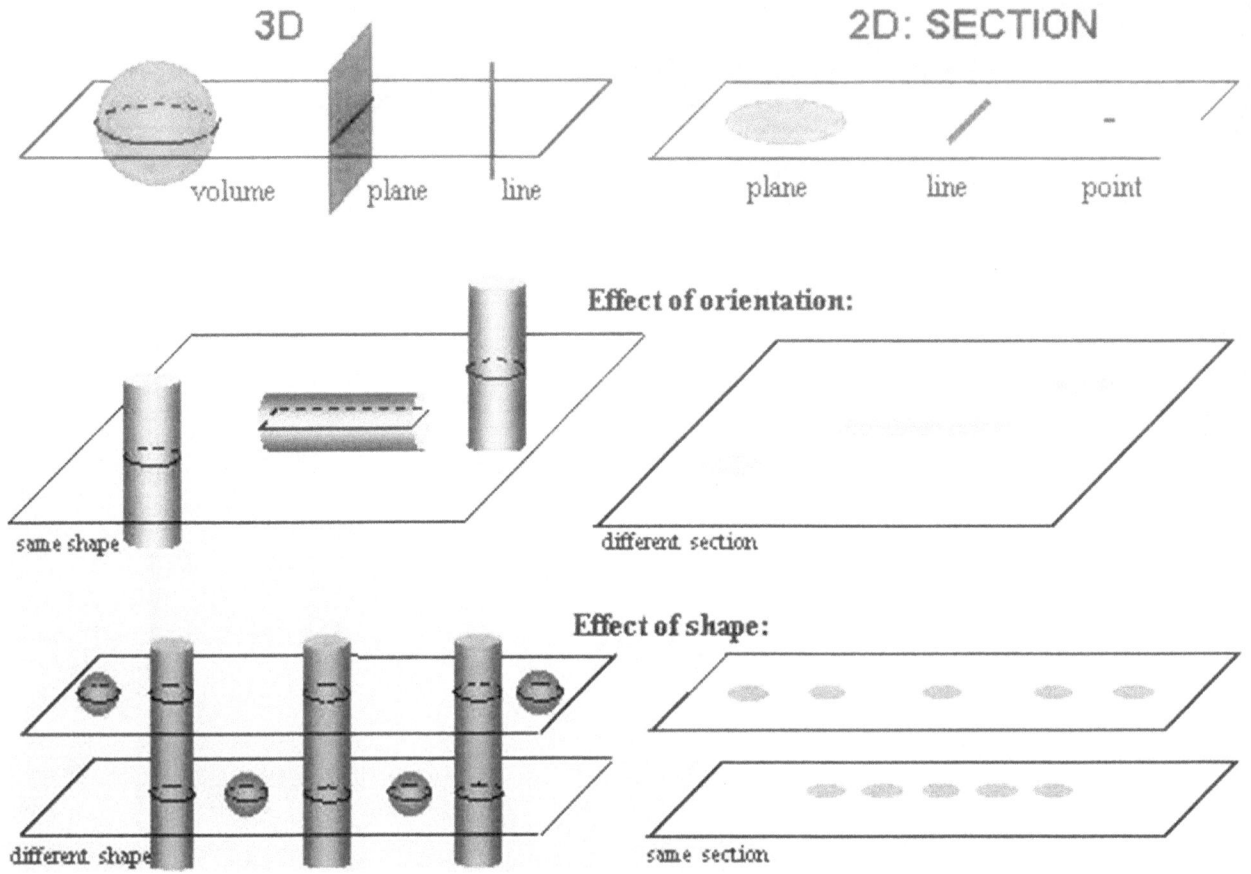

Fig. 1.6. The effect of cutting. Samples have to be cut, or sectioned, to allow observation with transmission microscopes, optic as well as electronic. In a tissue section, the third dimension is lost. This can produce surprising effects, which have to be taken into account while interpreting observations. Variations in the orientation of identical objects can result in different section shapes. Alternatively, different objects can produce identical section shapes.

relatively slow process that only works over short distances. For obvious reasons, fixation must be rapid and homogeneous. Fixation can be done by immersion, but to obtain satisfactory results the sample has to be small and large volumes of fixative have to be used. A better method is perfusion, whereby fixative is injected via the blood vessels.

Most microscopes are transmission microscopes, making use of radiation that penetrates the object under observation. Obviously, this won't work when the object is too thick to allow penetration of radiation. Cutting the biological sample into thin slices or **sections** circumvents this problem. In light microscopy, section thickness varies between 5 and 10 micrometers. Electrons have even less penetrating power than light has, and to prepare samples for electron microscopy, sections of about 50 nanometers in thickness have to be cut. Sectioning is done with a **microtome**, a device that allows a sample to be moved up and down against the cutting edge of a knife. After each cycle of the sample's movement, the knife advances a fixed distance, so that a thin slice is cut during the next cycle. As such, fixated material is usually not hard enough to allow cutting of sufficiently thin sections. Worse, it is often not equally hard throughout. Therefore, samples are submerged in a fluid which pervades them and which subsequently solidifies or polymerizes, hardening as it does so. When samples are embedded in this way, the embedding material confers sufficient overall hardness to the sample for it to be sectioned. In light microscopy, the most popular embedding media are based on paraffin. Sections are cut with a steel knife. In electron microscopy, where much thinner sections have to be cut, harder embedding media, resins or plastics, are used. Sections are cut with glass or diamond knives. You can't just dump a sample in embedding medium, though, because most of them don't mix with water. Prior to embedding, the fixated material has to be dehydrated in ethanol and toluene. Cut sections are mounted on a glass slide for light microscopy or on a minute copper grid, handled with tweezers, for electron microscopy.

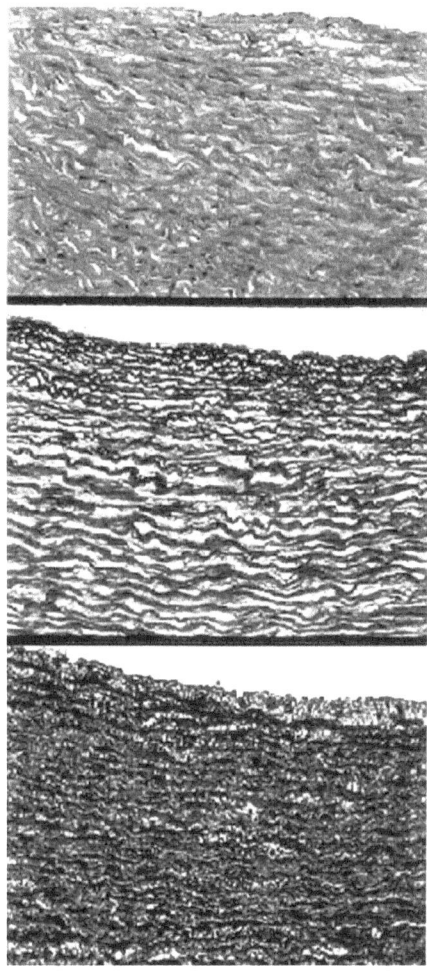

Fig. 1.7. The effect of staining. Tissue sections are stained for improved visualization of their structure. What can be observed depends on the type of stain used. This principle is illustrated by three sections of an elastic artery, stained with different methods. The section at the top was stained with hematoxylin and eosin. Hematoxylin is a dark stain that selectively reacts with cell nuclei, which show up as small dark dots. The cytoplasm of the cells, and the intercellular material, are stained more lightly with eosin. The middle section has been stained with Van Gieson's method. This stain demonstrates dark, wavy objects, which are not that prominent in the other images: elastic fibers. Masson's method, at the bottom, stains another type of fibers, collagen fibers, dark. Each staining method demonstrates another tissue component and by comparing them, a much more complete picture is obtained than is possible on the basis of a single method.

It is possible to simplify the above procedure by rapidly freezing a biological sample in carbon dioxide snow, or in liquid nitrogen. This eliminates the need of chemical fixation and makes the sample hard enough for cutting.
We still don't have a histologic section that is suited to microscopic observation. Such thin sections are not only transparent, but virtually colorless as well. In order to see something, they have to be stained. Since most **stains** come in the form of watery solutions, sections for light microscopy have to be deparaffinized and rehydrated. Then they are submerged in one or several color baths. A routinely used combination of pigments is **hematoxylin** (dark violet, reacts with acid tissue components) and **eosin** (pink red, reacts with alcalic tissue components). After staining, the sections are rinsed, and again dehydrated. They are sealed in Canada balsam or a comparable substance, and covered with a thin glass coverslip. Sections for electron microscopy have to be treated with substances that absorb or deflect electrons. These are oxides or salts of heavy metals: osmium, uranium, and lead. Osmium, in the form of tetroxide, was already applied during fixation. Uranium is applied as acetate, lead as citrate. Tissue components that absorb one or more of these metals will not allow electrons to come through and will appear dark on the electron microscope's fluorescent screen. Other components will light up.

Now we have histologic sections that can be studied with a microscope. But while we are observing, and trying to interpret what we observe, we have to keep in mind a number of things. What we are looking at is a very thin section, which has, to all practical purposes, only two dimensions (Fig. 1.6.). It is not always easy to extrapolate to the third dimension, because loss of the third dimension can play tricks on us (Fig. 1.6.). It is not necessarily so that two identical two-dimensional shapes derive from identical three-dimensional structures. Neither is it always true that different two-dimensional shapes must be of different three-dimensional objects. Fortunately, we can compensate for loss of the third dimension by looking at a large number of two-dimensional shapes, which are usually not all sectioned under the same angle, or at sections from successive levels.
Another important fact is that, as we have seen, biological material has to undergo a whole series of treatments before it is ready for microscopic observation. This inevitably means that what we eventually observe, greatly differs from the living material. So we have to be careful when we extrapolate to the living condition. The staining method, for example, determines which tissue component can be observed and which cannot (Fig. 1.7.). It is not because a certain component cannot be seen that it is not there. It may just not be stained. In a way, histologic sections are a very limited means to study the living world, but we have to make do. Some structures that appear in sections were certainly not there in the fresh sample, but are a consequence of preparation, maybe uncareful preparation. Examples

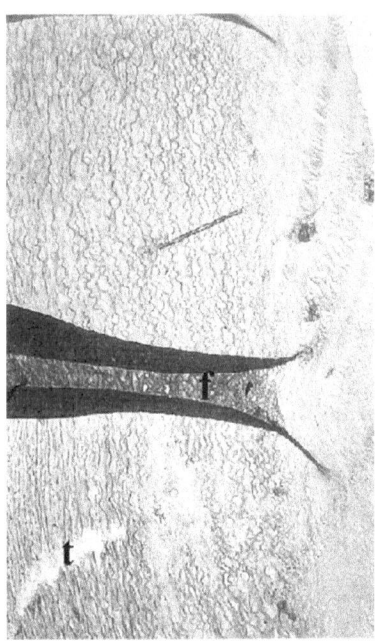

Fig. 1.8. Artefacts. Preparation of material for microscopic observation renders it into something artificial or artefactual. Sometimes, objects show up which were not formed in a controled way. These are artefacts in the narrow sense of the word. In this image, several examples of artefacts are seen, among them a tear (t) and a fold (f).

of such **artefacts** (in the narrow sense of the word, since the whole section is an artefact) are tears, folds, dirt, precipitation or elution of substances, etc. (Fig. 1.8.). Preparation techniques have been perfected to such a degree that such artefacts are avoided as much as possible, or at least standardized. Nevertheless, the preparation of histologic sections calls for great care and professionalism. It is a job requiring skilled technical personnel.

I.3. Histochemistry.

Histology studies the microscopic morphology of the body. The link with cell biology is made with **histochemistry** (or cytochemistry). This discipline attempts to locate, in their original context, specific substances in histologic sections. This may give valuable information about the function of a cell or tissue. Many techniques exist whereby specific substances can be labeled in situ, so that their presence, and their location, can be demonstrated. We will look somewhat closer at two relatively modern techniques: immmunochemistry and hybridochemistry.

Immunochemistry is based on immunologic principles. A section wherein a specific substance is to be demonstrated is treated with a solution containing an **antibody** directed against that substance. This antibody has been produced by certain immune cells, called plasma cells (II.2.1.1.4.), of an animal that was exposed to this substance. A substance against which an antibody is directed is an antigen. If a particular antigen is present in a tissue, the antibody will complementary bind with it. In theory, a molecule must have a complex, variable structure to be able to function as an antigen, which is why many antigens are proteins. Thousands of structural proteins, enzymes, peptides and hormones have been demonstrated with this method, as well as many non-protein molecules, even relatively simple ones.

Hybridochemistry is based on another type of specific binding: that between complementary strands of nucleic acid (II.1.2.). A strand of nucleic acid, called the **probe**, will bind to (hybridize with) a complementary strand in a section. In this way, activated genes and their transcription products can be demonstrated, which is an indirect indication that certain proteins are present.

Antibodies or probes are not visible as such, but are tagged with a label that is visible, or can be made visible, in a section. Labels include fluorescent molecules, radioactive molecules, heavy metals (in electron microscopy) or enzymes, such as peroxidase (Fig. 4.7.5.). In this last case, the tissue has to be treated, additionally, with a chromogen. This is a soluble, colorless substance, which the enzyme will convert to an insoluble pigment.

II. CELLS.

The body may be composed of cells, but they do not constitute its lowest level of organization. Cells contain less complex components, the **organelles** or cellular "organs". These constitute the least complex parts of the organism that can be observed directly by means of microscopy. The organelles themselves are composed of complex macromolecules: proteins, lipids, carbohydrates and nucleic acids. The organelles are embedded in a featureless, gel-like mass, the **cytosol**. Cytosol and organelles form the cell's **cytoplasm**.

The different organs of the body each have their own

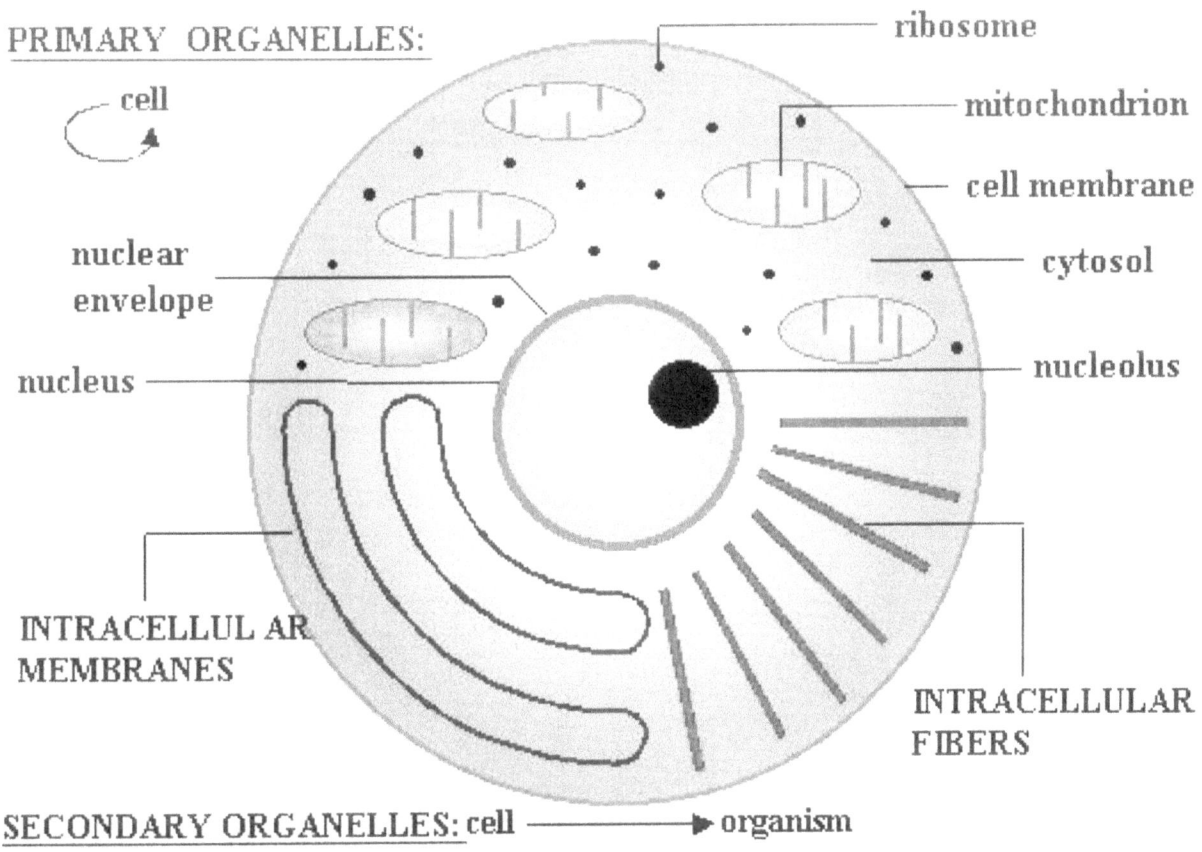

Fig. 2.1. The organelles or cellular "organs". Certain organelles ensure the cell's own survival. They can be called primary organelles. The most important ones are the cell membrane (the cell's "skin"), the cell nucleus (the genetic archive, containing the blueprint of proteins) and nucleolus, the ribosomes (which synthesize proteins) and the mitochondria (energy suppliers). Most cells contain additional organelles, which they need to exert a function that is necessary to the survival of the organism of which the cell is part: secondary organelles. The particular set of secondary organelles a cell is observed to contain, indicate the function it happens to be specialized in. Two major types of secondary organelles may be distinguished. Intracellular membranes take part in the synthesis of various substances, which the cell will liberate. The intracellular fibers support and strengthen the cell, or give it contractile properties.

specific function, and so have the organelles. In this respect, we can distinguish two fundamentally different types of organelle (Fig. 2.1.). In the first place, there are organelles that accomplish the cell's primary life functions, such as storage and use of genetic information, energy supply, and synthesis of the cell's own substances. The cell needs these organelles to stay alive, to maintain itself. These can be called the **primary organelles**. In the second place, there are organelles which are not necessary for the cell's survival, but which enable the cell to carry out a specific function. This function is essential, not to the cell's own existence, but to the functioning of the organism of which this cell is part. These kinds of organelles can be called the **secondary organelles**.

In principle, every cell possesses the primary organelles mentioned above. Embryonic cells, which have as yet no specific function, only possess primary organelles. In a fully developed organism, the cells are differentiated, i.e. they are adapted to specific functions. In order to exercise a particular function,

9

they need a specific set of secondary organelles. A large number (more than 200 according to certain estimates) of different cell types can thus be distinguished, each specifically adapted to a certain function. An overview of these various types is somewhat simplified by the fact that most cells can be classed under a few fundamental types and subtypes.

II.1. Primary organelles.

The primary organelles assure the cell's own survival. They are the **cell membrane**, the **cell nucleus**, the **ribosomes**, the **mitochondria** and the **peroxisomes**.

II.1.1. Cell membrane.

The cell membrane is the cell's "skin" and forms the boundary between the cytosol and the cell's outside world. It is by no means an inert envelope. The cell membrane is sensitive to various stimuli and controls the transport of substances between the cytoplasm and the extracellular space. The cell membrane is slightly less than 10 nanometers thick. Consequently, it can only be observed with the electron microscope.

The macromolecules building the cell membrane (Fig. 2.2.) cannot be observed directly with microscopy and, as such, strictly do not belong to this text's subject matter. Yet a basic understanding of the function of these molecules is relevant, since the typical

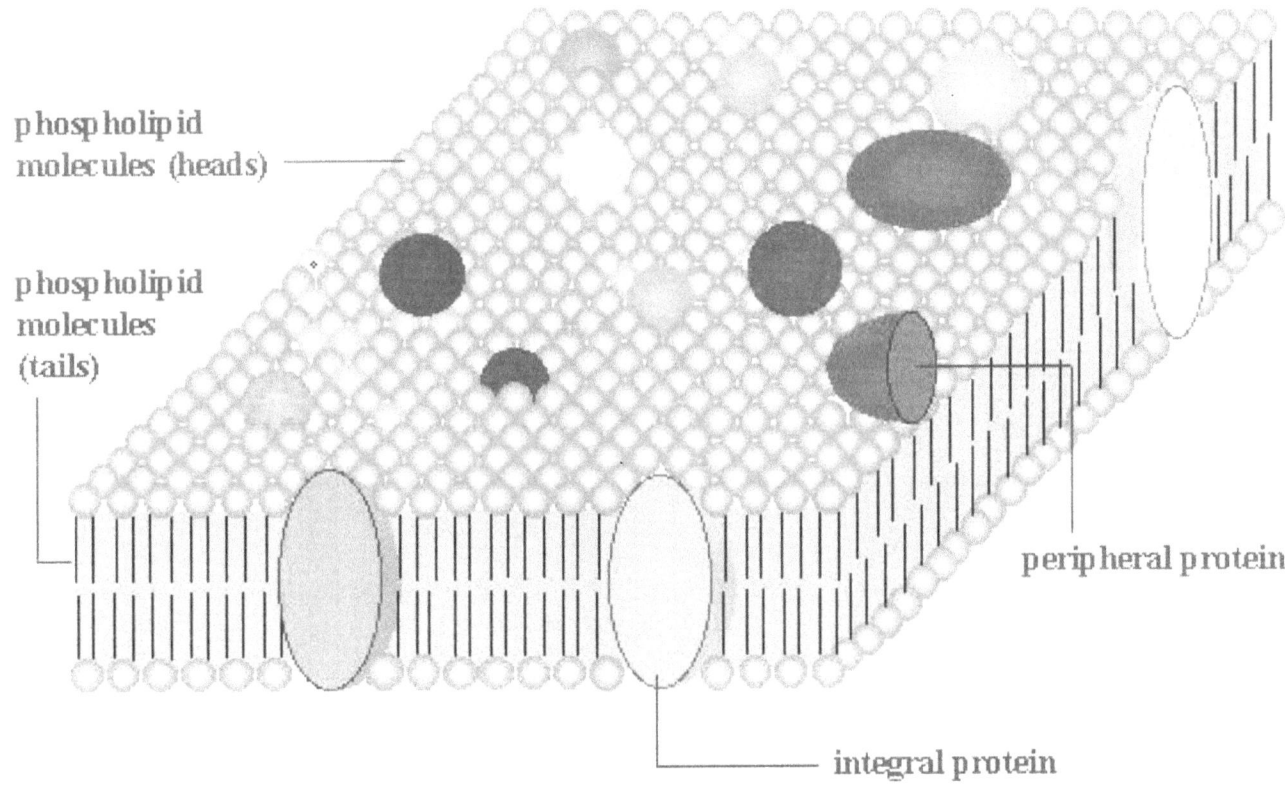

Fig. 2.2. The molecular structure of the cell membrane. The cell membrane consists of two layers of phospholipid molecules, with the hydrophobic tails of both layers touching. Embedded in this phospholipid bilayer are integral proteins. Peripheral proteins are more loosely associated with the bilayer surface.

characteristics of the cell membrane, many aspects of which can be observed microscopically, directly depend on them. The most important macromolecules of the cell membrane are **lipids** and **proteins**.

The lipids building the cell membrane belong to several categories, among which are the **phospholipids**. These molecules can be visualized as having a "head" and a "tail". The head is a phosphate-group, esterified with a glycerol molecule. The tail consists of two fatty acid molecules, also esterified with the glycerol molecule. Due to the presence of oxygen atoms, the phospholipid's head has an electron distribution resembling that of the water molecule, enabling water molecules to closely associate themselves with it: the head "attracts" water, i.e. it is hydrophilic. The phospholipid's tail only contains carbon and hydrogen atoms and its electron distribution is very different from that of water molecules. Consequently, water molecules cannot associate themselves in a stable configuration with this tail: the tail "rejects" water, i.e. it is hydrophobic. In a watery environment, there is only one stable configuration that these phospholipid molecules can form. This is a **bilayer**, which is the basic structure of the cell membrane. In the bilayer, the phospholipid molecules arrange themselves into two planes. In each plane, they lie parallel to one another and assume the same head-tail orientation. In the one plane, the orientation of the phospholipids is opposite to that in the other plane, and the tails in both planes face one another. In this way, the hydrophobic tails avoid contact with the watery environment inside and outside the cell, while the hydrophilic heads are exposed to it (Fig. 2.2).

Other kinds of lipids found in the cell membrane are glycolipids and cholesterol.

Glycolipids are found mainly in the outer layer of the cell membrane, facing the cell's exterior. Like the phospholipids, they have a hydrophilic head and a hydrophobic tail. The tail's structure is similar to that of a phospholipid tail. The head is a polysaccharide

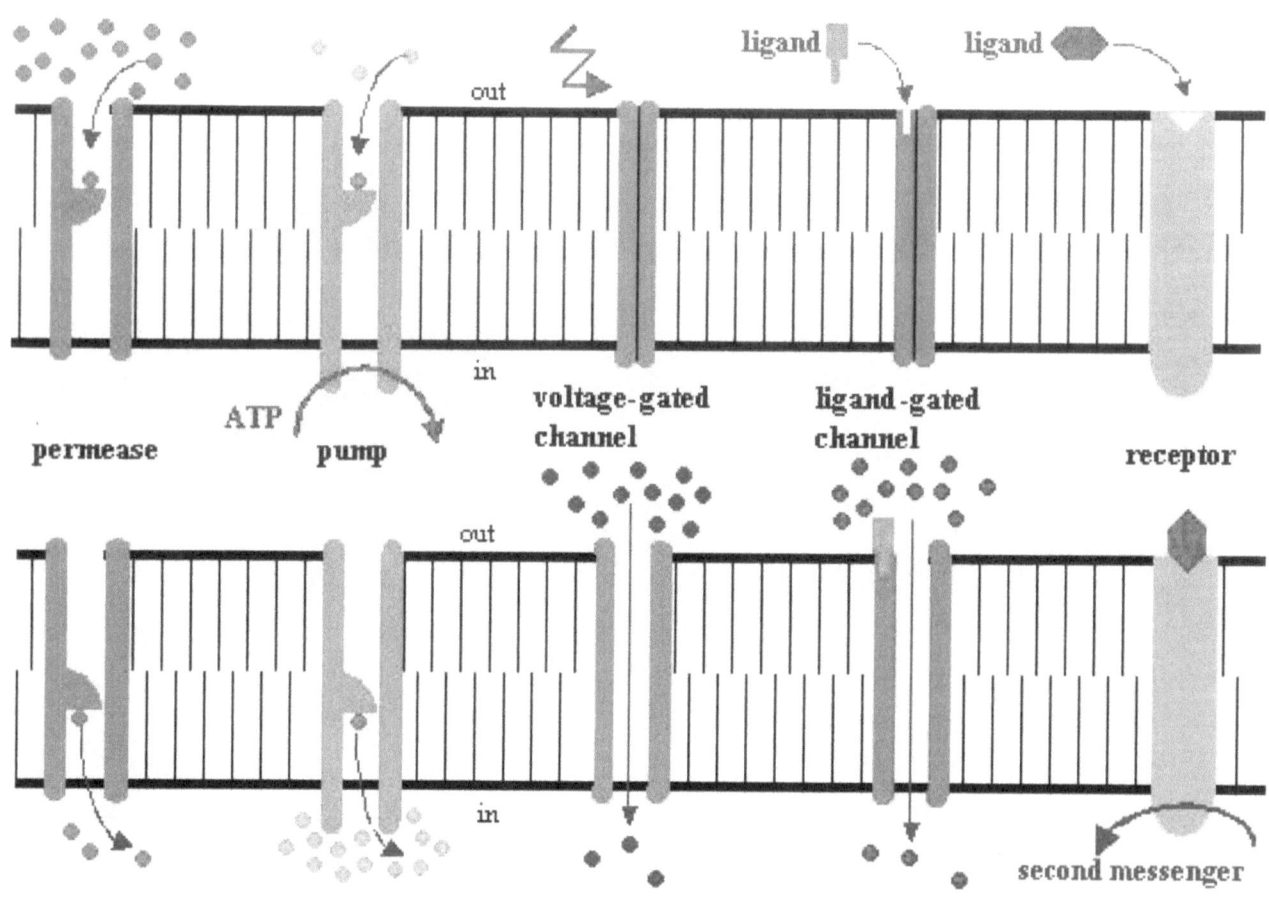

Fig. 2.3. Integral proteins. This section of the cell membrane shows various kinds of integral proteins, each having a particular function. Permeases ferry hydrophilic organic molecules across the cell membrane, driven by a concentration gradient. Pumps also ferry small hydrophilic molecules, mostly ions, across the cell membrane, but this transport is against a concentration gradient, and consequently necessitates the expenditure of energy, in the form of ATP. Pores are tubular proteins which, when opened, allow gradient driven transport of ions across the cell membrane. Voltage gated pores open upon depolarization of the cell membrane, ligand gated pores open when a specific messenger molecule, a ligand, binds with them. Strictly speaking, ligand gated pores answer to the definition of a receptor. In practice, this term is reserved for integral proteins that, upon binding of a specific ligand, induce the formation of second messenger molecules in the cell's interior.

molecule, a very complex string-like carbohydrate, often branched. The glycolipid molecule's tail is arranged parallel to those of the surrounding phospholipid molecules; the head rises above the plane of the cell membrane.

Cholesterol is a small, flat molecule, composed of a number of carbon pentagons and hexagons with common sides. The molecule is hydrophobic and it is inserted between the hydrophobic tails of the other lipid molecules.

The lipid molecules are the building blocks of the cell membrane. They form a coherent, stable bilayer that separates the cytosol from the cell's outside world. They do not form covalent chemical bonds among each other. This is what makes the cell membrane extremely pliable and plastic. Moreover, it is self-sealing, because, when its structure is disrupted, the lipid molecules can do nothing else but reassume their only stable configuration, the bilayer. These characteristics are beautifully demonstrated by the amoeboid movements of macrophages (II.2.1.4.), the complex shapes of certain cells, such as nerve cells, and the fusions and fissions that the cell membrane often shows. Examples of these are, on a small scale, exo- and endocytosis (Fig 2.12.) and on a larger scale, cell division (Fig. 2.59.) and fertilization.

Similarly important in the composition of the cell membrane are **proteins**. A protein molecule is derived from a polypeptide chain, composed of up to hundreds of amino acid residues. A functional protein is obtained by folding this polypeptide chain in a three-dimensional shape, often a very complex one. Some amino acids carry hydrophilic atom groups, others carry hydrophobic groups. Interactions between hydrophobic or hydrophilic groups from different regions of the chain provide a means by which the shape of the folded polypeptide is stabilized. The unique distribution of the amino acid residues in the polypeptide chains thus provides each kind of protein with a folding pattern that yields a distinct 3-dimensional structure, the latter being essential for function. Some proteins are loosely associated with the cell membrane, especially on its inside, and are called **peripheral proteins**. Others are deeply embedded in the cell membrane and can even span it. These are the **integral proteins**. Integral proteins, in particular, have a shape that brings hydrophobic amino acids to their exterior, so that they can associate with the tails of the lipid molecules making up the cell membrane (Fig. 2.2.).

Integral membrane proteins (Fig. 2.3.) are often implicated in the transport of substances across the cell membrane. Because of the hydrophobic nature of the bilayer, the cell membrane is, in principle, impermeable, in particular to hydrophilic molecules. This is both an advantage and a disadvantage. On the one hand, an impermeable cell membrane retains the cell's contents, but on the other hand, it may prevent movement of substances the cell needs or must get rid of. These problems are solved by the presence of integral proteins, which allow the cell to exchange specific substances between the cytosol and its exterior in a controlled fashion.

One kind of integral membrane protein is the **permeases** (Fig.2.3.). Permeases, as their name implies, confer permeability to the cell membrane, but selectively, only to specific substances. Most substances ferried by permeases are relatively small, hydrophilic organic molecules. Permeases transport substances passively down a concentration gradient. At one side of the cell membrane, the permease binds to a substance that is at a relatively high concentration. Binding induces shape changes of the permease, which result in transfer of molecules across the membrane and release of the transported molecules. The permease then returns to its original shape, allowing the cycle to be repeated. The energy needed for this change of shape is supplied by the concentration gradient. Permeases carry low molecular weight food molecules, such as glucose and amino acids, into the cell and waste substances, such as urea, out of it. The necessary concentration gradients across the cell membrane are maintained by continuous supply or production of molecules at one side and removal or break down at the other side.

Pumps (Fig. 2.3.) are integral proteins which function in a manner similar to permeases, but with one essential difference: a pump moves molecules up a concentration gradient and consequently requires a source of chemical energy, ATP (II.1.4.). In typical cases, pumps transport ions, such as sodium, potassium, chlorine, and calcium. Because of their small size and considerable thermal agitation, these ions are able, to a limited extent, to penetrate the cell membrane in spite of their extremely hydrophilic character. Consequently, the concentrations of these ions on both sides of the cell membrane should be equal. This, however, is not the case, and is due to the fact that the cell membrane contains pumps which maintain their concentration gradients. The sodium pump, for example, ferries sodium ions to the cell's exterior. Three ions are transferred each cycle. When the pump, after discharging the sodium ions, reverts to it original shape, it carries two potassium ions, transporting these to the cytosol. Both ions carry a net positive charge. For each cycle, the sodium pump (or more precisely, the sodium-potassium pump) carries a surplus of one positive charge to the cell's exterior. As a result, the cell's exterior is positive in comparison to the cytosol. Across the cell membrane, an electrical gradient or potential is maintained which, depending on the type of cell, varies between -50 to -100 millivolts. This **resting potential** is of paramount significance, as it enhances the sensitivity of the cell to a variety of stimuli.

Pores (Fig. 2.3.) are integral membrane proteins with

an internal canal, which may be either closed or open, depending on the type of pore. When the protein molecule forming them changes shape, closed canals open and open canals close. This change of shape can either take place when the resting potential changes (voltage-gated canals) or when a specific messenger molecule, a ligand, binds at the exterior face of the protein (ligand-gated canals). When a normally closed canal opens, a stream of specific ions rushes through, driven by their concentration gradient. In this way, sodium ions can enter the cell in large numbers. When a normally open canal closes, certain species of ions can no longer leave the cell. In this way, potassium ions can accumulate in the cytosol. Obviously, this has consequences for the resting potential of the membrane. When positive ions such as sodium enter the cell or, as is the case with potassium, can no longer leave it, the cytosol becomes less negative and may even change to positive in comparison with the exterior. The resting potential gradually decreases (depolarization), until a threshold value is reached. Then, very suddenly, the membrane potential reverses. During a very short time (milliseconds), the resting potential changes to an **action potential**. The action potential has a value of about +35 millivolts. One characteristic of an action potential is that it can spread. The presence of voltage-gated canals enables the action potential to induce depolarization of adjacent regions of the membrane and to run along the cell membrane at great speed (meters per second), a characteristic that enables nerve cells to conduct signals.

An integral membrane protein to which a specific molecule, a ligand, can bind is called a **receptor** (Fig. 2.3.). Strictly speaking, all integral membrane protein types discussed so far, with the exception of the voltage-gated canal, are receptors. Permeases and pumps even transport a bound molecule. A molecule, bound to its receptor, can also be transported by endocytosis (Fig. 2.12.). This mechanism, **receptor-mediated endocytosis**, allows the cell to take up specific high molecular weight molecules.

In a stricter sense, a receptor is an integral membrane protein able to bind messenger molecules, such as hormones or neurotransmitters, enabling the cell to react to stimuli. A ligand-gated canal can thus be regarded as a receptor. In other types of receptor, the binding of a messenger molecule at the outside of the cell induces formation of a "second messenger", such as cyclic AMP (Adenosine Mono-Phosphate) in the cytosol. This is the first link in a complex chain of events that ultimately leads to a reaction of the cell.

In contrast to phospholipids, the exposed "heads"of

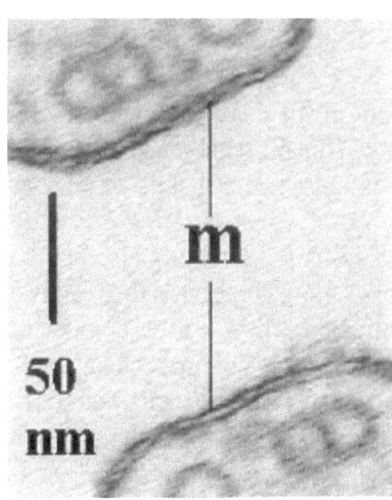

Fig. 2.4. In microscopic sections, the cell membrane shows up as a trilaminar complex (m). The light middle layer is probably hydrophobic, and coincides with the interior of the cell membrane, made up of phospholipid tails and integral proteins. The dense peripheral layers would then be hydrophilic, being made up of phospholipid heads and peripheral proteins. Cilium (Fig. 2.38.), airway epithelial cell, human, TEM.

which are very uniform, the exposed regions of membrane proteins display an unending variety of shape and form. In addition, many membrane proteins are in fact glycoproteins, which carry complex polysaccharide chains on their exposed parts. Glycolipids also present complex polysaccharide chains to the exterior of the cell. The presence of numerous, complex and variable proteins and polysaccharides on the cell membrane's exterior face makes it possible for it to carry a specific molecular signature, in part genetically determined and consequently unique to a particular individual. In this way, every cell of a certain individual has a "fingerprint" which is unique to that individual and identical in all the cells of that individual. In addition, the organism contains defender or immune cells, which carry membrane receptors enabling them to "read" this fingerprint. In this way they can distinguish between the cells of the body and those of an intruder's. This ability to distinguish between "self" and "foreign" is essential for the defense of the body against infection. A molecular pattern that can be recognized by an immune cell is an antigen. The antigens making up the cell's unique fingerprint are called **histocompatibility** or **transplantation antigens**. The cells making up the body must be compatible for the body to function as a unit. Transplantation or transfusion is only possible when donor and receptor are sufficiently compatible. The simplest example of histocompatibility antigens is to be found in the ABO blood group system.

What, finally, is there to tell about the microscopic structure of the cell membrane? In the electron microscope, and at extreme magnifications, the cell membrane shows a layered, trilaminar structure (Fig. 2.4.), which is considered a direct consequence of its molecular makeup. The translucent middle layer is regarded as largely hydrophobic: it contains the tails of the lipid molecules and the embedded parts of the integral proteins. The opaque superficial layers are taken to be hydrophilic: they correspond to the heads of the lipid molecules and the exposed parts of the integral and peripheral proteins.

II.1.2. Cell nucleus.

The most striking morphological feature of the cell is the presence of a nucleus (Fig. 2.5.). Apart from an occasional indentation, the typical cell nucleus has a smooth contour. Its diameter is 5 to 10 micrometers. The cell nucleus typically has a volume of one twentieth to one tenth of the total cell volume. In spherical or polyhedral cells, the nucleus is spherical as well. In distinctly elongated cells, such as muscle fibers, the nucleus is ellipsoid, its long axis lying parallel to the cell's longitudinal axis. In rarer cases, the cell nucleus can assume a very irregular shape, as in granulocytes (Figs. 3.1.9.-12.). Most cells contain a single nucleus, which can occupy a central or an eccentric position, depending on the cell type. Some cell types have no nucleus at all, such as erythrocytes, the red blood cells. Multinuclear cells exist as well, such as the skeletal muscle fibers (Figs. 3.3.3.-4.) and the osteoclasts of the bone (Fig. 3.2.21.). The nucleus has an envelope and contains miscellaneous darkly staining material.

The nucleus may be regarded as an archive or library storing and handling the cell's genetic information. The genetic information is a set of instructions for the construction of proteins. Proteins not only constitute the cell's building blocks, but also function as enzymes needed to synthesize various substances and to regulate the chemical reactions of the body's metabolism. A set of instructions for the construction of a single protein is called a gene.

The physical carrier of the genetic information is a **nucleic acid** molecule - more precisely **DNA** (Deoxyribo-Nucleic Acid). DNA consists of two strands that are held together with transverse connections, not unlike a ladder. The ladder has "rungs", each consisting of a pair of two bases. The base sequence attached to one strand is complementary to the base sequence attached to the other one, meaning that one type of base in one strand is always opposed to a fixed other kind in the other strand. This explains how a DNA molecule can make identical copies of itself. Both strands can be separated from each other by splitting up the base pairs making up the rungs. Each half of the structure now serves as a template for a new half. By complementary pairing of new bases to the original ones, the structure of the original DNA molecule is restored. The end result is that there are now two DNA molecules where there was originally only one, identical to each other and to the original molecule. This duplication process is the essence of cell multiplication. In this way, a single cell (for instance the fertilized ovum) can give rise to countless daughter cells, genetically identical to it and to each other.

The base sequence in a DNA molecule can be "translated" into an amino acid sequence. In other words: a particular base sequence in the DNA molecule determines the amino acid sequence in a polypeptide chain and consequently a protein's structure and function. The base sequence in a DNA molecule constitutes the genetic information proper. Two mechanisms take part in the construction of a polypeptide: transcription and translation. Transcription is essentially the same process as duplication, with a few minor differences. In transcription, only one strand of the DNA molecule is duplicated. Furthermore, it is a very local process, with only a short stretch of DNA, corresponding to a single gene, being duplicated. The complementary single-strand molecule thus formed is a copy of the original, non-duplicated DNA strand, except for a few details that must not concern us here. The newly formed stretch of nucleic acid is made of **RNA** (Ribo-Nucleic Acid). This RNA molecule detaches and is now an independent carrier of genetic information. It leaves the cell nucleus and enters the cytosol, where translation, the construction of a specific polypeptide determined by the RNA 's base sequence, takes place. This RNA molecule can be regarded as a messenger, transferring genetic information from the nucleus to the cytosol. It is in fact called messenger RNA.

Additional kinds of RNA are found in the nucleus. These include transfer RNA and ribosomal RNA, which are also transferred to the cytosol and perform essential parts of the translation mechanism. By complementary base pairing, as with messenger RNA formation, transfer RNA links amino acid molecules in a particular sequence to the messenger RNA molecule. The linked amino acid molecules form bonds that result in a polypeptide chain, the precursor of a protein, which detaches from the messenger RNA. This process is controlled by ribosomal RNA that forms a complex body, the ribosome (II.1.3.).

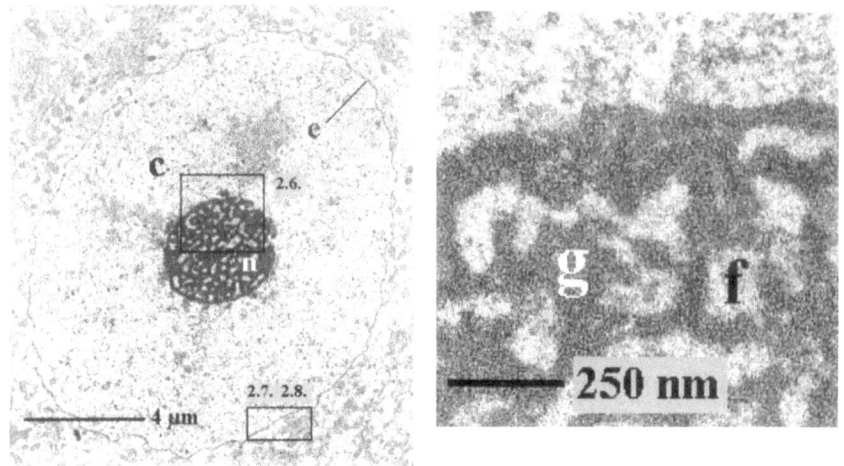

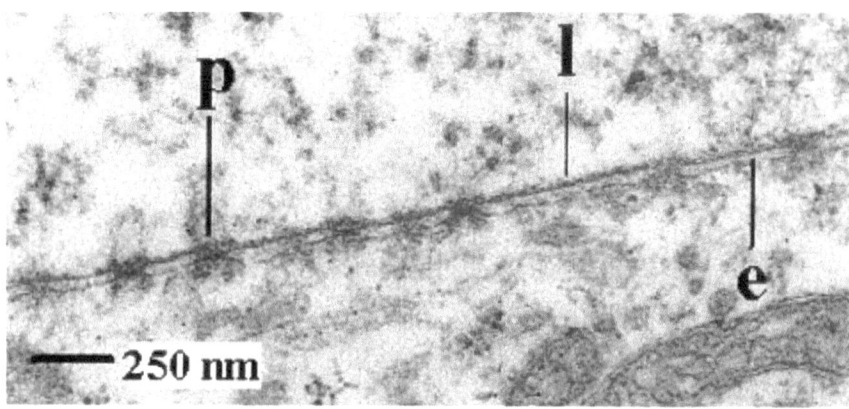

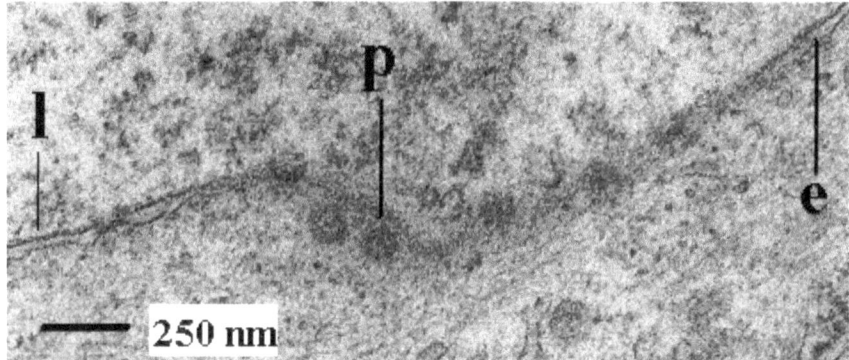

Fig. 2.5. (top left) The cell nucleus is separated from the rest of the cytoplasm by an envelope (e). The nuclear interior contains granular, dense material, chromatin (c), which is made up of DNA strings and proteins. If the chromatin is finely granular, as it is here, the nucleus has a clear aspect, and it is called euchromatic. In the center of the nucleus, the nucleolus (n) is visible as a dense, round object containing a maze of lighter cavities. The euchromatic character of this nucleus and the rather strong development of the nucleolus indicate that the cell containing this nucleus is intensely involved in protein synthesis. Motor nerve cell, spinal cord, rabbit, TEM. **Fig. 2.6.** (top right) The nucleolus consists of several components, of which the dense granular component (g) and the hollow fibrillar centers (f) can be made out in this picture. Sensory nerve cell, spinal ganglion, rabbit, TEM. **Fig. 2.7.** (left) The nuclear envelope in vertical section. The nucleoplasm is at the top. The nuclear envelope (e) consists of two membranes, separated by a narrow space. The inner membrane is thicker than the outer one because it is coated, on its inside, with a dense layer, the nuclear lamina (l). In many places, the two membranes fuse, producing nuclear pores (p). Sensory nerve cell, spinal ganglion, rabbit, TEM.

Fig. 2.8. (above) The nuclear envelope (e) in horizontal section. The nucleoplasm is at the top. l = nuclear lamina. The nuclear pores (p) have a dense circular rim and contain a diaphragm carrying a dense central dot. Sensory nerve cell, nodose ganglion, rabbit, TEM.

Electron microscopic observation shows that the nuclear substance, the karyoplasm, contains a granular material, which stains darkly because it absorbs heavy metals. In the light microscope, the karyoplasm shows a basophilic reaction: it can be differentially stained with alcalic pigments such as hematoxylin (I.2.), giving the nucleus a dark, granular aspect. This dark material assumes two forms: chromatin and the nucleolus.

Chromatin (Fig. 2.5.) consists of DNA and specific proteins. It can appear more or less opaque depending on the extent of activation of the genetic material. Loose chromatin, called **euchromatin**, represents uncoiled DNA strands, which are accessible to the enzymes regulating transcription and is thus actively involved in polypeptide synthesis. Euchromatin absorbs little pigment or heavy metals and consequently appears pale. Less active chromatin, called **heterochromatin**, represents tightly coiled DNA strands that are inaccessible to translation enzymes and are not involved in polypeptide synthesis. Such chromatin traps large amounts of pigment or heavy metals and appears dark. Heterochromatin is irregularly distributed, but often accumulates at the inner face of the nuclear envelope.

The **nucleolus** (Fig. 2.6.) is a dense body that, in a number of cell types, is more or less characteristic with regard to shape, size and texture. It often has an eccentric position, lying close to the nuclear envelope. In this "small nucleus", DNA is transcribed to ribosomal RNA, which is used to assemble ribosomes (II.1.3.), which in turn are essential for translation in the cytosol. The nucleolus consists of a dense, granular structure, the **granular component**, the interior of which is riddled with spaces with a fibrillar content, the **fibrillar centers**. The fibrillar centers are often enveloped with fibrous material, the **dense fibrous component**. The fibrillar centers may be open to the karyoplasm and allow uncoiled, euchromatic DNA to enter the nucleolus, where it is transcribed to ribosomal RNA. Transcription and the first steps of ribosome synthesis take place in the dense fibrillar component. Later steps take place in the granular component. Here, ribosomal RNA and specific proteins from the cytosol are assembled into ribosomal subunits that later, in the cytosol, will build complete ribosomes.

The relative amounts of euchromatin and heterochromatin and the degree of development of the nucleolus allow a rough estimation of the intensity of protein synthesis in the cell. In cells with a high level of protein synthesis, such as nerve cells (Fig. 2.5.), the nucleus is predominantly euchromatic and contains a well-developed nucleolus. Occasionally, more than one nucleolus can be present. Heterochromatic nuclei, wherein the nucleolus is underdeveloped or even missing, are found in cells synthesizing little or no protein.

The nucleus is surrounded by an **envelope** (Figs. 2.7.-8.) consisting of two parallel membranes with the same structure as the cell membrane. The narrow space separating both membranes is 20 to 50 nanometers wide. The inner face of the inner membrane, bordering the karyoplasm is coated with a thin, dense layer, the **nuclear lamina**. In several places, the outer membrane is continuous with the rough endoplasmic reticulum (II.2.1.1.). Filaments bridge the intermembranous space. These filaments and the nuclear lamina probably reinforce the envelope and stabilize the shape of the nucleus. Locally, the membranes of the nuclear envelope fuse, obliterating the space between them. In this way, **nuclear pores** are formed, which control exchange of particles and substances between cytoplasm and karyoplasm. Nuclear pores are circular, with a diameter of about 60 nanometers. The fused membranes form a diaphragm with a central knob-like thickening. The pore's rim is formed by a dense ring or annulus. Messenger RNA, transfer RNA and ribosomal subcomponents leave the nucleus via this route. Certain hormones use it to enter the karyoplasm.

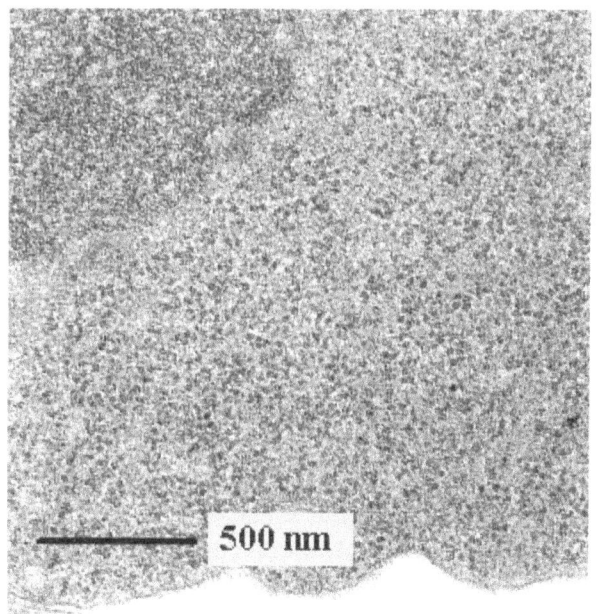

Fig. 2.9. Ribosomes look like dense, irregular granules, filling the cytosol. The cell nucleus is partly visible at the upper left. Hematopoietic cell, bone marrow, rat, TEM.

II.1.3. Ribosomes.

In the electron microscope, ribosomes appear as dense granules, about 15 nanometers in diameter, which are dispersed throughout the cytosol (Fig. 2.9.) or are attached to the membranes of the rough endoplasmic reticulum (Fig. 2.13.). They are very slightly elongated, because they consist of two subunits. In the light microscope, they cannot be observed directly because of their minute size. Since they contain nucleic acid, cytoplasm loaded with ribosomes shows a basophilic reaction, meaning that it stains with pigments such as hematoxylin (I.2.). A single cell may contain hundreds of thousands of ribosomes.

Ribosomes are essential in polypeptide synthesis, during translation to be precise. One end of a messenger RNA strand fits in a groove at the junction of both subunits and slides through it. Transfer RNA molecules bind to the stretches of the messenger RNA strand that successively pass through this groove. This binding, like the processes of duplication and transcription, relies on pairing between complementary base sequences. Each transfer RNA molecule carries a specific amino acid. The base sequence with which it will pair with the messenger RNA strand determines the nature of this amino acid. After pairing, each amino acid is covalently bound to the previously attached amino acid residue, after which the transfer RNA detaches and the ribosome moves on to the next section of the messenger RNA strand, where the cycle is repeated. As the ribosome slides along the messenger RNA strand, a chain of amino acids is generated - a polypeptide - which will fold into a protein.

II.1.4. Mitochondria.

Mitochondria (Fig. 2.10.) are more or less circular to distinctly elongated organelles. Their length can reach several micrometers, with a maximal thickness of about 1 micrometer. Their width is too small for them to be clearly made out with light microscopy, in which case they appear as dots or rods forming strings or "granular threads". Mitochondria are membranous corpuscles, having an outer and an inner membrane, both of which have the same structure as the cell membrane. The narrow space between them is 10 to 20 nanometers wide. The outer membrane has a smooth contour. The inner membrane locally protrudes into the mitochondrion 's interior, forming narrow **crests**. Usually, these crests are oriented more or less at right angles to the mitochondrion's longitudinal axis, but orientations parallel to this axis

are also observed, as for example in the processes of nerve cells. The bases of the crests may be constricted. Occasionally, the inner membrane does not form crests, but **tubes**. This occurs in steroid hormone secreting cells (Fig. 4.7.11.). The interior of the mitochondrion, enclosed by the inner membrane, is the matrix. The matrix appears slightly denser than the cytosol and contains dense granules. These may represent reserve material that can be used to produce extra internal membrane in case of a sudden increase in cellular energy requirements. A single cell may contain several hundred mitochondria.

Factors such as the number of mitochondria, their length, and the number and length of their crests, all positively correlate with the cell's level of energy expenditure. This is not surprising, since mitochondria are the cell's power plants. Cells requiring a lot of energy for contraction, such as muscle fibers (Figs. 3.3.8.-9.), of for transport of substances (Fig. 3.4.3.), show numerous, elongated mitochondria with a large number of tall crests.

To carry out their vital functions (movement, transport, synthesis, etc.) cells need energy. This energy is supplied by cellular fuel: **ATP** (Adenosine Tri-Phosphate), a molecule that carries a string of three phosphate groups. The chemical bond between the two terminal phosphate groups is unstable and thus energy-rich. The energy that is liberated upon rupture of this bond, which converts ATP to ADP (Di-Phosphate) plus phosphate, drives virtually every energy-consuming reaction in the cell.

The mitochondria generate ATP from ADP and phosphate. They need energy to do this and obtain it from the breakdown of another energy-rich compound, which is supplied by an external food source. This compound can be a carbohydrate, such as glucose, but fatty acids and even amino acids can also be used.

The energy contained in these compounds can be liberated by stripping them of electrons, which results in their breakdown, a process known as oxidation.

This is a complex process, the first steps of which do not take place in the mitochondria, but rather occur in the cytosol. A glucose molecule, for example, is broken down, in several steps, to two pyruvate molecules. This breakdown, or **glycolysis**, involves two oxidations which both liberate a pair of electrons, and supplies sufficient energy for direct generation of two ATP molecules.

The pyruvate molecules are fed into a cyclic reaction sequence, the Krebs or **citrate cycle**, which churns out carbon dioxide molecules (= breakdown of pyruvate) and electron pairs. The enzymes catalyzing this sequence are located in the mitochondrial matrix. The

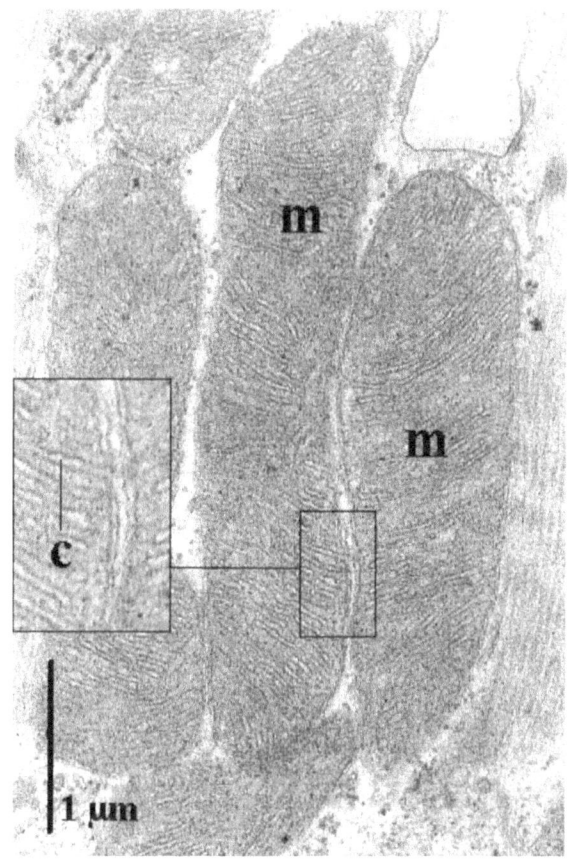

Fig. 2.10. Mitochondria (m) are oblong organelles, made up of a double membrane. The inner membrane forms a number of narrow, transverse, parallel folds, the crests or cristae. The one indicated (c) is seen to be in continuity with the inner membrane. Cardiac muscle fiber, rabbit, TEM.

two pyruvate molecules entering the cycle supply ten electron pairs (two times five) and, in addition, supply enough energy for the direct generation of another two ATP molecules.

The electron pairs supplied by glycolysis and the citrate cycle are transferred to the enzymes of the **respiratory chain**, which are integral proteins of the mitochondrion's inner membrane. These enzymes form units, in which they are arranged in increasing order of oxidative or electron-pulling power. They transfer electrons from the one to the next, "pulling" them through the membrane, and finally transfer them to the most powerfully oxidative substance of all, oxygen. This allows oxygen to bind protons, generating water. When the electrons enter the respiratory chain, they are associated with a proton, forming hydrogen. The enzymes of the respiratory chain are alternately located on the inside and on the outside of the mitochondrial inner membrane. While the enzymes on the inside accept both electrons and protons, those on the outside accept only electrons, the

accompanying protons being shed on the outside of the inner membrane. In this way, electron transfer to oxygen results in the transfer of protons to the outside of the inner mitochondrial membrane. Since this membrane is itself impermeable to protons, a proton gradient across the membrane is built up. Yet another kind of enzyme in the inner membrane is a pore that allows protons to enter. The energy of the proton gradient is used here to generate ATP. In this way, each original glucose molecule gives rise to an additional thirty-two ATP molecules. With the four ATP molecules directly generated by glycolysis and in the citrate cycle, this adds up to a total of thirty-six.

The net result is that glucose has been oxidized with oxygen, in a kind of slow burn. This process is called respiration. The thirty-six molecules of ATP formed upon breakdown of each glucose molecule represent about 50 per cent of the glucose molecule's total energy content, the rest being lost as heat. This is a very efficient energy transformation, far more efficient in fact than that which occurs in a modern combustion engine.

Originally, mitochondria were independent entities. Mitochondria are the descendants of bacteria that, at a certain stage in the development of life on earth, a few billion years ago, entered a host cell and took up permanent residence inside it. Bacteria, which are **prokaryotic** cells, have no nucleus, their DNA lying in the cytoplasm. The host cell that they entered, and which was the ancestor of the multicellular organisms of later times, was of a more complex type, possessing a nucleus: a **eukaryotic** cell. Thus, mitochondria are to be regarded as **endosymbionts**. Several of their characteristics indicate this. To begin with, they are bordered by a double membrane. This is a direct consequence of the way in which a host cell took them up: by phagocytosis (Fig. 2.12.). An object to be phagocytosed is enveloped by a fold of the cell's membrane and then internalized. Thus, the inner mitochondrial membrane is the original bacterial cell membrane. The outer membrane is the original host cell's. The host cell used phagocytosis as a means of obtaining food. To liberate the chemical energy of the food molecules and to use it to make ATP, the host cell only disposed of the relatively inefficient glycolysis, which only generates two ATP molecules per molecule of glucose. The free-living bacterial ancestor of the mitochondria, however, had developed a much more efficient mechanism for the breakdown of glucose: respiration, which generates no less than thirty-six molecules of ATP per glucose molecule. By establishing a symbiosis with these bacteria, instead of eating them, the host cell was able to exploit this efficient mechanism for its own benefit. This symbiosis proved to be so advantageous that natural selection made it permanent. Another observation indicating that mitochondria descend from bacteria is that the matrix still contains some bacterial genes, which are independent of the host cell's genome. Finally, mitochondria appear to act independently of the host cell. They seem to be able to move independently, to change their shape, to fuse, and to divide. Dividing mitochondria develop a transverse constriction, whereupon both parts separate. This process is highly reminiscent of cell multiplication and allows the mitochondria to increase in number independently of the cell.

II.1.5. Peroxisomes.

Peroxisomes (Fig. 2.11.) are membranous vesicles with a diameter of approximately 500 nanometers. Their interior has a homogeneous, moderately opaque aspect. In animals, but not in man, it often contains a crystalline structure, the nucleoid. They occasionally replicate by splitting, just like mitochondria do. For this reason, peroxisomes have been regarded as endosymbionts as well, but their case is not as strong as the mitochondria's.

Peroxisomes derive their name from their production of hydrogen peroxide, which they obtain from the

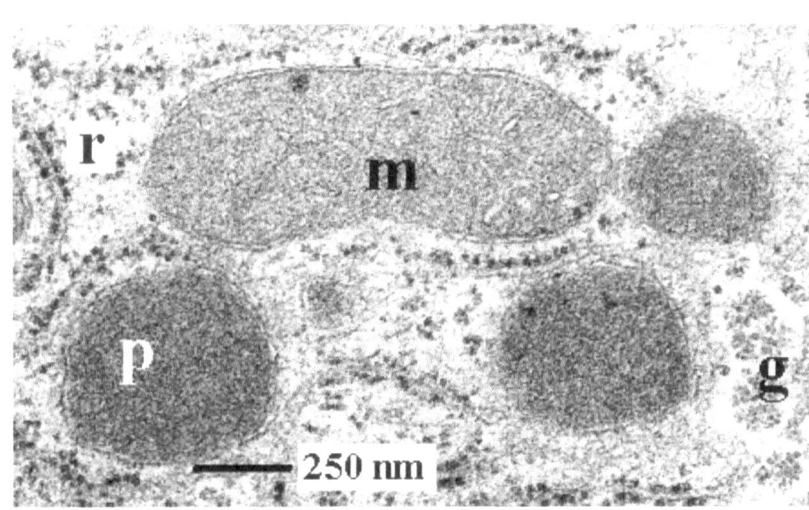

Fig. 2.11. Peroxysomes (p) are relatively small (compare with neighbouring mitochondria, m) round vesicles, bordered with a membrane. The dense granules are not ribosomes, but glycogen (g). Ribosomes dot the membranes of the rough endoplasmic reticulum (r). Hepatocyte, rabbit, TEM.

oxidation of organic molecules by means of oxygen. In contrast to mitochondria, they do not produce ATP as a result of this. The organic molecules they oxidize are, among others, fatty acids, the breakdown products of which can be recycled. Peroxisomes also enable the resulting hydrogen peroxide to be removed. They contain an enzyme, catalase, which speeds up the reaction of hydrogen peroxide with organic molecules. In this way, various toxic products of metabolism, such as ethanol, are eliminated. They also contain enzymes for the breakdown of urate. Hydrogen peroxide not only arises through the action of peroxisomes. During respiration, oxygen catches the electrons at the end of the respiratory chain and combines with protons, forming water. Occasionally, this process can give rise to hydrogen peroxide. Hydrogen peroxide is a very aggressive, highly toxic molecule, and consequently its concentration has to be kept low. Peroxisomes remove this peroxide by reacting it with organic molecules, and can be regarded as organelles whose function it is to protect the cell against toxic by-products of its metabolism.

References.

Baumgart E.: Application of in situ hybridisation, cytochemical and immunocytochemical techniques for the investigation of peroxisomes. Histochem. Cell Biol. 1997, 108: 185-210.
Bereiter-Hahn J., Vöth M.: Dynamics of mitochondria in living cells: shape changes, dislocations, fusion, and fission of mitochondria. Microsc. Res. Tech. 1994, 27: 198-219.
Jacob W.A., Bakker A., Hertsens R.C., Biermans W.: Mitochondrial matrix granules: their behavior during changing metabolic situations and their relationship to contact sites between inner and outer mitochondrial membranes. Microsc. Res. Tech. 1994, 27:307-318.
Lazarow P.B.: Peroxisome structure, function, and biogenesis - human patients and yeast mutants show strikingly similar defects in peroxisome biogenesis. J. Neuropathol. Exp. Neurol. 1995, 54: 720-725.

Perkins G.A., Frey T.G.: Recent structural insight into mitochondria gained by microscopy. Micron 2000, 31: 97-111.

Scheer U., Hock R.: Structure and function of the nucleolus. Curr. Opin. Cell Biol. 1999, 11: 385-390.

Schwarzacher H.G., Wachtler F.: The nucleolus. Anat. Embryol. 1993, 188: 515-536.

II.2. Secondary organelles and differentiated cells.

In addition to primary organelles, with which a cell is able to maintain itself, there are secondary organelles, which the cell uses to contribute to the proper functioning of the organism of which it is part. The presence and degree of development of such organelles indicate a cell's function. Two main groups of secondary organelles can be distinguished: **membranes** and **fibers** (Fig. 2.1.). In most cases, one kind is better developed than the other. There are numerous cell types in which membranes predominate. These are **membrane-bearing cells**. In other cell types, fibers predominate. These are **fiber-bearing cells**. Both groups can be divided further into subtypes. Naturally, it would be unwise to cling too tightly to this classification, which is only meant as an aid to description of the structure of cells. Nature herself is utterly indifferent to man-made classifications. Many cell types which we will meet

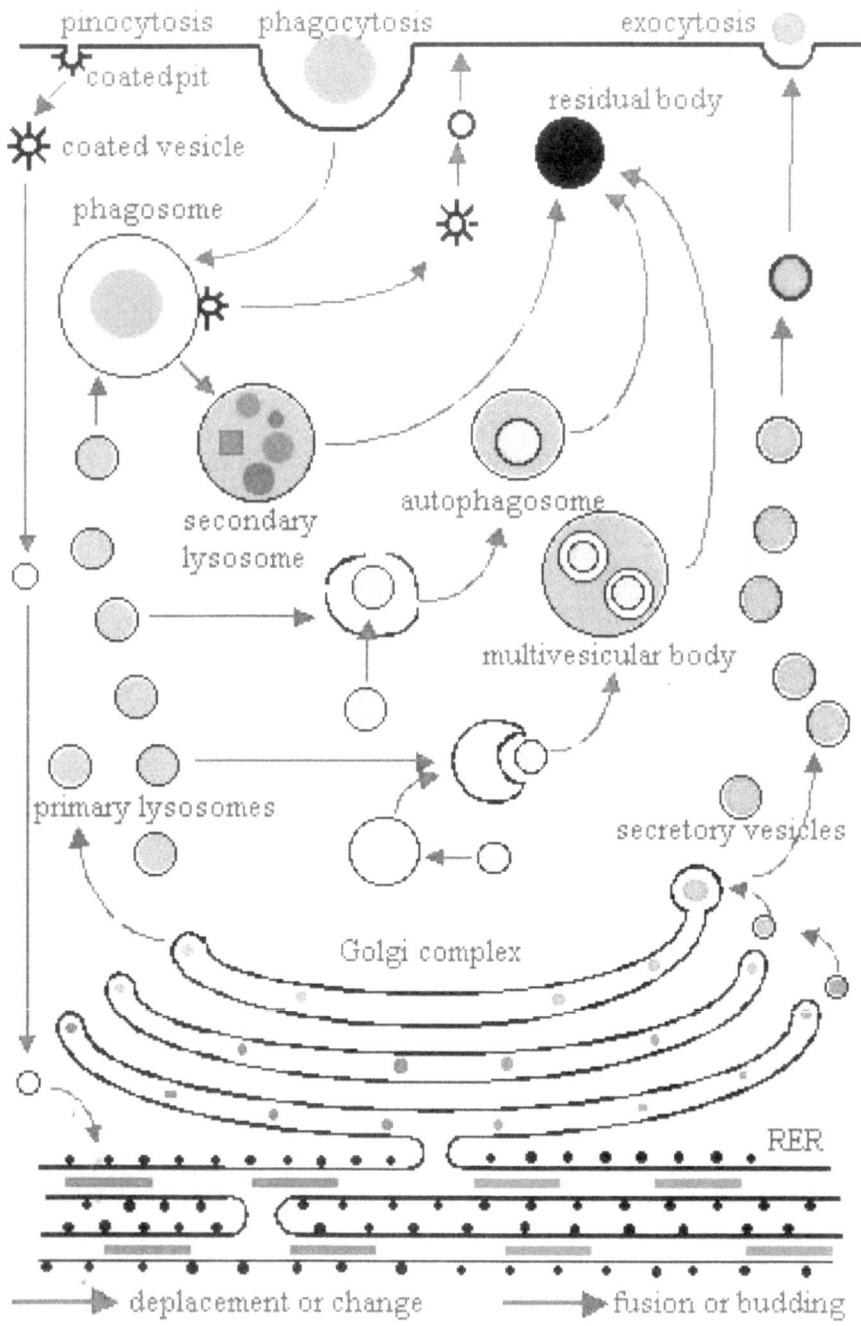

Fig. 2.12. The GERL-complex (Golgi-Endoplasmic Reticulum-Lysosomes) is a collection of morphologically diverse, but closely cooperating intracellular membranes. The rough endoplasmic reticulum (RER) synthesizes polypeptides. In the Golgi-complex, these polypeptides are processed, converted to biologically active proteins, and stored in secretory vesicles. Through exocytosis, the vesicles are emptied into the extracellular space. Lysosomes are vesicles that do not show exocytosis. They fuse with phagosomes, which are formed through phagocytosis, a form of endocytosis, and contain material from outside the cell. Alternatively, they fuse with multivesicular bodies, which contain intracellular material. The hydrolytic enzymes carried by the lysosomes digest the phagosomal or vesicular content, which results in the formation of secondary, tertiary, etc. lysosomes, and ultimately of residual bodies. Low molecular weight raw materials for synthetic purposes are taken up by pinocytosis, a form of endocytosis. In the same way, surface membrane is reinternalized and recycled. Pinocytotic vesicles, like secretory vesicles and lysosomes, but unlike phagosomes, have relatively standard dimensions. To form a vesicle, the cell membrane must bulge into the cell's interior. This change in shape is accomplished by contractile proteins, which coat the cytosolic face of the cell membrane. The bulge, with its protein coat, separates from the cell membrane, forming a coated vesicle.

later on, can be assigned to one of the groups on the basis of their predominating features, yet will be found to display, in smaller measure, features of the other group. Cell types also exist which are almost perfectly intermediate between both groups, i.e. they appear to equally contain membranes as well as fibers. These are referred to as **composite cells**. Finally, very eccentric cell types will be encountered occasionally, which fit into neither group. These cell types will be discussed with the tissue or organ in which they are found.

II.2.1. Membrane-bearing cells.

Many differentiated cells typically contain a well-developed system of cytosolic membranes. These membranes have the same structure as the cell membrane, although their chemical composition may be somewhat different. They are actively involved in the synthesis of biologically active substances, which the cell does not need for its own purposes, but which have a particular function in the body. Several types of cytosolic membranes exist, so that several subtypes of membrane-bearing cells can be distinguished, each of them dominated, to a certain extent, by another kind of membrane.

Most of these membranes work in co-operation, forming a structural and functional unit. This unit includes the **rough endoplasmic reticulum**, the **Golgi-complex**, the **secretory vesicles**, the **lysosomes** and the endosomes. The acronym GERL (Golgi-Endoplasmic-Reticulum-Lysosome) is occasionally used in referring to the entire system (Fig. 2.12.).
The rough endoplasmic reticulum's function is the synthesis of polypeptides. Its membrane is continuous with that of the Golgi-complex, in which most of the conversion of polypeptides to proteins takes place. The Golgi-complex also synthesizes a number of substances, including carbohydrates. The finished products end up in secretory vesicles that bud from the Golgi-complex. By means of secretory vesicles, the synthesized substances can be transported out of the cell. Their membrane fuses with the cell membrane, whereupon their lumen becomes continuous with the extracellular space and they are emptied. This process is called **exocytosis**. Membranous material may be "recycled" by the reverse process, endocytosis, in the form of small **pinocytotic vesicles**.
Apart from expelling substances, cells can also take them up. This is carried out by means of **endocytosis**, in which the cell membrane forms a depression, which deepens and is pinched off as a vesicle, an **endosome**.

Phagosomes are endosomes that contain substances or particles that, once internalized, have to be broken down. Specific enzymes are needed to break down the phagosome's contents. These are produced, as other proteins are, in the rough endoplasmic reticulum and the Golgi-complex, and stored in vesicles. These particular vesicles are lysosomes. Their membrane fuses with the phagosome's, mixing their enzymes with the phagosome's contents.

Another important membrane system, which is in principle independent from the GERL-complex, is the **smooth endoplasmic reticulum**.

II.2.1.1. Rough endoplasmic reticulum.

The rough endoplasmic reticulum (Fig. 2.13.) consists of parallel membranes that border a number of narrow, flattened spaces or cisterns, about 20 nanometers wide. Often, many of these cisterns are present, building extensive complexes, most often in the region of the nucleus. In several places, the membranes of two adjoining cisterns form a narrow interconnecting canal, so that the whole complex is in fact a network or reticulum. The cytosolic face of these membranes is studded with ribosomes, giving the complex a granular, or rough, look. Sometimes, the cisterns can be dilated or irregularly shaped. At the level of the nucleus, the membrane of the rough endoplasmic reticulum is continuous with the outer membrane of the nuclear envelope.

The ribosomes of the rough endoplasmic reticulum synthesize polypeptides in the same way as free ribosomes (II.1.3.) do. As they are formed, the polypeptide chains enter the interior of the reticulum's cisterns through pores in the membrane. These polypeptides, in contrast to those that are formed by the free ribosomes of the cytosol, will eventually leave the cell by way of the Golgi-complex and the secretory vesicles. They give rise to proteins which are not needed by the cell itself, but will be used elsewhere in the organism. In cell types that do not produce such export proteins, the rough endoplasmic reticulum is much less developed. Its function here is mainly the production of proteins that are to be incorporated into the cell membrane. Such proteins are not admitted into the interior of the rough endoplasmic reticulum's cisterns, but are incorporated into its membrane. Vesicles that bud from the rough endoplasmic reticulum carry the proteins, locked in their membrane, to the Golgi-complex. Secretory vesicles carrying these proteins bud from the Golgi-complex

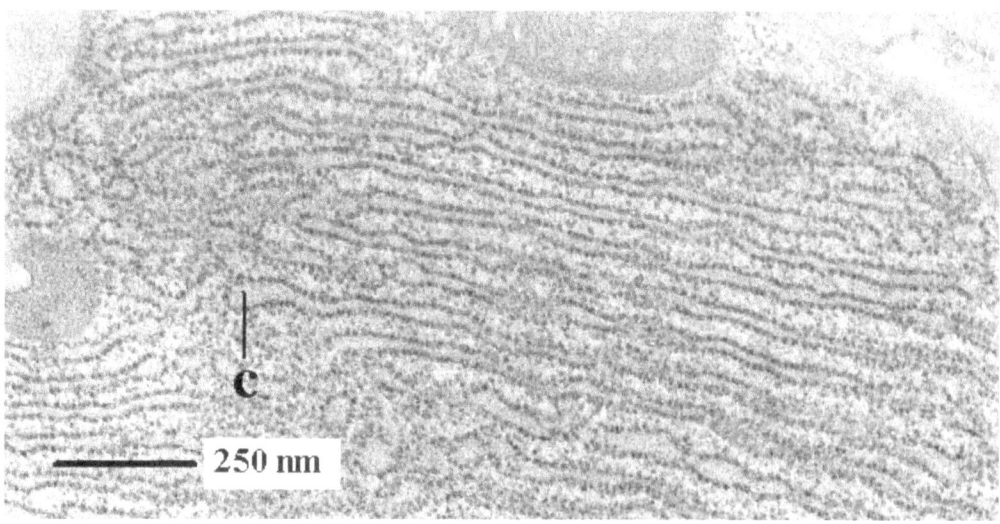

Fig. 2.13. The rough endoplasmic reticulum, in its most developed form, consists of a large number of flattened, parallel spaces or cisterns (c), bordered by a membrane, the cytosolic face of which is dotted with ribosomes. Zymogen cell, gastric fundus gland, rabbit, TEM.

and fuse with the cell membrane.

Cells with a strongly developed rough endoplasmic reticulum are specialized in the production of export proteins. Many types of gland cells belong to this category. The function of gland cells is the synthesis and secretion of biologically active substances. Some proteins, produced by gland cells, are enzymes that are necessary for the digestion of food. These are formed by **enzyme-secreting gland cells**. Other proteins serve as messenger molecules, called hormones. These are produced by **peptide hormone-secreting gland cells**. Still other proteins accumulate in the local extracellular space, forming a matrix that is an essential part of interstitial, connective, and supportive tissues. These are produced by **matrix-secreting cells**. Finally, certain proteins, the antibodies, are essential for the immunologic defense of the body: They are produced by **antibody-secreting cells**.

II.2.1.1.1. Enzyme-secreting gland cells.

Most enzyme-secreting gland cells, such as those of the pancreas (Fig. 2.14.), form part of the digestive system. They contact the lumen of the gut, either directly, or indirectly, by way of a duct, and their secretory products are released into this lumen. The gut's lumen is a space that is continuous with the outside world of the body. Gland cells that secrete into the outside world, or into an interior space in continuity with it, are **exocrine**, being involved in external secretion. This function imposes certain limitations to their structure. Exocrine gland cells

have to be constructed in such a way that they can secrete in a particular direction, i.e. into a lumen. As a consequence of this, they are distinctly asymmetrical or polarized, i.e. their basal and apical parts are clearly different. They are prismatic or pyramidal cells. Their top or apical part contacts the lumen. The nucleus lies in the basal part and the biosynthetic organelles (particularly the rough endoplasmic reticulum) occupy a perinuclear position. The Golgi-complex lies "above" the nucleus, towards the cell apex, and finally the secretory vesicles occupy the apical part of the cell. Exocytosis occurs at the exposed apical cell membrane.

In enzyme-secreting gland cells, the rough endoplasmic reticulum occupies a dominant position. It consists of numerous narrow and parallel cisterns, arranged in concentric layers around the nucleus. In extreme cases, it is so extensively developed that it occupies virtually all available space in the basal, perinuclear part of the cell. Consequently, such cells show a distinct basophilic reaction (I.2.). The apical part of the cell is filled with globular secretory vesicles. Depending on the particular cell type, these vesicles have a diameter of a few hundred to almost 2000 nanometers. Their content's electron density is also variable. Depending on the kind of enzyme they contain, the apical cytoplasm develops a basophilic or eosinophilic reaction. The vesicles are emptied by individual exocytosis. Gland cells secreting in this fashion are called **merocrine**.

Upon secretion, the liberated enzymes participate in the digestion of food in the gut's lumen. They are

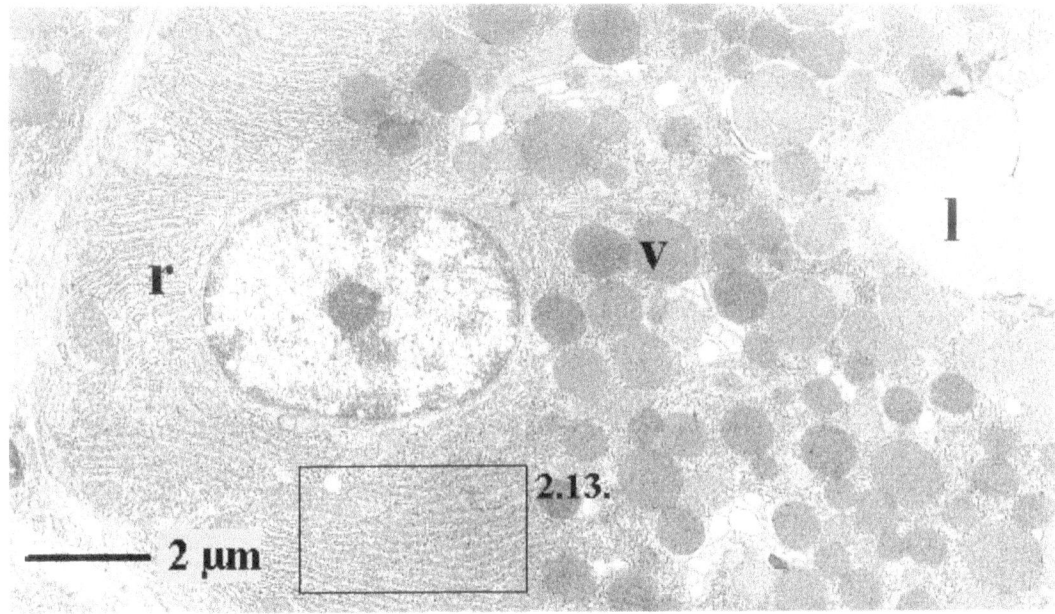

Fig. 2.14. An exocrine, enzyme-secreting gland cell. The top, or apex, of this cell borders a space or lumen (l) that, via the intestinal lumen, eventually opens into the body's exterior. Into this lumen, this cell secretes digestive enzymes. The enzymes are stored in globular secretory vesicles (v), which fill the apical cell part. Formation of these enzymes starts in the rough endoplasmic reticulum (r), which envelopes the basal nucleus. This cell is strongly polarized, i.e. its apical and basal ends, or poles, are different. Serous cell, exocrine pancreas, rabbit, TEM.

secreted as a clear fluid, a serum. Cells which secrete enzymes, i.e. **zymogen cells**, are therefore also called **serous cells**, examples of which include the cells forming the acini of the salivary glands (IV.15.1.2.) and the pancreas (IV.15.4.), and the zymogen cells found in the stomach's fundic glands (Figs. 4.15.29.-30.).

II.2.1.1.2. Peptide hormone-secreting gland cells.

Like all hormones, peptide hormones are secreted in the extracellular spaces and from there reach the blood circulation, which distributes them to the rest of the body. Thus, they are not released into the outside world or into an internal space in continuity with it. Therefore, hormone-secreting cells are **endocrine**, being involved in internal secretion. Upon secretion, the hormones either act in the immediate surroundings of the producing cell (paracrine secretion), or alternatively at some distance, being transported there by the circulation (endocrine secretion in the strict sense).

A typical endocrine cell is surrounded on all sides by the small blood vessels or capillaries that pervade the body, and thus does not need to be constructed so that its secretions are directed in a certain sense. In principle, therefore, endocrine cells are symmetrical

(Fig. 2.15.). These cells are globular or polyhedral and the nucleus occupies a central position. In peptide hormone-secreting cells, the nucleus is surrounded by concentric cisterns of the rough endoplasmic reticulum and one or several Golgi-complexes. The rough endoplasmic reticulum may confer basophilic properties to the cytoplasm. Particularly in cells that produce a glycopeptide hormone, the Golgi-complex is well developed. Secretory vesicles are distributed in the peripheral cytoplasm. Consequently, exocytosis (merocrine secretion) takes place along its entire circumference, where the hormone molecules can enter the ubiquitous capillaries.

Cells that belong to this category are usually grouped into glandular tissue that forms endocrine glands. Examples are the **organotroph cells** of the anterior pituitary gland (IV.7.1.), the thyroid's **parafollicular cells** (Figs. 4.7.5.-6.), the parathyroid's **principal cells** (IV.7.3.) and **Langerhans's islet cells** of the pancreas (IV.15.4.).

Alternatively, and similar to exocrine cells, endocrine cells that secrete peptide hormones can be polarized. In this case, they occur as solitary cells in the lining of the lumen of the respiratory and digestive tracts (IV.15.2.1.). In contrast to exocrine gland cells, however, their polarization is reversed (Fig. 2.16.). The nucleus and the perinuclear cisterns of the rough

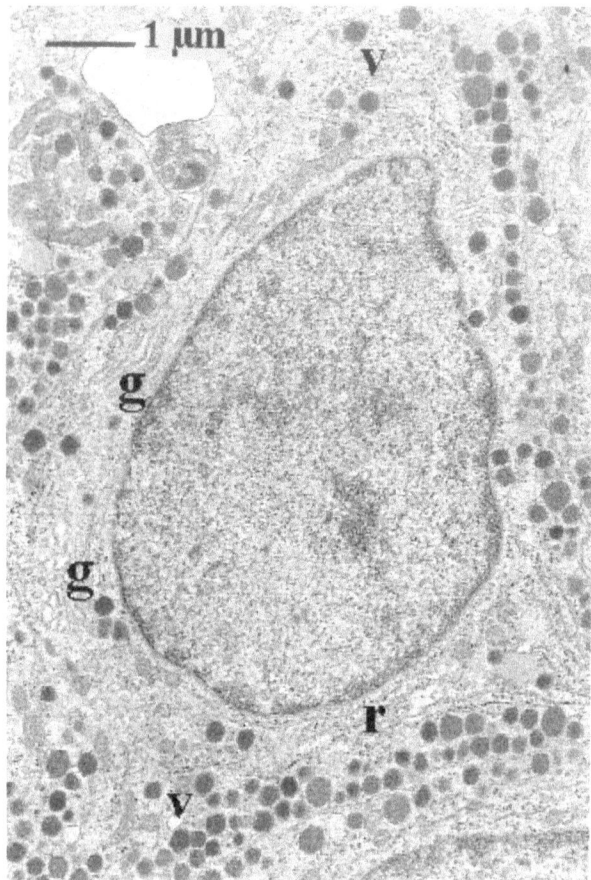

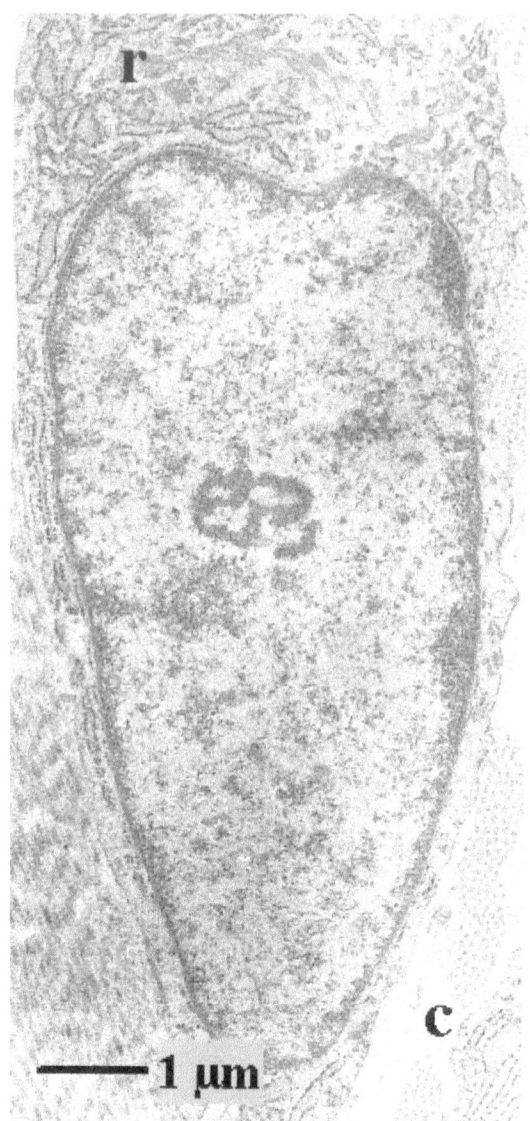

Fig. 2.15. An endocrine, peptide hormone-secreting gland cell. In this cell, the organelles have a symmetrical arrangement (compare with 2.14.). The nucleus occupies a central position, and is surrounded on all sides by, consecutively, rough endoplasmic reticulum (r) and secretory vesicles (v). A few Golgi-complexes (g) are also seen. Organotroph cell, anterior pituitary, rabbit, TEM.

Fig. 2.17. A matrix-secreting cell. This image shows a symmetric cell, the nucleus of which is completely surrounded by rough endoplasmic reticulum (r). The small volume of the cytoplasm, relative to the nucleus, as well as the absence of secretory vesicles, may indicate that this cell has entered a period of rest. The matrix contains collagen fibrils (c). Fibroblast, dermis, rabbit, TEM.

endoplasmic reticulum occupy the relatively expanded middle or basal parts of the cell, while the secretory vesicles are stored mainly in the basal portion of the cell. Exocytosis takes place at the basal cell membrane, not into the lumen. Close to the basal surface of the cell are capillaries, where the liberated hormone molecules enter the blood stream. The apical cell pole is tapered and may or may not contact the lumen. In the first case, the cell is accessible to stimuli from the lumen and is called an **open cell**. In the second case, the cell is **closed**.

II.2.1.1.3. Matrix-secreting cells.

Matrix-secreting cells (Fig. 2.17.) are in fact endocrine cells, the secretions of which remain close to the cell, and consequently accumulate in large amounts. Most

often, the cells end up by being enclosed by their own secretions. The secreted substance is rich in proteins. This so-called matrix is an essential part of interstitial, connective, and supportive tissues and contains two components, fibers and ground substance (III.2.2.-3.).

The cytoplasm of matrix-secreting cells is dominated by rough endoplasmic reticulum, which often shows dilated cisterns that vary in form and orientation. In principle, the cytoplasm shows basophilia, as

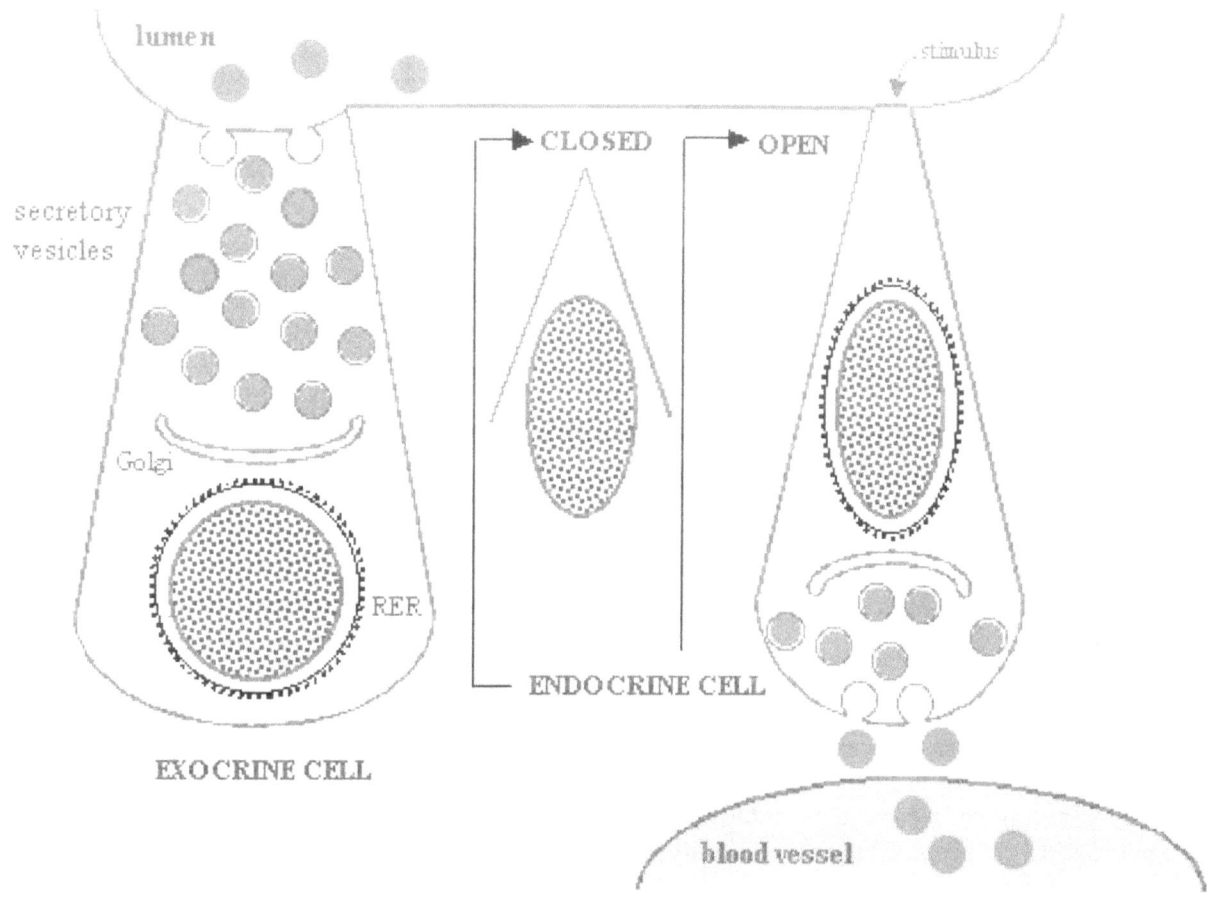

Fig. 2.16. Endocrine cells may be polarized, as exocrine cells are. Both cell types border a lumen, in which the exocrine cell liberates secretory products. The endocrine cell liberates its substances at the basal cell pole, away from the lumen. Nevertheless, an open cell remains exposed to this lumen, and may receive stimuli from it. A closed cell does not contact a lumen.

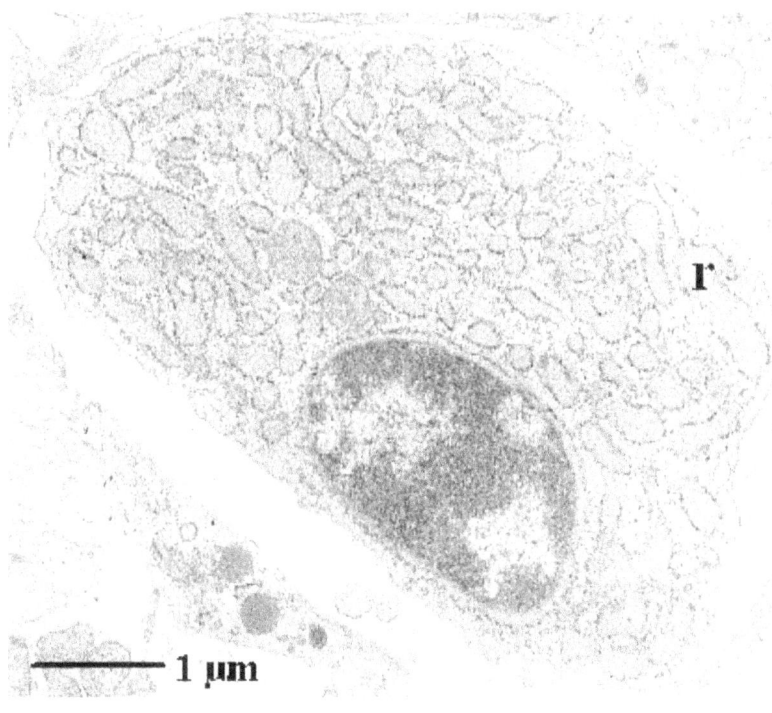

Fig. 2.18. An antibody-secreting cell. Synthesis of antibodies starts in the strongly developed rough endoplasmic reticulum (r), the cisterns of which are dilated. The absence of secretory vesicles and the heterochromatic aspect of the nucleus may indicate that this cell has entered a period of rest. Plasma cell, jejunal villus, rabbit, TEM.

serous gland cells do (II.2.1.1.1.). In addition, one or more well developed Golgi-complexes are found. The mechanism of secretion is merocrine, i.e. by exocytosis of individual vesicles. The spatial arrangement of the cell's organelles determines in which way the matrix is deposited. Sometimes, the cell is more or less symmetrical and the matrix is deposited all around it. In other instances, the cells are distinctly polarized and the matrix is deposited at one cell pole only.

The most typical members of this group are the **fibroblasts** (Fig. 2.17.). These are involved in the formation of all kinds of fibrous (III.2.4.2.) and elastic (III.2.4.3.) tissues. They develop processes, into which cisterns of the rough endoplasmic reticulum penetrate. More specialized matrix-secreting cells are the **chondroblasts** and the **osteoblasts**, which produce the matrices of cartilage (III.2.4.4.) and bone (III.2.4.5.), respectively.

II.2.1.1.4. Antibody-secreting cells.

Antibody-secreting cells participate in the defense of the body against invaders, which are generally called antigens. After being secreted, the antibodies specifically bind with a complementary type of antigen and thus initiate its elimination.

Antibodies are proteins and the cells that produce them, the **plasma cells** (Fig. 2.18.), have a strongly basophilic cytoplasm because of the well-developed rough endoplasmic reticulum, often with dilated cisterns. They are endocrine cells, but their symmetry is often disrupted by the eccentric position of the nucleus, which gives the cell an oval shape. The nucleus contains rough clumps of heterochromatin, which sometimes form more or less clear patterns, like a chessboard or the spokes of a wheel. Plasma cells are merocrine: the antibodies are secreted by individual exocytosis of vesicles.

II.2.1.2. The Golgi-complex and mucus-secreting gland cells.

The membranes forming the Golgi-complex line a number of flattened, parallel cisterns that are often arched and somewhat dilated at their periphery (Fig. 2.19.). A cell can number one or several Golgi-complexes, which are most frequently located in the vicinity of the nucleus. Due to the parallel arrangement of the arched cisterns, the whole complex has a convex pole and a concave one. Either pole can point towards the nucleus. The Golgi-complex collects the polypeptides, synthesized by the rough endoplasmic reticulum. While moving through the complex, they are converted to proteins, and packed into secretory vesicles that will bud from the Golgi-complex and eventually discharge the proteins into the extracellular space (Fig. 2.12.). The face where substances enter is called the cis-side, the face where they leave the trans-side. Usually, the cis-side is the convex one, the trans-side the concave one. The cisterns in the middle of the stack, often called mid-saccules, tend to appear uninterrupted. The cisterns on both the cis- and the trans-side are often perforated in many places. In sections, they will appear as rows of flattened vesicles. These perforations transform the cisterns into a network: a cis–Golgi network and a trans-Golgi network, respectively. The trans-Golgi network in particular is variable and its structure depends on the types of secretory material to be handled.

Vesicles, which bud from the rough endoplasmic

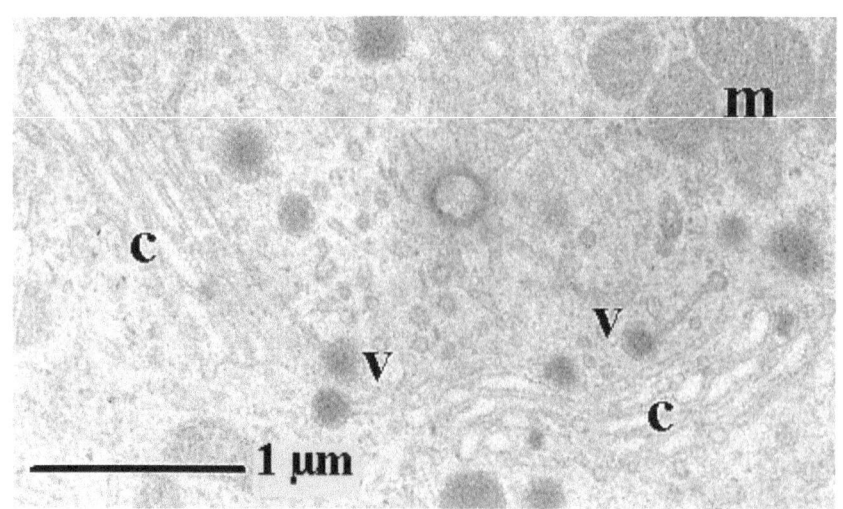

Fig. 2.19. The Golgi-complex is made up of a number of flattened, parallel cisterns (c), bordered by a membrane. The complex may be arched, having a concave and a convex side. The rim of the cisterns may be dilated and contain dense material. These dilated parts are the precursors of secretory vesicles (v), which are liberated by budding. m: mitochondria. Thyroid parafollicular cell, rat, TEM.

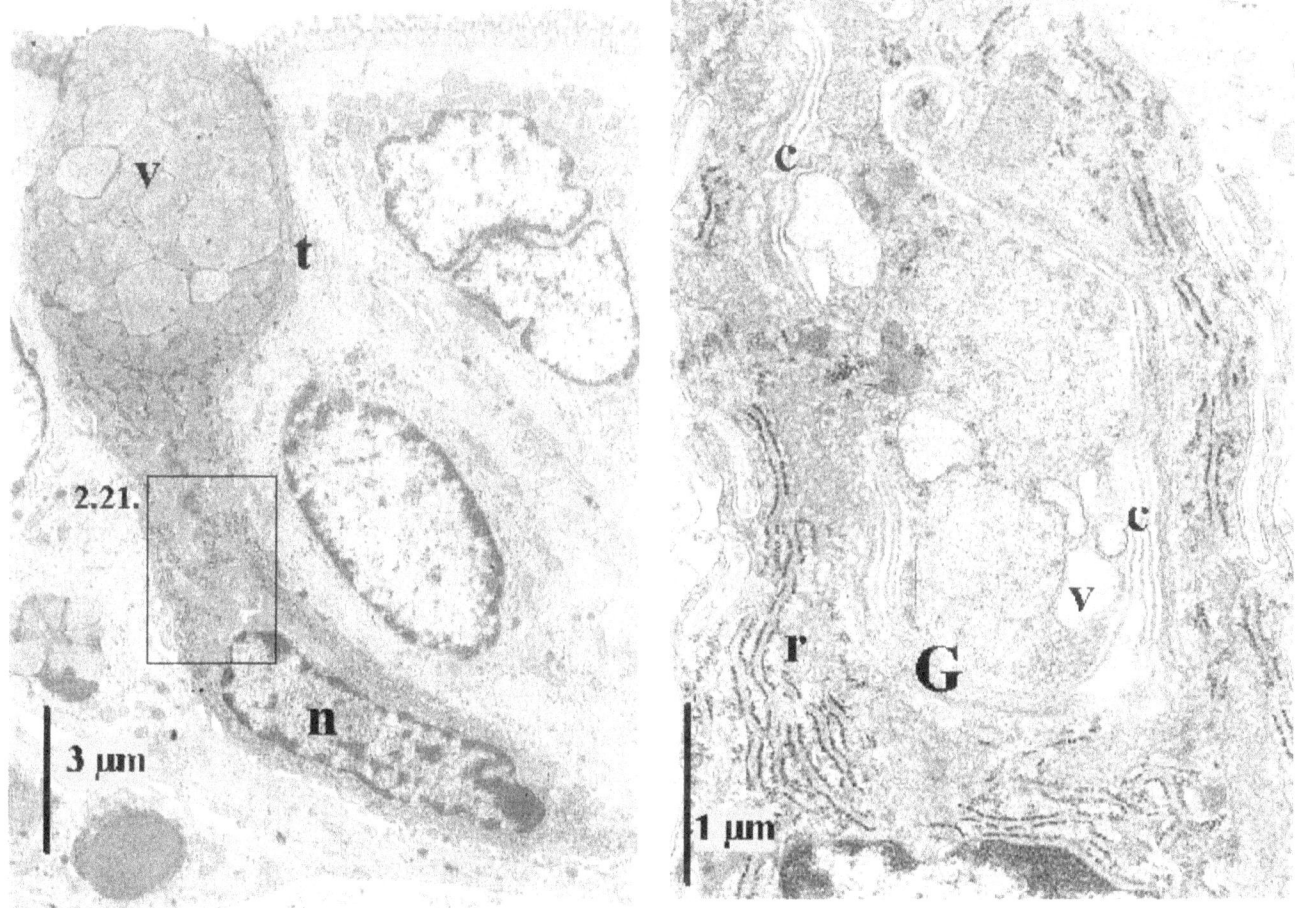

Fig. 2.20. (left) The Golgi-complex may be particularly well developed in mucus-secreting gland cells, such as goblet cells. These are polarized, exocrine gland cells. The basal cell pole contains the nucleus (n), surrounded by rough endoplasmic reticulum. The apical pole, bordering a lumen, is loaded with mucus-filled secretory vesicles (v). These vesicles are squeezed together, and tend to coalesce into a single mucus bubble, which appears as if resting in the expanded, cup-shaped apical cell part or theca (t). The strongly developed Golgi-complex occupies a supranuclear position, indicated by the rectangle. Goblet cell, small intestine, rabbit, TEM. **Fig. 2.21.** (right) Enlargement of the approximate area indicated in Figure 2.20. The Golgi-complex (g) of a goblet cell is very large and numbers several narrow, parallel cisterns (c). The concave side of the complex points away from the nucleus, and is associated with incipient secretory vesicles (v). It can be safely regarded as the trans side, where secretory vesicles originate. Rough endoplasmic reticulum (r) can also be seen. Goblet cell, small intestine, rabbit, TEM.

reticulum, are ferried to the cis-Golgi network and fuse with the cisternal membrane, discharging their polypeptide content in its interior. Inside the Golgi-complex, the polypeptides are unidirectionally transported towards the trans-Golgi network. A well-established means of transport (evidence exists for alternative means) is by vesicles that detach from the edge of a cis-cistern and fuse with a trans-cistern. Vesicle formation and detachment is made possible by proteins with the same function as clathrin (II.2.1.4.), which associate themselves with the cytosolic face of the cisternal membranes. Eventually, at the trans-Golgi network, secretory vesicles bud which are ferried to the cell membrane. The material that will end up in secretory vesicles may be opaque. In this case, it can already be made out in the cisterns of the Golgi-complex (Fig. 2.19.). This vesicular transport mechanism forms a beautiful illustration of the plastic and self-sealing properties of cytosolic membranes (II.1.1.).

During transport of the polypeptides, the Golgi-complex converts them to biologically active proteins.

Polypeptides are just chains of amino acids and have to undergo a whole range of modifications before they are functional proteins. These modifications include folding of the polypeptide chains, clipping of certain parts, formation of links between different parts of a chain, and attachment of carbohydrate molecules, forming glyco- or mucoproteins. These carbohydrates are partly synthesized in the Golgi-complex.

The Golgi-complex can even sort different kinds of proteins. This is accomplished by means of specific receptor proteins in its membranes. In this way, the Golgi-complex of the same cell can form different kinds of vesicles, such as secretory vesicles and lysosomes, each with their own content.

The Golgi-complex reaches its most extreme level of development in **mucus-secreting gland** cells, which are often encountered in the lining of the lumen of various internal organs. Mucus, a complex mixture of glyco- and mucoproteins, has a lubricating and protective function.

The most typical examples of mucus-secreting gland cells are the **goblet cells**, found in the linings of the gut lumen and the airways. They show the typical characteristics of exocrine cells. They are distinctly polarized (Fig. 2.20.). The rough endoplasmic reticulum occupies a perinuclear position in the cell basis. The Golgi-complex is excessively developed (Fig. 2.21.) and occupies a supranuclear position. The cell apex or theca, contacting the lumen, is filled with secretory vesicles. They are large, up to 1 micrometer in diameter, and have an electron lucent content. They are closely squeezed together, forcing them into polyhedral shapes, and have a strong tendency to fuse with their neighbours, giving rise to ever-larger vesicles. In extreme cases, this may result in a single apical mucus bubble. This bubble is so large that it is visible by light microscopy. Because of the bubble's large size, the theca is dilated. In the electron microscope, the cell appears as a goblet with a narrow stem and a cup-like apex in which the mucus bubble appears to be resting. The cytoplasmic wall of the theca is reinforced with intermediate filaments and microtubules.

Goblet cells are continuously active, releasing mucus through exocytosis of single vesicles: merocrine secretion. Occasionally, they may be spurred to more intense bouts of activity. In the most extreme case, the entire mucus bubble is discharged into the lumen upon disruption of the apical cell membrane. Thus, the complete apical cell part, which may even include fragments of cytoplasm, is lost. Such a secretory mechanism, which involves loss of the cell's top part, is called **apocrine**. The remaining basal cell half can

regenerate a new top half, starting a new cycle of synthesis and discharge. Between both extremes, intermediate forms of secretion have been observed. Several vesicles may fuse into a larger one, which undergoes exocytosis: compound exocytosis. Small fragments of cytoplasm may separate from the cell apex, enclosing one or more mucus vesicles: micro-apocrine secretion.

Other types of mucus-secreting cells occur elsewhere in the gut and respiratory tract. Examples are the mucous cells of the gastric mucosal glands (Fig. 4.15.28.), the mucous cells of the submucosal glands of oesophagus, cardia, duodenum (Fig. 4.15.35.) and airways (Fig. 4.14.14.), and the mucous acinar cells of the salivary glands (Figs. 4.15.16.-17.). In general, and compared to goblet cells, these cells are less polarized and their secretory vesicles show less tendency to fuse. The degree of development of rough endoplasmic reticulum and Golgi-complex depends on the chemical composition of the mucus produced.

II.2.1.3. Secretory vesicles and amine hormone-secreting gland cells.

Amine hormone-secreting gland cells are endocrine cells in which, of all GERL components, the secretory vesicles are most prominent.

Amine hormones are small, relatively simple messenger molecules that contain nitrogen atoms. A few well-known examples are adrenaline, noradrenaline, dopamine, and serotonin. These molecules are produced by decarboxylation of a precursor amino acid, such as phenylalanine or tryptophan. Decarboxylation, as well as the subsequent reaction steps leading to the formation of the messenger molecule, is catalyzed by cytosolic enzymes. Consequently, the finished amine hormone molecules accumulate in the cytosol. The action of pumps in the membrane of the secretory vesicles concentrates the hormone molecules in the vesicular interior, where they are bound to a carrier protein, chromogranin. In amine hormone-secreting gland cells, neither the rough endoplasmic reticulum nor the Golgi-complex are well developed, since they are not involved in the production of secretory product, which is not a protein. Their only task is the production of vesicular membrane with integral proteins (pumps) and of carrier protein. The enzymes needed to produce amine hormone molecules are made by free ribosomes.

Amine hormone-secreting gland cells can be of the

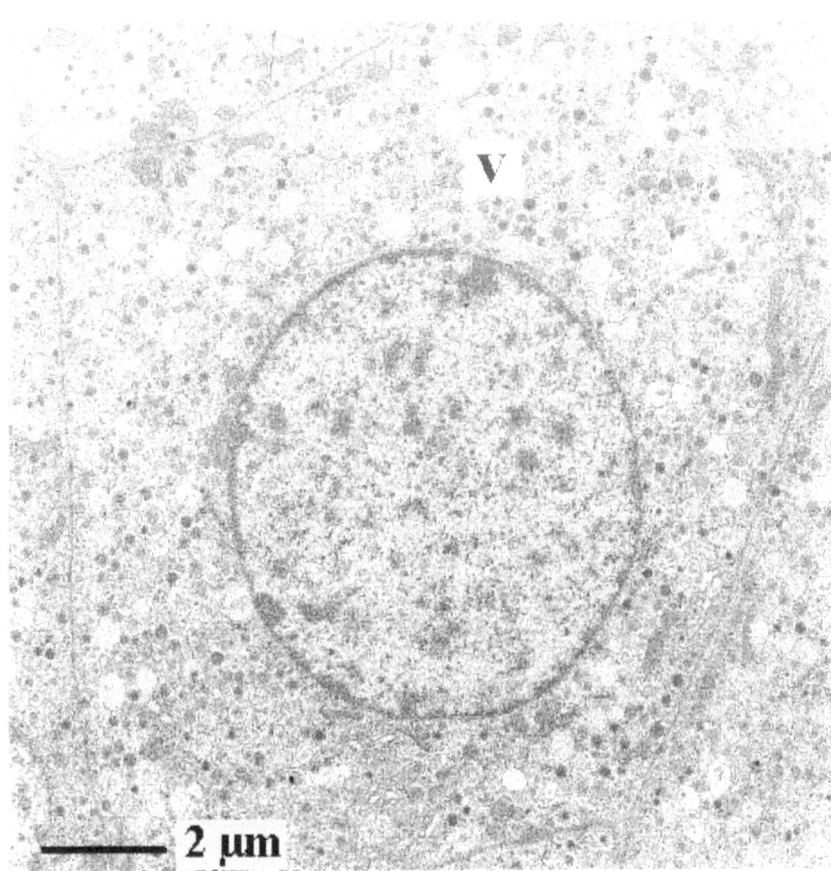

V

—— 2 μm

Fig. 2.22. An amine hormone-secreting gland cell. This is a symmetric cell with a central nucleus, surrounded by secretory vesicles (v), which are very numerous and almost completely fill the cytosol. Other GERL components are not well-developed and only show up sporadically. Adrenal medulla, rabbit, TEM.

symmetric or the asymmetric type, similar to peptide hormone-secreting gland cells.

In the symmetric type, the best-known example of which are the **chromaffin cells** of the adrenal medulla (Fig. 2.22.), the secretory vesicles are distributed evenly, surrounding the central nucleus. With a diameter of only a few tens of nanometers, the secretory vesicles are relatively small. Usually, there is a narrow, translucent halo between the vesicle's opaque content and its membrane. The cells have a merocrine secretory mechanism, the vesicles discharging their content by individual exocytosis.

In the asymmetric, polarized type, which is found primarily in the interior lining of the gut (IV.15.2.1.) and the airways (IV.14.1.2.), the secretory vesicles accumulate in the cell basis and their content is discharged in the subcellular space. Their apex may or may not contact the lumen, the cells being of the open or the closed type, respectively.

II.2.1.4. Endosomes, lysosomes, and macrophages.

Endosomes arise from a local depression in the cell membrane, which deepens and is finally pinched off.

This process, **endocytosis** (Fig. 2.12.) is the reverse of exocytosis. In this way, various substances can be carried into the cell's interior.

In many cells, the endosomes have fairly standard dimensions, with a diameter of about 50 nanometers, and these are called **pinocytotic vesicles**. The particular process of endocytosis that forms them is called pinocytosis. Pinocytosis is a way of recycling of membrane, which has been inserted into the cell membrane by exocytosis. In the rough endoplasmic reticulum and Golgi-complex, a certain amount of neoformation of membrane takes place, but in cells where exocytosis is intense, this does not suffice to maintain the amount of cytosolic membrane. Looked at from another perspective, exocytosis increases the area of the cell membrane, and this too cannot continue indefinitely. By pinocytosis, superfluous cell membrane is re-internalized, whereupon it can be incorporated into some component of the cytosolic membrane system (Fig. 2.12.). Pinocytosis also occurs in cells regulating the exchange of fluid between two compartments of the organism, such as endothelial and mesothelial cells (III.4.2.). In these cells, pinocytotic vesicles shuttle between the luminal (apical) and the abluminal (basal) cell membranes, carrying fluid between two compartments, such as the

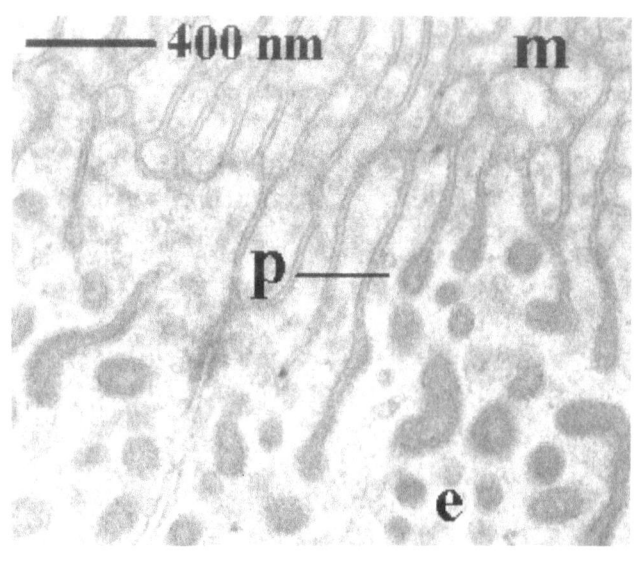

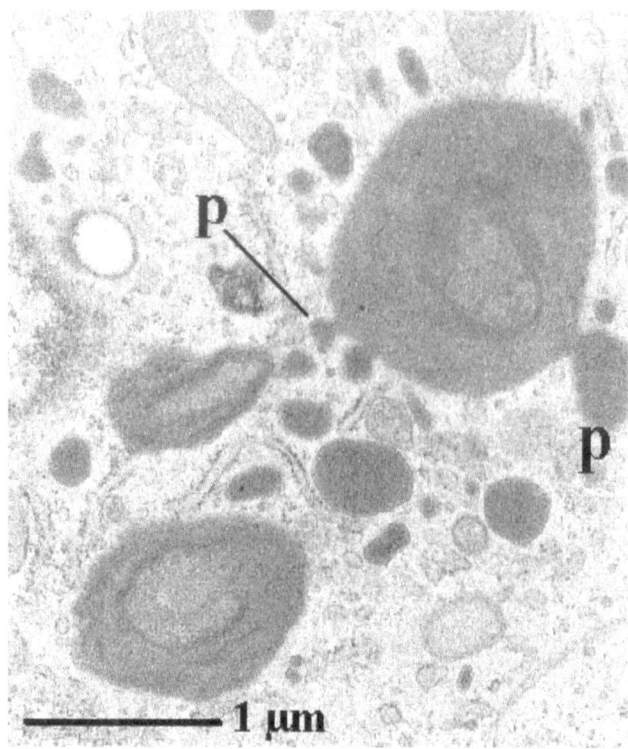

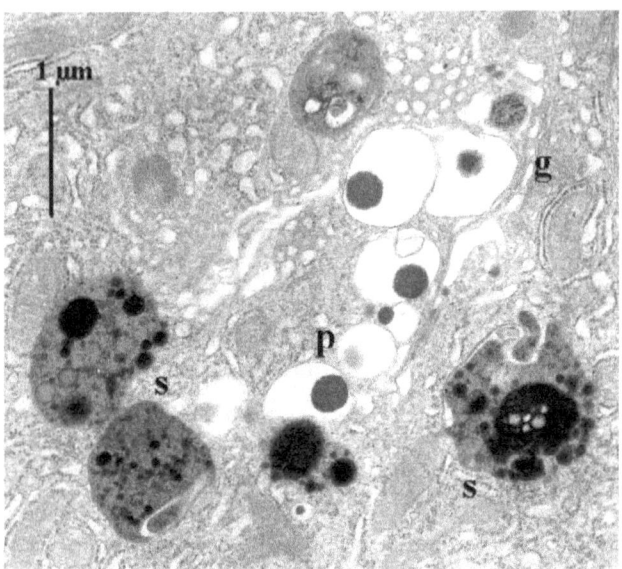

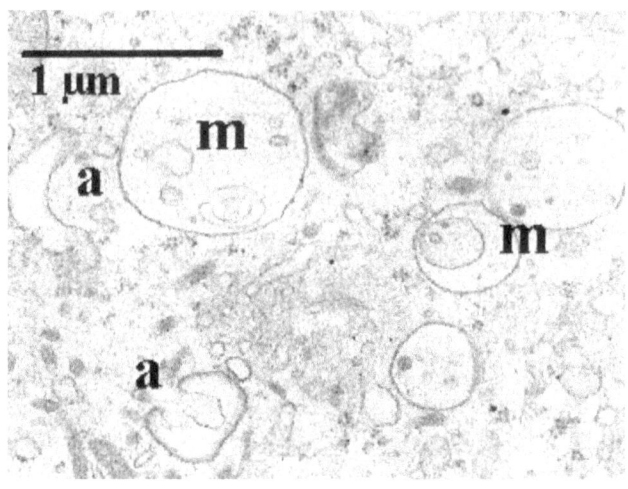

Fig. 2.23. (top left) Endosomes. This picture shows the apex of an epithelial cell of a kidney proximal convoluted tubule (compare with Figure 4.8.10.). It carries numerous microvilli (m), sectioned transversely. At the bases of the microvilli, the cell membrane forms inpocketings, the cytosolic face of which is lined with a fibrillar coat: coated pits (p). The coated pits detach from the cell membrane and are converted to coated vesicles. When these shed their coat, they are called endosomes (e). Endosome formation allows these cells to absorb substances from the tubular lumen. Kidney proximal contorted tubule, rabbit, TEM. **Fig. 2.24.** (bottom left) Primary lysosomes (p) lie next to the Golgi-complex (g) they have budded from. The larger bodies with variable content are probably secondary lysosomes (s), because they contain dense round inclusions resembling the content of the surrounding primary lysosomes. Probably, these bodies have recently fused with primary lysosomes. Epithelial cell, seminal vesicle, hamster, TEM. **Fig. 2.25.** (top right) Primary lysosomes (p) fuse with a larger body in a macrophage's cytoplasm. This body does not contain material resembling the primary lysosomal content, making it unlikely that it has already undergone fusion with primary lysosomes. For this reason, it can be regarded as a phagosome. Macrophage, spleen, rabbit, TEM. **Fig. 2.26.** (bottom right) Autophagosomes (a) engulfing parts of the cytosol, and multivesicular bodies (m) form in an epithelial cell. Kidney proximal convoluted tubule, cat, TEM.

vascular lumen and the intercellular spaces.

At the spot where endo- or pinocytosis is about to take place, the interior face of the cell membrane gets coated with a dense protein layer. This protein is a contractile one, the coat protein or **clathrin**. Contraction in this protein layer produces a local bowl-like depression of the cell membrane. In a tissue section studied with the electron microscope, this depression looks like the Greek letter omega, coated on its convex face with clathrin: a **coated pit**. The pit deepens, its rim is constricted, and a vesicle is pinched off, still coated on its cytosolic face with clathrin: a **coated vesicle** or **acanthosome** (Figs. 2.12., 2.23.). An endosome or pinocytotic vesicle proper is formed upon shedding of the coat. Proteins similar to clathrin participate in the vesicular transport mechanism in the Golgi-complex (Fig. 2.12.), and acanthosomes can be observed here as well.

A much less specific form of endocytosis is **phagocytosis**, by which large particles (cell debris, micro-organisms, etc.) can be internalized. Phagocytosis amounts to engulfment of a particle by the cell, and is the hallmark of macrophages, cells that are specialized in the removal of debris. The uptake of large particles naturally gives rise to larger endosomes, or **phagosomes**.

Substances and particles taken up by endocytosis will be degraded. In this process, **lysosomes** participate. Similar to secretory vesicles, lysosomes bud from the Golgi-complex (Fig. 2.24.) and contain enzymes produced by the rough endoplasmic reticulum. The major distinction between lysosomes and secretory vesicles is that the former, in principle at least, never fuse with the cell membrane and consequently never take part in exocytosis. Instead, they fuse with endosomes. Lysosomes contain a cocktail of hydrolytic enzymes, suited for degradation of the most diverse macromolecules. Fusion with endosomes discharges these enzymes into the endosome's interior, whereupon they mix with and degrade the contents. Thus, endosomes may function as cellular "stomachs", the digestive enzymes being supplied by lysosomes.

A newly formed lysosome is called a **primary lysosome** (Figs. 2.12., 2.24.-25.). Primary lysosomes have a diameter of a few hundred nanometers and a homogeneous, moderately opaque content. They are most frequent in the vicinity of the Golgi-complex. After fusion with an endosome (Fig. 2.25.), initiating the degradation of its contents, the resulting vesicle is referred to as a **secondary lysosome** (Figs. 2.12.,

2.24.). Secondary lysosomes have a variable appearance, due to several reasons. First, there can be considerable variation in the chemical composition of the material to be degraded. Second, the appearance of the secondary lysosomes changes as degradation progresses. In general, secondary lysosomes contain irregular bits and pieces of variable density. Since they arise from the fusion of two vesicles, they are distinctly larger than primary lysosomes. Secondary lysosomes may fuse with a new endosome or with a new primary lysosome. The latter will contribute a fresh supply of enzyme. This can continue for a while, but eventually the secondary lysosome's supply of enzymes will be exhausted. At the same time, indigestible residues gradually accumulate. The end result is a **residual body** (Fig. 2.12.) that has lost all enzymatic activity. Older cells may accumulate such residual bodies in growing numbers, giving rise to light optically visible lipofuchsin pigment, the so-called wear and tear pigment. The cells making up multicellular organisms have lost the faculty of "defecation" and, consequently, cannot discard these remains. The reason for this is that, in multicellular organisms, digestion of foodstuffs is largely an extracellular process, taking place in the gut lumen. Only low molecular weight food molecules, the end products of this digestion, are taken up by the cells. These molecules produce little or no indigestible leftovers. Therefore, cells that engulf large amounts of particulate matter (cell debris, micro-organisms), such as macrophages, do not live long, because they soon suffer from "constipation" and die.

In a more general sense, lysosomes contribute to cell maintenance and rebuilding. Damaged or worn out organelles, or organelles that are no longer needed at a particular stage of cell development, have to be cleared away. This can be done in two ways (Fig. 2.12.). One way is neoformation of membrane in the cytosol, surrounding the organelle, which thus ends up in a closed vesicle: an **autophagosome**. Subsequently, lysosomes will fuse with it. This mechanism is used primarily to degrade the larger organelles or even substantial parts of the cytoplasm as a whole. Another way is engulfment of an organelle by a vesicle or endosome, giving rise to a complex vesicular body: a vesicle enclosing a smaller vesicle enclosing the organelle to be degraded. This process may be repeated a number of times, giving rise to a **multivesicular body** (Fig. 2.26.), with which lysosomes fuse. In these ways, cells can degrade or "eat" parts of themselves, a process referred to as **autophagocytosis**.

Malfunctioning of lysosomes is at the root of so-called

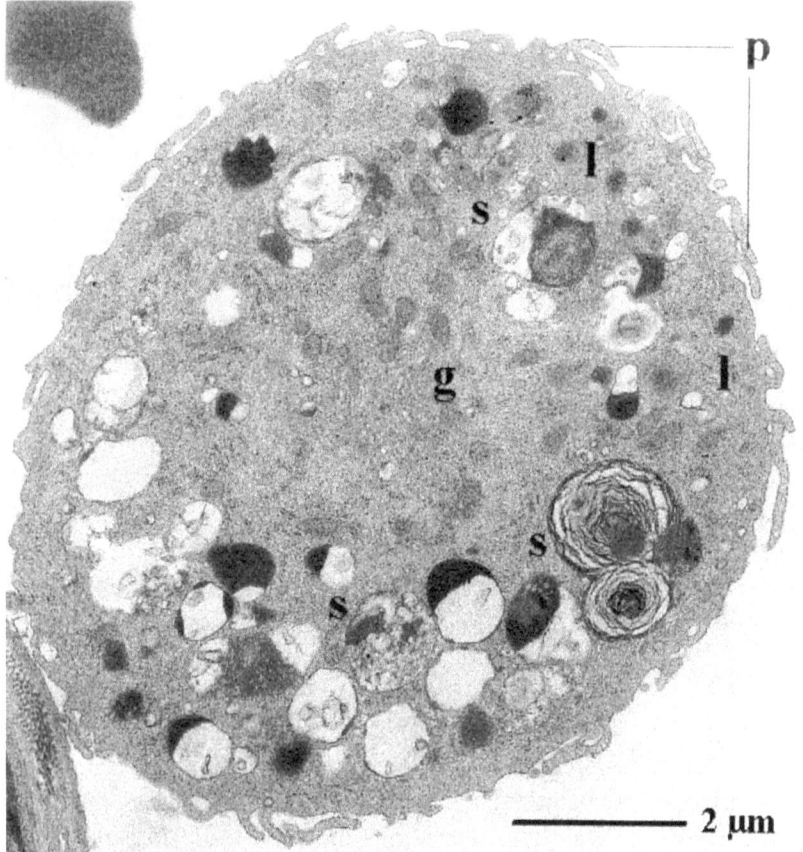

p

Fig. 2.27. The nucleus of this macrophage, which in principle occupies a central position, lies outside the section plane. In the center of the cell, a few Golgi-complexes (g) are seen. The cellular periphery is dominated by primary lysosomes (l) and numerous phagosomes and secondary lysosomes (s). The cell membrane shows slender outpocketings: pseudopodia (p). Pulmonary macrophage, human, TEM.

——————— 2 μm

storage diseases. When they lack a specific enzyme, the corresponding substance can no longer be degraded and accumulates inside the cell.

Lysosomes are most conspicuously present in cells called **macrophages**. Macrophages (Fig. 2.27.) are, in principle, symmetrical cells with a central nucleus, surrounded by a strongly developed rough endoplasmic reticulum for synthesis of lysosomal enzymes and several Golgi-complexes. At the cell's periphery, the cytoplasm is loaded with lysosomes and phagosomes that have a variable appearance, depending on their contents and the progress of its degradation.

Macrophages often have very irregular shapes, which is a consequence of their active mode of life. Macrophages not only phagocytose, but also are continuously on the move, searching for material to engulf. The means by which macrophages move and phagocytose all depend on amoeboid movements, which refers to the mechanism of movement of the well-known unicellular organism. The peripheral layer of cytosol contains a network of actin molecules and has a gel-like consistency, while the deeper cytosol is more fluid, or sol-like. Locally, by reversible dismantling of the actin network, the gel-phase can change into the sol-phase. When the remaining gel-layer contracts, a protrusion forms and the cell "flows" in its direction, displacing itself. The gel's contraction is made possible by the interaction of actin molecules with myosin molecules (II.2.2.2.). By continuation of this process, a macrophage can "crawl" along. On a smaller scale, this mechanism gives rise to protuberances, with which the macrophage can engulf particles. Depending on their shape, distinction is made between rather short, blunt **pseudopodia** and longer, more slender **filipodia**.

Macrophages are found throughout the organism. By swallowing foreign invaders, they contribute vitally to the body's defense against infection. After phagocytosis and digestion of foreign material, parts of it are incorporated in their cell membrane, like trophies. Specific kinds of immune cells interact with these fragments and are stimulated by this contact to perform their own immunological reactions. It appears as though the macrophages show them their trophies: antigen presentation. Another important function of macrophages is the removal of waste and sick and dead or dying cells. The most typical kinds of macrophages are the **alveolar macrophage** of the lungs (Fig. 2.27.) and the **histiocyte** of the interstitial tissues (Fig. 3.2.6.). The **neutrophilic** and **eosinophilic granulocytes** of the blood and the interstitial tissues (Figs. 3.1.9.-10.) are rather specialized macrophages. The **osteoclast** of the bone (Fig. 3.2.21.) is another specialized kind of macrophage.

II.2.1.5. Smooth endoplasmic reticulum.

The smooth endoplasmic reticulum consists of cytosolic membranes, lining a network of cisterns (Fig. 2.28.). In contrast to the rough endoplasmic reticulum, these cisterns are not plate-like, but tubular. They ramify intensively. Since they do not carry ribosomes, they appear smooth. The smooth endoplasmic reticulum is not clearly integrated in the GERL (II.2.1.) and appears to function independently.

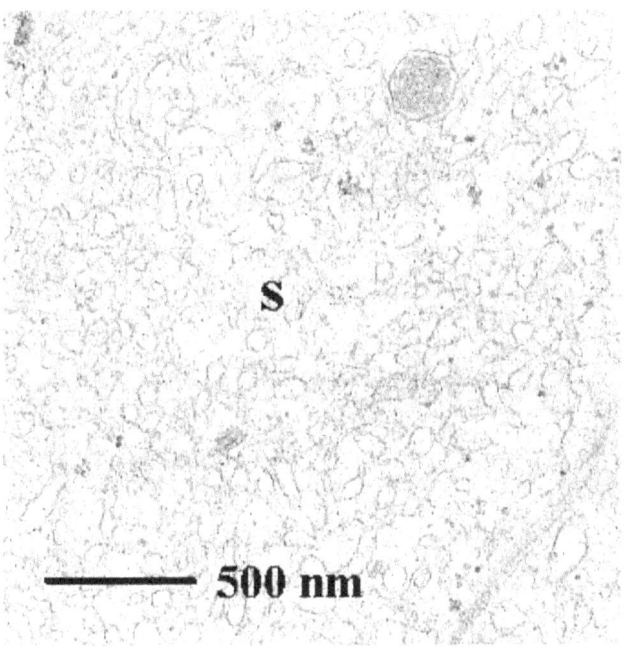

Fig. 2.28. Smooth endoplasmic reticulum (s) is made up of a maze of tubular membranous cisterns that, in section, show circular to elongated shapes. Leydig cell, testis, mouse, TEM.

The smooth endoplasmic reticulum carries some of the enzymes that are required for the synthesis of fats and carbohydrates. These substances accumulate in the cytosol, at the outside of the smooth endoplasmic reticulum, implying that they are not surrounded by a membrane. The fats synthesized by the smooth endoplasmic reticulum include lipids (esters of fatty acids and glycerol) and steroids (derivatives of cholesterol). Lipids can be expelled in exocrine secretion or stored in the cell, a process that occurs in the specialized lipocytes or fat cells (III.2.1.2.). Steroids function as hormones and are expelled in endocrine secretion.

In some instances, continuity between the membranes of the smooth and the rough endoplasmic reticuli is found, implying that both reticuli can cooperate in the production of substances such as lipoproteins.

The most important carbohydrate synthesized by the smooth endoplasmic reticulum is glycogen, a polymer of glucose. Glycogen stores take the form of dense particles with a diameter of 15 to 30 nanometers, which accumulate in the cytosol (Fig. 2.11.). A number of particles may aggregate to form larger complexes, called rosettes. Glycogen is a reserve energy store that can be used, when needed, to supply glucose to the mitochondria.

The smooth endoplasmic reticulum's interior is also a storage site for calcium ions, particularly in the case of muscle fibers, since calcium is an important agent that regulates the muscle fiber's contractility (II.2.2.2.2.2.).

II.2.1.5.1. Lipid-secreting gland cells.

Lipid-secreting gland cells have an exocrine secretory mechanism. The most important members of this group are found in the respiratory tract and in the skin. Since lipids are synthesized at the outside of the smooth endoplasmic reticulum, they are not surrounded by a membrane. Rather they accumulate as droplets.

In the respiratory tract, **Clara cells** (Fig. 2.29.) line the distal airways. They are clearly polarized, as are many exocrine cells (II.2.1.1.1., II.2.1.2.). Their nucleus occupies the cell basis, while the smooth endoplasmic reticulum and lipid droplets are found in the apical part of the cell. Clara cells secrete a complex mixture of phospholipids. The secretory mechanism is **apocrine**, i.e. the cell apex, or parts of it, is lost. The phospholipids coat the interior of the smallest airways and have a stabilizing effect on their surface tension, preventing them from collapsing. The lining of the pulmonary alveoli also contains lipid-secreting cells, the **type II alveolar epithelial cells** (Fig. 4.14.6.). Their function is analogous to that of the Clara cells.

The **sebum gland cells** of the skin are also lipid-secreting (IV.9.1.4.3.). They belong to the rare exocrine gland cells that are not polarized, but symmetrical. This is a direct consequence of their secretory mechanism. Smooth endoplasmic reticulum is only present during lipid synthesis, after which the cells enter a period of rest. Lipid droplets accumulate in the cytosol surrounding the nucleus until they fill the whole cell. They are set free at the skin's surface by disruption of the cell. This method of secretion, whereby the whole cell is lost, is called **holocrine**.

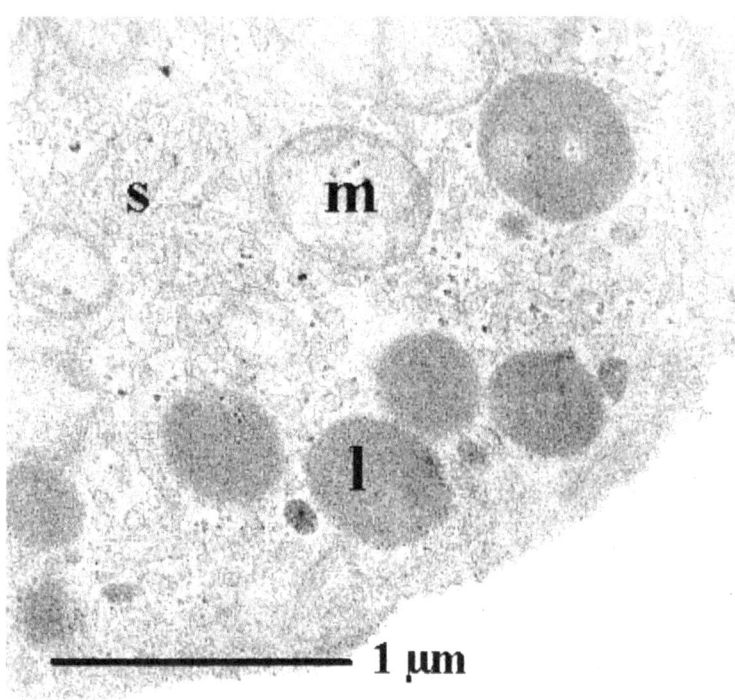

Fig. 2.29. Smooth endoplasmic reticulum is strongly developed in lipid-secreting gland cells, such as the Clara cells of the airways. These are polarized exocrine cells with a basal nucleus. This image shows the apex of a Clara cell. In between the smooth endoplasmic reticulum's cisterns (s), lipids accumulate into droplets (l), which may have a fibrillar coat, but lack a membrane. m = mitochondria. Airway epithelium, rabbit, TEM.

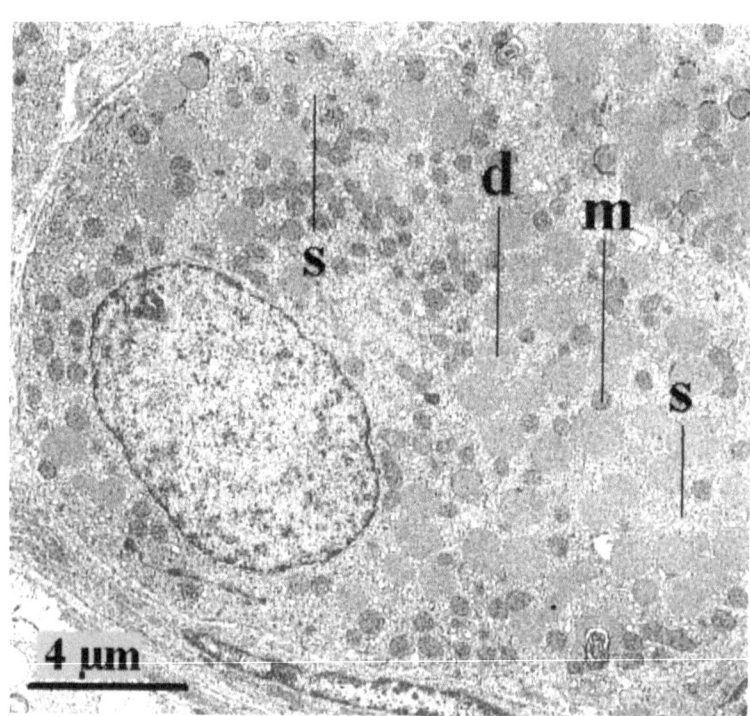

Fig. 2.30. Smooth endoplasmic reticulum is also strongly developed in steroid hormone-secreting gland cells. Smooth endoplasmic reticulum (s) and steroid droplets (d) surround the central nucleus. The small dark objects are mitochondria (m). Interstitial cell, ovary, rabbit, TEM.

II.2.1.5.2. Steroid-secreting gland cells.

Steroid-secreting gland cells are endocrine and always symmetrical (Fig.2.30.). A prominent smooth endoplasmic reticulum surrounds the centrally located nucleus. Some of the enzymes needed for steroid synthesis are carried in the reticulum's membrane, while the others are located in the mitochondria's inner membrane. The inner mitochondrial membrane typically does not form crests, but tubules. Steroid-secreting gland cells take in cholesterol by means of receptor-mediated endocytosis. Cholesterol is the precursor molecule from which steroids are derived. It is stored in the cytosol, not inside vesicles, but in the form of droplets, with a diameter of up to a micrometer or more. These steroid droplets may be coated, but lack a membrane. It must be stressed that these droplets do not contain finished product, but only precursor molecules, which is a fundamental difference with lipid-secreting cells. In actively secreting cells, the number and size of these droplets can decrease dramatically, not as a consequence of secretion, but due to depletion of precursor molecules during synthesis. Preparation of tissues for light microscopy necessitates the use of dehydrating fluids, such as ethanol, which dissolve steroids. As a consequence, steroid-secreting cells may appear as vacuolated, spongy cells and are called spongiocytes (Fig. 4.7.10.). The finished steroids enter the cytosol, but do not accumulate. They are only produced to the extent that they are needed. Their chemical structure enables them, in principle, to leave the cell by diffusion through the cell membrane. The exact secretory mechanism is still debated.

The most important cell types of this category are the **adrenal cortical cells** (IV.7.4.), the interstitial **Leydig cells** of the testes (IV.10.1.2.), the **ovarian interstitial cells** (Fig. 2.29.), the **theca interna cells** of the ovarian follicles (IV.11.1.2.) and the **granulosa lutein** and **theca lutein cells** of the corpus luteum (IV.11.1.3.).

II.2.2. Fiber-bearing cells.

Many cell types contain massive amounts of cytosolic fibers that belong to one of three categories: **microtubules**, **microfilaments** and **intermediary filaments**. In general, these fibers contribute to the **cytoskeleton**, which supports the cell and gives it the shape it needs to function. Cells have a strong tendency to assume a spherical shape because of the

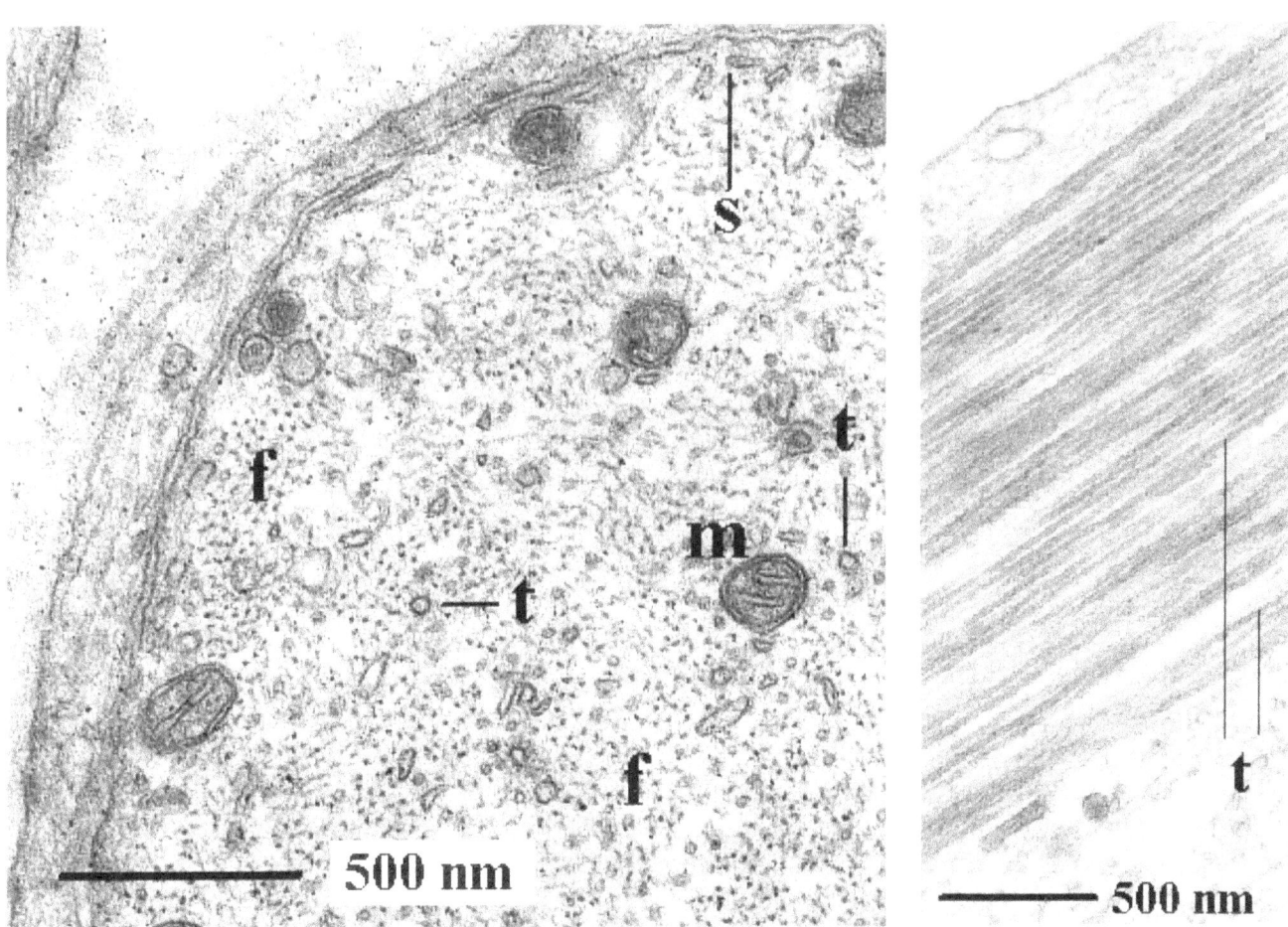

Fig. 2.31. (left) A transverse section of an axon, a process of a nerve cell. The minute circles are transversely sectioned microtubules (t). The dots are intermediary filaments, the neurofilaments (f). Smooth endoplasmic reticulum (s) and mitochondria (m) are also present. Spinal ganglion, cat, TEM. **Fig. 2.32.** (right) A bundle of longitudinally sectioned microtubules (t) in a supporting cell of Deiters. Corti's organ, cat, TEM.

pressure exerted by the cytosol. Deviations from this shape cannot be permanent unless they are supported by a cytoskeleton. Cytosolic fibers may confer motile or contractile properties either to the whole cell, or to

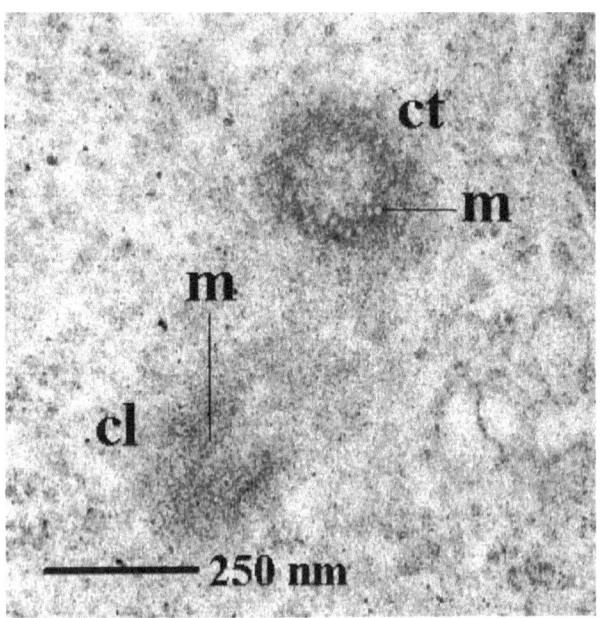

Fig. 2.33. A centrosome is composed of 2 tubular centrioles at right angles to each other (ct = transversely sectioned centriole, cl = longitudinally sectioned centriole). Each centriole is made up of 9 inclined triplets of microtubules (m). Compare with a ciliary root, Figure 2.36. Nerve cell, hamster, TEM.

parts of it. They can strengthen the cell, enabling it to protect or to support other cells.

Either type of cytosolic fiber may predominate, so that several types of fiber-bearing cells can be distinguished.

II.2.2.1. Microtubules, cilia, and ciliated cells.

Microtubules are hollow, tubular fibers, varying in length, and with a diameter of about 25 nanometers (Figs. 2.31., 2.32.). They are assembled from building blocks, consisting of the protein tubulin. Microtubules are an important part of the cytoskeleton, the cell's internal scaffolding. They fix bulky membrane systems, the endoplasmic reticula and the Golgi-complex, to more or less permanent positions in the cell's interior. They are conspicuously present in cells with complex shapes. We see this, for example, in nerve cell processes (Fig. 2.31.), which contain numerous, parallel microtubules.

Microtubules are dynamic structures which, depending on the circumstances, may be built up or broken down quickly. In these construction and demolition processes, the role of the **centrosome** (Fig. 2.33.) turns out to be crucial. In the cytosol next to the centrosome, tubulin building blocks are either added to existing microtubules, causing them to lengthen and appear to grow from the centrosome, or removed, shortening them. The most spectacular manifestation of this mechanism is seen in the formation and operation of the mitotic spindle during cell multiplication (II.3.1.). Usually the centrosome occupies a position adjacent to the nucleus, close to the cell's center, which explains the origin of its name. Starting at the centrosome, microtubules radiate towards the cell's periphery.

The centrosome is actually a double body, composed of two **centrioles** at right angle to each other. A centriole is itself composed of microtubules arranged in **triplets**. Each triplet contains three short (length: 0.5 micrometers) microtubules. Nine such triplets form a cylinder, with a diameter of about 0.25 micrometers (Fig. 2.37.). The triplets are inclined with regard to the cylinder's circumference. The microtubule which is closest to the central axis is complete (circular in cross section), while the two others are incomplete (c-shaped in cross section) and closely adhere with their open side to the adjacent tubule. The outer tubule of one triplet is connected to the inner tubule of the next one by means of filaments.

Combined with an ATPase, **dynein**, microtubules enable movement (Fig. 2.34.). The dynein molecules, carried by a microtubule, can attach their free end to various particles, such as vesicles, and subsequently bend by means of the energy liberated upon breakdown of ATP, which transfers the vesicle to the next dynein molecule. By repetition of this cycle of attachment, bending and release, vesicles can be transported over considerable distances, the microtubule serving as a guiding rail.

This mechanism of movement based upon microtubules is best developed in the actively moving, thread-like appendages of certain cells: **flagella** and **cilia**. These appendages are motile because they contain microtubules that can slide longitudinally past one another. There are only quantitative differences between both appendages. Flagellae ("whips") are very long and fairly thick and no cell has more than a single one. It is carried by the male gamete, the spermatozoon (Fig. 4.10.7.). The beating of the flagellum propels the cell. Cilia ("lashes") are much

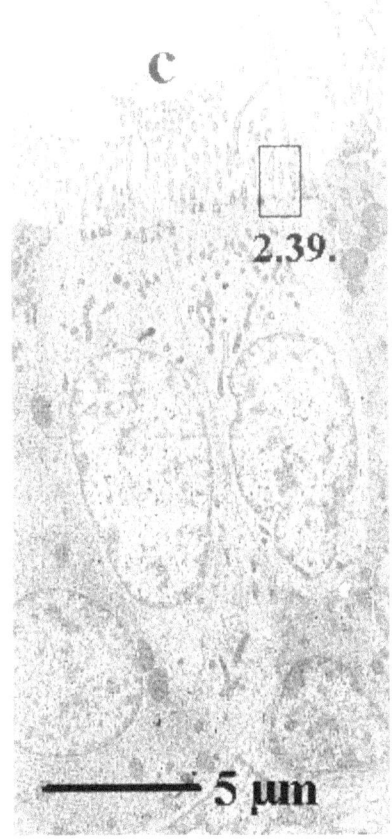

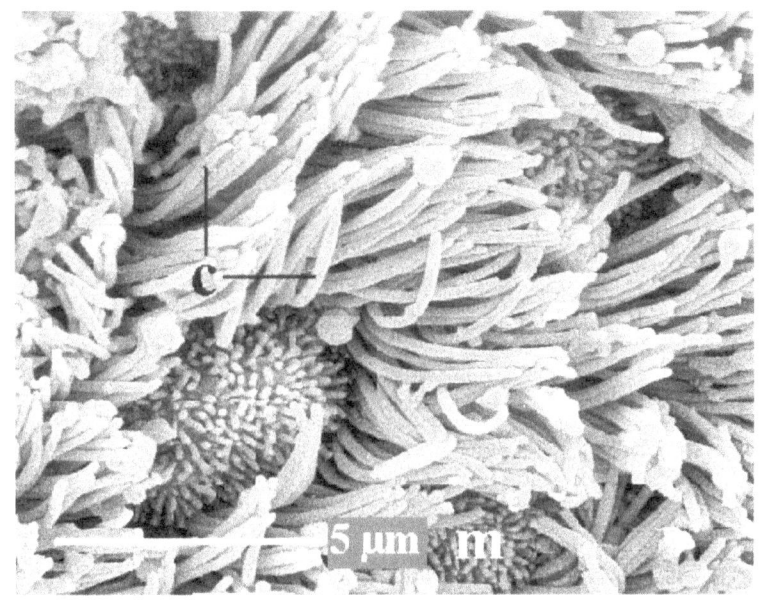

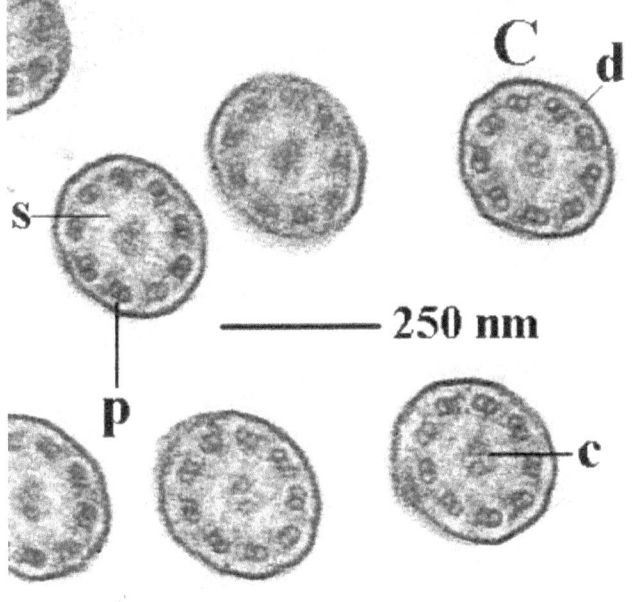

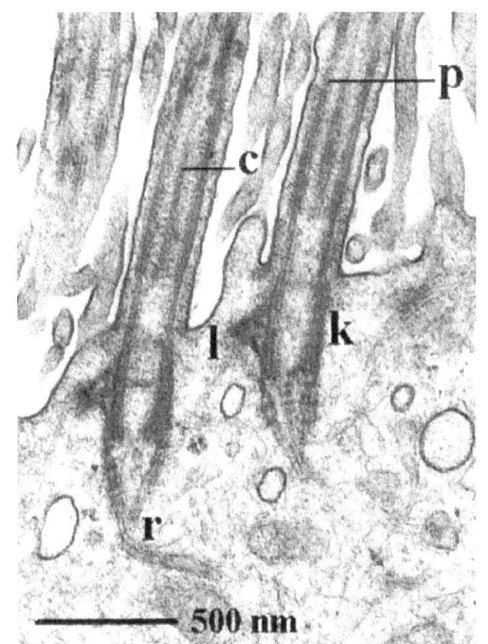

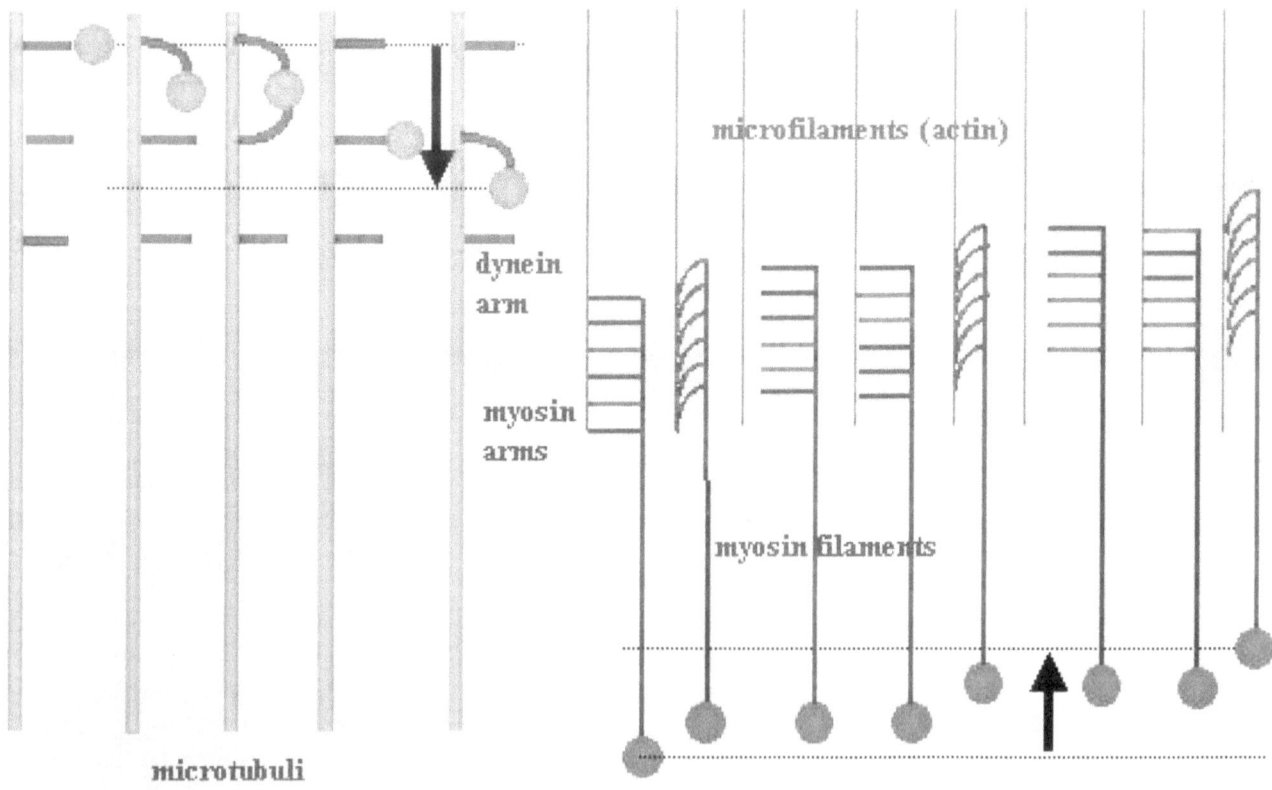

microtubuli

microfilaments (actin)

dynein
arm

myosin
arms

myosin filaments

Fig. 2.34. Microtubules and microfilaments allow transport (arrows) of various particles in the cytoplasm. Microtubules carry dynein arms, which can attach to particles and move them. Myosin filaments, towing a particle, move along microfilaments with the help of their "heads".

shorter, thinner, and much more numerous, up to many thousands per cell. Their beating does not move the cell, which is connected to other cells, but displaces fluids or particles relative to the cell, whereby these cells participate in transport processes.

Cilia are appendages of the apical cell membrane of a specialized cell type: the **ciliated cell** (Figs. 2.35.-36.). The apical cell membrane is exposed to a lumen. Ciliated cells line the larger airways, the oviducts

(IV.11.2.) and the brain's ventricles. These last cells are called **ependyma cells** (IV.4.7.).

The resolving power of the light microscope is just sufficient to visualize cilia as thread-like appendages of the apical cell membrane, not unlike the fringe of a carpet (Fig. 4.14.12.). Ultrastructurally, they appear as tubular appendages, lined with cell membrane and supported by microtubules (Figs. 2.38.-39.). Cilia reach lengths of up to 20 micrometers and over most

Fig. 2.35. (top left) Microtubules are an essential component of cilia (c), which are found at the apex of ciliated cells. Airway epithelium, rabbit, TEM. **Fig. 2.36.** (top right) Cilia (c) are thread-like appendages of the apical cell membrane of ciliated cells, exposed to a lumen. Other cells, studded with much shorter microvilli (m), are also seen. Airway epithelium, luminal surface, rabbit, SEM. **Fig. 2.38.** (bottom left) Enlargement of an area similar to the one indicated in Figure 2.35.. Transverse sections of cilia (C) show the typical arrangement of microtubules: 2 single ones in the center (c), and 9 peripheral (p) doublets (compare with Figure 2.37.). Traces of dynein arms (d) and spokes (s) can be made out. Ciliated cell, airway epithelium, human, TEM. **Fig. 2.39.** (bottom right) Longitudinal sections show how cilia are implanted at the apex of a ciliated cell. The peripheral microtubules (p) lengthen into a kinetosome (k), which has the same structure as a centriole (compare with Figures 2.33. and 2.37.). The central microtubules (c) do not continue into the apical cytoplasm. The kinetosome ends in a tapering ciliary root (r). A lateral process (l) anchors the cilium to cytoplasmic fibers. Ciliated cell, airway epithelium, human, TEM.

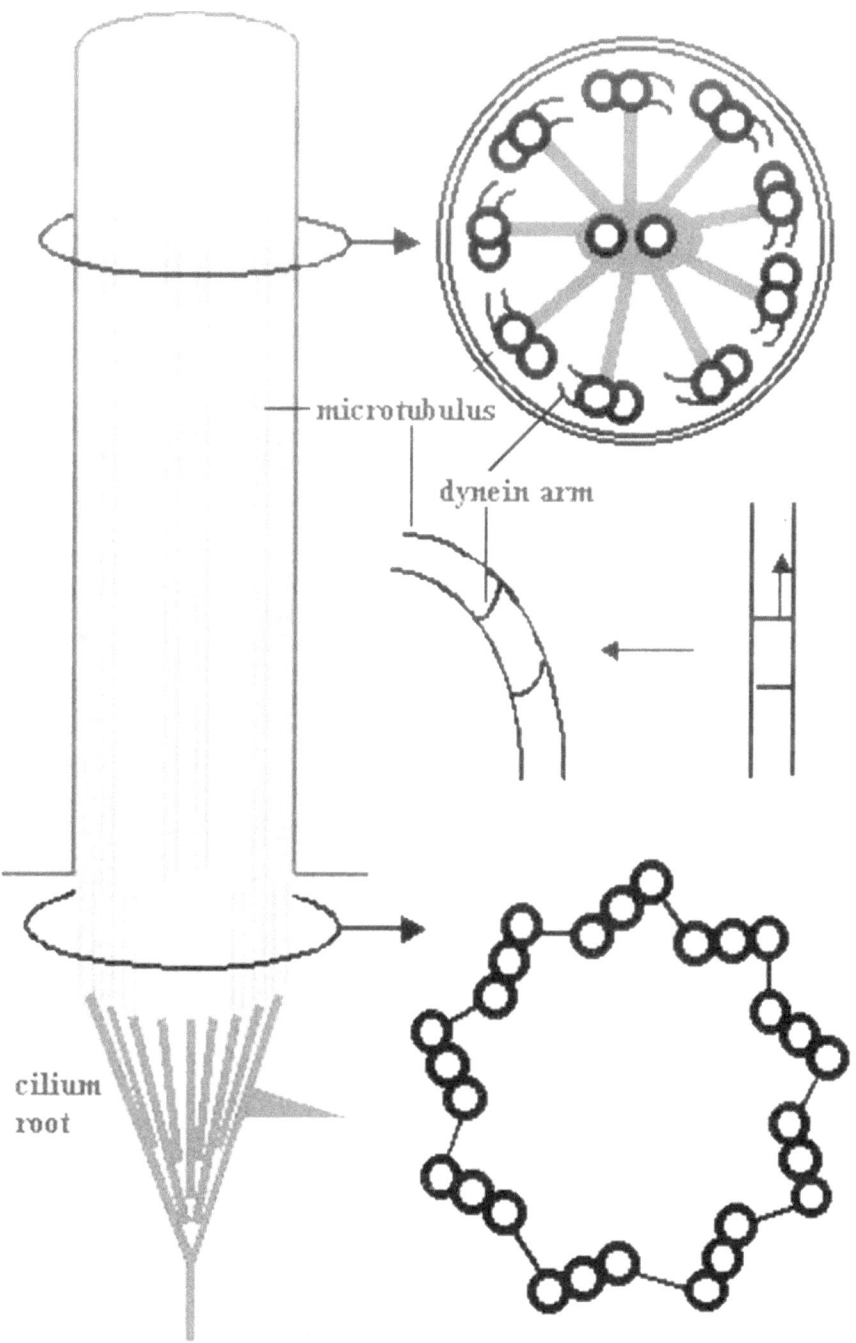

Fig. 2.37. The structure of a cilium. A transverse section (upper right), shows 2 central microtubules, embedded in a protein sheath, which sends a "spoke" to the "complete" microtubule of each of the 9 peripheral doublets. Except for an "incomplete" microtubule, this microtubule also carries 2 dynein arms. These arms may form links with adjoining tubules. By bending, they move the microtubular doublets relative to one another, causing the whole cilium to beat (middle right). The "complete" microtubule of each doublet continues into the central microtubule of a centriole-like structure, the kinetosome, by means of which the cilium is implanted in the apical cytoplasm of a ciliated cell (lower part).

microtubulus

dynein arm

cilium root

of this length, their diameter is about 0.2 micrometers. They taper at their top.

In cross section, a cilium is seen to contain two central microtubules, which presumably serve as purely supportive elements. At the periphery, the microtubules form nine **doublets**, one tubule of which is complete, the other, adjoining one, c-shaped. At the opposite side from the adjoining tubule, the complete tubule carries two "arms", consisting of dynein. These nine doublets form a circle, concentric with the cilium's membrane and with a constant orientation, the dynein arms pointing clockwise. The central

microtubules are embedded in a dense, fibrous sheath. There are cross-links between the fibrous sheath and the complete tubules of each peripheral doublet, not unlike the spokes of a wheel. The basis of the central doublet is situated at the junction of the cilium and the cell's apex. The peripheral doublets reach into the apical cytosol (Fig. 2.39.). They are continuous with a basal body or **kinetosome**, out of which they grow during the cell's development. The kinetosome has the same structure as the centriole. The two "central" microtubules of each triplet are continuous with cilium's doublets. The base of the kinetosome tapers to a cone-shaped root, which carries a lateral, fibrous appendage. Both structures anchor the cilium to fibers in the cell's cytoplasm.

The peripheral doublets are the cilium's motor (Fig. 2.37.). The dynein arms of one doublet can attach their free ends to the adjoining doublet. Breakdown of ATP supplies chemical energy, which is transformed to mechanical energy: the dynein arms bend, causing the two linked doublets to slide past each other. By coordination of the movements of all nine doublets, the whole cilium can be made to move. Each cilium "beats" with a fast power stroke, and is pulled back with a slower recovery stroke. During the power stroke, it is fully extended, while during the recovery stroke it bends wave-like so as to reduce drag. This cycle is repeated 5 to 10 times per second. In ciliated cells, the movement of the cilia themselves is also coordinated. They all beat in the same direction. This coordinated beating enables the cell to propel a layer of fluid or mucus, in which trapped particles are carried along. This is how ciliated cells contribute to various transport processes.

II.2.2.2. Microfilaments.

Microfilaments are the thinnest cytosolic fibers, having a diameter of only 5 nanometers. They are mainly composed of the protein **actin**. Microfilaments tend to aggregate in a thin layer close to and parallel to the cell membrane. Since they also participate in support and movement, their function shows some similarity to that of microtubules. They are also dynamic structures.

Since microfilaments contribute to the cytoskeleton's structure, they are conspicuously present in irregularly shaped cells and in cellular appendages. Microfilaments support **microvilli**, the hallmark of **brush border cells**.

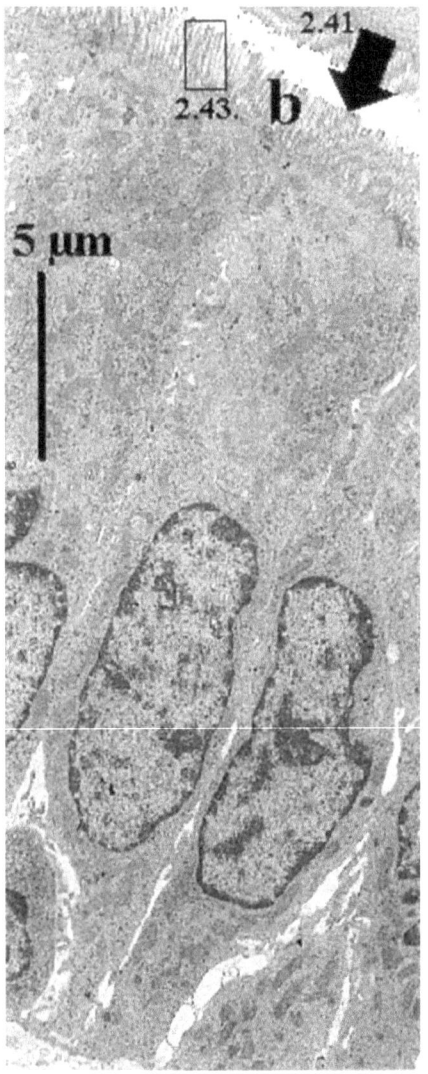

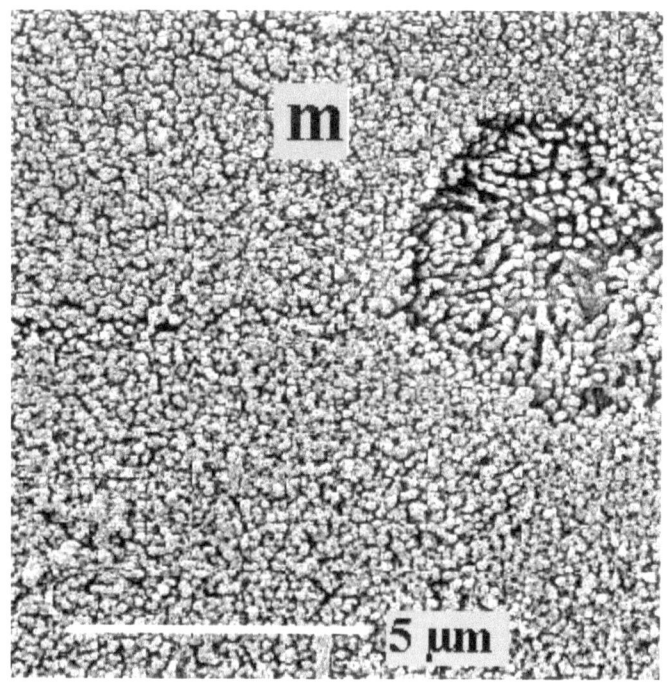

Fig. 2.40. (left) Large numbers of regularly arranged microvilli form a brush border (b) at the cell apex of brush border cells, which contacts a lumen. Enterocytes, jejunum, rabbit, TEM. **Fig. 2.41.** (above) The brush border's microvilli (m) are like the hairs of a brush, lying so closely together that only their tips are visible from the lumen. Enterocytes, jejunum, rabbit, SEM.

In combination with the filamentous ATPase **myosin**, microfilaments enable movement (Fig. 2.34.). Along its length, a myosin-filament carries "heads" which can attach themselves to a parallel microfilament. ATP breakdown causes these heads to bend, whereupon both filaments slide past each other. When a myosin filament is linked with a vesicle, this vesicle can be propelled along a microfilament in continuous cycles of attachment of myosin heads, ATP breakdown, bending of the heads and detachment. In **muscle fibers**, microfilaments (actin filaments) and myosin filaments are present in overwhelming numbers and arranged in a very specific, orderly fashion, in such a way that their sliding past one another causes the whole fiber to contract.

II.2.2.2.1. Brush border cells.

Brush border cells are cells whose apical membrane,

exposed to a lumen, carries a **brush border** composed of large numbers of parallel **microvilli**. By their large numbers, the microvilli enormously extend the apical membrane's surface, creating ample space for integral membrane proteins involved in various transport processes. This explains how brush border cells are able to absorb or secrete various low molecular weight substances.

Microvilli are extremely thin (diameter a little less than 0.1 micrometers) and short (length about 1 micrometer) appendages, lined with cell membrane, and supported by an axial bundle of microfilaments (Figs. 2.42., 2.43.). The microfilamentous axis enters the apical cytosol and merges with the **terminal web**, a layer of microfilaments parallel to the cell membrane. With the light microscope, microvilli, in contrast to cilia, cannot be made out separately. Their diameter happens to be smaller than the mean wavelength of visible light (I.1.). Consequently, the

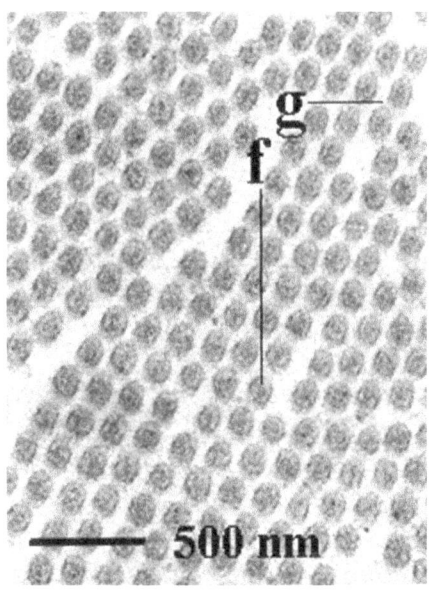

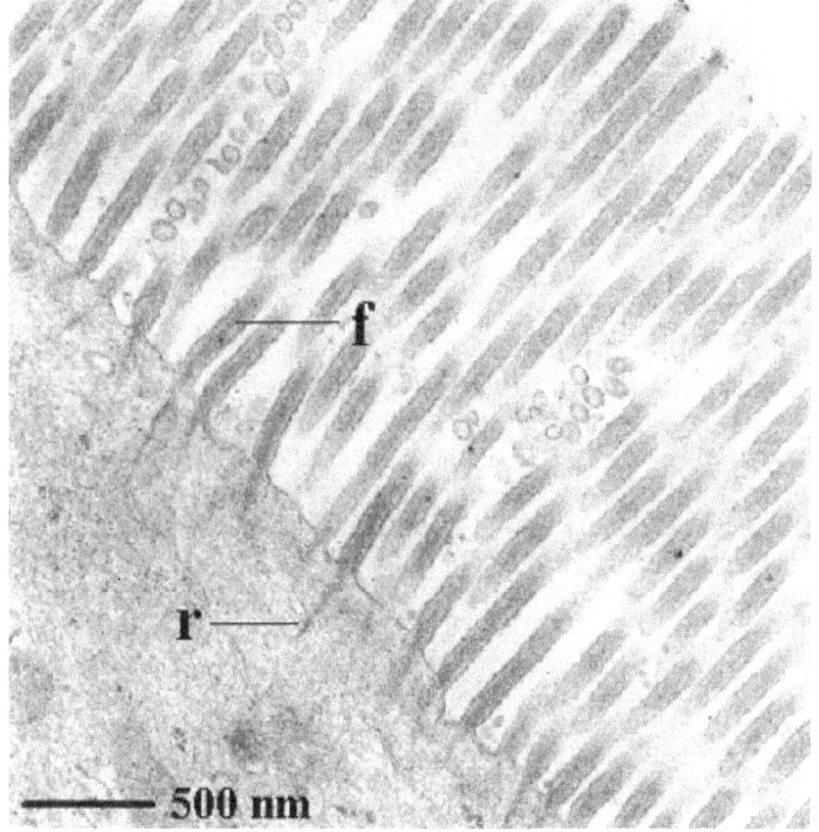

Fig. 2.42. A transverse section shows the closely packed, hexagonal arrangement of microvilli in a brush border. The center of each microvillus is occupied by a dense microfilamental axis (f). Some fuzzy material, the glycocalyx (g), is seen to coat the microvilli. Enterocyte, jejunum, rabbit, TEM. Fig. 2.43. A longitudinal section of microvilli shows their microfilamental axis (f). This axis continues into the brush border cell's apical cytoplasm, where it forms a kind of root (r), which is anchored to the terminal microfilamental web. Enterocyte, jejunum, rabbit, TEM.

brush border looks like a clear, amorphous layer along the exposed cell surface (Fig. 4.15.33.). Frequently, the brush border is coated with a layer of carbohydrate molecules that contains various hydrolytic enzymes, the **glycocalyx**.

The most common type of brush border cells are the **enterocytes**, which line the greater part of the small intestine's lumen (Figs. 2.40.-41., 4.15.33.). Enterocytes perform the final stages of digestion of carbohydrates and proteins (most of which has already taken place in the intestinal lumen). They do this by means of maltases and peptidases, associated with their glycocalyx. The end products of digestion of carbohydrates and proteins, monosaccharides and amino acids, respectively, are taken up by means of permeases in the brush border's membrane. Another important type of brush border cell is that of the **proximal convoluted tubules** in the kidneys (IV.8.1.1.2.). These actively participate in the absorption of sodium ions from the tubular lumen.
Apart from these absorbing brush border cells, secreting brush border cells exist as well. The most typical example of these is the **choroid plexus cells** (IV.4.7.). In a few localized places, these cells line the lumen of the brain ventricles. By secretion of ions through the brush border, they contribute to the formation of cerebrospinal fluid.

II.2.2.2.2. Muscle fibers.

Muscle fibers derive their contractile properties from a very specific arrangement of actin microfilaments and myosin filaments. They are more often called fibers rather than cells, because of their elongated shape. There are two fundamentally different kinds of muscle fibers: **smooth muscle fibers** and **striated muscle fibers**.

II.2.2.2.2.1. Smooth muscle fibers.

Smooth muscle fibers are found in greatest number in the walls of hollow, tube-like internal organs, such as the gut, the airways, the blood vessels and the urogenital system. They form concentric layers, and their degree of contraction determines the diameter of the lumen.

Muscle fibers of this type are spindle-shaped to extremely elongated, and have a spindle-shaped, central nucleus. Typically, smooth muscle fibers attain lengths of 100 micrometers and diameters of 10 micrometers. These dimensions, however, are variable and depend on the organ in which the fibers are found and their state of contraction. The nucleus has a length of up to 25 micrometers. When the fibers contract, the nucleus develops deep, transverse furrows. By light microscopy, the cytoplasm is featureless, or smooth.

Ultrastructurally, the cytosol is crowded with filaments (Figs. 2.44.-45.). They are generally arranged more or less longitudinally, adapting themselves to the shape of the muscle fiber and the nucleus. Filaments with an oblique course occur as well. The filaments are not all the same. Apart from thin actin microfilaments, and much rarer, thick myosin filaments, there is a third, intermediate type of fiber, which is a member of the intermediate filament category (II.2.2.3.), and consists of desmin or vimentin. Between the filaments and at the inner face of the cell membrane, spindle-shaped fibrous bodies are distributed. These are the **fusiform densities**. They are approximately 0.5 micrometers thick and several micrometers long and consist of the protein actinin. They serve as anchoring places for the filaments.
Membranous organelles are rather scarce and are limited to two cap-like zones of cytoplasm at both poles of the nucleus. The cell membrane shows numerous small dents, referred to as **caveolae intracellulares**, or simply caveolae, as if endosomes are forming there. Some pinocytotic vesicles and smooth endoplasmic reticulum are also found in the peripheral cytosol.

Myosin fibers are less apparent then in striated muscle fiber types. Nevertheless, myosin's enzymatic activity (ATP breakdown) is the essence of the smooth muscle fiber's contractile mechanism. It enables the myosin filaments to pull on the actin microfilaments. The force thus generated is transmitted, through the fusiform densities, to the whole muscle fiber, which contracts. The crucial attachment of myosin heads to actin is only possible in the presence of calcium ions. These seem to be preferentially taken in at the caveolae. The third type of fiber is not directly involved in contraction, it is part of the cytoskeleton. Actin filaments may partly serve as cytoskeletal elements as well.

A curious property of smooth muscle fibers is that they can reversibly turn into matrix-secreting cells and become involved in synthetic activities. In this case, they partly lose their cytosolic fibers and develop a rough endoplasmic reticulum.

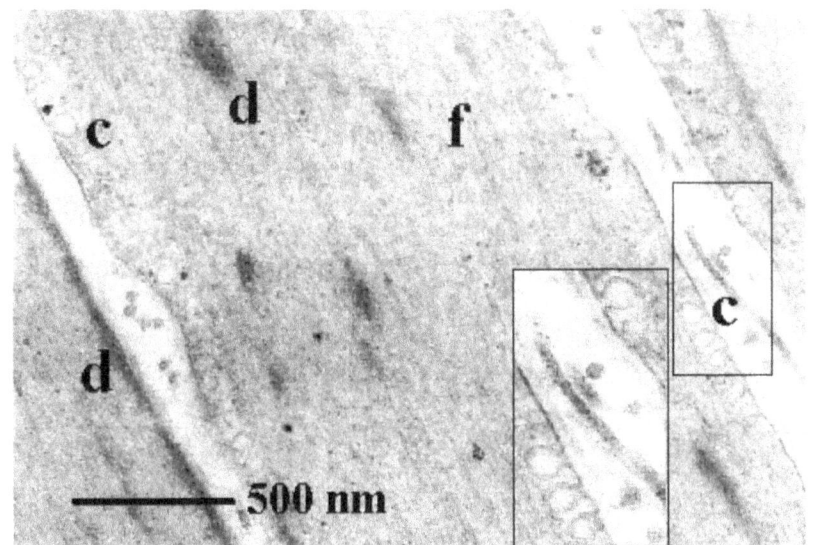

Fig. 2.44. A longitudinal section of a smooth muscle fiber (and parts of two adjoining ones) shows parallel filaments (f) and a number of fusiform densities in the cytosol, as well as on the cytosolic face of the cell membrane (d). Mark the presence of caveolae (c) in the peripheral, filament-free cytoplasm. Musculosa urine bladder, cat, TEM.

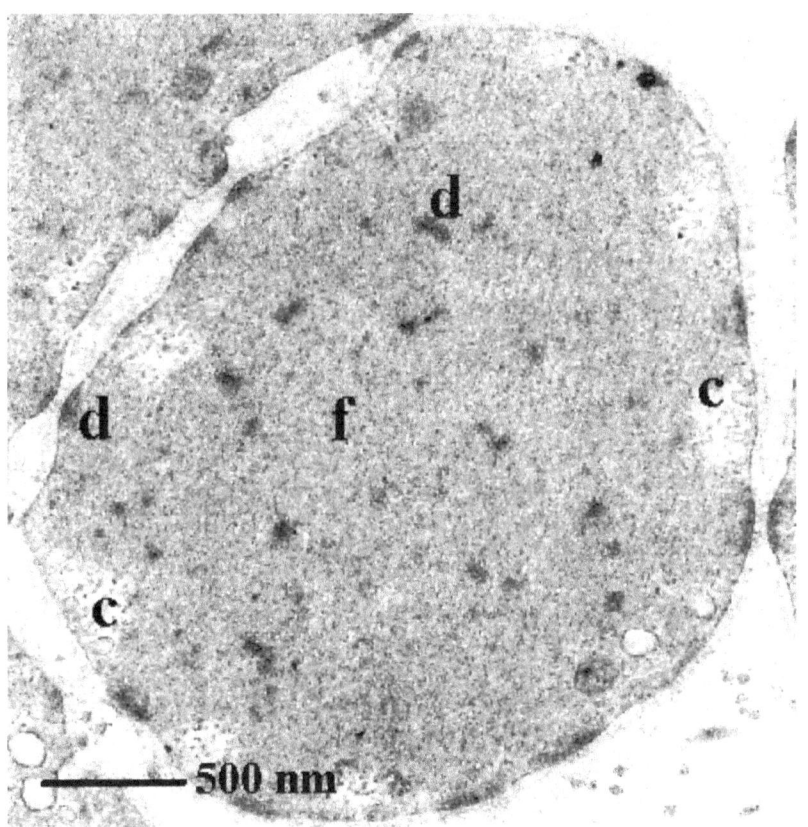

Fig. 2.45. A transverse section of a smooth muscle fiber, see Figure 2.44.

II.2.2.2.2.2. Striated muscle fibers.

Striated muscle fibers are quantitatively the most important muscle fibers. Distinction must be made between the skeletal muscle fibers, building the skeletal muscles, and the cardiac muscle fibers of the heart.

Skeletal muscle fibers are cylindrical and exceedingly long. Their length can attain several centimeters, while their diameter is in the range of 20 micrometers. This extreme length is explained by their embryonic development. Skeletal muscle fibers are formed by fusion of a long string of embryonic muscle cells called myoblasts. Thus, a skeletal muscle fiber is not a cell in the strict sense, but a supercell, or a **syncytium**. A direct consequence of this fusion is the large number of cell nuclei found in a single fiber, each individual myoblast having contributed one. The nuclei occupy a peripheral position, making room for a number of longitudinal filament bundles, the **myofibrils**, in the center. The myofibrils have a distinctive transverse striation (Fig. 2.46.), consisting of alternating dark **A-bands** and light **I-bands**. The myofibrils are arranged so that the bands of neighbouring myofibrils line up. This explains the distinctive transverse striation of the skeletal muscle

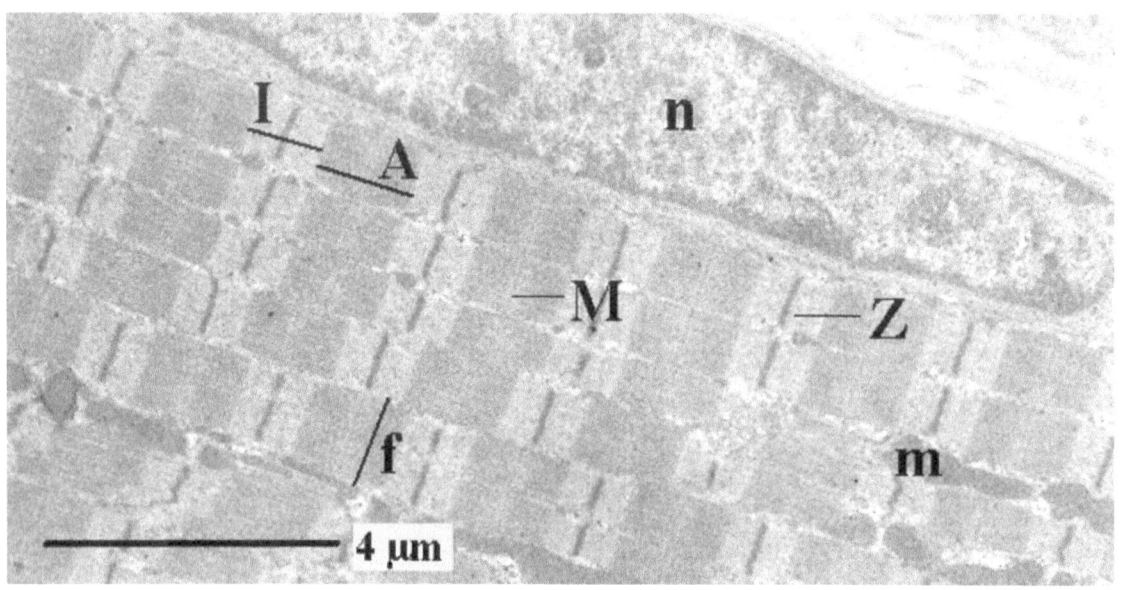

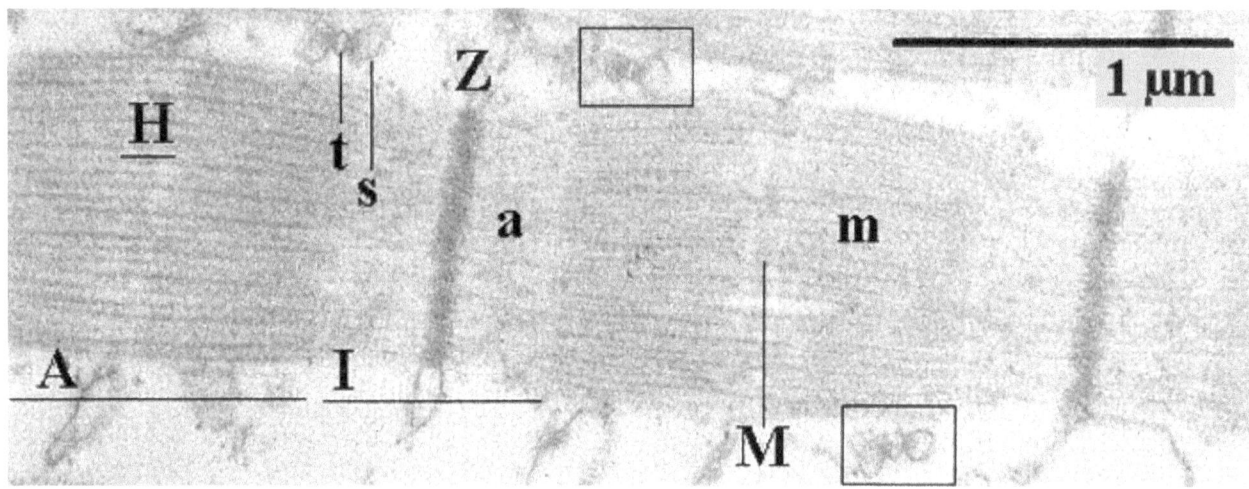

Fig. 2.46. (top) A longitudinal section of a skeletal muscle fiber, an example of a striated muscle fiber, shows a peripheral nucleus (n) and a number of longitudinal myofibrils (f), separated from one another by filament-free cytoplasm with mitochondria (m). Each microfibril shows a regular succession of dark A-bands (A) and light I-bands (I), in the middle of which lies a Z-membrane (Z). The H-bands with their M-line (M) can be faintly made out. The myofibrils tend to line up in such a fashion that their striations coincide. This confers a cross striated aspect to the whole fiber. Skeletal muscle, rabbit, TEM. **Fig. 2.47.** (bottom) At a higher magnification of a single myofibril, its cross striation is seen to be a consequence of the partial overlap of microfilaments or actin filaments and myosin filaments. The I-bands (I) contain actin filaments (a) only. The actin filaments continue into the A-bands (A) and penetrate between the myosin filaments (m) which occur there. Midway in the A-band, an actin-free zone remains, the H-band (H). In the middle of the H-band is an M-line (M), on both sides of which myosin filaments are attached. The actin filaments attach to the Z-membrane (Z). Where A- and I-bands meet, groups of 3 "vesicles" lie in the cytoplasm, the triads (rectangle). The central "vesicle" is in fact a tubular inpocketing of the cell membrane, a T-tubule (t). Both lateral "vesicles" are cisterns of the smooth endoplasmic reticulum (s). Skeletal muscle fiber, rabbit, TEM.

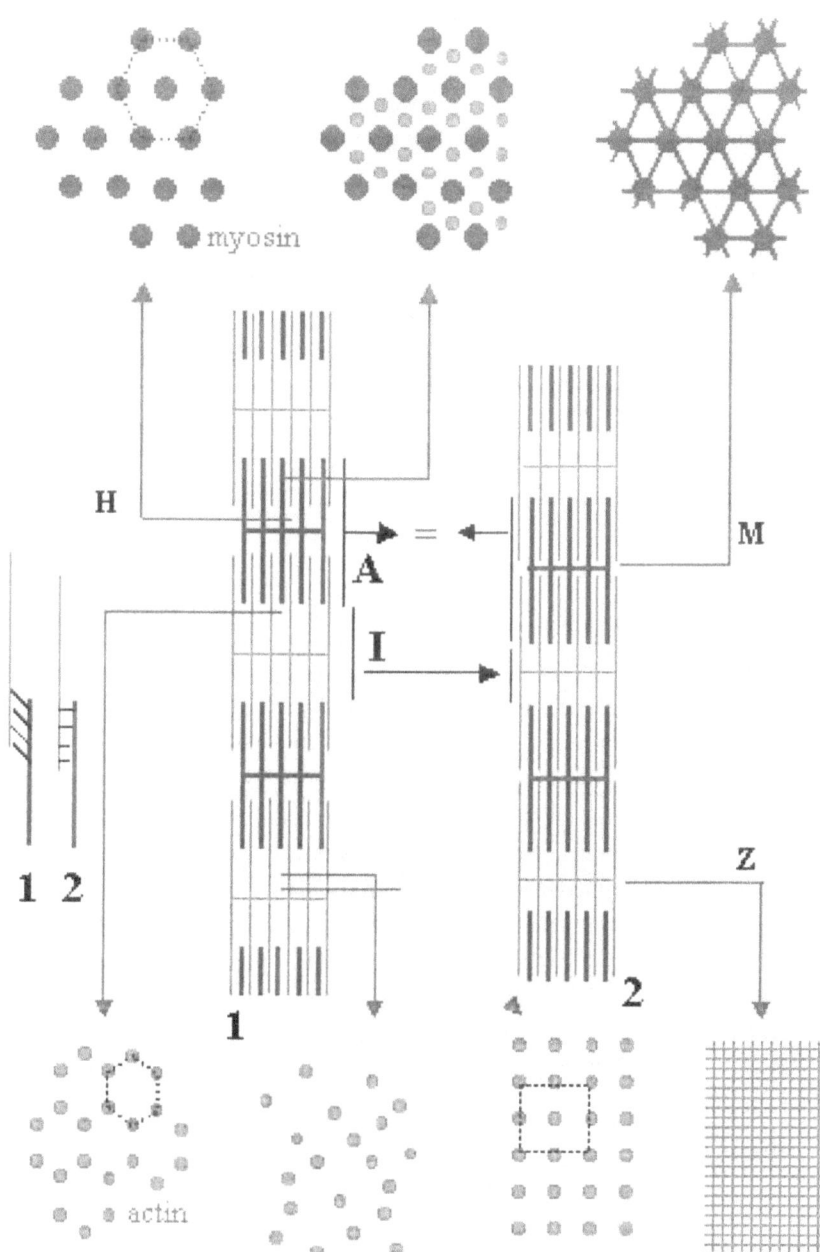

myosin

actin

H

A

=

I

M

1 2

1

4

2

Z

Fig. 2.48. A myofibril is a highly regular arrangement of myofilaments. In cross section, myosin filaments are arranged hexagonally. At the level of the M-line, they show cross links. The H-band only shows myosin filaments. The rest of the A-band contains actin filaments that penetrate between the myosin filaments. The hexagonal pattern of the actin filaments changes into an orthogonal one near the Z-membrane. Between the two regions is a transitional zone. In the actual Z-membrane, the actin filaments form subfilaments that will link with the actin filaments of the next I-band. They keep an orthogonal, but denser, pattern. Myofibrils (1) contract when actin and myosin filaments slide between one another (2). The myosin filaments pull at the actin filaments by means of their "arms" (see Fig. 2.34.). As a consequence of this (2), the H-bands and I-bands narrow, while the other zones keep their width.

fiber's cytoplasm, as observed by light microscopy. The myofibrils are bundles of **myofilaments**: relatively thin actin microfilaments and thicker myosin filaments. The transverse striation of the myofibrils is seen to be the consequence of the partial overlap of actin and myosin filaments (Fig. 2.47.). Where both filaments overlap, A-bands are formed. I-bands are stretches of actin microfilaments that do not overlap with myosin filaments. The actin microfilaments do not quite reach the center of the A-bands, leaving a short stretch of myosin filaments without overlap. Thus, a light transverse band is formed in the center of an A-band: the H-band or **Hensen's disk**. Myosin

filaments run uninterrupted through the center of the H-band, and are connected there by transverse links or M-bridges, which give rise to a thin transverse line in the middle of the H-band, the **M-line** (German: Mitte, middle). In the center of the I-bands, the actin microfilaments terminate and are connected with the microfilaments of the next segment of myofibril. Each microfilament end is frayed and forms four subfilaments, each of which merges with a subfilament of another microfilament of the next section. In this way, a dense transverse line is formed in the middle of the I-band, the **Z-membrane** (German: Zwischen, between two A-bands). By light microscopy, the H-band and particularly the M-line and the Z-membrane, which are approximately 0.1 micrometers thick, can only be observed well under ideal conditions.

This highly ordered configuration of the myofilaments is even more evident when the myofibrils are observed in cross section (Figs. 2.48.-49.). The exact structure of such a cross section depends on its location along the myofibril. At the level of Hensen's disk, only myosin filament sections can be seen. They look like dense dots with a diameter of about 10 nanometers and are arranged in a highly regular pattern. They are at the corners and in the center of adjoining hexagons. At the exact level of the M-line, the M-bridges are seen as connections between the myofilaments. They form the sides of the hexagons and connect the central myosin filament with the peripheral ones. In the A-band proper, the hexagonal pattern of the myosin filaments continues, and actin microfilament sections are added to it. In each hexagon, delineated by six myosin filament sections, lie six actin filament sections. With reference to the central myosin filaments, each hexagon can be thought of as partitioned in six triangles. The actin microfilament sections, which look like smaller, 5 nanometer diameter dots, occupy the center of these triangles. In the I-band, the hexagonal pattern typical of the A-band is at first conserved, the actin microfilament sections occupying the corners of hexagons, but without a

central dot. Somewhat deeper in the I-band, this arrangement is lost and the microfilaments are randomly distributed. Close to the Z-membrane, a new ordered configuration appears. The microfilament sections now occupy the corners of adjoining squares. In the Z-membrane proper, this orthogonal pattern is conserved, but is now much denser due to the fraying of the microfilament ends.

It is evident that the A-band in particular has a highly regular, periodic, almost crystalline, structure. This explains its particular optical properties. A-bands are anisotropic, I-bands isotropic. Anisotropy, or birefringence, is an optic phenomenon well known in crystallography. It is a consequence of the strict, orderly arrangement of atoms in a crystal grid. A light wave cannot pass through a crystal unless its plane of polarization, i.e. the plane in which it vibrates, has a precise orientation, so that it can pass between planes of precisely arranged atoms. When a beam of unpolarized light, in which the individual waves vibrate in various planes, enters a crystal, it is often split into two beams of polarized light. Both beams are refracted to a different degree and leave the crystal at a different angle relative to the entering beam. The polarization plane of one beam is at right angles to that of the other one. It takes special equipment to demonstrate this, since the human eye is insensitive to light's plane of polarization.

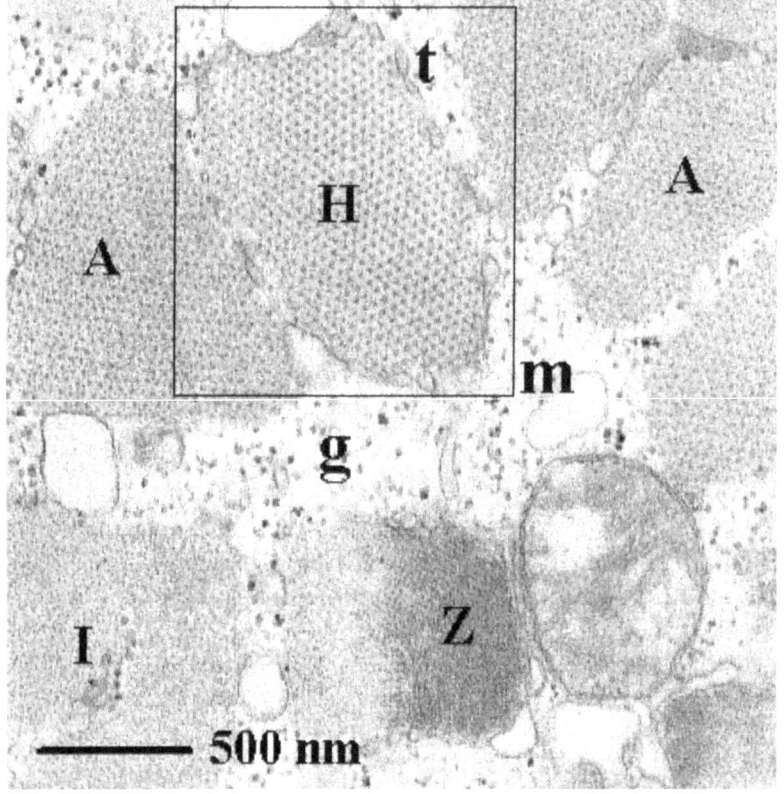

Fig. 2.49. The myofibrils (m) in this image are transversely sectioned, but at different levels, which may indicate that they do not lie exactly in phase, or that the section plane is not exactly transverse. The presence of myofibrils showing two patterns, such as the one at the bottom, argues in favor of the second alternative. Most myofibrils contain coarse dots, arranged hexagonally: myosin filaments. Most often, actin filaments show up between the myosin filaments, looking like much finer dots. Consequently, these myofibrils have been sectioned at the level of the A-band (A). Where only myosin filaments show, the section plane passes through the H-band (H). Sections showing only actin filaments are through I-bands (I). In the Z-membrane, actin filaments have an orthogonal arrangement and are connected through cross-links (Z). Compare with Figure 2.48. Between the myofibrils lie mitochondria, smooth endoplasmic reticulum and T-tubules (t), and glycogen granules (g). Skeletal muscle fiber, hamster, TEM.

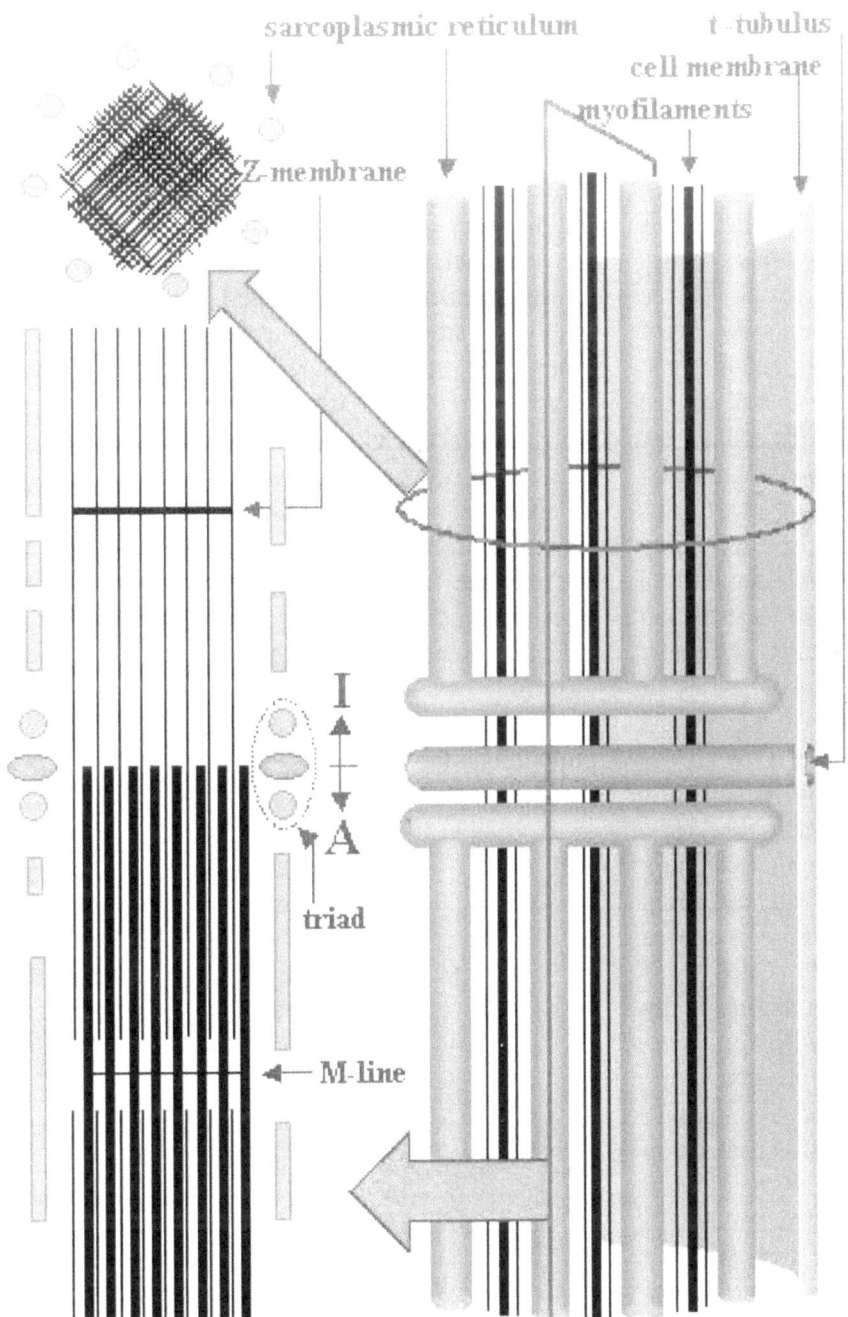

sarcoplasmic reticulum

t-tubulus

cell membrane

myofilaments

Z-membrane

I

A

triad

M-line

Fig. 2.50. The triad system. To the left, the triad system is schematically represented as it appears in a longitudinal section (horizontal filled arrow) of a skeletal muscle fiber. In the threedimensional representation to the right, the T-tubule is seen to be an inpocketing of the cell membrane. The T-tubulus is only represented over a very short length. The smooth endoplasmic reticulum forms tubular cisterns, which run parallel to the bundles of filaments or myofibrils (also see at the upper left). When they meet a T-tubule, they coalesce into an annular cistern, surrounding the myofibril.

It has already been described how myosin filaments can pull at actin microfilaments to move particles in the cytoplasm (Fig. 2.34.) or to contract smooth muscle fibers. This same phenomenon is also the basis of the striated muscle fiber's contractile mechanism. The regular configuration of the myofilaments in the A-bands optimizes the interaction between both types of filaments: each myosin filament, by bending its "heads", can pull at six actin microfilaments, while each actin microfilament can be pulled at by three myosin filaments. Contraction of the myofibril means that the actin microfilaments penetrate further between the myosin filaments,

narrowing the I-bands and the H-bands. This shortens the myofibrils. This process is coordinated over the whole length of the myofibril and between the myofibrils of the muscle fiber, so that the muscle fiber can contract as a whole.

In the cytoplasm surrounding the myofibrils, numerous mitochondria and dense glycogen granules are found. Glycogen is a polysaccharide, a polymer of glucose, and represents a reserve energy store.

A few membranous components are found as well. The cell membrane forms deep tubular depressions, the **T-tubules**, which bifurcate and merge extensively and penetrate between the myofibrils. The T-tubules lie in a plane that is at right angles to the axis of the myofibrils, and encircle them at the transition between A-band and I-band. Parallel with the myofibrils are cisterns of the smooth endoplasmic reticulum. On both sides of the T-tubules encircling the myofibrils, they form a local circular expansion. In sections, this configuration gives rise to so-called **triads** (Figs. 2.47., 2.50.). The triad is a central vesicle at the junction of A- and I-bands (the T-tubule), sandwiched between two lateral vesicles (the smooth endoplasmic reticulum). The triad system is essential to the contractile mechanism of the myofibrils and to the coordination of the contraction along the length of an individual myofibril and between different myofibrils. A skeletal muscle fiber only contracts after being stimulated by a motor nerve fiber, which depolarizes the fiber's cell membrane and gives rise to an action potential. The action potential propagates extremely rapidly. The T-tubules ensure that it encompasses all but instantly the whole triad system of the muscle fiber. This ensures that all the segments of all the myofibrils of the fiber will contract at virtually the same time. At the triads, the action potential releases calcium ions from the smooth endoplasmic reticulum. The calcium ions bind with the myofibrils, causing a change in shape of particular proteins and thus expose binding sites for the myosin "heads". Once these heads bind, the contraction mechanism automatically starts.

Cardiac muscle fibers (Figs. 3.3.5.-9.) closely resemble skeletal muscle fibers, the differences being relatively minor. With lengths of 60 to 70 micrometers and a diameter of approximately 15 micrometers, they are much shorter than skeletal muscle fibers. They are not cylindrical, but form a few short, broad processes at either end. They contain a single to a small number of nuclei, which occupy an axial position. They have exactly the same type of transverse striation as do skeletal muscle fibers. Only, their myofibrils accommodate themselves to the presence of axial nuclei and to the shape of the terminal processes. The triads are associated with the Z-membrane. There is much less cytoplasm between the myofibrils, making it difficult to distinguish individual myofibrils. What little interfibrillar cytoplasm there is, is occupied by mitochondria, which are often crowded so tightly that they are forced into polygonal shapes. Cardiac muscle fibers are not innervated by motor nerves. They contract under the influence of the cardiac pacemaker system.

II.2.2.3. Intermediary filaments, lining cells, and supporting cells.

The diameter of intermediary filaments, as their name implies, is intermediate between those of microtubules and microfilaments, being 10 to 12 nanometers. Intermediary filaments are rather static components of the cytoskeleton and are not clearly involved in transport and movement. Their function seems to be purely to strengthen the cell, making it suited to protect or support other cells. Their chemical composition differs depending on the cell type in which they are found. Unlike the other cytosolic fiber types, they do not form a homogeneous group. Thus, in epithelial cells (II.4.1.3.5.), **cytokeratin** is most commonly found, which forms **tonofilaments**. Other intermediate filaments are made of **vimentin** and are typical of matrix secreting cells. Muscle fibers also contain intermediary filaments that are made of **desmin**. Finally, the glia cell's (III.6.1.2.-2.2.) **gliofilaments**, composed of glial fibrillary acidic protein, and the nerve cell's (II.2.3.) **neurofilaments**, are intermediary filaments.

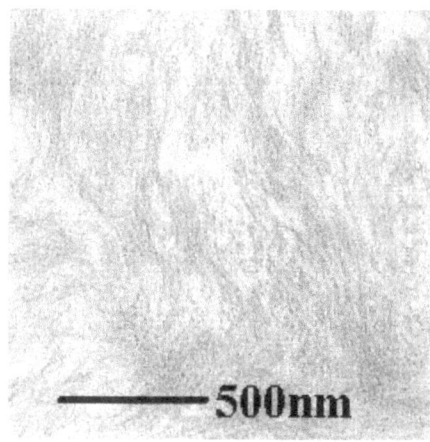

Fig. 2.51. The cytoplasm of a keratinized epidermal cell or keratinocyte, crammed with bundles of intermediary filaments, made of keratin. Compare their thickness with that of microtubules (Fig. 2.31.) and microfilaments (Figs. 2.43., 2.49.). Epidermis, human, TEM.

Lining cells form the boundary between the body and the external world, and are also found lining the body's cavities, which may or may not open into the outside world. The lining cells exposed at the surface of the body, or at the lumen of cavities that are open to the exterior (e. g. the gut) are called **epithelial cells**. Their primary function is to protect the underlying cells and tissues. In the body's interior cavities, epithelial cells may also control the transport of substances or may develop into gland cells.

At the surface of the body, the protective function predominates. These cells are the **keratinocytes** (Fig. 2.51.). They form the horny, protective layer of the skin. They are flattened cells with undulating margins, allowing them to closely adhere to neighbouring cells. Their cytoplasm contains nothing but tightly packed bundles of filaments, embedded in an amorphous matrix. These filaments are made of the protein **keratin**, and are derived from tonofilaments. All other organelles, the nucleus included, have been eliminated. This means that, strictly speaking, keratinocytes are not functional cells, only dead scales. They are descended from deeper, living cells that undergo, as we shall see, a complex process of differentiation or keratinization (III.4.1.3.4.).

Lining the body cavities that open directly into the exterior, such as the oral cavity, the pharynx, the oesophagus and the rectum are other types of epithelial cells, in which the keratinization process is much less

advanced. Apart from primary organelles, these cells contain bundles of tonofilaments.

Supporting cells do not line the exterior surface or the cavities of the body, but are found in the interior of various tissues and organs, where they support other cells.

Tissues that contain matrix, such as the interstitial, connective, and supportive tissues, or that consist of fiber-bearing cells, such as muscle tissue and epithelia, are relatively firm. Other tissues are weak. They can be reinforced to some extent by supporting cells. The best example of a soft tissue is the nerve tissue of the central nervous system. Apart from nerve cells, it contains supporting glia cells. These come in several varieties, and have a number of other functions beyond support. From a morphological viewpoint, the support function seems to dominate in a particular class of glia cells, the **astrocytes** (III.6.1.2., III.6.2.2.). As their name implies, these are star-shaped cells (Fig. 3.6.2.). They form a number of processes that are supported by gliofilaments. On the basis of number, length,

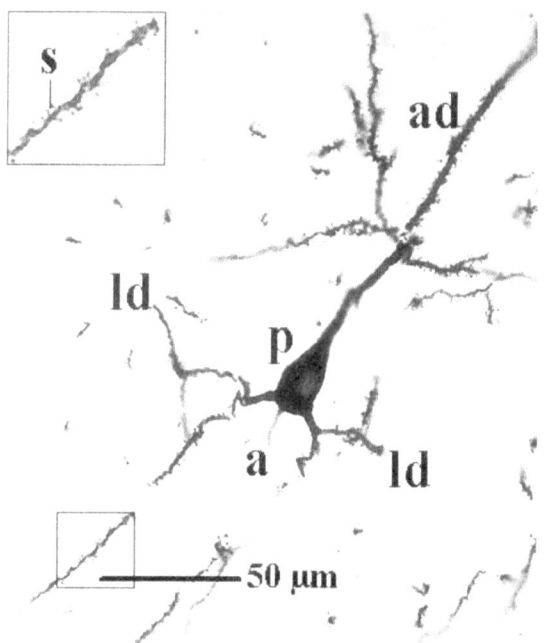 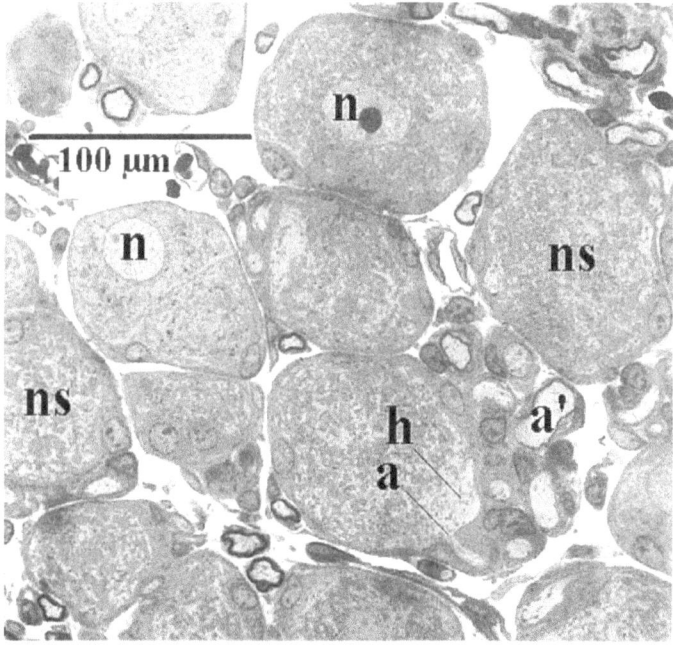

Nerve cells typically carry processes. **Fig. 2.52.** (left) Pyramidal nerve cells are multipolar: they carry multiple processes. All but one of these are the relatively thick and short, highly branched dendrites. Pyramidal nerve cells have a stout apical dendrite (ad) and several more slender lateral ones (ld). The bases of these dendrites give the nerve cell perikaryon (p) its polygonal, pyramidal shape. Mark the minute thorns, or spines (s), dotting the dendrites. Opposed to the apical dendrite is another kind of process, much thinner than a dendrite, of which a multipolar nerve cell carries only a single one, the axon. In this particular slide, it is disappearing from the section plane (a). Cerebral cortex, cat, silver impregnation (Golgi stain). **Fig. 2.53.** (right) Pseudounipolar nerve cell bodies have a smooth contour because they only form a single process, an axon. These cell bodies are filled with granules, the Nissl substance (ns) and contain a relatively large, rounded, euchromatic nucleus (n) with a dense nucleolus. One perikaryon shows an axon emerging from it (a). Next to it, a group of thicker axonal sections (a') is seen. This indicates that, shortly after it emerges from the cell body, the axons thickens and coils, prior to splitting in two branches (not visible). Note how the Nissl substance tends to disappear in the region where the axon emerges. This is the axon hillock (h). Spinal ganglion, cat, 1-micrometer plastic section, toluidin blue.

degree of ramification and amount of filaments of the processes, several subcategories of astrocytes have been recognized. In so-called sensory epithelia, such as the retina (IV.12.4.), the maculae and Corti's organ (IV.13.3.3.), supporting cells are found which are regarded as highly modified astrocytes, such as Müller's cells of the retina.

II.2.3. Composite cells: nerve cells.

Cell types exist which are composite types, i.e. they show characteristics, in more or less equal measure, of both membrane-bearing and fiber-bearing cells. The most important members of this group are the **nerve cells**.

Nerve cells show typical characteristics of **fiber-bearing cells**. They form **processes** that are implanted on the cell body or **perikaryon** and are supported by a filamentous cytoskeleton. Most nerve cell types even have two kinds of process (Fig. 2.52.). One is relatively short and highly branched, like a shrub: a **dendrite**. A nerve cell can carry numerous dendrites. The second kind is very long and has fewer branches, usually perpendicular to the process and at some distance from the cell body: the **axon**. Most types of nerve cell carry a single axon.

The nerve cell's processes function as conductors of signals. Nerve cells collect signals, in many cases from other nerve cells, at their dendrites. As a result of this, the perikaryon's membrane depolarizes (II.1.1.). Depolarization is a gradual process, but once a critical value is reached, it gives rise to an all or nothing response, an action potential. Action potentials arise at the **axon hillock**, the basis of the axon, and are conducted away from the perikaryon by the axon.

A nerve cell carrying multiple processes, i.e. a single axon and numerous dendrites, is called a **multipolar nerve cell** (Fig. 2.52.). In tissue sections, only the bases of these processes are visible. They give the perikaryon a polygonal shape. Most nerve cells are multipolar and can be subdivided between a large number of types, differing from one another in the shape of their perikaryon and the architecture of their dendritic tree.

Another, much rarer, kind of nerve cell has only two processes, on opposite sides of the perikaryon. These are **bipolar nerve cells**. Both processes have the shape and the internal structure of an axon. One axon conducts action potentials towards the perikaryon, the other one away from it. During embryonic development, most bipolar nerve cells are transformed into unipolar nerve cells. The bases of both processes

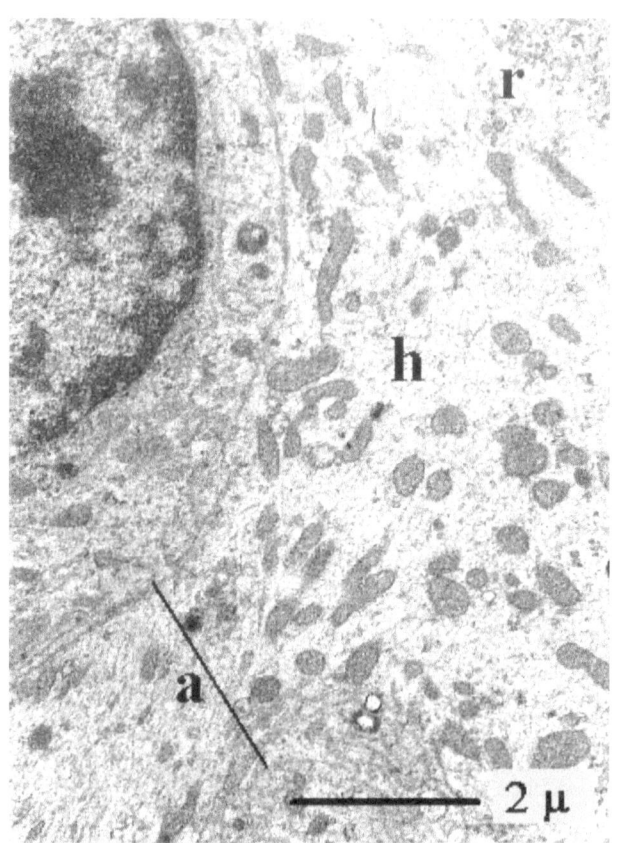

Fig. 2.54. Nerve cell processes, such as this axon (a), emerging from the cell body of a pseudounipolar nerve cell, are rich in cytoplasmic fibers. They are supported by microtubules, neurofilaments, and microfilaments. In the cell body, membranes predominate. It contains accumulations of rough endoplasmic reticulum (r), the Nissl substance. The actual zone of emergence of the axon is free of Nissl substance, and is called axon hillock (h). Spinal ganglion, rabbit, TEM.

migrate towards one another and merge. Thus, a unipolar nerve cell has a single process, the initial segment, which, at a certain distance from the perikaryon, splits into two axons, an afferent one (conducting in the direction of the perikaryon) and an efferent one (conducting away from the perikaryon). The action potential no longer passes via the perikaryon, bypassing it completely. The initial segment may be fairly long and follow a tortuous course. Strictly speaking, unipolar nerve cells are not truly unipolar. They are modified bipolar ones. Thus the term **pseudounipolar nerve cell** is preferred (Fig. 2.53.). Because of the small number of processes, both bipolar and pseudounipolar nerve cells have a rounded perikaryon.

Both dendrites and axons are supported by a well-developed cytoskeleton, the most prominent components of which are microtubules and intermediary neurofilaments (Fig. 2.54.). This type of cytoskeleton is also well developed in the perikaryon.

In addition, nerve cells are **membrane-bearing cells**. Light optical examination shows that the perikaryon contains a granular, basophilic substance, the **Nissl substance** (Figs. 2.53., 2.56.), the texture of which differs in various nerve cell types. Ultrastructurally, this granulation corresponds to extensive accumulations of ribosomes and rough endoplasmic reticulum (Fig. 2.55.). The Nissl substance is absent in the axon hillock and in the axon proper (Figs. 2.54., 2.56.), but invades the dendrites. In the perinuclear region, up to several well-developed Golgi-complexes can be found. In addition, the perikaryon contains vesicles and lysosomes. Running longitudinally down the axon are tubular cisterns of smooth endoplasmic reticulum. It appears that the nerve cell is specifically adapted to the synthesis of proteins. The reason for this is not clear at first, but becomes apparent when a number of points are taken into account.

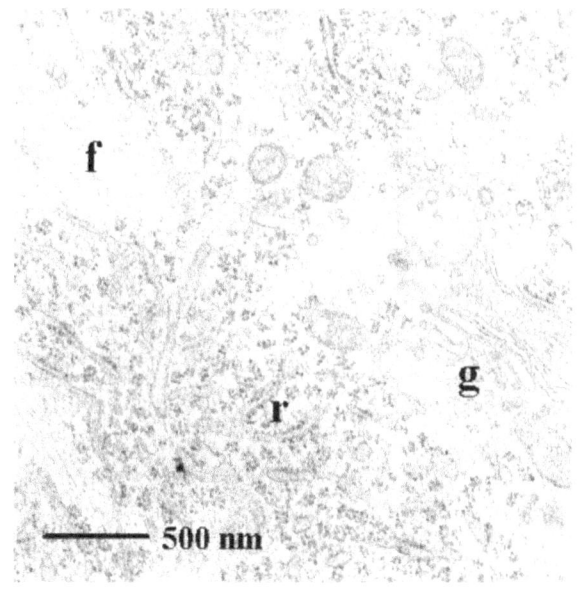

Fig. 2.55. The cytoplasm of a nerve cell body shows characteristics of both membrane-bearing and fiber-bearing cells. It is rich in rough endoplasmic reticulum (r) or Nissl substance, and contains a well-developed Golgi-complex (g). On the other hand, it is rich in neurofilaments (f). Pseudounipolar nerve cell, nodose ganglion, rabbit, TEM.

To begin with, the axon has a large volume and is intrinsically unable, because of the lack of ribosomes and rough endoplasmic reticulum, to synthesize the proteins it requires. With a diameter of only a few tenths of a micrometer, the axon may be very thin, but it is also very long. In fact, it can be extremely long: up to tens of centimeters. Consequently, the axon's volume may be very large, larger even than the perikaryon's volume. In some cases, it might be more precise to describe the perikaryon as an appendage of the axon, rather than vice versa. For protein synthesis, the axon is completely dependent upon the perikaryon. This dependence is so extreme that the axon is unable to survive in isolation. If the axon is cut, the severed part degenerates. The perikaryon is the so-called trophic center of the nerve cell. Proteins are produced in the perikaryon and, packaged in vesicles or via the smooth endoplasmic reticulum, transported along the axon, by anterograde transport. Waste substances travel in the opposite direction to be degraded by means of lysosomes in the perikaryon, by retrograde transport. Older nerve cells may accumulate lipofuchsin or wear and tear pigment. Vesicular transport depends upon the axon's cytoskeleton, both the tubulin-dynein and the actin-myosin systems being operative.

In neuroanatomical research, clever use is made of the axon's trophic dependence upon the perikaryon. Neuroanatomists try to find out where particular nerve cells send their axons or, alternatively, where particular axons have their cell bodies of origin. Because of the enormous numbers of nerve cells in the body, and the extreme lengths of their axons, this seems to be an all but impossible task. To appreciate the magnitude of the problem, one look at a section of brain tissue suffices. If, however, a specific axon (or a whole bundle of them) is transected, the severed stretch degenerates. The same result is obtained if the cell bodies of origin are destroyed. Experiments of this kind can only be done in experimental animals, but in the human body, the consequences of injuries, infections, or tumors may be similar. Degenerating axons may make their presence felt by precisely localized losses of function or paralyses or may be demonstrated at autopsy. Degenerating axons have a distinctive morphology (fragmentation, breakdown by macrophages) and can be specifically stained.

The perikaryon will usually survive severing of its axon and may even attempt to regenerate it. In doing this, the perikaryon swells, assumes a rounded shape (in case it is a multipolar one) and disperses its Nissl substance. As a result of this, the perikaryon loses its specific staining properties, a phenomenon called **chromatolysis** (Fig. 2.57.). If a particular group of nerve cells develops chromatolysis, this proves that they are the cell bodies of origin of the affected axons. Should the regenerating axon succeed in recontacting its original target, chromatolysis subsides and the perikaryon assumes its original aspect.

Apart from transection of axons, less dramatic ways exist to demonstrate axonal transport and trophic dependence of the axon. Substances exist which can

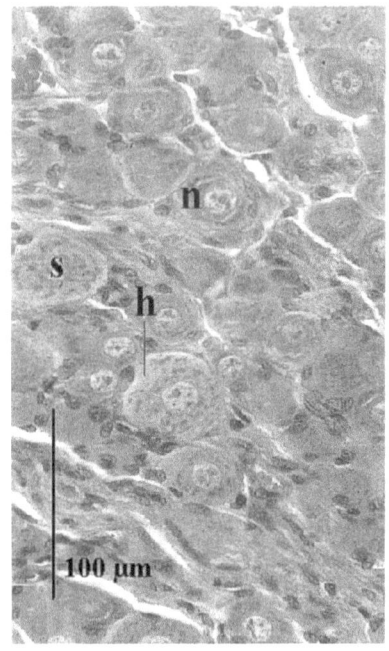 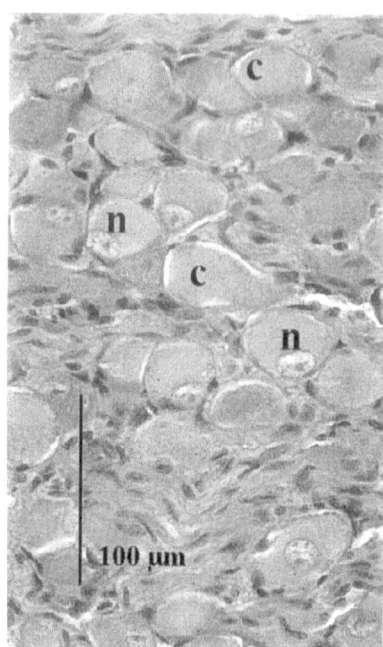

Fig. 2.56. (left) Intact pseudounipolar nerve cells have a rounded, central, euchromatic nucleus with a prominent nucleolus (n), and coarsely granular Nissl substance (s). Mark the nerve cell that looks as if something took a bite from it: it displays its axon hillock, which lacks Nissl substance (h). Nodose ganglion, rabbit, cresyl violet. **Fig. 2.57.** (right) The same kind of nerve cells as in Figure 2.56., some time after sectioning of their peripheral axon. The nuclei have shifted to an eccentric position (n) and the Nissl substance appears to have been dissolved, a phenomenon called chromatolysis (c).

be taken up by nerve cells and be demonstrated in tissue sections. Should such a substance be applied to the perikaryon, the axon will be labeled by anterograde transport. If it is applied at the axon terminals, it will be transported retrogradely and the perikarya will be labeled.

References.

Allen R.D.: The microtubule as an intracellular engine. Sci. Am. 1987, february: 26-33.

Carmichael S.W., Winkler H.: The adrenal chromaffin cell. Sci. Am. 1985, august: 30-39.

Chapman M.J., Dolan M.F., Margulis L.: Centrioles and kinetosomes: form, function, and evolution. Quart. Rev. Biol. 2000, 75: 409-428.

Chen D., Zhao C.M., Andersson K., Meister B., Panula P., Hakanson R.: ECL cell morphology. Yale J. Biol. Med. 1998, 71: 217-231.

Clermont Y, Rambourg A., Hermo L.: Trans-Golgi network (TGN) of different cell types: three-dimensional structural characteristics and variability. Anat. Rec. 1995, 242: 289-301.

Cole N.B., Lippincott-Schwartz J.: Organization of organelles and membrane traffic by microtubules. Curr. Opin. Cell Biol. 1995, 7: 55-64.

Cuervo A.M., Dice J.F.: Lysosomes, a meeting point of proteins, chaperones, and proteases. J. Mol. Med. 1998, 76: 6-12.

Dannies P.S.: Protein hormone storage in secretory granules: mechanisms for concentration and sorting. Endocr. Rev. 1999, 20: 3-21.

Deyrup-Olsen I., Luchtel D.L.: Secretion of mucous granules and other membrane-bound structures: a look beyond exocytosis. Int. Rev. Cytol. 1998, 183: 95-141.

Fath K.R., Mamajiwalla S.N., Burgess D.R.: The cytoskeleton in development of epithelial cell polarity. J. Cell Sci. 1993, Suppl. 17: 65-73.

Fuchs E., Cleveland D.W.: A structural scaffolding of intermediate filaments in health and disease. Science 1998, 279: 514-519.

Fujimoto T., Hagiwara H., Aoki T., Nomura R.: Caveolae: from a morphological point of view. J. Electron Microsc. 1998, 5: 451-460.

Gunst S.J., Tang D.D.: The contractile apparatus and mechanical properties of airway smooth muscle. Eur. Resp. J. 2000, 15: 600-616.

Hardin J.A., Gall D.G.: The regulation of brush border surface area. Ann. NY Acad. Sci. 1992, 664: 380-387.

Hermo L., Smith C.E.: The structure of the Golgi apparatus: a sperm's eye view in principal epithelial cells of the rat epididymis. Histochem. Cell Biol. 1998, 109: 431-447.

Hirokawa N.: Kinesin and dynein superfamily proteins and the mechanism of organelle transport. Science 1998, 279: 519-526.

Kimelberg H.K., Norenberg M.D.: Astrocytes. Sci. Am. 1989, april: 66-76.

Kobayashi N., Mundel P.: A role of microtubules during the formation of cell processes in neuronal and non-neuronal cells. Cell Tissue Res. 1998, 291: 163-174.

Motta P.M., Macchiarelli G., Nottola S.A., Correr S.: Histology of the exocrine pancreas. Microsc. Res. Tech. 1997, 37: 384-398.

Orci, L., Vassalli J.D., Perrelet A.: The insulin factory. Sci. Am. 1988, september: 50-61.

Rogers D.F.: Airway goblet cells: responsive and adaptable front-line defenders. Eur. Respir. J. 1994, 7: 1690-1706.

Rothman, J.E.: The compartmental organization of the Golgi apparatus. Sci. Am. 1985, september: 84-95.

Rothman J.E., Orci, L.: Budding vesicles in living cells. Sci. Am. 1996, march: 50-55.

Satir P.: Mechanisms of ciliary movement: contributions from electron microscopy. Scanning Microsc. 1992, 6: 573-579.

Small J.V., Fürst D.O., Thornell L.E.: The cytoskeletal lattice of muscle cells. Eur. J. Biochem. 1992, 208: 559-572.

Small J.V., Gimona M.: The cytoskeleton of the vertebrate smooth muscle cell. Acta Physiol. Scand. 1998, 164: 341-348.

Stossel T.P.: The machinery of cell crawling. Sci. Am. 1994, september: 40-47.

Tandler B., Phillips C.J.: Structure of serous cells in salivary glands. Microsc. Res. Tech. 1993, 26: 32-48.

Toth I.E., Szabo D., Bruckner G.G.: Lipoproteins, lipid droplets, lysosomes, and adrenocortical steroid hormone synthesis: morphological studies. Microsc. Res. Tech. 1997, 36: 480-492.

Walker C.A., Spinale F.G.: The structure and function of the cardiac myocyte: a review of fundamental concepts. J. Thorac. Cardiovasc. Surg. 1999, 118: 375-382.

Yamashina S.: Dynamic structure and function of Golgi apparatus in the salivary acinar cells. J. Electron Microsc. 1995, 44: 124-134.

II.3. The cell cycle.

Multicellular organisms arise and grow through cell multiplication during their embryonic development. But multiplication is not enough. Cells must also differentiate, i.e. specialize in different functions. During embryonic development, cells that are destined to certain functions migrate and arrange themselves into tissues and organs and subsequently differentiate. Multiplication and differentiation of cells are not the only factors that are operative in a multicellular organism. Sometimes it is as important to the organism that cells die as that they thrive and function.

II.3.1. Cell multiplication.

Cells grow in numbers by repeatedly dividing themselves, so that a single cell gives rise to two daughter cells. Multiplication through division (what a contradiction in terms) is primarily important in periods of growth, in the first place the embryonic period. Multiplication is first and foremost a characteristic of immature, unspecialized cells, which have as yet not taken the path of differentiation. In the mature organism, which consists largely of specialized, differentiated cells, cell multiplication is less frequent. Notable exceptions are those organs that produce cells, such as the bone marrow, lymphoid organs, and reproductive organs, or tissues that continuously lose cells, such as the epidermis and the intestinal epithelium.

Actually, the term cell division is not very accurate, because it conveys the impression that it is simply a matter of splitting a cell in two equal parts. Something much more fundamental happens during cell multiplication. Proper functioning of the body implies, at least in principle, that all its cells carry the same genetic information, and thus act according to the same instructions. This is particularly important in tissues, which often consist of identical cells. The mechanism of cell division ensures that the daughter cells that arise from it are genetically identical to one another and to the original cell. They are identical twins, and all the cells of the body are clones.

Genetically identical daughter cells are obtained by preliminary duplication of the original cell's genetic material, so that it contains two copies of it, and one of

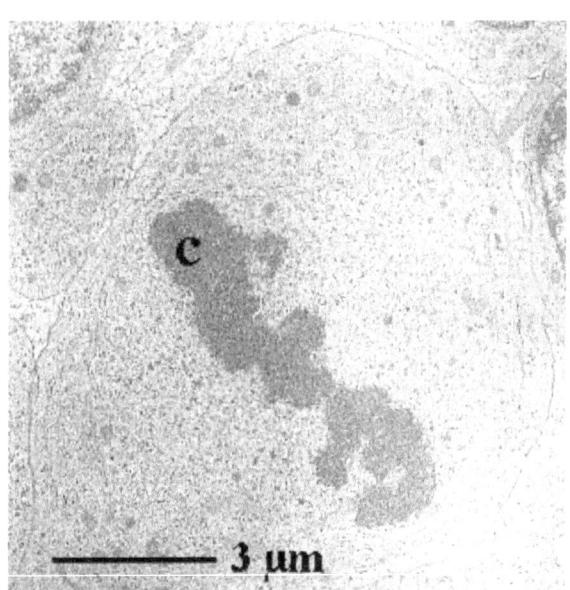

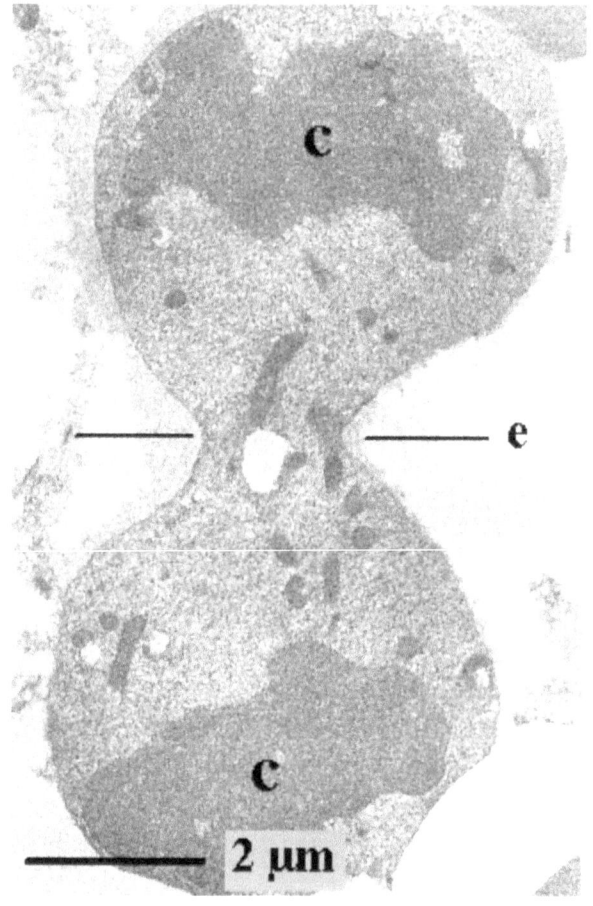

Fig. 2.58. (above) The mitotic nuclear division during metaphase. Prior to nuclear division, the nuclear envelope has been degraded and chromatin (c) has condensed and aggregated in the cell's equatorial plane. This mass of chromatin represents the chromosomes. Follicular granulosa cell, ovary, rabbit, TEM.
Fig. 2.59. (right) The mitotic nuclear division during the transition from anaphase to telophase. Two chromatin masses (c), each carrying a copy of the original cell's genetic archive, have been moved towards the opposite poles of a dividing cell. In its equatorial plane (e), this cell is constricting, giving rise to 2 genetically identical daughter cells. Hematopoietic cell, bone marrow, rabbit, TEM.

each will be received by each daughter cell. The genetic material is stored in the cell nucleus. The microscopic structure of a dividing cell is dominated by what happens with the cell nucleus, so much so that it would be better to speak of nuclear division instead of cell division.

In a cell that is about to divide, the nuclear envelope and the nucleolus are dismantled. The centrioles (Fig. 2.33.) separate. The chromatin condenses into several masses. With suitable techniques, these can be visualized as intensely staining, thread-like bodies, the **chromosomes**. Since chromosomes look like threads, nuclear division is also called **mitosis**. Chromosomes may be regarded as a particular organization of the chromatin, facilitating its displacement. Chromatin consists of extremely lengthy strands, which might easily get tangled. In a chromosome, these strands are compacted, making them easier to handle. All these phenomena are included in the term **prophase**, the first phase of mitosis.

During the subsequent **metaphase** (Fig. 2.58.), the chromosomes, or the chromatin masses of histologic sections, are moved to the cell's equatorial plane. The centrioles have arrived at opposite cell poles, and have doubled again to make up complete centrosomes. Between both centrosomes, a cell-bridging microtubular complex has formed, the **mitotic spindle**. Some of its microtubules extend uninterruptedly between both centrosomes, others are also attached to a chromosome. Shorter microtubules extend into the peripheral cytoplasm. At this stage, the chromosomes can be visualized as double bodies, each consisting of two **chromatids**, connected to each other somewhere along their length. This structure is a direct consequence of DNA duplication during interphase, the time period between successive mitoses. Both chromatids of a chromosome are identical copies.

During the **anaphase**, the chromatids of each chromosome separate and are moved to opposite cell poles by the mitotic spindle.

The **telophase** (Fig. 2.59.) is largely the opposite of prophase. At both cell poles, the chromatids lose their dense structure and convert to chromatin. A new nuclear envelope and nucleolus are assembled and two nuclei form. They are genetically identical. The cell lengthens and forms an equatorial belt of microfilaments, enabling it to constrict and giving rise to two daughter cells, each with a single nucleus.

II.3.2. Differentiation.

All cells of a single individual, no matter how different they may look, descend from a single cell, a fertilized ovum, and have the same genetic make up, thanks to the mechanism of mitosis. During embryonic development, the cells start to differentiate, becoming different. Generally, undifferentiated cells contain little cytoplasm, in which primary organelles predominate (Fig. 3.1.16.). In a histological sense, differentiation is the gradual appearance of a specific set of secondary organelles, membranes and fibers, which enable the cell to carry out its task. In the end, differentiation comes about by selective inhibition and activation of genes during development.

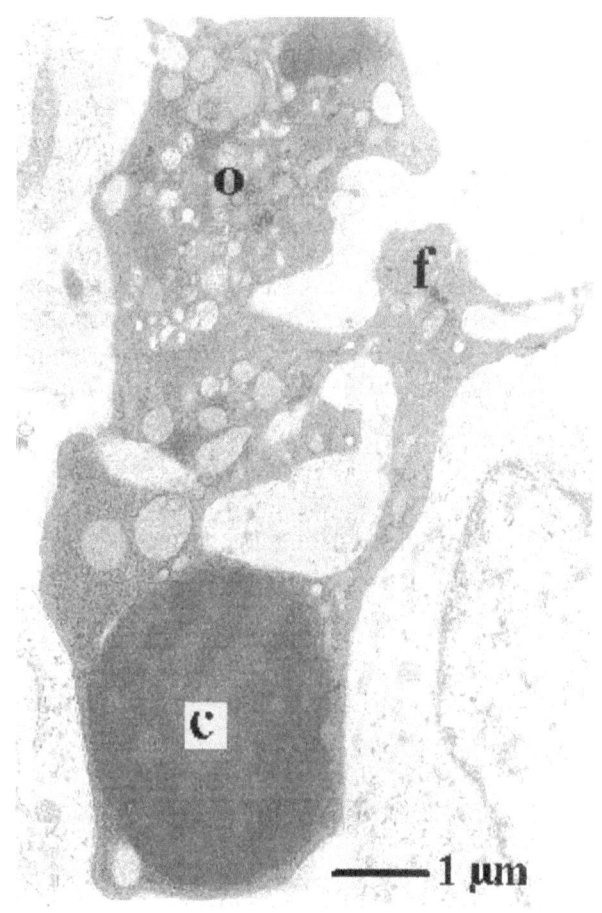

Fig. 2.60. An apoptotic cell shows extremely condensed nuclear chromatin (c), degradation of the organelles (o), and fragmentation of the cytoplasm (f). Spleen, rabbit, TEM.

III.3.3. Cell death.

Sometimes, cells must be prepared to the ultimate sacrifice, and commit suicide for the benefit of the organism. During embryonic development, cells are often superfluous and must be eliminated to the advantage of others. Cell death is particularly important in the embryonic nervous system, which has to get rid of nerve cells that have not formed the right connections with other cells, or in the developing lymphoid organs where lymphocytes, which happen to react against the organism itself, must be eliminated.

In its physiologic form, as a counterpart to mitosis, cell death is a genetically programmed phenomenon called **apoptosis**. In apoptosis, cells never die in large numbers, as often happens in pathological forms of cell death. The cells that die are rare and far between, a bit like autumn leaves, which are shed one by one.

In the nucleus of apoptotic cells (Fig. 2.60.), the chromatin gradually condenses, starting at the periphery. Eventually, a **pycnotic** nucleus, small and extremely heterochromatic, results. All this points at irreversible inactivation of the genetic material. The nucleus will also fragment. The cell as a whole starts to shrink. It loses any junctions it has with other cells and assumes a spherical shape. In the end, the cell fragments, giving rise to a number of **apoptotic bodies**. The organelles degenerate gradually. The cell membrane remains intact, resulting in neatly wrapped packages of junk, which remain in the intercellular space, or are ejected into a nearby cavity. Eventually, they are ingested and degraded by macrophages.

In the postnatal organism, apoptosis or apoptotic phenomena occur during the life cycle of certain blood cells, such as erythrocytes (III.1.1.) and granulocytes (III.1.3.), in the cartilaginous growth plate of long bones (IV.2.2.1.), and during oogenesis (IV.11.1.1.). Not infrequently, cell death is an integral part of differentiation, so that many differentiating cells show aspects of apoptosis. Examples include the stratified epithelium of the epidermis (III.4.1.3.4.), and the eye lens (IV.12.6.).

References.

Duke R.C., Ojcius D.M., Young J.D.E.: Cell suicide in health and disease. Sci. Am. 1996, december: 48-55.

Fahimi H.D., Baumgart E. : Current cytochemical techniques for the investigation of peroxisomes : a review. J. Histochem. Cytochem. 1999, 47: 1219-1232.

Häcker G.: The morphology of apoptosis. Cell Tissue Res. 2000, 301: 5-17.

Majno G., Joris I.: Apoptosis, oncosis, and necrosis. An overview of cell death. Am. J. Pathol. 1995, 146: 3-15.

McIntosh J.R., McDonald K.L.: The mitotic spindle. Sci. Am. 1989, oktober: 26-34.

Wyllie A.H., Kerr J.F.R., Currie A.R.: Cell death: the significance of apoptosis. Int. Rev. Cytol. 1980, 68: 251-306.

III. TISSUES

In multicellular organisms, cells with identical morphological characteristics, and consequently identical functions, or cells with complementary functions, form a structure with a higher level of organization: a **tissue**. A tissue is a collection of identical, or at least complementary, cells. The proper functioning of a tissue often requires that its cells be in some specific way connected or associated. They may even pass explicit messages among one another. These are the two morphological aspects we have to consider when discussing the morphological characteristics of a tissue: the kind of cells that participate in it, and the kind of contact these cells maintain.

Cells can be combined to tissues in several ways (Fig. 3.1.). A logical sequence in which tissues can be discussed suggests itself when the complexity of this arrangement is considered. In a purely structural respect, the least complex tissue is one that consists of loose, **independent cells**. **Lymphoid** and **myeloid tissue**, and the closely related **blood**, are the first examples of this kind of tissue that come to mind. The **interstitial**, **connective** and **supportive tissues** equally consist of cells that have, at least in principle, no direct physical contact. They are separated from each other by an intercellular matrix. Elongated cells can be joined to **bundles**. These cells can touch, but are usually not interconnected. Skeletal **muscle tissue** is an example of such a tissue, as is conductive nerve tissue, which consist of bundles of axons. In **lining tissues**, the cells are arranged in one or more layers or **sheets**, and tightly joined. Exocrine **glandular tissue** is formed in the same way; the structure of endocrine glandular tissue is derived from this pattern. The most complex association between cells is a **network**. The most obvious example of this is **nerve tissue**, but some types of muscular tissue (cardiac, visceral) and supportive tissue (the osteocytes in bone) show this pattern of organization as well.

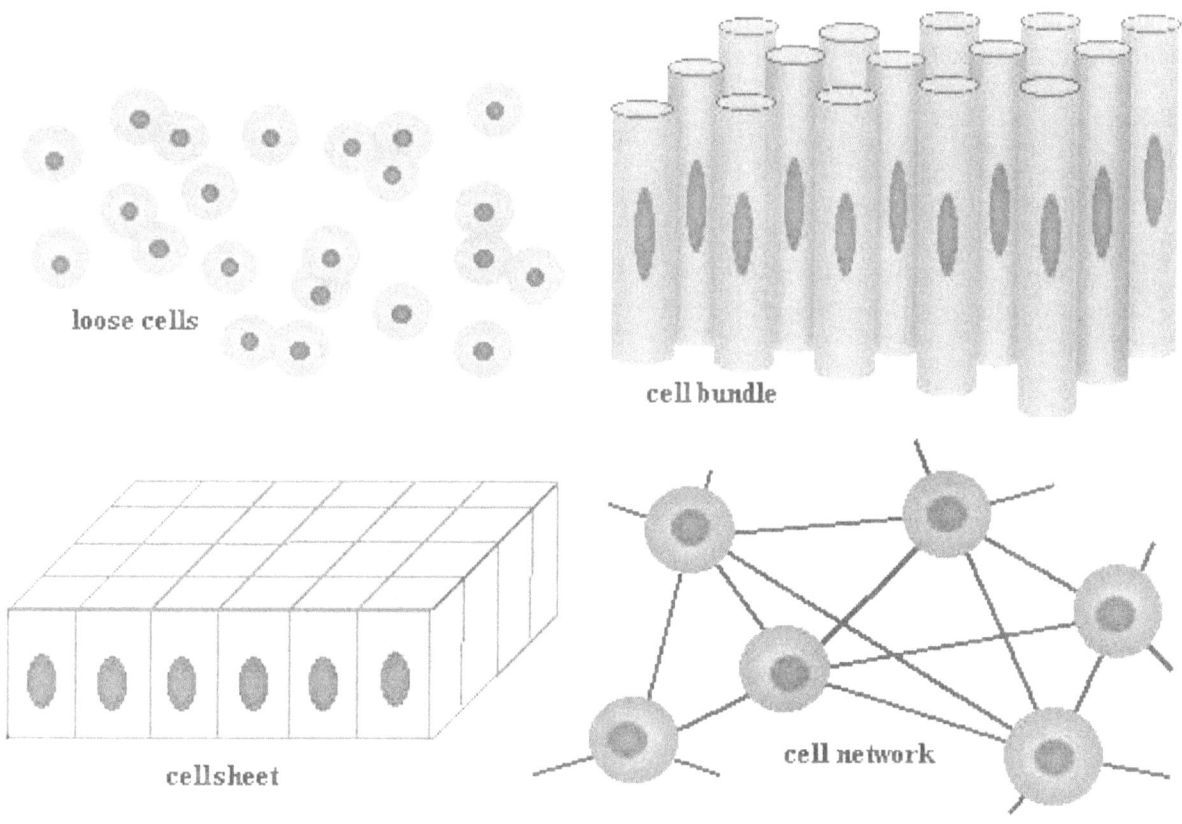

loose cells

cell bundle

cellsheet

cell network

Fig. 3.1. A tissue is an aggregation of identical, or at least closely cooperating, cells. Tissues differ from one another in the kind of cells they are made of and the way in which those cells are arranged and interconnected. The simplest tissues consist of loose cells. Elongated cells often aggregate into bundles. Cells can adhere tightly, and form plates or sheets. The most complex tissues consist of cells with processes, which are interconnected to form a network.

III.1. Myeloid and lymphoid tissues, and blood.

Myeloid tissue, lymphoid tissue and blood can be mentioned in a single breath because they consist of closely related cells. The cells that are encountered in the **blood** are either differentiated or undifferentiated. Of the differentiated cells, the erythrocytes and the thrombocytes function locally, in the blood itself. In this way, they are the only true blood cells. The granulocytes and the undifferentiated cells, the lymphocytes and the monocytes, use the blood as a transport medium on their way to the interstitial tissue of the organs (granulocytes, monocytes), or to the secondary lymphoid organs (lymphocytes), where they will terminally differentiate and become functional. On becoming functional, or even before this, all these cells loose their capacity of mitotic division and multiplication. Their numbers can only be maintained by the continuous maturation of precursor cells, which do have the capacity of multiplication. These precursor cells occur in impressive numbers and form the **myeloid tissue** of the bone marrow and the **lymphoid tissue**, which is distributed over the body and occasionally participates in the formation of discrete lymphoid organs. The myeloid (or hematopoietic) and lymphoid (or lymphopoietic)

tissues belong to the rather rare type of tissue that, even in the postnatal organism, retains embryological characteristics. They form disorderly masses, containing undifferentiated cells, rich in primary organelles, which multiply intensively. Part of them gradually differentiate to functional cells.

The different cell types of the myeloid tissue, lymphoid tissue and blood ultimately descend from a single type of primitive, pluripotent stem cell, which probably resides in the myeloid tissue, but has not yet been identified morphologically. This stem cell's descendants differentiate along three lines of descent. One line leads to the lymphocytes, another one to the monocytes. Both are still very incompletely differentiated cells, which migrate from the myeloid tissue at an early stage to continue their differentiation elsewhere: the lymphocytes in the lymphoid tissues and the monocytes in the interstitial tissues. The third cell line starts at the **hemocytoblast**. Hemocytoblasts are relatively large cells with a diameter of about 20 micrometers. Their cytoplasm is rich in ribosomes, which confer basophilic properties on it. The relatively large nucleus is euchromatic and contains one or more well developed nucleoli. Hemocytoblasts are multipotent in the sense that they still retain the

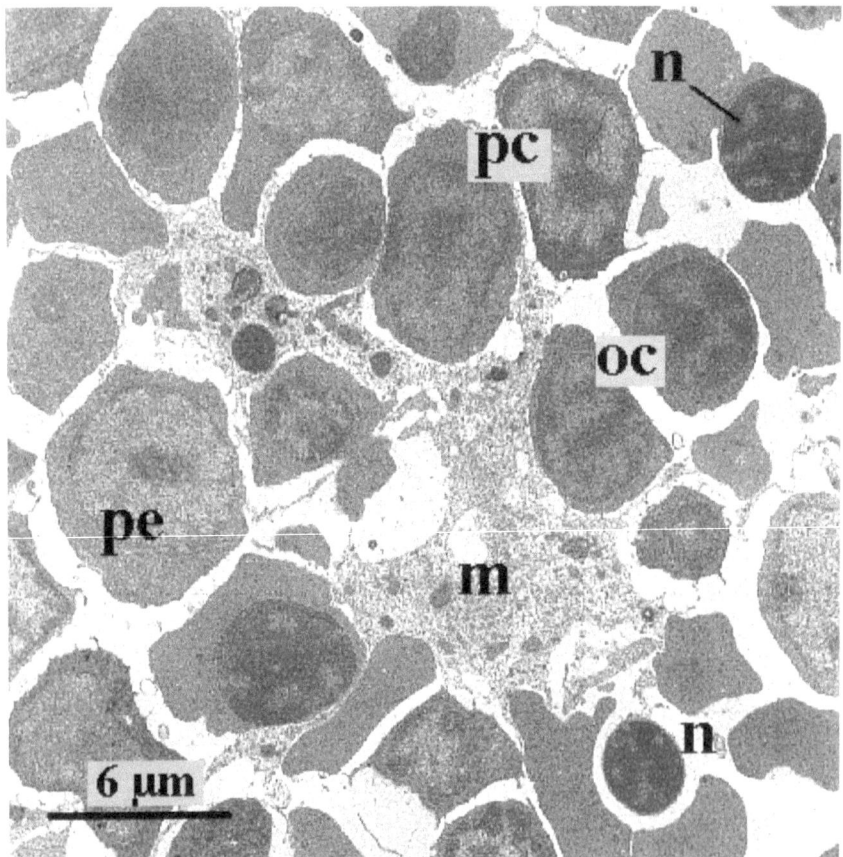

Fig. 3.1.1. A collection of developing erythrocytes, with a macrophage (m) in the center, in the myeloid tissue of bone marrow. Most of these cells represent relatively advanced maturation stages, such as polychromatophilic (pc) and orthochromatic erythroblasts (oc), which are characterized by dense, heterochromatic nuclei and a featureless, dense cytoplasm. At the end of development, the nucleus is ejected (n). This and other cell debris is engulfed by the macrophage. A few representatives of early stages in erythrocyte development are also present, probably proerythroblasts (pe), characterized by a euchromatic nucleus. Bone marrow, rat, TEM.

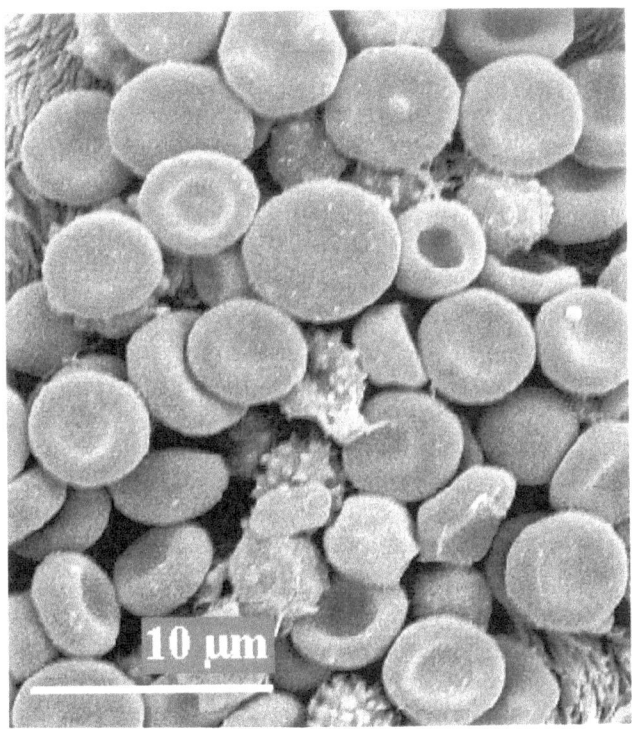
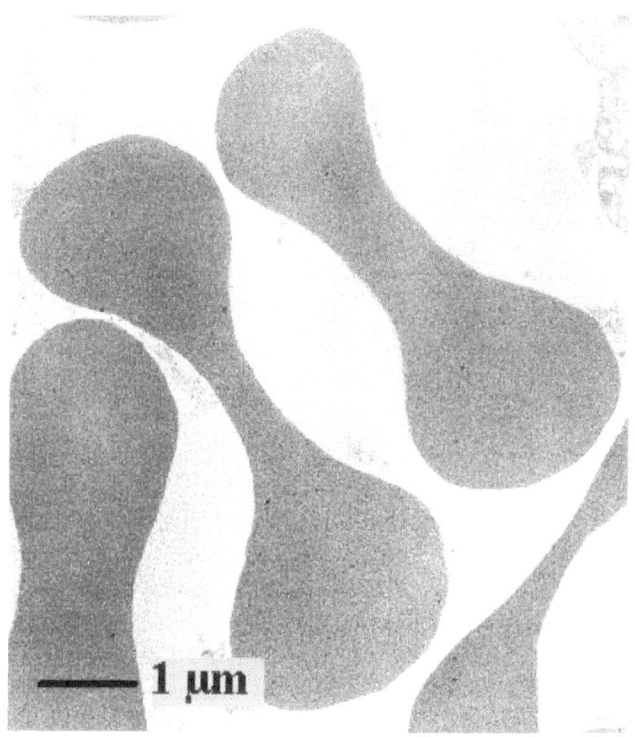

Fig. 3.1.2. (left) Ripe erythrocytes look like biconcave disks. Blood, rabbit, SEM. Fig. 3.1.3. (right) Vertical sections show the erythrocyte's typical biconcave shape. Their cytoplasm, or matrix, is featureless. Bone marrow, hamster, TEM.

capacity of gradual differentiation into several other cell types: erythrocytes, thrombocytes, and granulocytes. These cells, in their successive stages of differentiation, form the myeloid tissue. Hemocytoblasts still are mitotically active, a capacity their descendents quickly loose.

Morphologically, blood is a suspension of cells in a clear fluid, the plasma. The plasma can be considered analogous to the matrix of interstitial, connective and supporting tissues. It can in fact form fibrils, made of fibrin, in the process of blood clotting. The defense function of interstitial tissue also has a counterpart in the blood plasma: it contains globulins, secreted by plasma cells, which are the antibodies, vital to the immunological defense of the organism. Most often, blood is microscopically studied as a smear.

III.1.1. Erythrocytes and their precursors.

The erythrocyte's precursors mature in the myeloid tissue (Fig. 3.1.1.). The most primitive cell type that is a direct precursor of the erythrocyte is the **proerythroblast**. This cell is somewhat smaller than the hemocytoblast, but its diameter is still almost double that of the ultimate erythrocyte. The voluminous, euchromatic nucleus leaves room for only

a rather narrow rim of basophilic cytoplasm, rich in free ribosomes. These are the telltale characteristics of an undifferentiated cell involved in large-scale synthesis of RNA and proteins (hemoglobin) for its own use. The cytoplasm may contain vesicles, called siderosomes, in which iron, bound to protein, is stored in the form of ferritin or transferrin. Iron is a vital component of the hemoglobin's oxygen-carrying heme prosthetic group. At an early stage, RNA synthesis is discontinued and the process that will lead to the elimination of the nucleus is initiated. The proerythroblast nucleus begins to shrink and to condense, as in apoptosis. As the nucleus shrinks, the relative amount of cytoplasm increases, although the total cell volume diminishes. This stage is called the **basophilic erythroblast**. In the cytoplasm, hemoglobin synthesis continues. Hemoglobin has eosinophilic staining properties, and gradually masks the basophilic reaction of the ribosomes. The nucleus and the cell as a whole continue to shrink. This stage is the **polychromatophilic erythroblast**. The succeeding **orthochromatic erythroblast** has eosinophilic cytoplasm and a diminutive, densely heterochromatic, eccentric nucleus. Ribosomes have largely disappeared and the cell is filled with a homogeneous mass of hemoglobin. Eventually, the nucleus, surrounded with a narrow rim of cytoplasm, is pinched off from the rest of the cell. What results is

61

technically not a cell, since it contains neither a nucleus nor organelles. It is a membranous container, packed with the highly specific protein hemoglobin, an **erythrocyte**. Fully differentiated erythrocytes are released into the blood, where they can be thought of as forming a tissue, consisting of loose cells.

Erythrocytes are by far the most common blood "cell" type. A milliliter of blood contains about five billion of them. Erythrocytes are one of the cell types that cannot be incorporated in any of the proposed categories. They only consist of a homogeneous matrix of hemoglobin, bordered by a cell membrane (Fig. 3.1.3.). Because of the presence of iron, the matrix is electron opaque. The fact that erythrocytes occur as loose cells does not imply that they are globular. In fact, their most distinctive feature, in a morphological sense, is their shape. They are biconcave disks with a diameter of about 7 micrometers (Fig. 3.1.2.). The biconcave shape is very apparent on an axial section (Fig. 3.1.3.). In the light microscope, erythrocytes may appear as rings (Figs. 3.1.11.-15.) because their center is much thinner than their rim. The biconcave shape is actively maintained by a cytoskeleton of spectrin, of the intermediate filament category, which forms a supporting layer underneath the cell membrane. The cytoskeleton is rigid, but does allow changes of shape. This facilitates passage of the erythrocytes through even the narrowest of capillaries, the diameter of which hardly exceeds that of the erythrocyte.

Hemoglobin reversibly binds oxygen, enabling the erythrocytes to play their vital role in the transport of oxygen by the blood. The biconcave shape is not without significance in this respect. Given an identical volume, the sphere has the smallest surface area of all geometric shapes. Consequently, any deviation from the perfect spherical shape increases the relative surface area. In the specific case of the erythrocyte, its shape exposes more hemoglobin to the exterior than would be possible in a spherical cell and consequently facilitates exchange of oxygen between the cell's interior and its surroundings.

The specializations of the erythrocytes, involving the loss of organelles, imply that they are doomed. They cannot sustain themselves indefinitely, because they have lost the capacities of synthesis and multiplication. The lack of mitochondria means that their energy supply is likewise limited. After about 120 days after they were liberated into the circulation, it is over. Worn out, senescent erythrocytes are trapped in the spleen, the liver and the bone marrow, and ingested by macrophages. The hemoglobin's protein fraction is excreted by the liver in the form of bilirubin, bile pigment. The iron is recuperated in the form of ferritin and taken up by maturing erythrocytes.

III.1.2. Thrombocytes and their precursors.

The biggest cell type in the myeloid tissue, the **megakaryocyte** (Fig. 3.1.4.), happens to be the precursor of the smallest cellular element of the blood, the thrombocyte. Megakaryocytes attain diameters of 100 micrometers and more and have abundant cytoplasm. Their nucleus is multilobed and polyploid: it contains multiple copies, up to 32, of the genome. The immediate benefit for the cell is that multiple copies of the same genes enable it to intensify the synthesis of certain proteins, thus forming large amounts of cytoplasm and growing to a large size. Polyploidy is a consequence of repeated endomitosis: successive cycles of genome replication and chromatid separation without intervention of cell division.

Megakaryocytes descend from the hemocytoblast through the **megakaryoblast**, a large cell with a diameter of up to 40 micrometers, but with an unlobed nucleus and without specific organelles. At a certain stage in megakaryoblast development, the normal mitotic cycle is interrupted. Anaphase is no longer followed by telophase and cell division, but the genetic material is duplicated and a new cycle starts. In the course of successive cycles, as the number of genome copies goes up, a complex multipolar mitotic spindle is generated. Several microtubule bundles radiate from each pole, indicated by its centrosome, and connect it to several sets of chromosomes, creating a spherical complex, which resembles a geodesic dome. During anaphase, several sets of chromatids are pulled towards each pole. Eventually, endomitosis stops and a new nuclear envelope forms. At each mitotic spindle pole, where chromatids have aggregated, the envelope bulges, resulting in a multilobed nucleus.

Megakaryocytes are clearly membrane-bearing cells. A Golgi-complex and rough endoplasmic reticulum are found in a perinuclear position. The peripheral cytoplasm is loaded with dense cored membranous vesicles and an extensive network of membranous tubules (Fig. 3.1.5.). These tubules are in fact narrow lamellar spaces, continuous with the extracellular space, and bordered by so-called **demarcation membranes**. They delineate parts of the cytoplasm, eventually separating them from the megakaryocyte. These fragments are the immediate precursors of the thrombocytes. Similar to erythrocytes, thrombocytes are not true cells: they are cytoplasmic fragments. In principle, the cytoplasm lost by fragmentation can be replenished. Eventually though, the cell does not recuperate any longer. What remains of it undergoes apoptosis and is removed by macrophages.

A milliliter of blood may contain several hundred

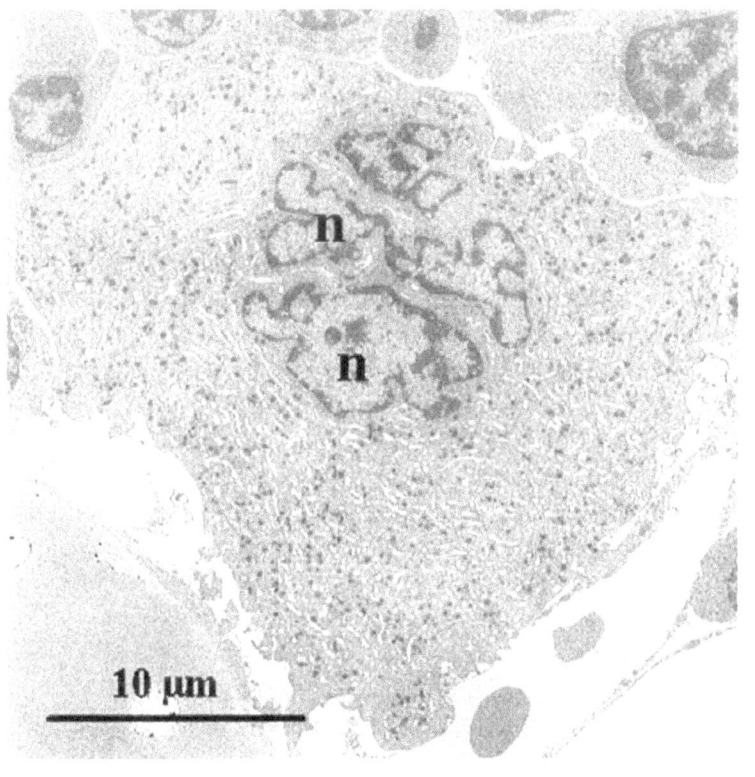

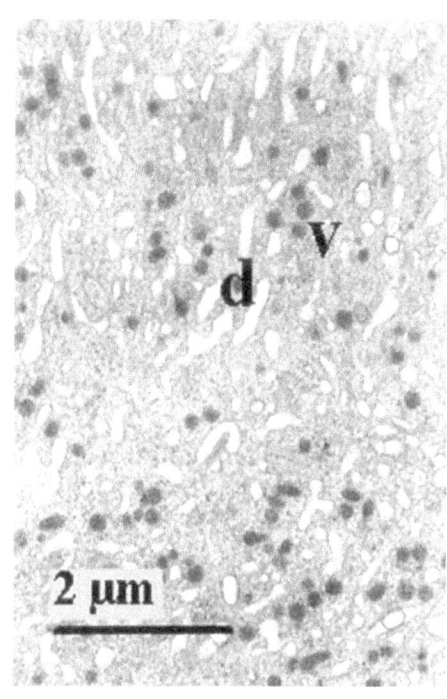

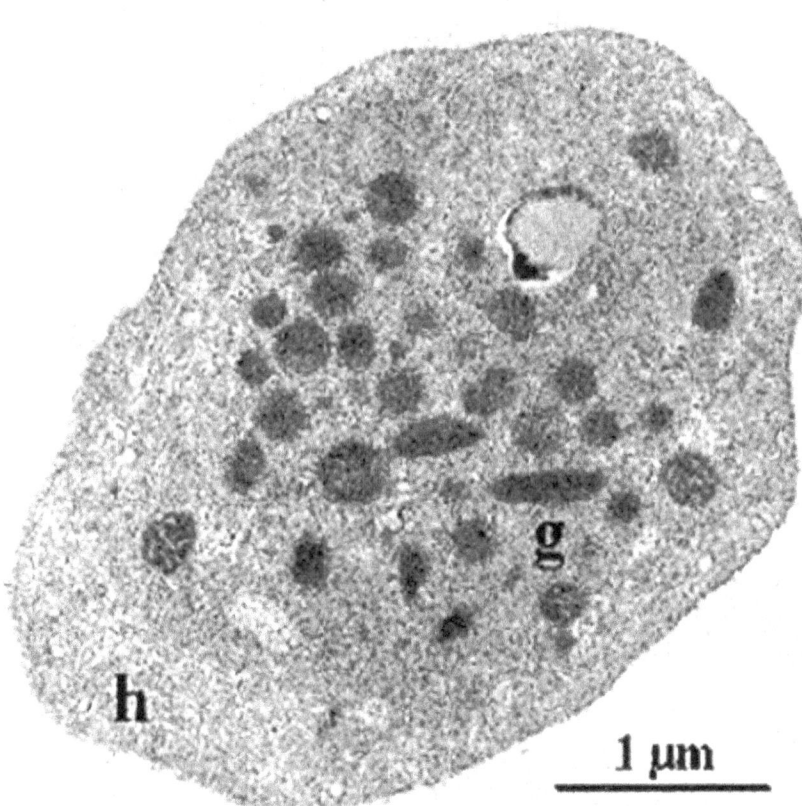

Fig. 3.1.4. (top left) A megakaryocyte is a giant cell with a lobed nucleus (n), the cytoplasm of which is filled with membranes and dense vesicles. Bone marrow, rabbit, TEM. **Fig. 3.1.5.** (top rigt) An enlarged view of the megakaryocyte of Figure 3.1.4.. The cytoplasm contains numerous demarcation membranes (d), which will allow it to fragment, giving rise to thrombocytes. It is loaded with dense vesicles (v) as well. Bone marrow, rabbit, TEM. **Fig. 3.1.6.** (left) A thrombocyte or platelet is a cytoplasmic fragment of a megakaryocyte. The central part, containing the dense vesicles that were already present in the megakaryocyte, is the granulomere (g). The periphery, or hyalomere (h), is fibrous. These intracellular fibers reinforce the platelet and enable it to maintain its flattened shape (only visible in side view). Blood, cat, TEM.

thousand **thrombocytes** or **platelets** (Fig. 3.1.6.). Like erythrocytes, they can be thought of as constituting a tissue of loose cells. They are the smallest cellular elements of the blood (Fig. 3.1.13.). They look like round, biconvex disks with a maximal diameter of 3,5 micrometers. Their center, in the light microscope, has a granular look. Ultrastructurally, it contains the same dense cored vesicles as the megakaryocyte cytoplasm. The edge is often difficult to make out in the light microscope for lack of

63

granular material and because of its thinness. The center and the edge of the platelet are called the **granulomere** and the **hyalomere**, respectively. The hyalomere may be largely free of inclusions, but it does contain a ring of microtubules, making two to four loops. This cytoskeleton, the **marginal band**, maintains the thrombocyte's shape. Thrombocytes survive in the circulation for only about ten days.

The granulomere vesicles contain various proteins, among them clotting factors. The single most important function of the thrombocytes is the induction and regulation of blood clotting. Upon rupture of a vessel wall, thrombocytes aggregate to form a plug. Actual clotting involves the formation of fibrin fibrils out of circulating fibrinogen. Fibrin fibrils display regular transverse striations, as collagen fibrils do (III.2.3.1.). This striation's periodicity is only 24 nanometers, compared to collagen's 64 nanometers. They don't aggregate to larger fibers, but form a disorderly mass. The vesicles are similar to those of the amine hormone-secreting gland cells (II.2.1.3.) and in fact store an amine, serotonin, a vasoconstrictor substance that can contribute to stemming of the blood flow through a vessel wall rupture. Serotonin is not synthesized by the thrombocytes, but taken up from the blood.

III.1.3. Granulocytes and their precursors.

The most primitive direct precursors of the granulocytes are the **myeloblasts**. They resemble hemocytoblasts, but their basophilia is more pronounced. Myeloblasts develop into **promyelocytes** (Fig. 3.1.7.): rough endoplasmic reticulum and a Golgi-complex appear, followed by membranous vesicles. Light optically and with specific staining procedures for studying blood smears, these appear as azurophilic granules. These granules will disappear in every other granulocyte cell line but only partly so in the one that leads to the neutrophilic granulocytes. They are called primary granules because they are the first ones to appear in the course of granulocyte development.

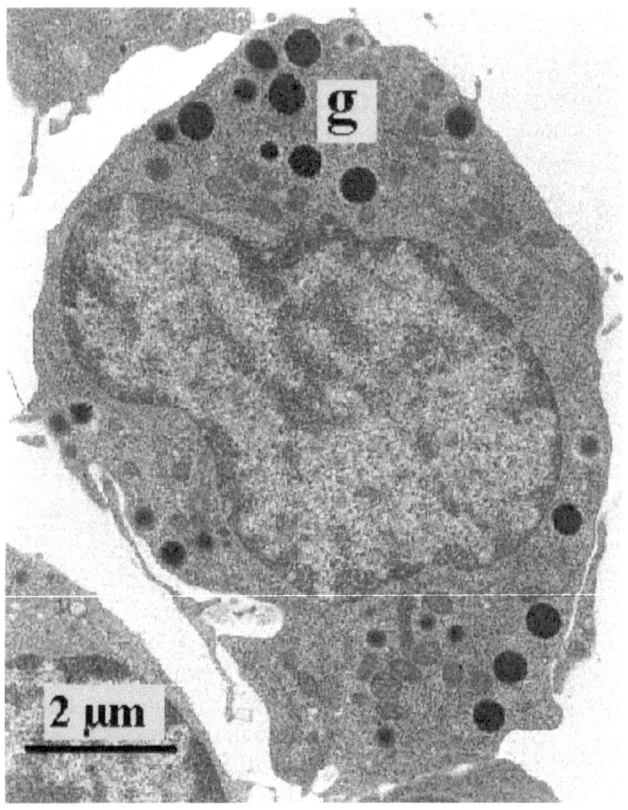
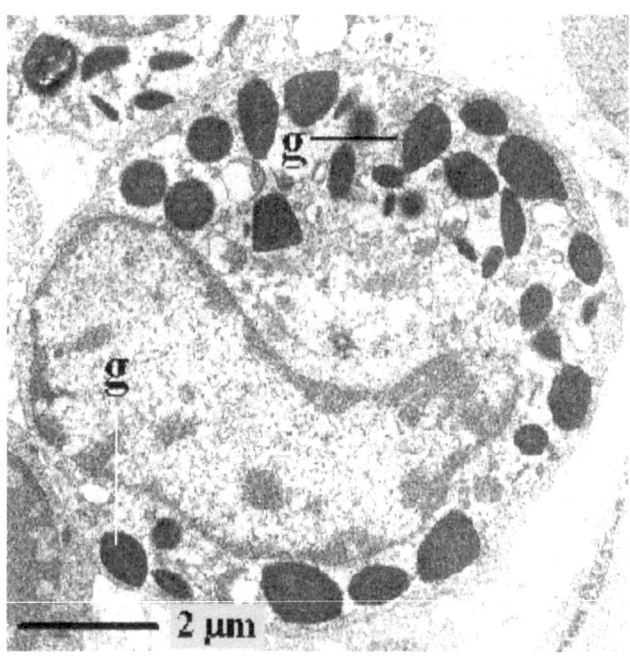

Fig. 3.1.7. (left) The promyelocyte is an early stage in the development of granulocytes and contains only a single type of relatively large granules (g). Bone marrow, rat, TEM. Fig. 3.1.8. (right) The myelocyte is a later stage in granulocyte development. Myelocytes develop the specific types of granules that characterize the 3 types of mature granulocytes, but their nucleus is not yet segmented. This particular myelocyte is eosinophilic, as it contains granules with a crystalline matrix (g), typical of the later eosinophilic granulocyte. Bone marrow, rabbit, TEM.

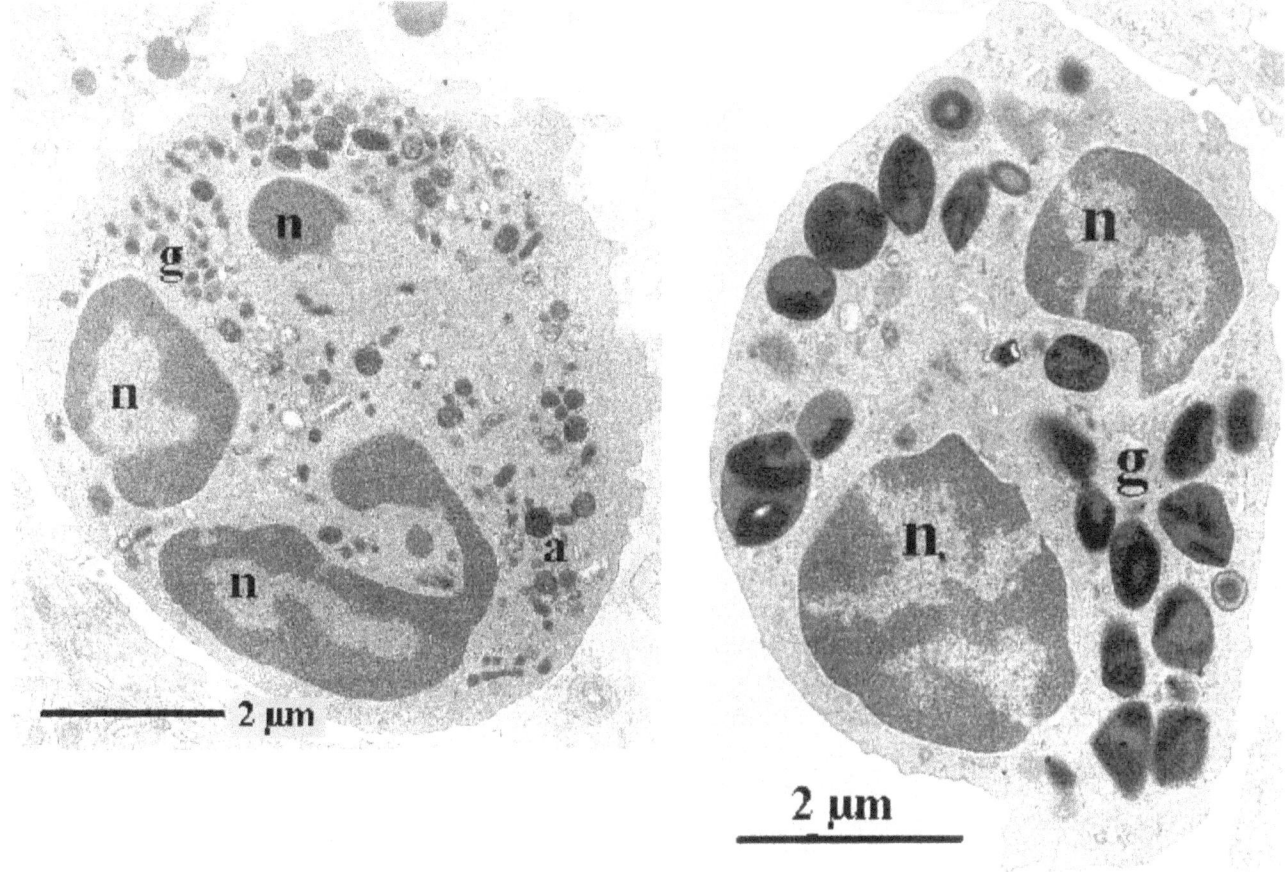

Fig. 3.1.9. (left) A mature neutrophilic granulocyte contains, apart from a few large, aspecific granules (a), numerous small, specific, or neutrophilic, granules (g). The nucleus is strongly segmented and multilobed (n). Pulmonary interstitial tissue, human, TEM. **Fig. 3.1.10.** (right) A mature eosinophilic granulocyte, recognizable by its typical granules with their crystalline matrix (g), and a bilobed nucleus (n). Blood, cat, TEM.

Promyelocytes develop into **myelocytes** (Fig. 3.1.8.) when neutrophilic, eosinophilic, or basophilic granules are produced and accumulated at the expense of the primary azurophilic granules. These granules are called secondary or specific. The myelocyte is the last stage in granulocyte development that is capable of mitosis. Gradually, the nuclei become multilobed, and the resulting cells are called **metamyelocytes**. At the same time, the rough endoplasmic reticulum and the Golgi-complex involute and the amount of heterochromatin increases. The cells are released in the blood stream as fully developed granulocytes.

Granulocytes have a multilobed, heterochromatic nucleus and numerous cytoplasmic vesicles, which light optically appear as granules. Three types of granulocytes can be distinguished on the basis of the appearance of the cell nucleus and the staining properties of the specific granules: **neutrophils**, **eosinophils**, and **basophils**.

III.1.3.1. Neutrophils.

Neutrophils (Figs. 3.1.9., 3.1.11., 3.1.15.) are the most common type of granulocyte: a milliliter of blood contains a few million. They are spherical cells, with a diameter of 12 to 14 micrometers. The nucleus is divided into three to five lobes, which are interconnected by very thin strands. The cytoplasm contains two kinds of granules. The relatively large (diameter about 400 nanometers) and rare primary granules are azurophilic. The smaller (diameter below 300 nanometers) and more numerous secondary or specific granules are neutrophilic. The secondary granules, in particular, do not form a homogeneous population. At least three subsets are distinguished and the tendency is to reserve the term secondary for only one of these. These vesicles have different contents and appear at different times and in different circumstances. Consequently, neutrophils may show variation in their vesicle population.

The large primary granules are lysosomes. They store acid hydrolases, and bactericides, such as myeloperoxidase. Myeloperoxidase, by the reduction of oxygen, gives rise to the extremely reactive hydrogen peroxide and superoxide. The smaller vesicles contain proteinases, bactericidal enzymes, and plasma proteins.

Neutrophils circulate in the blood for only a few hours after their release from the myeloid tissue. Soon, they migrate into the interstitial tissues of the body, where they function as defender cells. They show pronounced chemotactic properties in response to chemicals generated by foreign invaders and by debris of the body's own cells and have a strongly developed tendency to amoeboid movement. At the level of the capillaries, they leave the blood by diapedesis: they crawl in between the lining endothelial cells of the capillary, locally degrade the basement membrane by secretion of proteinases, and move into the surrounding tissue. There, they actively seek out bacteria and cellular debris and remove them by phagocytosis. Neutrophils have a pronounced taste for opsonized bacteria, which have been coated with specifically bound antibody proteins. Neutrophils contain few mitochondria and produce their energy mainly by glycolysis. They also have few ribosomes and their nucleus is heterochromatic, which implies a low level of protein synthesis, insufficient for maintaining their stock of lysosomes. Once their lysosomal enzymes have been depleted and they have become loaded with indigestible remains, they die. Most probably, they only live for a few days after their release. In pathological circumstances, such as inflammation, dead neutrophils can accumulate in excessive numbers, forming pus.

III.1.3.2. Eosinophils.

A milliliter of blood contains a few hundred thousand eosinophils (Figs. 3.1.10., 3.1.12.). They are somewhat larger than neutrophils: their maximal diameter is about 17 micrometers. They are easily distinguished by their numerous, relatively large (diameter up to 1 micrometer), eosinophilic granules. Most often, the nucleus is bilobed. It can be partially masked by the granules. Ultrastructurally, these granules, or vesicles, have a very distinctive aspect. They are ovoid and contain a matrix. A dense crystalloid, with a diskoid to irregular shape, is embedded in this matrix. These vesicles are lysosomes. The crystalloid is made of a very basic protein, the major basic protein. In addition, several other types of hydrolytic enzymes and peroxidases are stored in the matrix and the crystalloid.

Eosinophils are macrophages, with a specific taste for antigen-antibody complexes. They are less bactericidal than neutrophils. They show distinct chemotactic properties under the influence of histamine and eosinophil chemotactic factor of anaphylaxis, substances liberated by basophils and mast cells. They are also activated by the presence of multicellular parasites. Just like neutrophils, eosinophils migrate from the blood to the interstitial tissues of the body. They contain more organelles than neutrophils, and live somewhat longer. The actual age they can reach is unknown.

III.1.3.3. Basophils.

Basophils (Fig. 3.1.13.) are the rarest type of granulocyte: a milliliter of blood contains only a few ten thousand. They have virtually the same dimensions as the eosinophils. Likewise, their nucleus is bilobed and their specific, basophilic granules are very distinctive with light microscopy. The granules almost completely mask the nucleus. The basophilic granules are somewhat larger and less numerous than eosinophilic granules. They also show metachromatic staining properties, like those of mast cells (III.2.1.3.3.). There are other points of resemblance between basophils and mast cells and this is taken as an indication that basophils and mast cells share a common precursor cell in the myeloid tissue. Ultrastructurally, the granules correspond to membranous vesicles with a homogeneously opaque content, separated from the membrane by a narrow, translucent halo.

The vesicles are secretory vesicles. Their content is liberated upon simple exocytosis (merocrine secretion) or by compound exocytosis or piecemeal degranulation, similar to mast cell secretion. The secretory vesicles contain the same substances as those of mast cells and it is assumed that basophils and mast cells have similar functions (III.2.1.3.3.). It is not well understood where basophils perform their function: in the blood or in the peripheral interstitial tissues. Like the eosinophils, they contain relatively numerous organelles and live for a comparatively long time. Exactly how long is not known.

III.1.4. Monocytes.

A milliliter of blood contains a few hundred thousand monocytes (Fig. 3.1.14.). They are large blood cells, their diameter may attain up to 20 micrometers. The nucleus is relatively large, bean or kidney shaped, and occupies an eccentric position. Light optically, the

66

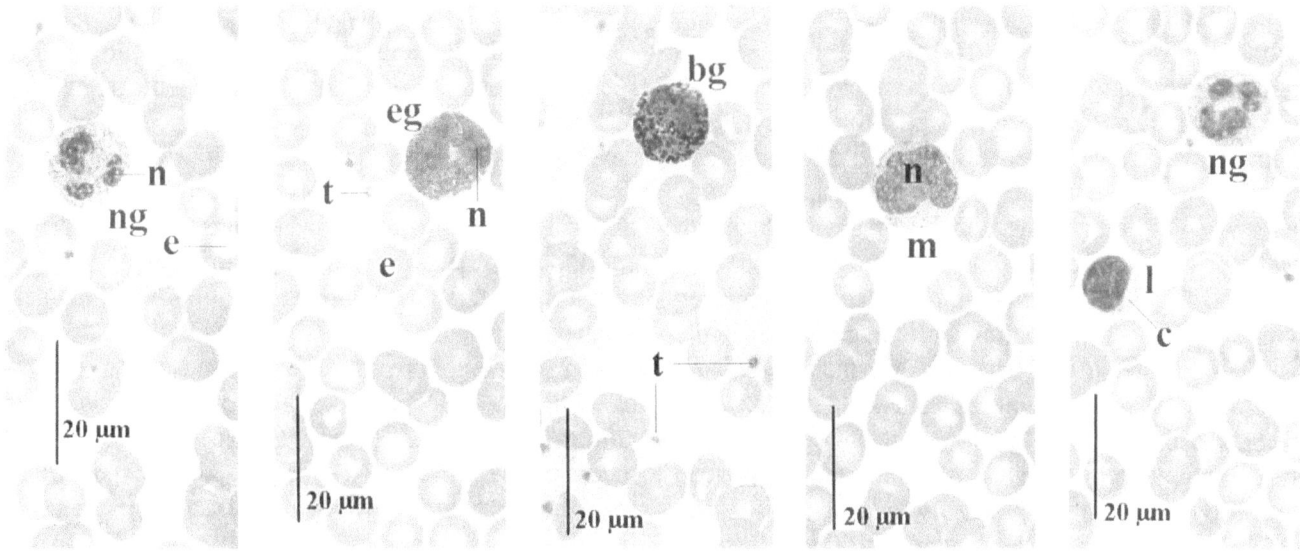

Left to right: **Fig. 3.1.11.** A neutrophilic granulocyte (ng), characterized by a multilobed nucleus (n) and a very fine, neutrophilic, granulation. Mark the translucent center of the surrounding erythrocytes (e). Blood smear, cat, Giemsa stain. **Fig. 3.1.12.** An eosinophilic granulocyte (eg) is characterized by a bilobed nucleus (n) and a coarse, eosinophilic granulation. e = erythrocyte, t = thrombocyte. Blood smear, cat, Giemsa stain. **Fig. 3.1.13.** A basophilic granulocyte (bg). Its nucleus is masked by a very coarse, basophilic granulation. A few thrombocytes are present (t). Blood smear, cat, Giemsa stain. **Fig. 3.1.14.** A monocyte (m) has a relatively large, kidney-shaped nucleus (n) and scanty cytoplasm. Blood smear, cat, Giemsa stain. **Fig. 3.1.15.** A lymphocyte (l) can be recognized by its small size (compare with surrounding erythrocytes), its rounded, dense nucleus and its narrow rim of cytoplasm (c). A neutrophilic granulocyte (ng) is also seen. Blood smear, cat, Giemsa stain.

cytoplasm is basophilic. Ultrastructurally, the cytoplasm contains ribosomes, a relatively well-developed rough endoplasmic reticulum and Golgi-complex, and lysosomes. The cell membrane forms pseudopodia.

Monocytes are the precursors of histiocytes (III.2.1.3.1.) and other types of macrophages. Just like the granulocytes and lymphocytes, they use the blood as a means of transport. They are chemotactic and capable of amoeboid movement. They enter the interstitial tissues by diapedesis, as granulocytes do. In the interstitial tissues, they differentiate to macrophages that remove cellular debris and foreign invaders.

III.1.5. Lymphocytes.

The lymphocytes are the most important defender cells of the body, forming the backbone of the immune system. Functionally, distinction is made between T- and B-lymphocytes. Morphologically, these hardly differ from each other. Lymphocytes arise in the myeloid tissue of the bone marrow. Via the blood, the T-lymphocytes migrate, at an early stage, to the thymus (IV.1.2.), where they complete a further stage of their development. T stands for thymus dependent. Subsequently, they migrate to the peripheral lymphoid organs (lymph nodes and spleen) and to the mucosal lymphoid tissues, associated mainly with the intestine and the airways (tonsils, Peyer's patches, etc.). In birds, B-lymphocytes continue their development in a large gut-associated lymphoid organ, Fabricius's bursa. Thus, B-lymphocytes are bursa dependent. In mammals, B-lymphocytes remain somewhat longer in the myeloid tissue and undergo most of their development there. Eventually, they also migrate to the peripheral lymphoid organs and mucosal lymphoid tissues. It is here, in the first place, that both T- and B-lymphocytes may come in contact with specific antigens and become activated. Activated lymphocytes multiply and may transform themselves (in case of B-lymphocytes) and migrate, via the lymph and blood circulation, to the interstitial tissues, where they will attack the antigen that has activated them.

A milliliter of blood contains 2 to 3 million lymphocytes (Figs. 3.1.15.-16.). Most of them are hardly bigger than erythrocytes, having a diameter of 6 to 9 micrometers. These are inactive lymphocytes, on their way to the peripheral lymphoid organs and mucosal lymphoid tissues. A small fraction, a few percent, of the circulating lymphocytes is bigger, with a diameter of 9 to 15 micrometers. These are activated lymphocytes, mostly B-lymphocytes, undergoing lymphoblastic transformation while on their way to the peripheral interstitial tissues. Lymphocytes are spherical and have a heterochromatic nucleus. The nucleus occupies most of the available space within the cell so that lymphocytes, especially the small ones, have little cytoplasm left. The cytoplasm is basophilic and contains ribosomes. Secondary organelles are virtually absent. These are all telltale signs indicating that the lymphocytes of the blood are undifferentiated cells.

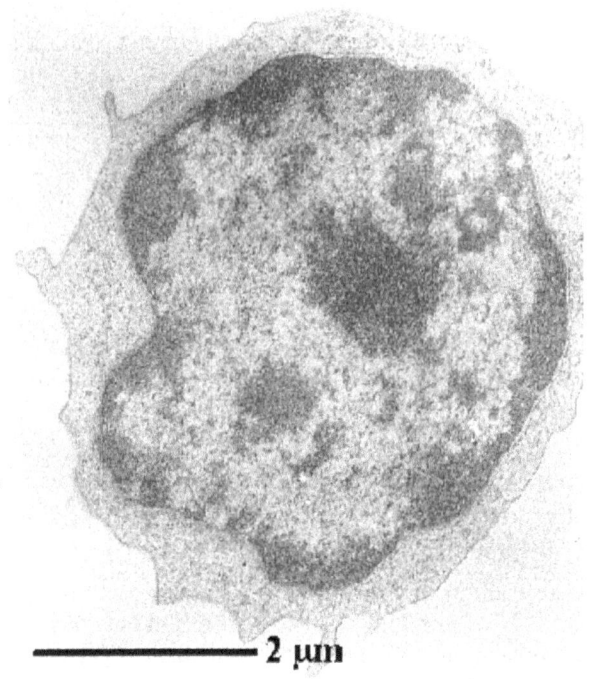

Fig. 3.1.16. A lymphocyte has a rather heterochromatic nucleus and scanty cytoplasm with few organelles. Lymph node, rabbit, TEM.

In a purely morphological sense, lymphocyte activation and interaction with antigen is not dramatic. It's functional aspects, on the other hand, are very complex.

T-lymphocytes interact with antigens by means of complementary membrane receptors. They are activated by antigens that are carried by antigen presenting cells, mostly macrophages and dendritic cells. Unimaginably numerous types of antigen specific receptors are in circulation, each carried by a different T-lymphocyte. During lymphocyte development, the genes responsible for receptor protein synthesis are split up and recombined in ever changing combinations, which accounts for the enormous repertoire of T-lymphocyte antigen receptors in existence. Upon activation by an antigen, a relatively small number of specific T-cells, carrying a fitting membrane receptor, start to multiply, a phenomenon called clonal expansion. In this way, the number of available antigen specific membrane receptors is dramatically increased, so that the antigen can be efficiently neutralized. Activated T-lymphocytes differentiate in various ways, but hardly so in a morphological sense. **Cytotoxic T-cells** physically contact cells carrying the antigen by which they were activated and kill them. **Helper T-cells** contribute to the activation of cytotoxic cells and B-lymphocytes. **Suppressor T-cells** regulate the immune response by inhibiting other immune cells. **Memory T-cells** do not engage the antigen, but remain in circulation, ensuring that a future attack by the same antigen will be met with much more quickly. This is what makes the body immune to certain diseases. This kind of immunity is mediated by cells: it is called cellular immunity.

B-lymphocytes only interact with antigens if these are carried by specific T-lymphocytes: helper T-cells. Upon activation, B-lymphocytes undergo clonal expansion, similar to T-lymphocytes. They also undergo lymphoblastic transformation, in a much more pronounced fashion than do T-lymphocytes. Lymphoblastic transformation involves growth of the cytoplasm and, eventually, transformation to **plasma cells**. Immature B-lymphocytes interact with antigens by means of membrane receptors of the immunoglobulin type. Plasma cells also synthesize immunoglobulins, but secrete them as antibodies. Antibodies will specifically bind to the antigen present, contributing to its neutralization and eventual elimination. Innumerable different types of receptors and antibodies may be synthesized. This is explained in the same way as the formation of different receptors by the T-lymphocytes: recombination in the relevant part of the genome during lymphocyte development. In each immune response, a fraction of the activated B-lymphocytes does not transform to plasma cells, but remains as **memory B-cells**, contributing to the body's immunity. This aspect of immunity is mediated by secretions of cells, or humors. It is called humoral immunity.

As far as their mechanism of defense is concerned, T-lymphocytes may be compared to the infantry, which directly confronts the enemy. B-lymphocytes, on the other hand, are the immune system's artillery, which fires projectiles, or better still guided missiles, to far away targets.

References.

Borregaard N., Lollike K., Kjeldsen L., Sengelov H., Bastholm L., Nielsen M., Bainton D.: Human neutrophil granules and secretory vesicles. Eur. J. Haematol. 1993, 51: 187-198.

Breton-Gorius J., Reyes F.: Ultrastructure of bone marrow cell maturation. Int. Rev. Cytol. 1976, 46: 251-321.

Cramer E.M.: Megakaryocyte structure and function. Curr. Opin. Hematol. 1999, 6: 354-361.

Dvorak A.M.: Similarities in the ultrastructural morphology and developmental and secretory mechansisms of human basophils and eosinophils. J. Allergy Clin. Immunol. 1994, 94: 1103-1134.

Dvorak A.M., Ishizaka T.: Human eosinophils in vitro. An ultrastructural morphology primer. Histol. Histopathol. 1994, 9: 339-374.

Jelinek D.F.: Regulation of B lymphocyte differentiation. Ann. Allergy Asthma Immunol 2000, 84: 375-386.

Nurden P., Poujol C., Nurden A.T.: The evolution of megakaryocytes to platelets. Baillière's Clin. Haematol. 1997, 10: 1-27

III.2. Interstitial, connective, and supportive tissues.

Interstitial, connective, and supportive tissues differ from all other tissues in that they not only consist of cells, but of a substantial amount of intercellular material as well. This intercellular material, or **matrix**, is a complex mixture of proteinaceous substances, produced by specialized matrix-secreting cells. Not infrequently, the amount of matrix is so large that the cells themselves constitute only a minor fraction of the whole tissue volume. Consequently, and contrary to other tissues, it is not the cells that determine the typical properties of this particular tissue, it is the matrix that does. The primary function

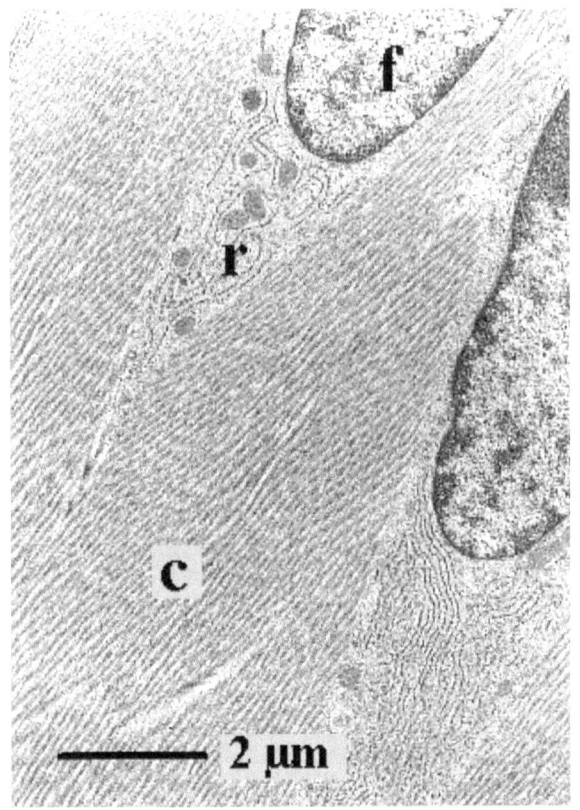

Fig. 3.2.1. The closely related interstitial, connective, and supportive tissues are the only tissue type that contains large amounts of intercellular material, the matrix. In this image, the matrix happens to be rich in collagen fibrils (c). The matrix is produced by matrix-secreting cells, fibrocytes (f), characterized by the presence of rough endoplasmic reticulum (r). Epineurium, vagus nerve, rabbit, TEM.

of the matrix is to confer firmness to the tissue. Notwithstanding the presence of a cytoskeleton, cells are little more, in a mechanical respect, than lumps of watery gel. Relatively big organisms, certainly so when they live on dry land and are under the full influence of gravity, simply cannot exist without a supplementary reinforcement of their body, supporting

it and enabling it to withstand fatal compression and deformation.

Analogous to reinforced concrete, which is composed of cement and steel wire, the matrix has two components: ground substance and fibrils. While the **ground substance** is amorphous, the **fibrils** have a distinct microscopic structure. The relative share of both is variable and can be adapted to specific local requirements, so that several types of matrix containing tissues can be distinguished. The least specialized ones are the **interstitial tissues**, which can be regarded as just filling the spaces, or interstices, between other tissues. The mesenchymal, mucous, and loose fibrous tissues are examples of this category. They are not just passive stuffings of any available spaces, though. Their relative firmness lends support to the surrounding tissues, and enables them to bind or hold them together. Starting from the interstitial tissues, it is either the connective function or the supportive function that can be developed to greater extremes. The most widespread of the interstitial tissues, loose fibrous tissue, is composed of about equal amounts of ground substance and fibrils. When the relative amount of fibrils is increased, the connective function predominates, since fibrils are well suited to withstand traction, especially so when they all have the same orientation. Thus, **connective tissues** are formed. The dense fibrous, as well as the elastic, tissues are specialized in this way. When the matrix is made resistant to compression, the supportive function predominates. Thus the highly specialized **supportive tissues**, cartilage and bone, are formed.

It must be mentioned that some of these tissues have other functions besides conferring firmness. Bone also serves as a calcium store for the body's metabolism. Loose fibrous tissue also stores substances in various specialized cells, such as fat in lipocytes. Loose fibrous tissue is the most important field of action of the body's defender cells: monocytes, histiocytes, granulocytes, plasma cells, lymphocytes, and plasma cells.

III.2.1. Cell types.

III.2.1.1. Matrix-secreting cells.

The most typical cells of the interstitial, connective and supportive tissues are the matrix-secreting cells (II.2.1.1.3.). Active matrix-secreting cells have a euchromatic nucleus and a well-developed rough endoplasmic reticulum, sometimes with dilated cisterns. Resting cells have rather heterochromatic nuclei and less abundant cytoplasm with relatively little rough endoplasmic reticulum. Several types of matrix-secreting cells exist, each secreting their own typically composed matrix. **Fibroblasts** are spindle-shaped cells which secrete the matrix of the fibrous and elastic connective tissues. When the deposition of matrix is completed, fibroblasts reversibly revert to a resting stage, the fibrocyte (Fig. 3.2.1.). **Reticuloblasts** are a specialized fibroblast variant, distinctly star shaped. They secrete a particular type of collagen fibrils, which form reticulin fibers. **Chondroblasts** secrete the matrix of cartilage. Chondroblasts can rest on the surface of existing cartilage and deposit additional layers of matrix at their interface with the cartilage. Alternatively, they can be located in the interior of cartilage and deposit matrix all around them. In the first instance, the chondroblasts are prismatic and polarized, cytologically similar to exocrine cells. In the other instance they are globular and symmetrical, similar to endocrine cells. Resting chondroblasts are called chondrocytes. **Osteoblasts** secrete the matrix of bone. They occur exclusively at the surface of existing bone, where they deposit additional layers of matrix. They are prismatic, polarized cells. When they enter a resting stage, they are walled in by the secretions of neighbouring osteoblasts. These osteocytes normally do not revert to active synthesis again.

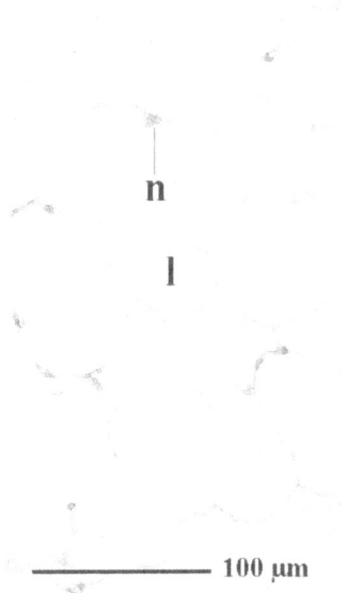

Fig. 3.2.2. The "empty" aspect of white adipose tissue is a consequence of the use of lipid solvents during tissue preparation. White, or unilocular, lipocytes accumulate large amounts of lipid in a single intracellular lipid droplet (l), which inflates them like balloons. They end up tightly crowded, as a consequence of this, and acquire a polygonal shape. Thus, white adipose tissue resembles a honeycomb. Expansion of the intracellular lipid droplet flattens the nucleus, which ends up at the cell's periphery (n). Testis, rat, HE.

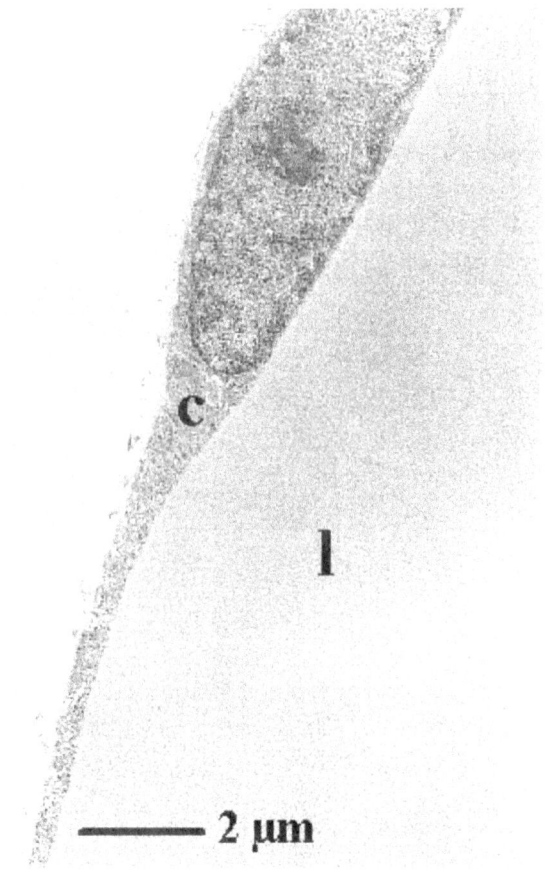

Fig. 3.2.3. A single giant lipid droplet (l) occupies virtually the entire volume of a white lipocyte. At the cell's periphery, only a narrow rim of cytoplasm (c) remains, containing the nucleus. Retroperitoneal adipose tissue, hamster, TEM.

III.2.1.2. Lipocytes.

Loose fibrous connective tissue, in particular, serves as a depot for the storage, temporary or permanent, of various substances. Among these belong lipids (predominantly triglycerides: esters of fatty acids and glycerol), which are stored in specialized fat cells, called adipocytes or **lipocytes**. Lipocytes have a wide distribution. Locally, they can accumulate in such numbers that they form real **adipose tissue**. Adipose tissue can be subdivided by fibrous tissue septa, giving rise to aggregates with a deceptive gland-like appearance.

Lipocytes develop from unspecialized interstitial tissue cells, the mesenchymal cells, which change into lipoblasts by accumulating lipid droplets. In the course of their development, lipoblasts may accumulate excessive amounts of lipid, which occupy most of their cytoplasm, changing them into lipocytes. Lipoblasts take up fatty acids and glycerol from the blood and tissue fluid, and use them to synthesize triglycerides. They can also synthesize triglycerides from glucose. The enzymes needed for synthesis are located on the smooth endoplasmic reticulum, although this is never very strongly developed. Triglycerides accumulate in the cytoplasm as droplets, not vesicles, i.e. they are not enclosed by a membrane. At most, they are surrounded by a thin layer of microfilaments.

III.2.1.2.1. White or unilocular lipocytes.

In **white lipocytes** (Fig. 3.2.2.), most lipid droplets eventually coalesce into a single central lipid droplet, which displaces the nucleus towards the cell's periphery. White lipocytes are also called **unilocular**

lipocytes because of this single droplet. The droplet further accumulates lipid, and it attains a quite impressive size. Mature white lipocytes are large cells, with a diameter of up to 200 micrometers. The cytoplasm is almost exclusively occupied by a single gigantic lipid droplet. The nucleus is flattened and lies against the cell membrane (Fig. 3.2.3.). The nucleus is heterochromatic and the narrow peripheral ring of remaining cytoplasm contains few organelles, all of which indicates that the cell has entered a resting phase. Lipocytes that lie in groups press firmly against one another, forcing them into polyhedral shapes. White adipose tissue therefore resembles a honeycomb. In preparations for light microscopy, this impression is strengthened further by the dissolution of the lipid droplet, which makes the lipocytes appear empty. With electron microscopy, the lipid droplet appears homogeneously opaque.

White adipose tissue has a number of important functions.
As **structural tissue**, it functions as a kind of supportive tissue. The lipid droplets are resistant to compression, and act as an intracellular matrix. In this

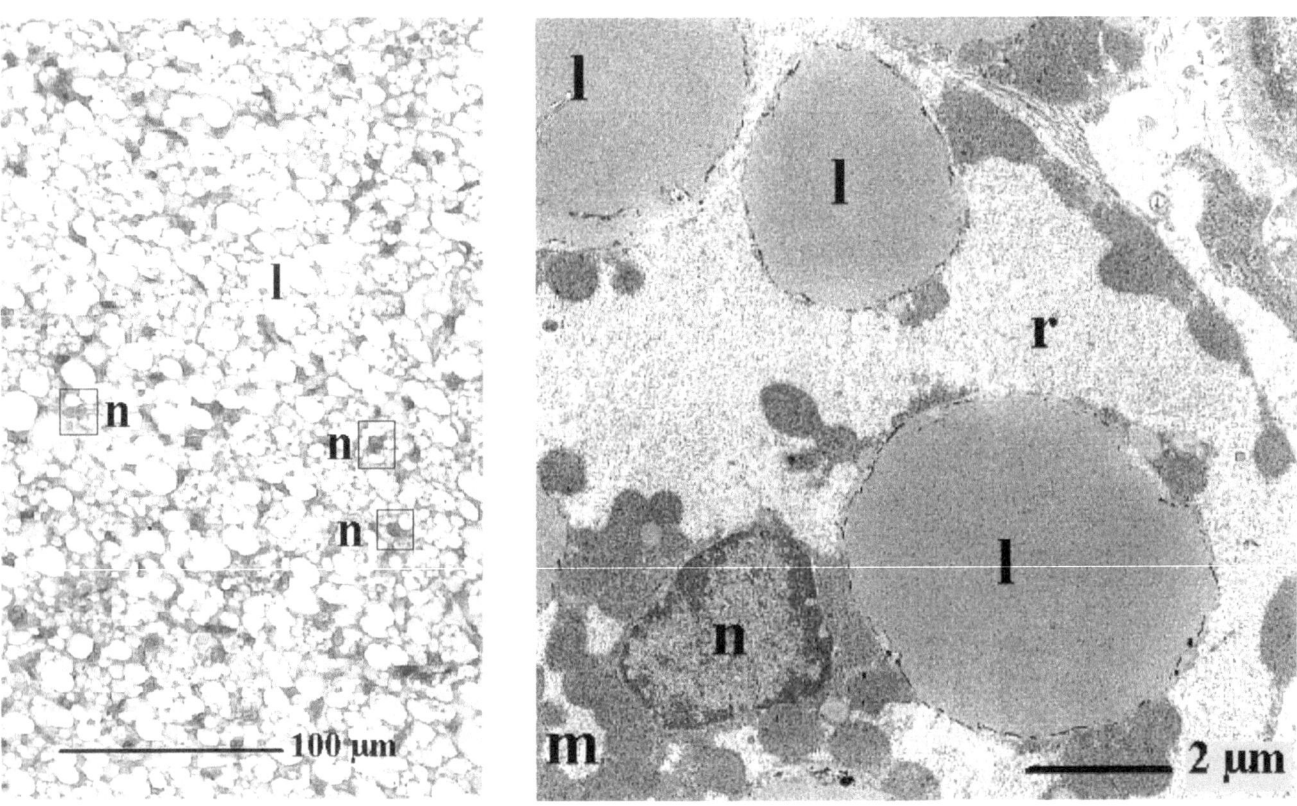

Fig. 3.2.4. (left) Brown adipose tissue has multilocular lipocytes. They contain numerous small lipid droplets (l), which surround the central nucleus (n). Kidney hilus, cat, HE. **Fig. 3.2.5.** (right) A brown lipocyte contains numerous lipid droplets (l), coated by a fibrous layer, which surround the nucleus (n). The cytoplasm is rich in mitochondria (m) and ribosomes (r). Hypodermal adipose tissue, hamster, TEM.

way, adipose tissue helps to support the body and even determines the shape of certain body parts, such as the breasts. It is also found abundantly in the cheeks, the eye sockets, the buttocks, the palm of the hand and the sole of the foot. Structural adipose tissue is not readily influenced by the energy demands of the body.

Storage tissue, on the other hand, serves as an energy store, which helps the organisms to survive periods of scarcity. When levels of food intake are high, fatty acids and glycerol are taken up from the blood, triglycerides are synthesized, and storage tissue forms and extends. In the reverse condition, lipid reserves are mobilized, and the storage tissue involutes. Triglycerides are hydrolyzed, under hormonal influence, liberating fatty acids and glycerol, which can be oxidized to liberate energy. These substances leave the cell through a not completely understood mechanism; they may diffuse through the cell membrane. During the mobilization of fat reserves, the lipid droplet may fragment and the smooth endoplasmic reticulum may proliferate. Storage tissue is found in the hypodermis of the skin of certain body regions such as the belly, in the bone marrow, and in the retroperitoneum and the mesenterium of the abdominal cavity.

There is no sharp distinction between both adipose tissue types. In addition, both types can function in thermal isolation.

III.2.1.2.2. Brown or multilocular lipocytes.

In **brown** or **multilocular lipocytes** (Fig. 3.2.4.), lipid synthesis and storage is less extreme and the lipid droplets do not coalesce. Brown lipocytes are relatively small. Their nucleus occupies a central position and their cytoplasm is richer in organelles, such as mitochondria (Fig. 3.2.5.). The numerous lipid droplets give brown adipose tissue a spongy look, not unlike the steroid-secreting cells of the adrenal cortex. It is more densely vascularized than white adipose tissue and its mitochondria are richer in cytochromes, hence its darker color, which explains its name.

Brown adipose tissue occurs almost exclusively in the hypodermis of the shoulder and pelvic regions of neonates and in hibernating mammals. Its function is equivalent to white storage tissue, but there is a difference. White storage tissue releases glycerol and fatty acids, which are oxidized by the body cells that need energy to generate ATP. In brown adipose tissue, an important part of the glycerol and fatty acids is oxidized by the lipocyte itself, and the liberated energy is not used to generate ATP, but to produce heat. The dense vascularization of brown adipose tissue helps to evacuate this heat and to distribute it over the rest of the body. In periods of cold, nerves stimulate brown adipose tissue and it plays an important role in thermoregulation.

III.2.1.3. Defender cells.

Infectious agents or antigens invade the body by penetrating its lining tissues. They enter the underlying interstitial tissues, where various types of defender cells await them. These cells are, in principle, mobile. They move spontaneously, patrolling the tissues, or in response to chemicals secreted by the invaders or by other defender cells. In this way, they can concentrate in a threatened area. During infection, inflammation or allergic reactions, they can accumulate in great numbers. In normal circumstances, they are scarce. In principle, all defender cells descend from precursor cells in the myeloid tissue of the bone marrow. Some of them are found as such in the blood or interstitial tissues; others differentiate further on contacting an antigen. The **granulocytes**, **monocytes**, **lymphocytes** and **plasma cells** have been discussed already. This chapter will concentrate on the **histiocytes** and **mast cells**.

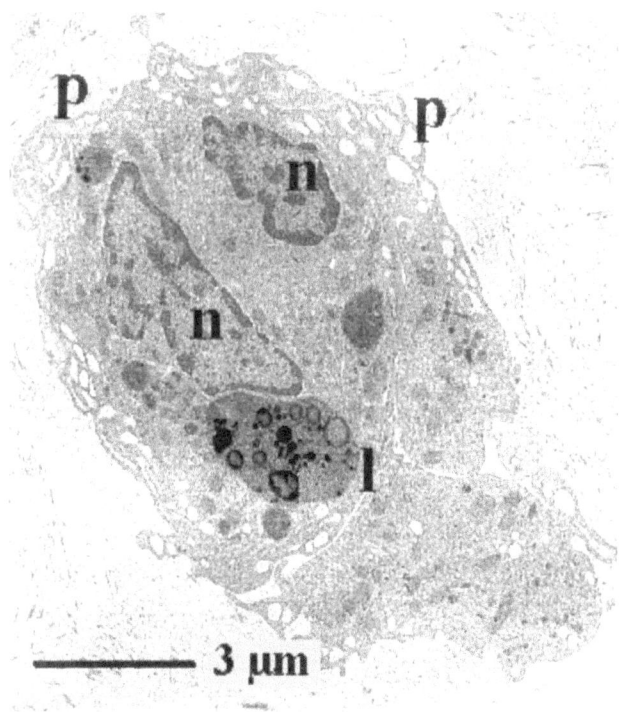

Fig. 3.2.6. A histiocyte or interstitial tissue macrophage. Mark the lobed nucleus (n), the secondary lysosome or phagosome (l), and the numerous pseudopodia (p). Pulmonary interstitial tissue, human, TEM.

III.2.1.3.1. Histiocytes.

Histiocytes (Fig. 3.2.6.) are macrophages. They are direct descendents of monocytes, which reach the interstitial tissues via the circulation, and can be found there as such. Inactive histiocytes are inconspicuous cells. They can be activated experimentally and made more conspicuous by supravital staining. Contrasting material, injected in the circulation, enters the interstitial tissue and is engulfed by histiocytes, making them easy to spot in histological sections.

Often, macrophages such as histiocytes are the first defender cells to encounter and be activated by antigenic material. After breaking it down, they incorporate parts of it in their cell membrane. They migrate to the peripheral lymphoid organs, where they activate T-lymphocytes with the bound antigen, a phenomenon called antigen presentation. Histiocytes also remove opsonized microorganisms and antigen-antibody complexes.

III.2.1.3.2. Mast cells.

Mast cells were named by their discoverer, the German physician Paul Ehrlich, who considered them as well fattened (German: masten = to fatten), because of their content of granules. They have a widespread distribution in the interstitial tissues, in particular those of the blood vessels, skin, airways, and intestine. Mast cells stand out after staining with basic pigments such as toluidin blue (Fig. 3.2.7.). They show up as rounded or elongated cells with a central nucleus, loaded with coarse cytoplasmic granules which stain metachromatically: the original blue color of the pigment is changed to reddish purple as a consequence of chemical modification.

Ultrastructurally, the cytoplasm is loaded with relatively large (diameter up to 2 micrometers), rounded membranous vesicles with a dense content (Fig. 3.2.8.), which may show a substructure of granules or spirally wound lamellae. The vesicles leave little room for other organelles, except for a rather well developed Golgi-complex. The cell membrane carries a varying number of irregular microvilli. The cytological structure of the mast cell is reminiscent of an endocrine, amine hormone-secreting gland cell (II.2.1.3.). The dense vesicles are in effect secretory vesicles, which undergo exocytosis. Because of the dense content, another term used is degranulation. Exocytosis or degranulation can take

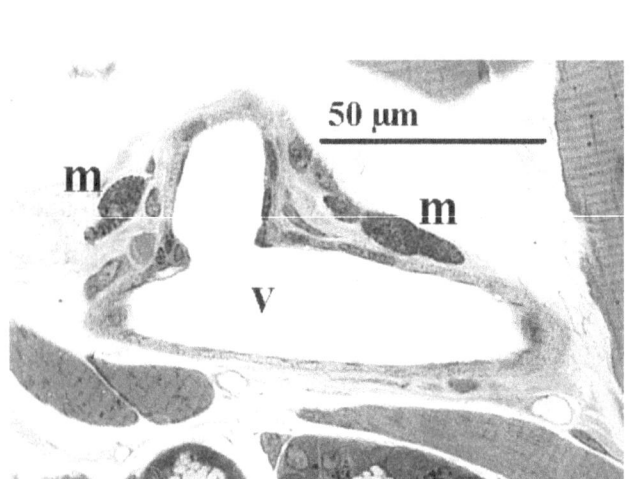
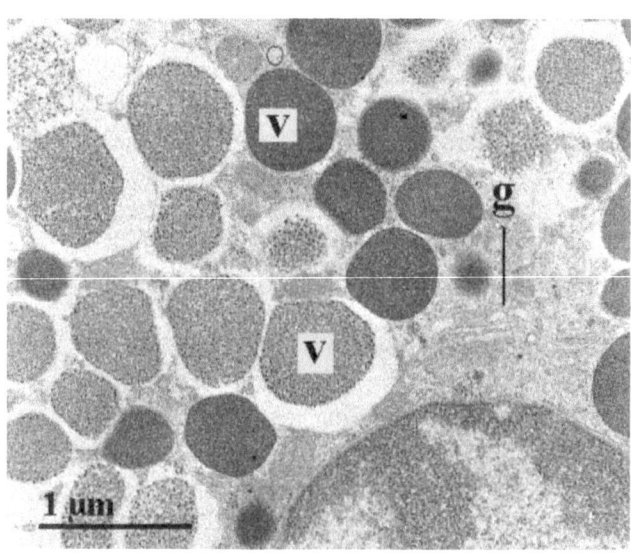

Fig. 3.2.7. (left) Mast cells (m) are widely distributed in the interstitial tissues of the body and in the walls of small blood vessels (v). They are loaded with granules, which stain metachromatically with toluidin blue. Dermal interstitial tissue, cat, 1-micrometer plastic section, toluidin blue. **Fig. 3.2.8.** (right) A mast cell is crammed with secretory vesicles (the granules of Figure 3.2.7.), with a variably dense content (v). Mark the Golgi-complex (g). Interstitial tissue of the tongue, cat, TEM.

place on a massive scale. Under such circumstances, many vesicles do not undergo exocytosis at the cell membrane, but fuse with another vesicle, which is itself in the process of exocytosis. By repetition of this process, a kind of regularly constricted tubes arise, or degranulation canals, which open into the extracellular space. Another mechanism of degranulation works with small vesicles that shuttle between the big ones and the cell membrane. In this way, the content of the dense vesicles is liberated in small portions at a time, a process called piecemeal degranulation.

The vesicular content is, at first sight, a very heterogeneous cocktail of chemical substances. Mast cells are not unlike dispensaries, storing various drugs. In addition to chondroitin sulfate, a component of the ground substance, they store heparin, a substance related to chondroitin sulfate, but functioning as an anticoagulative agent. Both substances are responsible for the metachromatic staining characteristic. Another substance stored by mast cells is histamine, a vasodilator amine. Various proteins are stored, such as the proteolytic enzymes chymase and tryptase, and chemotactic substances, such as eosinophil chemotactic factor of anaphylaxis. The common denominator of all of these substances is that they contribute, in one way or another, to the defense of the body against infection. By inhibiting blood clotting and dilating the blood vessels, heparin and histamine promote the local supply of blood and, carried by it, defender cells. The proteolytic enzymes affect the matrix of the interstitial tissue, facilitating movement of defender cells. The chemotactic substances attract defender cells. Mast cells are stimulated to release these factors by immunoglobulin E, produced by plasma cells.

III.2.2. Ground substance.

The ground substance is an amorphous, translucent material with a gel-like consistency. It consists of **proteoglycans**, giant molecular complexes of protein and carbohydrates. The carbohydrate molecules are very long, unbranched chains. They used to be termed, rather vaguely, mucopolysaccharides. Today, a much more specific designation is preferred: **glycosaminoglycans**. In addition to the usual carbon, hydrogen and oxygen atoms, they also contain nitrogen and, sometimes, sulfur.

Glycosaminoglycans are a very particular kind of polysaccharides. More exactly, they are repeating disaccharides, formed by linking a large number of identical disaccharides. The kind of disaccharide determines the type of glycosaminoglycan. Every disaccharide consists of an N-acetyl-hexosamine, such as glucosamine or galactosamine, and (in principle, for there are exceptions) a hexuronic acid, such as glucuronic acid or iduronic acid. If sulfur is present, it is in the form of sulfate groups.

The most common and longest glycosaminoglycan is **hyaluronic acid**. It is the only one that does not carry sulfate groups. It participates in every proteoglycan complex and forms its backbone. The proteoglycan complex looks like a lamp brush. Implanted on the hyaluronic acid backbone are hundreds of protein strands, each of which carries numerous glycosaminoglycan side chains. These do carry sulfate groups and their exact composition is typical to the location where they are found. **Chondroitin sulfate** is found in proteoglycans of cartilage ground substance, **dermatan sulfate** in the skin, **keratan sulfate** in the cornea, and **heparan sulfate** in the liver and the vessel wall. Hyaluronic acid is also found in isolation, as are the protein-glycosaminoglycan complexes, which used to be called mucoproteins.

Glycosaminoglycans carry negative charges because the hydroxyl, carboxyl, and sulfate groups they contain, being acids, eject protons. This implies that the ground substance, especially when plentiful, has basophilic properties, as is the case in cartilage and in the mucous tissue of the umbilical cord. Because like charges repel one another, the glycosaminoglycan within each proteoglycan complex will tend to move as far apart as they can. Thus, proteoglycans are voluminous molecules, occupying considerable space and, moreover, resistant to compression. Pressure will move the negative charges closer together, increasing electrostatic repulsion. The space filling capacity of the proteoglycans is increased even further by their intense hydration. Water molecules are polarized and carry partial charges, which enable them to bind electrostatically to the proteoglycans. Thus, the resistance of the ground substance to compression is explained by its particular chemical composition.

III.2.3. Fibrils.

Based on their microscopic structure, chemical composition and physical properties, two fundamentally different fibril types can be distinguished: the traction-resistant **collagen** and **reticulin fibrils** and the reversibly deformable **elastic fibrils**.

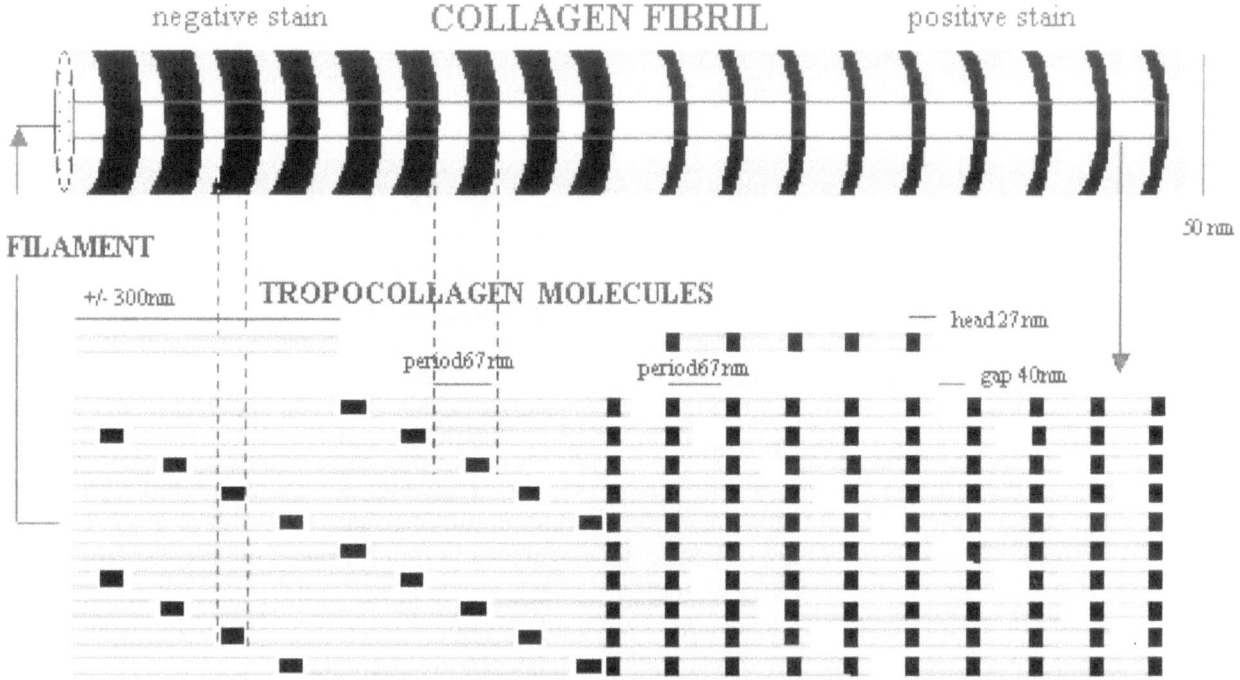

negative stain   COLLAGEN FIBRIL   positive stain

FILAMENT

+/- 300nm   TROPOCOLLAGEN MOLECULES

period 67 nm   period 67 nm   head 27 nm   gap 40 nm

50 nm

Fig. 3.2.9. The molecular structure of a collagen fibril. Collagen fibrils are made of rod-like tropocollagen molecules. Staining for electron microscopy, either positive or negative, gives them a cross striation with a typical periodicity. Tropocollagen rods are synthesized and secreted by fibroblasts and other matrix-secreting cells. In the extracellular space, they polymerize in such a fashion that their cross striations line up with those of adjoining rods. Each rod is shifted over a distance of one period relative to its neighbours. The gap between successive rods is also of constant width. As a consequence of this highly ordered aggregation, the entire fibril acquires the same cross striation as the individual rods.

III.2.3.1. Collagen and reticulin fibrils.

Quantitatively, collagen is the most important animal protein. Its name, literally "glue maker" is derived from the observation that collagen of bone and hides can be broken down, by boiling, to a sticky mixture which can be used as glue. Collagen and reticulin fibrils can be regarded as polymers of a fibrous protein, **tropocollagen**. Tropocollagen is synthesized by the matrix-secreting cells and secreted in the extracellular space. There, polymerization of tropocollagen molecules to fibrils takes place.

Tropocollagen is a rod-like molecule with a length of somewhat less than 300 nanometers. After release in the extracellular space, tropocollagen rods act like building blocks and spontaneously assemble into **fibrils** (Fig. 3.2.9) of indeterminate length and a diameter of 40 to 50 nanometers. In the fibril, tropocollagen rods line up to form filaments, with a gap of about 35 nanometers between successive rods.

In a given filament, the rods are shifted over a distance of 67 nanometers relative to those in the neighbouring filament.

Collagen fibrils can be negatively stained, i.e. heavy metals can accumulate in the gap between successive rods. In the electron microscope, the regular staggered arrangement of the rods results in a characteristic cross striation with a period (i.e. the total thickness of a dark band and its succeeding clear band) of 67 nanometers. The thickness of the dark bands is identical to the length of the gaps, 35 nanometers. The clear bands are a little narrower.

Collagen fibrils can also be stained positively. In this case, a tropocollagen rod, starting from one of its ends, displays five major electron dense bands, at regular intervals, and numerous minor ones in between. One major dense band plus the relatively clear zone following it occupy a length of 67 nanometers, the rod's periodicity. Each rod has four periods, which add up to a length of 268 nanometers. The remaining terminal stretch of about 30 nanometers, which starts

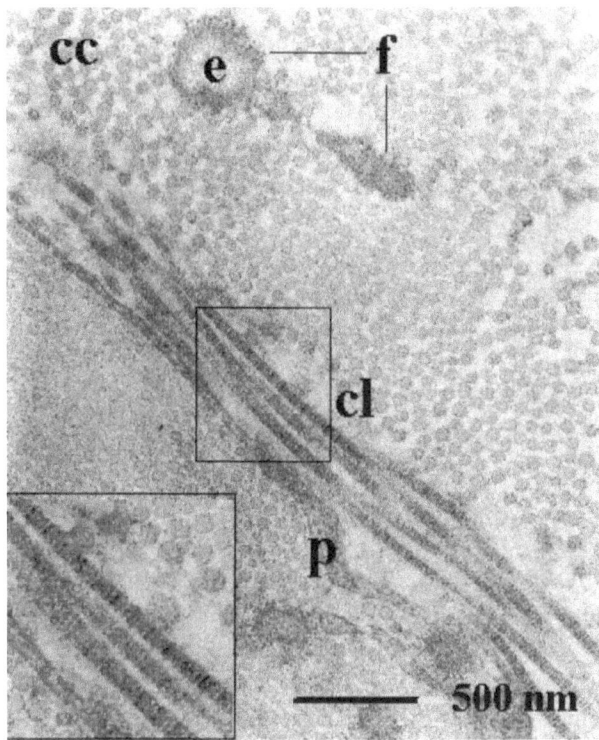

properties and shows birefringence (II.2.2.2.2.2.). Macroscopically, collagen is white.

Their regular cross striation, as well as their birefringence, are direct indications of the highly ordered structure of the collagen fibrils. In turn, this structure explains collagen's physical characteristics. Collagen fibrils are supple, but cannot be stretched. Their tensile strength is in the same order of magnitude as that of steel wires. Tropocollagen rods are strongly bound by covalent chemical bonds, which prevent any shifting between the rods. The overlap of tropocollagen rods ensures that the fibril is homogeneously strong over its entire length, without any weak spots. A chain is only as strong as its weakest link. It is very essential that the collagen fibril is not massive, but can be regarded as a bundle of filaments. In principle, a cable composed of many threads is stronger than a single massive wire of the same thickness. Moreover, the subdivision of the fibrils in substructures introduces an element of safety. Should one element fail, the break will be limited to that single element. In case of a massive fibril, the break would extend indefinitely and cause the whole fibril to collapse. All these are common engineering principles.

Fig. 3.2.10. Collagen and elastic fibrils each have a characteristic ultrastructure. In longitudinal section (cl), collagen fibrils have a distinctive cross striation. In cross section, they are circular (cc). Elastic fibrils are composed of an amorphous elastin core (e), enveloped with fibrillin fibers (f). Dura mater, hamster, TEM.

Tropocollagen rods consist of three tightly wound helical protein chains, the composition of which is variable. Consequently, several types of collagen can be distinguished. Of the types mentioned here, only I, II and III have cross striations. Type I collagen is the most common one and is found in interstitial and fibrous connective tissues, the cornea, and bone. It forms comparatively thick fibrils. Type II collagen is typical for cartilage and the eye's vitreous humor. Type III collagen forms the thin reticulin fibers and selectively stains with silver salts because of its association with polysaccharides. Therefore, reticulin fibers used to be regarded as fundamentally different from collagen fibers. Reticulin fibers are in fact rather thin collagen fibrils that do not form fibers, but a reticulum. They typically occur in the myeloid and lymphoid organs. Likewise, type IV collagen does not form fibers, but dense reticula, which build up the **dense lamina** of the basement membranes that support lining tissues and envelop muscle fibers and glia cells. This type of collagen is not secreted by matrix-secreting cells, but by lining cells and by the cells it envelops. Type VII collagen forms the **anchoring fibrils** that, beneath stratified epithelia, link the dense lamina to the collagen fibrils of the underlying interstitial tissue. Types IX and XII collagen participate in the junction of collagen fibrils into fibers.

with the fifth dense band, is called the head. The rest of the rod is the tail. In a filament, the rods line up with the same head-tail orientation. Their staggered arrangement results in overlap of the dark bands, and the total length of the head and the gap amounts to one period. Consequently, the fibril acquires a characteristic cross striation with a period of 67 nanometers. In this case, however, the dense bands are markedly narrower (about 8 nanometers) than the clear ones, and the fibrils show numerous minor striations in between the major ones.

Collagen fibrils can be bundled to fibers, much less sharply delineated than fibrils, which can attain a thickness of more than 10 micrometers. The lateral association of fibrils in the fiber is less ordered than that of the rods in the fibril. Consequently, collagen fibers do not show cross striations.

The regular cross striation is the most distinctive characteristic of collagen fibrils in the electron microscope (Fig. 3.2.10.). Light optically, collagen fibrils cannot be made out separately, but collagen can be stained specifically. Collagen has anisotropic

III.2.3.2. Elastic fibrils.

Elastic fibrils are made of the fibrous protein **elastin** and the glycoprotein **fibrillin**. Both molecules are synthesized and secreted by fibroblasts and excreted into the intercellular space, where they self-assemble to fibrils. Elastin and fibrillin can also be synthesized by smooth muscle fibers.

Ultrastructurally, elastin is an amorphous mass. It occupies the interior of the fibrils, and is enveloped by a thin layer of parallel, longitudinally oriented fibrillin filaments, which are 10 nanometers thick (Fig. 3.2.10.). Elastic fibrils can assemble into fibers of about 1 micrometer thick. Alternatively, they can form sheets.

Elastic fibers seldom occur in large amounts. Light optically, they are seldom conspicuous, except where they form sheets, as in the walls of large blood vessels. In this case, they look like thin, undulating layers of eosinophilic material (Fig. 4.5.6.) They can also be specifically stained (Fig. 1.7.). Macroscopically, their presence may give the tissue a yellowish color.

Elastic fibrils can be reversibly stretched, when subjected to forces, to up to one and a half times their original length. They confer elastic properties to the tissues and organs in which they occur, such as the larger blood vessels and the lungs.

The physical properties of the elastic fibers are explained, in principle, by their molecular structure, but the connection between the two has not yet been fully elucidated. It is assumed that the elastin core is the only truly elastic component of the elastic fibril and that it consists of a mass of randomly coiled protein strings that can reversibly be stretched.

III.2.4. Tissue types.

Leaving apart the adipose tissue, which can be regarded as deviating because of its intracellular matrix, distinction can be made between the more generalized interstitial tissues, with comparatively little matrix, and the specialized connective and supportive tissues. In the connective tissues, either collagen or elastic fibrils may dominate, forming dense fibrous and elastic tissues, respectively. It is in these specialized tissues that the matrix predominates and determines the specific properties of the tissues.

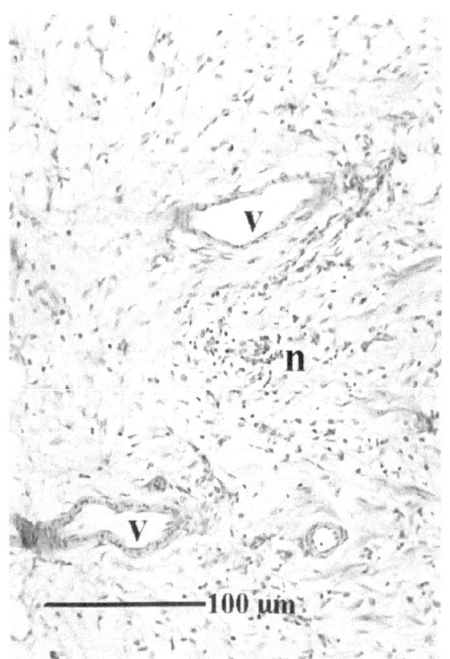
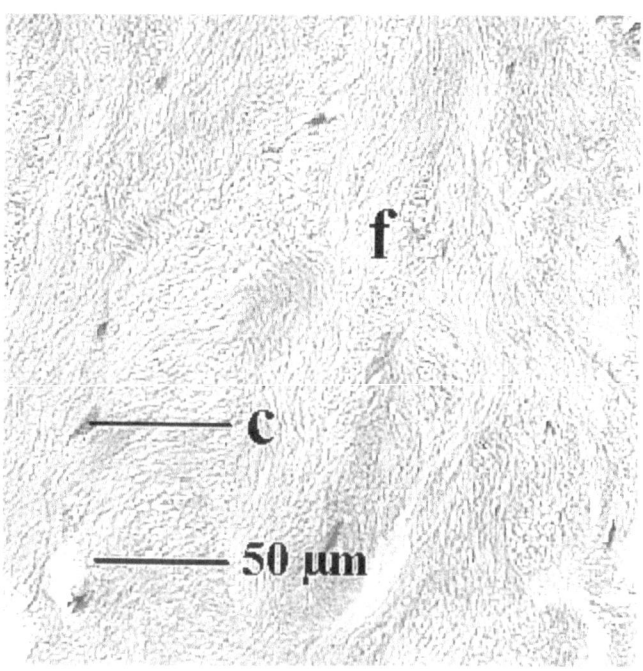

Fig. 3.2.11. (left) Loose fibrous tissue is an interstitial tissue wherein the cells are relatively numerous (mark the large number of nuclei, n), at the expense of the matrix. v = blood vessels. Kidney hilus, cat, HE. **Fig. 3.2.12.** (right) Dense woven fibrous tissue is a connective tissue characterized by an abundant fibrous matrix (f), and a small number of fibrocytes (c). Corpus albicans, ovary, human, HE.

III.2.4.1. Interstitial tissues.

Interstitial tissues fill the spaces between other tissues, support them and hold them together.

The most primitive form of interstitial tissue, from which all other types of interstitial, connective, and supportive tissue are derived, is **mesenchymal tissue**. Mesenchymal tissue, or mesenchyme, is at it most widespread during embryonic development. It consists of mesenchymal cells, star shaped cells that are interconnected through their processes and form a network. They can be regarded as primitive fibroblasts. They form little matrix, so that mesenchymal tissue is comparatively rich in cells, and practically no fibers. After embryonic development, mesenchymal tissue survives in places where growth is still going on, such as the periost of bones (Fig. 4.2.5.). In the adult organism, practically no organized mesenchymal tissue remains to be found. Solitary or small groups of mesenchymal cells have a wide spread distribution. If necessary, these cells can multiply and differentiate to replace (mostly to a limited extent) certain damaged tissues.

Mucous tissue is a somewhat more specialized form. In addition to primitive, star-like fibroblasts, it also contains histiocytes. There is abundant matrix with collagen fibers, in which the ground substance predominates. The ground substance confers a gel-like consistency to mucous tissue, which is also called **Wharton's jelly**. It is found mostly in the umbilical cord (Fig. 4.6.3.). It confers a certain amount of rigidity to the umbilical cord and supports its blood vessels. This way, excessive coiling and kinking, which would arrest the blood flow, are avoided. The interstitial tissue forming the tooth pulp (IV.15.1.1.) is also regarded as mucous tissue.

Loose fibrous tissue is the most wide spread form of interstitial tissue (Fig. 3.2.11.). It is comparatively rich in cells, because the matrix is not excessive. The matrix contains more or less equal amounts of fibers and ground substance. The fibers, collagen or elastic, are thin and homogeneously distributed. It is found supporting lining and glandular tissues and enveloping muscle and nerve fibers. The larger blood vessels, the airways and the intestine contain fairly thick sheets of loose fibrous tissue. Apart from fibroblasts, other cell types may be found: adipocytes, histiocytes, granulocytes, mast cells, lymphocytes, and plasma cells, implying that loose fibrous tissue has various metabolic and immunologic functions. The loose fibrous tissue of the bone marrow and the lymphoid organs is rich in reticular fibers and is often called **reticular tissue**.

III.2.4.2. Dense fibrous tissues.

When fibroblasts shift to synthesis of collagen fibers, a connective tissue is formed, which is poor in cells, but which has an abundant, fibrous matrix. This is **dense fibrous tissue**. It consists of tight bundles of collagen fibers, in which elongated, spindle shaped fibroblasts lie embedded, their long axis parallel with the collagen fibers. The collagen may be arranged in two ways.

In **woven fibrous tissue**, the collagen fiber bundles have many orientations (Fig. 3.2.12.). The presence of large amounts of collagen fibers makes this kind of tissue very tough. It is most often found in the fibrous capsules of various organs, such as the tunica albuginea of the testis and the sclera of the eye, to protect them. It also forms scar tissue, such as the corpora albicantia of the ovaries.

Fig. 3.2.13. In dense ordered fibrous tissue, the abundant collagen fibers (f) run parallel. This can be deduced from the elongated shape of the cell nuclei of the fibrocytes, also called tendinocytes (t), and their parallel and linear arrangement. Finger tendon, human, HE.

In **ordered fibrous tissue**, the collagen fiber bundles all course in the same direction (Fig. 3.2.13.). Thus, a tissue is formed with great tensile strength, admirably suited to a connective function. Ordered fibrous tissue forms **tendons**, which connect skeletal muscles to bones, and **ligaments**, which connect bones to one another. The fibrocytes themselves, sometimes called tendinocytes, form longitudinal rows, parallel to the collagen fiber bundles. In cross section, they appear star shaped, their processes or wings penetrating between the collagen fibers.

III.2.4.3. Elastic tissue.

Elastic tissue is analogous to dense ordered fibrous tissue, but it contains elastic fibers. Elastic tissue is rare as such. Here and there, ligaments are found which consist almost exclusively of elastic tissue: the ligamentum nuchae and the ligamenta flava of the spine, and in the vocal cords. Contrary to tendons, which are white, these ligaments are yellowish.

III.2.4.4. Cartilage.

Cartilage is made by specialized matrix-secreting cells, the chondroblasts (Fig. 3.2.14.), which, in addition to fibrils, abundantly synthesize proteoglycans. The composition of the matrix is variable, so that several types of cartilage can be distinguished.

The most common form of cartilage is **hyaline cartilage**. The most obvious light optical characteristic of hyaline cartilage is its abundant, basophilic matrix, in which chondroblasts lie embedded (Fig. 3.2.15.). Macroscopically, it has a turbid, milky look. The collagen fibers, although fairly abundant, have the same refractory index as the ground substance and, consequently, cannot be made out without some specific staining procedure. Ultrastructurally, they form a dense network of fine fibrils (Fig. 3.2.14.). The matrix immediately surrounding a chondroblast may stain more darkly than at greater distances, because of the higher concentration of proteoglycans. Thus, distinction can be made between the territorial matrix and the interterritorial matrix, respectively. As a consequence of cell multiplication, many chondroblasts are seen to lie in groups of two to four. By continued production of matrix, these cells will separate. In this way, hyaline cartilage can grow from within, by **interstitial**

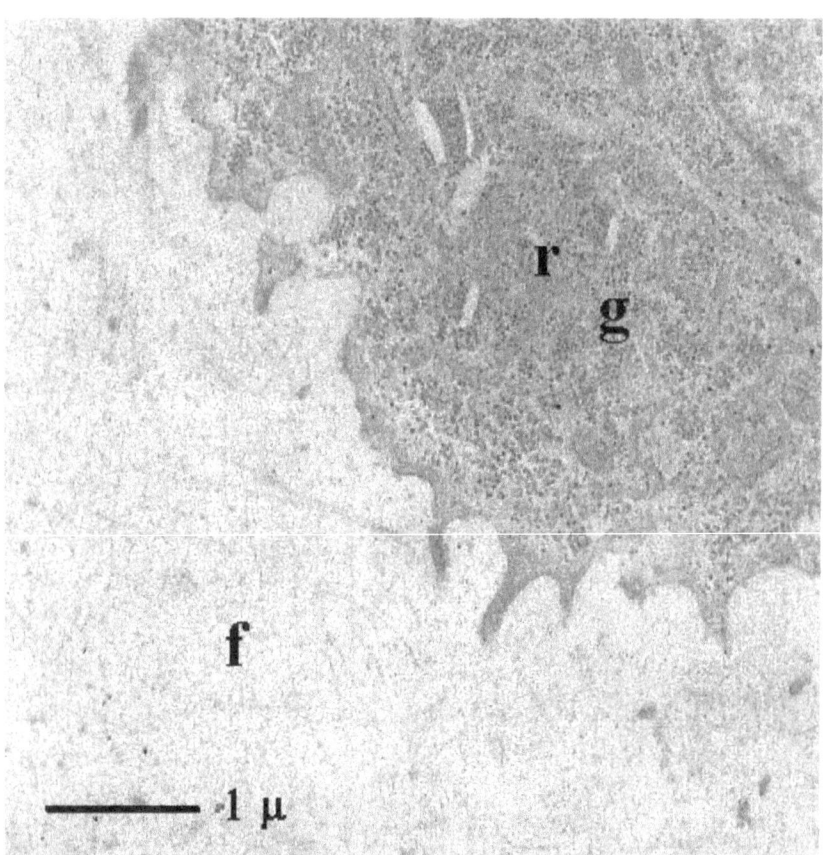

Fig. 3.2.14. This matrix–secreting cell of cartilage contains little rough endoplasmic reticulum and may be in a period of rest. Therefore, it may be called a chondrocyte. The granules in its cytoplasm are ribosomes and glycogen (r, g). The matrix is composed of very fine, diffuse collagen fibrils (f). Hyaline cartilage, bronchus, rabbit, TEM.

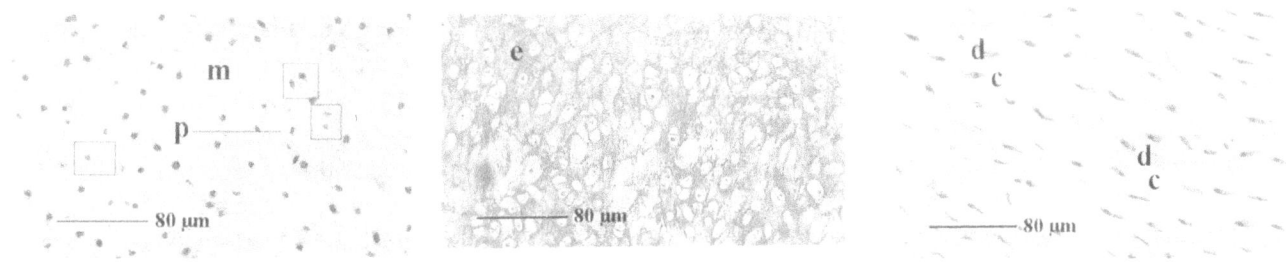

Left to right: **Fig. 3.2.15.** Typical of hyaline cartilage is its abundant, featureless, basophilic matrix (m). The chondrocytes show some shrinkage as a consequence of tissue preparation and appear to lie in cavities, the chondroplasts (p). The presence of groups of 2 adjoining chondrocytes (rectangles) indicates ongoing cell multiplication, and thus interstitial growth. Articular cartilage, foetal bone, human, HE. **Fig. 3.2.16.** The matrix of elastic cartilage is rich in eosinophilic elastic fibres (e). Epiglottis, human, HE. **Fig. 3.2.17.** Fibrous cartilage is actually a mixture of tissues. It consists of layers of hyaline cartilage (c) and dense fibrous tissue (d). Intervertebral disk, rat, HE.

growth. Another form of growth is **appositional** or subperichondrial growth, which adds layers to already existing cartilage. Usually, the surface of cartilage is lined with a fibrous connective tissue layer, the perichondrium, the deeper layers of which contain mesenchymal cells. Some of these can differentiate to chondroblasts, which deposit additional layers of matrix, and may get walled in.

Hyaline cartilage is not vascularized and can only be nourished and supplied with oxygen by diffusion from surrounding tissues. Consequently, chondroblasts have a low level of metabolism. They live in a relatively oxygen-poor environment and acquire their energy mainly by glycolysis. Their cytoplasm, apart from the usual organelles for protein synthesis, contains an energy reserve in the form of lipid droplets and glycogen granules (Fig. 3.2.14.). Lipids and glycogen are easily dissolved during preparation of histological sections, so that the chondroblasts have a tendency to shrivel. Artefactually, they may end up as lying loose in a cavity, the chondroplast (Fig. 3.2.15.).

The presence of a copious amount of ground substance in the interstices of a dense network of collagen fibrils, makes hyaline cartilage admirably suited to sustain pressure. It is a supporting tissue that serves as a buffer in places that are exposed to pressure, such as the articular surfaces of bones. It has other functions as well. When it is not lined with perichondrium, it provides a smooth articular surface that minimizes friction. It forms supporting rings in the airway walls and connects the ribs to the breastbone. The processus xiphosurus of the breastbone, and the nose septum, are equally made of hyaline cartilage. The embryonic skeleton consists almost entirely of hyaline cartilage, and it plays a vital role in the longitudinal growth of the bones.

Cartilage may contain large amounts of elastic fibers, making it reversibly deformable. This kind of

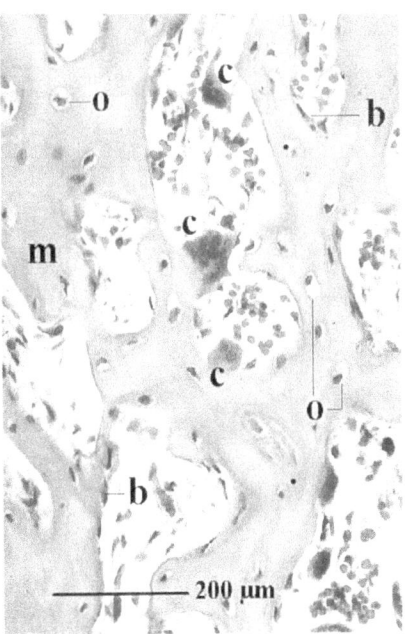

Fig. 3.2.18. Bone is characterized by an eosinophilic matrix (m) with walled-in osteocytes (o). Osteoblasts or bone-forming cells are somewhat flattened and lie at the edge of the matrix (b). The large multinucleated cells which usually rest on the matrix are bone-degrading cells or osteoclasts (c). Cancellous bone, femur, rat, HE.

cartilage, **elastic cartilage**, occurs in the external ear, the epiglottis (Fig. 3.2.16.), and the larynx. Elastic cartilage has less abundant matrix, compared to hyaline cartilage, and the eosinophilic properties of the elastic fibers contrast them with the ground substance.

In places that may be exposed to excessive loads, such as the intervertebral disks of the spine, cartilage is strengthened with additional collagen fibers: **fibrous cartilage** (Fig. 3.2.17.). Fibrous cartilage is in fact a composite of two tissues: hyaline cartilage, alternated with layers of dense fibrous tissue. Fibrous cartilage is also associated with the Achilles tendon, the patella, and the symphysis of the pubic bones.

III.2.4.5. Bone.

Bone is the most complex form of supporting tissue. It is deposited by specialized matrix-secreting cells:

osteoblasts. The matrix is relatively poor in ground substance, but rich in collagen fibers. The specific characteristic of bone is calcification: in the ground substance and on the collagen fibrils, calcium salts are deposited. This hardens the collagen and makes bone suited to sustain pressure. Contrary to intuition, the supportive abilities of bone do not reside in the ground substance, as they are in cartilage, but in the fibers. Collagen also makes bone resistant to tensile forces.

Contrary to cartilage, bone only grows through appposition. **Osteoblasts**, or bone-forming cells, lie at the surface of growing bone (Fig. 3.2.18.). Light optically, they may appear as a coherent layer of cuboidal cells, not unlike a simple epithelium. Ultrastructurally, this impression is strengthened by the presence of specialized junctions, such as gap junctions. Active osteoblasts (Fig. 3.2.19.) have abundant rough endoplasmic reticulum at the cell pole facing the bone tissue. They secrete additional, as yet

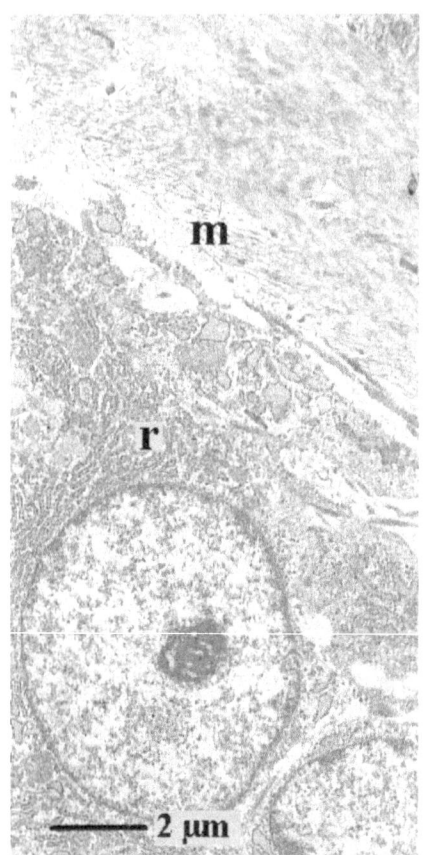
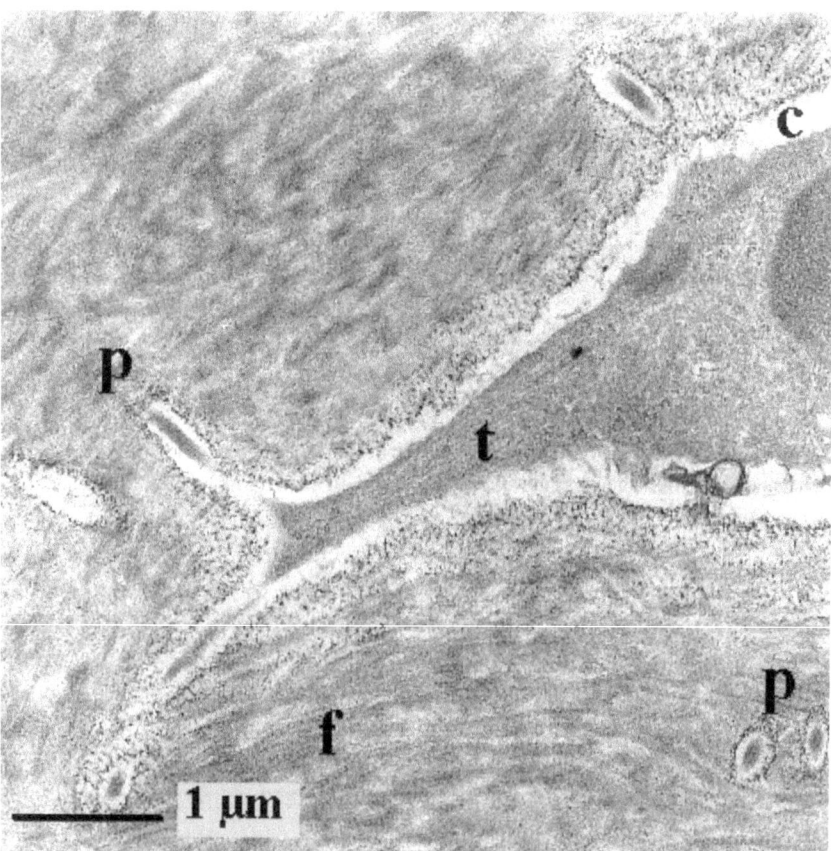

Fig. 3.2.19. (left) Osteoblasts have a euchromatic nucleus and contain abundant rough endoplasmic reticulum (r). They secrete the bone matrix (m), wherein collagen fibrils can be seen. Fibrous bone, rabbit, TEM. **Fig. 3.2.20.** (right) An osteocyte, embedded in bone matrix, rich in collagen fibrils (f). This cell carries branched processes (p), and is surrounded by a narrow space or canaliculus (c). The nucleus is heterochromatic and the cytoplasm is poor in rough endoplasmic reticulum (compare with Figure 3.2.19.), which indicates a very decreased synthetic activity. The processes are supported by bundles of microtubules (t). Skull bone, rat, TEM.

uncalcified matrix, called **osteoid,** and deposit it on top of older matrix, adding layer after layer. As long as the osteoid is not yet calcified, the osteoblasts retain the capability of reabsorbing it. At regular intervals, scattered osteoblasts stop secreting. As a consequence of this, they are overtaken and walled in by neighbouring osteoblasts. Alternatively, osteoblasts may get walled in because, at a certain moment, they assume a symmetric structure and start to secrete osteoid in all directions.

Walled in osteoblasts are called **osteocytes.** Osteocytes (Fig. 3.2.20.) are spindle shaped cells with a number of elongated, slender processes, which give them a spider-like appearance. Their cell body is relatively poor in organelles. Their processes lie in narrow canals or canaliculi in the matrix and come into contact with processes of other osteocytes. At the places of contact, gap junctions are formed. The processes are supported by a cytoskeleton of microfilaments and microtubules. Via their processes, osteocytes transfer metabolites, which may compensate for the circumstance that the calcified matrix allows little diffusion. They also signal changing load patterns, which may ultimately lead to the breakdown of old bone by osteoclasts and the deposition of new bone by the osteoblasts.

Bone is the only type of connective or supportive tissue that, in addition of matrix-secreting cells, contains cells that break down the matrix. The relatively inert, calcified matrix hinders adaptation of bone tissue to changing circumstances and necessitates the presence of specialized bone-removing cells, the **osteoclasts.** The bone-removing capability of the osteoclasts complements the bone-forming one of the osteoblasts. In cooperation, they form a mechanism that allows bone to adapt itself to changing load patterns as a consequence of growth. In addition, bone is an important calcium reserve and calcium may be mobilized by hormonal stimulation of osteoclast activity.

Osteoclasts are very distinctive cells because of their large size (diameter up to 100 micrometers) and because of their large number of nuclei: ten or more. Just like megakaryocytes, they are polyploid. They arise from normal, diploid, mononuclear precursor cells in the myeloid tissue, which fuse. The osteoclast's polyploid character enables it to synthesize proteins on a massive scale. These proteins are lytic enzymes. Osteoclasts may be found at bone tissue surfaces, where they displace themselves by amoeboid movements (Fig. 3.2.18.). As a consequence of their demolition work, they often lie in

a depression they have excavated: **Howship's lacuna.** The osteoclast's cytological structure is that of a macrophage, be it a polarized one (Fig. 3.2.21.). The cell's part facing away from the bone surface contains the nuclei and abundant organelles for protein synthesis and expedition: rough endoplasmic reticulum and Golgi-complexes. The part facing the bone matrix is very specialized. The central stretch of the cell membrane touching the bone surface recedes from it,

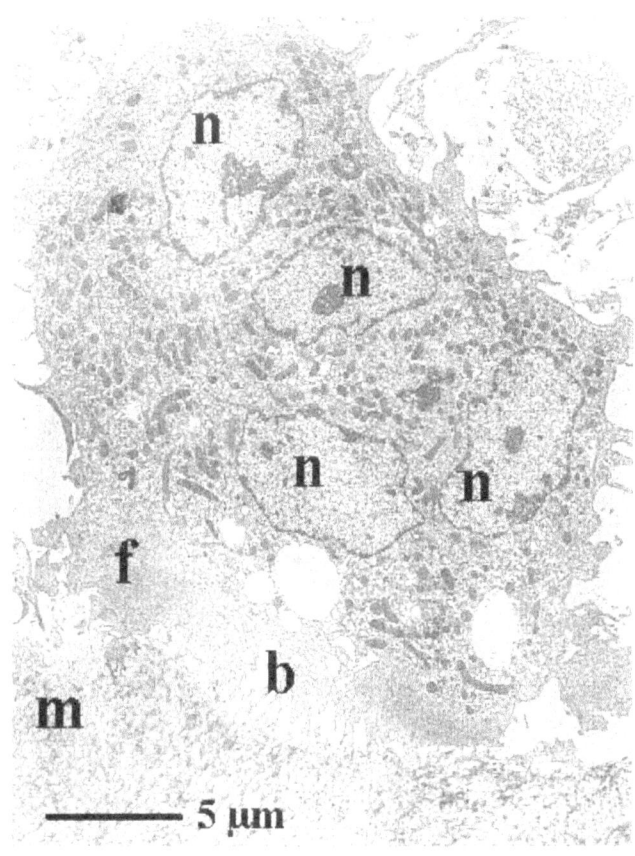

Fig. 3.2.21. A multinuclear (n) osteoclast adheres to the bone matrix (m) with the filamentous part of its cytoplasm, the clear zone (f), and creates a closed cavity, in which it secretes hydrolytic enzymes at the level of its (rather irregular) brush border (b). Bits and pieces of degraded bone matrix are subsequently engulfed. Bone tissue, rabbit, TEM.

so that a cavity is formed. It carries a brush border, or **ruffled border,** consisting of numerous microvilli, which project into the cavity. The cytoplasm surrounding the cavity is rich in microfilaments and forms what is called the **clear zone.** It is firmly attached to the bone surface. The cytoplasm above the ruffled border is loaded with lysosomes and phagosomes. It is a unique feature of the osteoclast that the lysosomes undergo exocytosis, discharging their enzymes in the cavity occupied by the ruffled border, which is extracellular space. The cavity appears to be hermetically sealed, however, by the clear zone. At the ruffled border, protons are pumped into the cavity (apart from being macrophages, osteoclasts are secreting brush border cells), acidifying it, which degrades the bone matrix by dissolving calcium salts. The lytic enzymes continue the break down process. Bits and pieces are engulfed by phagocytosis at the base of the ruffled border and further degraded intracellularly.

Bone tissue is rich in collagen fibrils. As a consequence of bone's appositional growth, they are deposited in lamellae, a few micrometers thick, so that bone acquires a layered structure: **lamellar bone**. Each lamella consists of five sublamellae of unequal thickness, in which the orientation of the collagen fibrils changes under a constant angle, which results in considerable mechanical strengthening. In growing bones, another type of bone tissue may temporarily be present: **fibrous bone**, or woven bone, in which collagen fibrils course in every direction. Fibrous bone is much weaker, mechanically, than lamellar bone, and is ultimately replaced by it. At the bone surface, lamellar bone forms layers that circumscribe the entire bone: **circumferential lamellae**. Deeper down, the lamella form a number of concentric cylinders around blood vessels, **Havers's columns**, which have a diameter of a few tens of micrometers and may reach lengths of a few centimeters. Circumferential lamellae and Havers's columns do not show large spaces, and are collectively called **compact bone**. In the center of bones, the lamellae form a complex network of trabecules: **cancellous** or **spongy bone** (Fig. 3.2.18.). In the interstices of this network, myeloid tissue is usually present.

Calcification is a complex process, to a certain extent reversible, and regulated by a number of hormones and calcium-binding proteins. Essentially, calcification is the deposition of calcium phosphate crystals in the matrix of bone. Cartilage can be calcified as well. As far as their structure and composition is concerned, these crystals are analogous to those of the mineral apatite. They start to form at so called nucleation centers. Two types of nucleation centers are known: matrix vesicles and collagen fibrils. **Matrix vesicles** (Fig. 3.2.22.) are membranous vesicles with a diameter of up to 200 nanometers. They form from microvilli-like extensions of the cell membrane of chondroblasts and osteoblasts, which are pinched off. The matrix vesicle membrane contains phosphatases, which can liberate phosphate from ATP and other substances, and calcium-binding phospholipids. These substances induce the formation of crystal germs in the vesicle's

interior. The germs grow, and penetrate the vesicular membrane. The crystals continue to grow in the matrix and soon obliterate the vesicles. Matrix vesicles are important in the calcification of cartilage and fibrous bone. In a more common mechanism of calcification, wherein collagen fibrils act as nucleation centers, crystal germs form in the gaps between successive tropocollagen rods. They are plate-like and orient themselves with their long axis parallel to the fibril's. In successive sublamellae of lamellar bone, the crystals are rotated under a different angle.

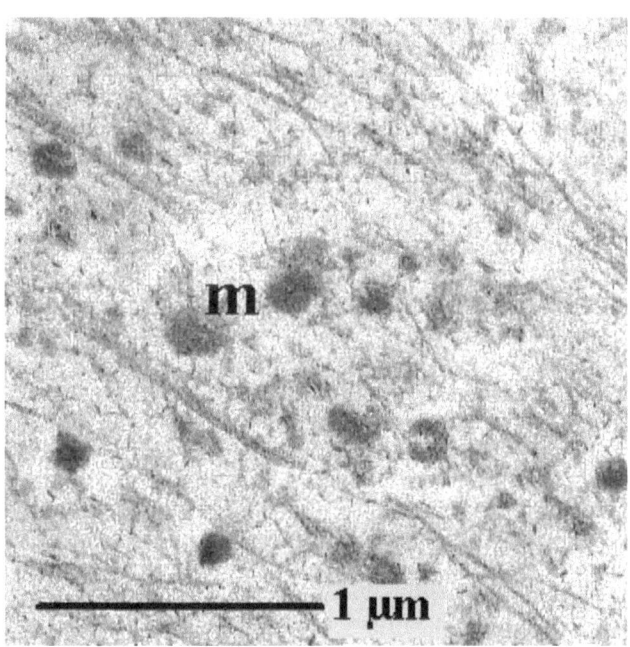

Fig. 3.2.22. Fibrous bone, showing diffuse and randomly distributed collagen fibrils, mixed with matrix vesicles (m). These serve as nucleation centers in the formation of calcium crystals, leading to matrix calcification. Bone tissue, rabbit, TEM.

Subsequently, the crystals grow in any available spaces of the collagen fibrils, gradually obscuring them. This process is regulated by osteopontin, osteonectin, and osteocalcin: negatively charged proteins that bind collagen and calcium. This mechanism of calcification is found in lamellar bone.

References.

Aarden E.M., Burger E.H., Nijweide P.J.: Function of osteocytes in bone. J. Cell. Biochem. 1994, 55: 287-299.
Boivin G., Anthoine-Terrier C;, Obrant K.J.: Transmission electron microscopy of bone tissue. Acta Orthop. Scand. 1990, 61: 170-180.

Boskey A.L., Posner A.S.: Bone structure, composition, and mineralization. Orthop. Clin. North Am. 1984, 15: 597-612.

Dijkgraaf L.C., de Bont L.G.M., Boering G., Liem R.S.B.: Normal cartilage structure, biochemistry, and metabolism: a review of the literature. J. Oral Maxillofac. Surg. 1995, 53: 924-929.

Dvorak A.M.: New aspects of mast cell biology. Int. Arch. Allergy Immunol. 1997, 114: 1-9.

Ito T., Tanuma Y., Yamada M., Yamamoto M.: Morphological studies on brown adipose tissue in the bat and in humans of various ages. Arch. Histol. Cytol. 1991, 54: 1-39.

Kadler K.E., Holmes D.F., Trotter J.A., Chapman J.A.: Collagen fibril formation. Biochem. J., 1996: 1-11.

Montes G.S.: Structural biology of the fibres of the collagenous and elastic systems. Cell Biol. Int. 1996, 20: 15-27.

Otani V., Raspanti M., Ruggeri A.: Collagen structure and functional implications. Micron 2001, 32: 251-260.

Pasquali-Ronchetti I., Fornieri C., Baccarani-Contri M., Quaglino D.: Ultrastructure of elastin. Ciba Found. Symp. 1995, 192: 31-50.

Pierce A.M., Lindskog S., Hammarström L.: Osteoclasts: structure and function. Electron Microsc. Rev. 1991, 4: 1-45.

Weiner S., Traub W., Wagner H.D.: Lamellar bone: structure-function relations. J. Struct. Biol. 1999, 126: 241-255.

Yong L.C.J.: The mast cell: origin, distribution, and function. Exp. Toxic. Pathol. 1997, 49: 409-424.

Zancanaro C., Poltronieri R., Sbarbati A., Merigo F., Cevese A.: Adipocyte morphology during hormone-induced lipid deposition and mobilization. An ultrastructural investigation in the perfused cardiac fat. Cell Biol. Int. 1995, 19: 1001-1009.

III.3. Muscle tissue.

Muscle tissue consists of muscle fibers. Smooth muscle fibers are very numerous in the internal organs or viscera: the intestine, the airways, the blood vessels, and the genital organs. There, they form layers of **visceral muscle tissue**. Striated muscle fibers are associated with the skeleton, where they form **skeletal muscle tissue**. They also form a large part of the heart: **cardiac muscle tissue**. In a purely structural sense, skeletal muscle tissue is the least complex type of muscle tissue, since it simply consists, in principle at least, of parallel bundles of muscle fibers, which are not interconnected. Visceral and cardiac muscle tissue are more complex. Their fibers are interconnected through specialized membrane junctions, so that they form a network.

III.3.1. Visceral muscle tissue.

Visceral muscle tissue consists of smooth muscle fibers. Light optically, these appear arranged in layers or bundles (Fig. 3.3.1.). The nuclei of the fibers are often larger and more clearly euchromatic than those of the surrounding fibrocytes. The relatively abundant

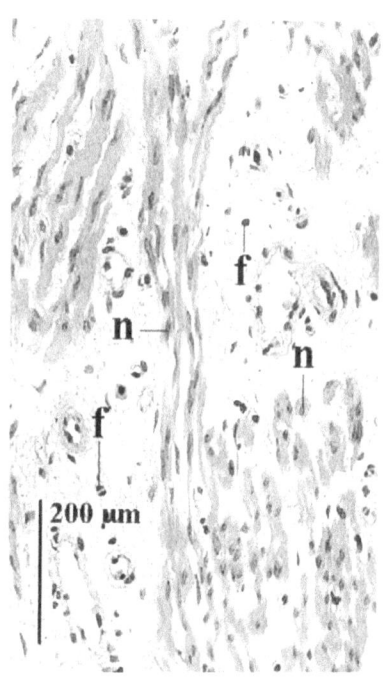
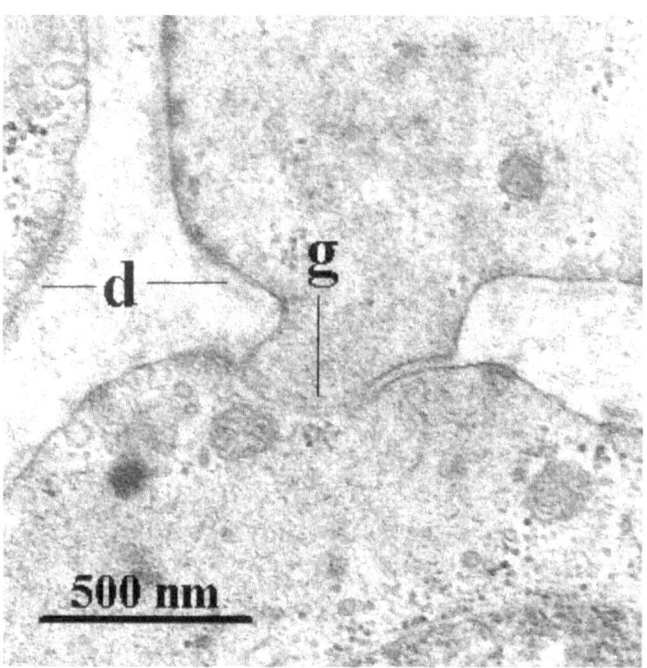

Fig. 3.3.1. (left) Visceral muscle tissue is composed of bundles of fusiform smooth muscle fibers, containing a central, oval nucleus (n). The nuclei have a paler aspect than those of the surrounding fibrocytes (f). In the center, and at the upper left, these bundles are sectioned longitudinally, at the lower right, transversely. Myometrium, human, HE. **Fig. 3.3.2.** (right) Smooth muscle fibers are enveloped in a basement membrane (lamina densa: d), and joined to one another in various places. This creates a network of fibers. Where 2 muscle fibers touch, gap junctions (g) are formed. At the level of these junctions, the individual cell membranes cannot be distinguished clearly, because they are joined and bridged by tubular integral membrane proteins. Musculosa of the urethra, cat, TEM.

eosinophilic cytoplasm contrasts with the surrounding, poorly staining interstitial tissue matrix. The fibers are spindle shaped and neighbouring fibers are shifted, relative to one another, so that the expanded middle part of a fiber joins the narrow ends of other fibers. This way, the available space is efficiently filled and tight layers or bundles are formed. In cross section, many fibers do not show a nucleus, since it lies outside the section plane. Electron microscopically, each smooth muscle fiber is enveloped by a basement membrane (Fig. 3.3.2.), which serves to anchor it to other fibers and to the surrounding collagen fibrils.

Electron microscopic observation reveals the presence of intercellular junctions, which implies that visceral muscle tissue forms a network.

The cytosolic face of the cell membrane carries **fusiform densities**, similar to those distributed in the cytoplasm (II.2.2.2.2.1.), which anchor the ends of actin microfilaments and intermediary filaments. Specialized membrane proteins connect the fusiform densities to the dense lamina of the basement membrane. These junctions enable the fibers to transmit tensile forces during contraction. They are the equivalent of the intermediate junctions and desmosomes of epithelial cells (III.4.1.1.).

A completely different type of junction is the **nexus** or **gap junction** (Fig. 3.3.2.). To form it, the membranes of two neighbouring muscle fibers locally approach each other to about 3 nanometers. The trilaminar aspect of two parallel cell membranes, in combination with the narrow intercellular space, gives rise to a septalaminar structure. In the gap junction, both membranes are connected by a series of tubular intramembrane proteins, the connexons, which bridge both membranes and form pores. Via these pores, the cytoplasm of two fibers is continuous and ions can stream from one fiber to the other. The pores form the gaps that give this kind of junction its name. The ion concentrations inside a muscle fiber change upon depolarization of the cell membrane and induction of contraction. Via the gap junctions, depolarization of one fiber may induce ion concentration changes, and thus depolarization, in another fiber. Consequently, smooth muscle fibers are electrically coupled and behave as a functional syncytium: if one fiber contracts, there is an increased probability that the others will do so as well. In this way, contraction waves arise which are at the basis of the peristaltic movements in the internal organs.

III.3.2. Skeletal muscle tissue.

In principle, skeletal muscle tissue is built from parallel striated muscle fibers, which are nowhere directly interconnected (Figs. 3.3.3.-4.). There are exceptions to both rules, however. Individual fibers may be arranged in other patterns. In so-called pennate muscles, for instance, the fibers have a fan-like arrangement. The resulting muscle has a narrow insertion point at one end, and a broad insertion zone at the other. In addition, myomuscular junctions have been described, although they may be relatively rare. Individual muscle fibers participating in such junctions usually have tapered ends, which overlap. In these zones of overlap, side-to-side as well as end-to-side junctions occur. The two fibers engaged in a junction closely appose and interdigitate their cell membranes. The basal laminae of their basement membranes usually merge. In sharp contrast to cardiac muscle tissue, there is no sign of gap junctions, indicating that this junction is entirely for force transmission, not for action potential propagation. The cytosolic faces of the membranes are coated with dense material, in which the actin filaments of the myofibrils are anchored.

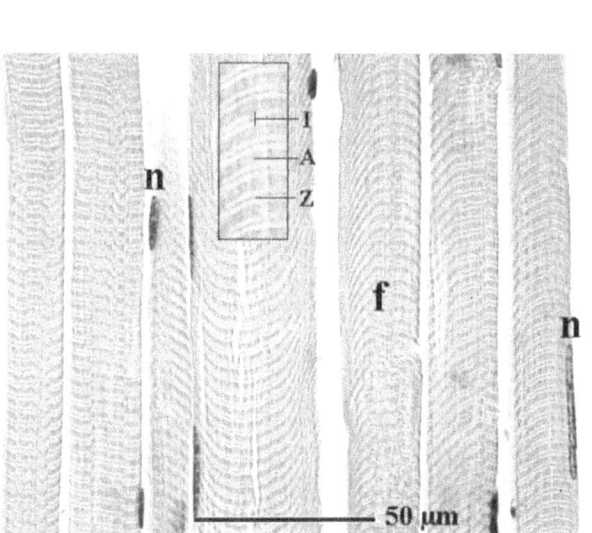
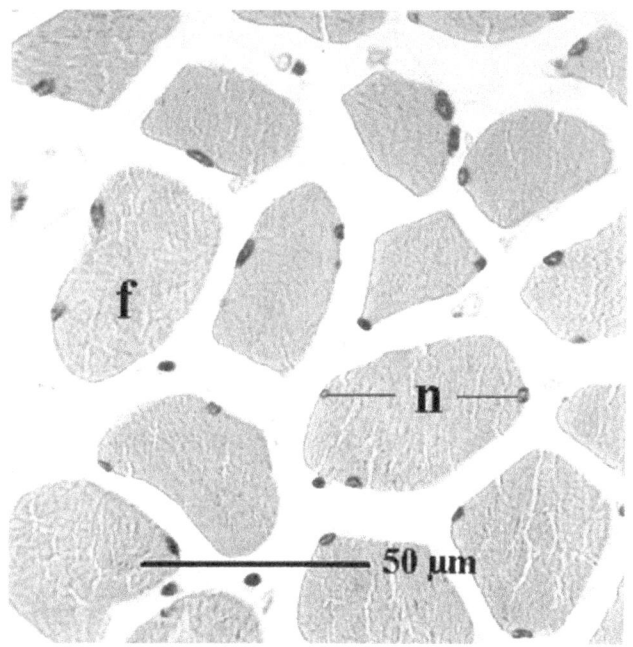

Fig. 3.3.3. (left) Skeletal muscle tissue consists of parallel, cylindrical, striated muscle fibers (f). Apart from the typical cross striation (inset: mark the dark A-bands, as well as the light I-bands with the Z-membrane), they are characterized by the peripheral position of their multiple nuclei (n). Skeletal muscle, human, HE. **Fig. 3.3.4.** (right) In transverse section, cross striation cannot be seen, but it is apparent that these muscle fibers (f) are skeletal from the presence of multiple nuclei (n), which occupy a peripheral position. The surface of these sections is granular, which is caused by the presence of myofibrils. Skeletal muscle, human, HE.

The striated fibers of skeletal muscle tissue do not form a completely homogeneous population. Distinction can be made between **white fibers** and **red fibers**. The distinction between the two is fundamentally metabolic. White fibers can contract fast, but get fatigued soon. Red fibers contract more slowly, but are better resistant to fatigue. White fibers contain relatively little myoglobin and abundant glycogen. In red fibers, the situation is reversed. Consequently, white fibers have a partly anaerobic metabolism and derive their energy to a large extent from glycolysis, breaking down glucose to lactate. Red fibers are more pronouncedly aerobic. They liberate energy by the much more efficient process of respiration and metabolize glucose completely to carbon dioxide. White fibers are relatively thick and contain thick myofibrils. Their mitochondria are small and rather few in number. Red fibers are thinner and contain thinner myofibrils. They have more numerous and larger mitochondria. Red fibers dominate in muscles that have to work under relatively light loads during prolonged periods of time, like the respiratory muscles of the diaphragm and the rib cage. White fibers dominate in muscles that have to work intermittently, during relatively short periods of time, and under variable loads. Many muscles consist of a mixture of red and white fibers.

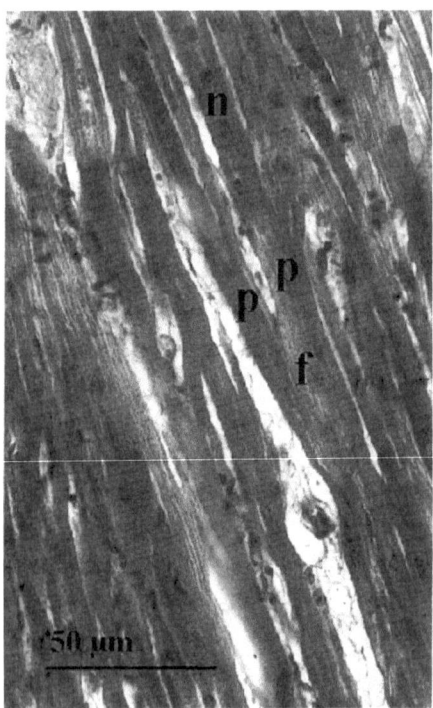

Fig. 3.3.5. Cardiac muscle fibers (f) are elongated, but have fairly irregular shapes because they bifurcate and develop processes (p). Mark the central position of the nuclei (n). Heart, human, Masson stain.

Occasionally, a satellite cell is included within the basement membrane enveloping an individual skeletal muscle fiber. Satellite cells are regarded as leftover embryonic cells, which have not participated in the formation of the muscle fiber syncytium. They may participate in the recovery of damaged muscle fibers by multiplication and merging. Light optically, these flattened cells are difficult to observe. The nucleus is heterochromatic and their cytoplasm is poor in organelles. Both characteristics testify to the undifferentiated nature of these cells.

III.3.3. Cardiac muscle tissue.

Cardiac muscle fibers are more irregularly shaped than skeletal ones and have centrally located nuclei (Figs. 3.3.5.-8.). In the light microscope, apart from the normal cross striation which can also be seen in skeletal muscle fibers, cardiac muscle fibers show an additional type of cross striations, the **intercalated disks** (Fig. 3.3.6.). Intercalated disks lie in groups, are oriented parallel to the traditional dark A bands, but are shorter and thicker. The position of individual disks in the group may evoke the image of a staircase. Originally, the intercalated disks were taken for just what they look like: additional cross bands, maybe A bands which are somewhat wider than others.

Ultrastructural observation has allowed a correct interpretation of the intercalated disks: they are specialized cell junctions. Before this was realized, cardiac muscle was regarded as a syncytium, as skeletal muscle fibers are. Intercalated disk are formed in places where the processes of successive cardiac muscle fibers touch. At these contact places, the cytosolic face of the cell membrane is locally coated with a dense material, the **fascia adhaerens**, in which the actin microfilaments of the myofibrils are anchored (Fig. 3.3.9.). Intercellular fibers connect the fasciae adhaerentes of adjoining muscle fibers. They are analogous to the intermediate junction of epithelial cells. The unequal length of neighbouring processes causes the fasciae to lie on successive levels, which is responsible for the step-like arrangement, light optically, of the intercalated disks. It is through the fasciae adhaerentes that tensile forces are transmitted when the muscle fibers contract.

A second kind of junctions consist of dense plaques on the cytosolic face of the cell membrane, which anchor the intermediate filaments of the muscle fiber's cytoskeleton, made up of desmin, and are connected by intercellular fibers to similar plaques in a neighbouring fiber. These are **desmosomes** or maculae adhaerentes. They effectively connect the cytoskeletons of adjoining fibers, allowing transmission and spread of

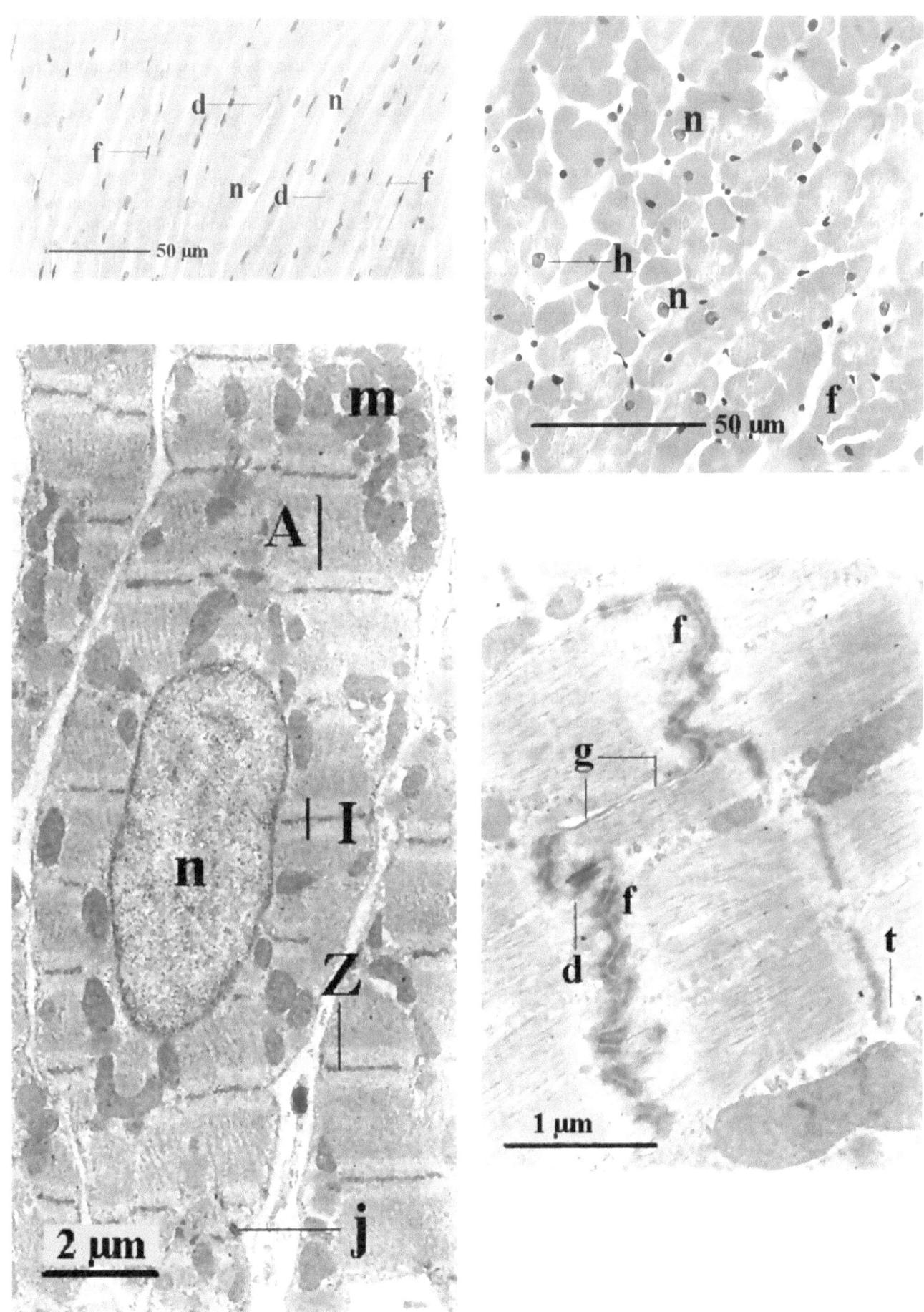

Fig. 3.3.6. (top left) In longitudinal section, cardiac muscle fibers have elongated shapes. The relatively large, euchromatic nucleus (n) occupies the clear, fibril-free axial part of the fibers (compare with Figure 3.3.7.). The smaller, slender, and heterochromatic nuclei (f) are those of fibroblasts, which lie between adjoining cardiac fibers. The cross striation typical of striated muscle fibers does not show clearly. Here and there, groups of thick and short cross stripes can be seen, which may be arranged like steps in a flight of stairs: the intercalated disks (d). Heart, dog, HE. **Fig. 3.3.7.** (top right) In cross section, the nucleus of cardiac muscle fibers (f) is seen to occupy a central, axial position (n). It is often surrounded by a clear, fibril-free halo (h). Some fibers do not show nuclei, since these lie outside the section plane. These sections have a granular look, caused by the presence of myofibrils. Heart, dog, HE. **Fig. 3.3.8.** (bottom left) A longitudinal section of a cardiac striated muscle fiber displays the same kind of cross-striated myofibrils as does a skeletal muscle fiber (compare with Figure 2.47.) A-bands (a), as well as I-bands (i) and Z-membranes (z) can be distinguished. The most obvious differences between both fiber types is that the nucleus (n) of a cardiac muscle fiber lies centrally. Cardiac muscle, cat, TEM. **Fig. 3.3.9.** (bottom right) The intercalated disks are in fact cell junctions, which are found at the tips of a cardiac fiber's processes, and which join them with other fibers. This implies that cardiac muscle tissue is a network, as visceral muscle tissue is. Because the lengths of succeeding processes differ, these junctions are increasingly shifted relative to one another, producing the effect of a flight of stairs. The tips of the processes, where the junctions are located, lie at right angles to the fiber's long axis. The cell membranes lining these tips are deeply folded to increase their available surface, and their cytosolic face is coated with a dense fibrous material, which anchors the actin filaments of the myofibrils: the fasciae adhaerentes (f). These junctions are analogous to the intermediate junctions of epithelial cells (compare with Figure 3.4.2.). They transmit contractile forces from one fiber to the next. Where the membranes run longitudinally, they are connected through gap junctions (g). Here, the cardiac fibers are coupled electrotonically, enabling the entire heart muscle to function as a syncytium. Mark the position of the triads: at the level of the Z-membranes (t). Compare this with their position in a skeletal muscle fiber, Figure 2.47.. Cardiac muscle, rabbit, TEM.

tensile forces, and adding to the mechanical strength of the tissue. They are analogous to the desmosomes of epithelial cells.

A third kind of junction is mainly found on the longitudinally oriented stretches of the cardiac muscle fiber's cell membrane. They are **gap junctions**, which link adjoining fibers, not in a mechanical sense, but electrically, as they do in visceral muscle tissue. Through these gap junctions, action potentials are transmitted, and contraction of a cardiac fiber induces contraction of the fibers that are connected with it. The resulting wave of contraction is vital to the heart's functioning. Like visceral muscle, cardiac muscle is a functional syncytium.

References.

Beyer E.C.: Gap junctions. Int. Rev. Cytol. 1993, 137: 1-37.
Severs N.J.: Cardiac muscle cell interaction: from microanatomy to the molecular make-up of the gap junction. Histol. Histopathol. 1995, 10: 481-501.

III.4. Lining tissues: epi-, meso-, and endothelium.

Lining tissues form the border between the outside world or a body cavity and the underlying tissue. Depending on the type of lining tissue and its position, it may shield and protect underlying tissue or control the exchange of substances between this tissue and a body cavity. Both functions imply the tight joining of lining cells into layers or sheets. Depending on the embryological derivation of the tissue, distinction is made between **epithelium** on one hand, and **meso-** and **endothelium** on the other hand.

III.4.1. Epithelium.

Epithelium is a lining tissue of mostly, but not exclusively, endo- or ectodermal origin (Fig. 4.1.). In practice, this means that epithelia line the surface of the body or of those body cavities (e.g. the gut lumen)

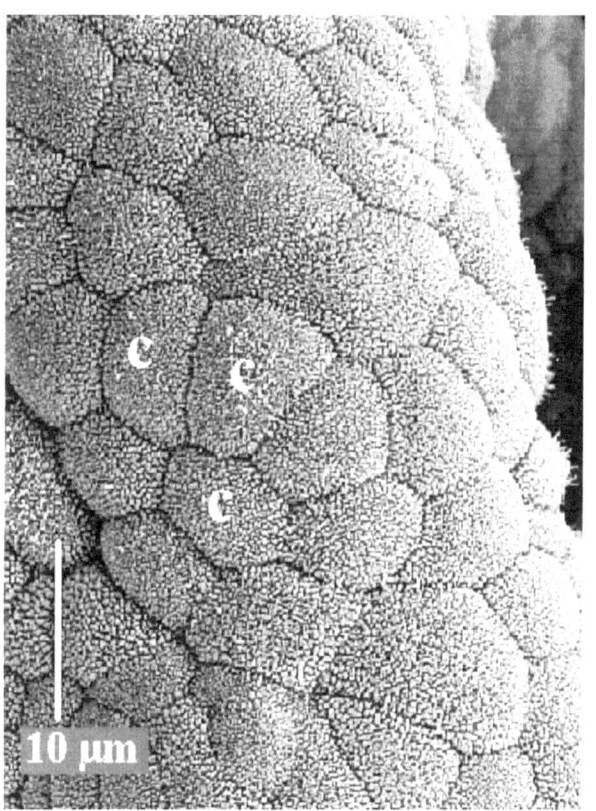

Fig. 3.4.1. The gall bladder's epithelium, viewed from the lumen, shows the tight adherence of cells (c) typical of an epithelium. As a direct consequence of this, they assume a polygonal (usually hexagonal) shape. The apical, exposed cell membrane carries microvilli. Gall bladder, rabbit, SEM.

that are in continuity with the outside world. Consequently, epithelia are found lining the skin, the

gut lumen and the airway lumen. In rarer cases, in the kidney and the reproductive organs, epithelium is derived from mesoderm.

An epithelium consists of one ore more layers of cells, so tightly joined that there is hardly any intercellular space left (Fig. 3.4.1.), and interconnected through **junctions**. The lateral, adjoining cell membranes may interdigitate, a specialization that promotes tight junction of the cells. In addition, the epithelium is anchored to the underlying, mostly interstitial, tissue via a **basement membrane**. Epithelium's primary function is to shield the underlying tissues and to protect them against mechanical damage, dessication, infection, harmful chemicals and ultraviolet radiation. A secondary task, which in many epithelia has become primary, is the exchange of substances between the underlying tissues and a body cavity, and its control. Exchange of substances may involve absorption of food substances or raw material for synthesis, or secretion of waste substances. Some epithelia specialize in the secretion of biologically active substances they have synthesized themselves. These are glandular epithelia. Since epithelial cells are often exposed to external influences, they may specialize as receptor cells, which receive stimuli.

Since an epithelium's primary function is the shielding of underlying tissues, it consists in principle of reinforced, fiber-bearing cells: lining cells. This is most clearly the case in epithelia that are exposed to the outside world. Lining cells derive their toughness from their intracellular fibrils, which form a cytoskeleton. The cytoskeleton of epithelial cells is mainly composed of intermediary filaments (Fig. 3.4.2.), the so-called **tonofilaments**, which are made of **cytokeratin**. In the most exposed epithelium of all, the epidermis of the skin, tonofilaments are chemically modified and present in such massive amounts that they completely fill the cell, to the exclusion of all other organelles (Fig. 2.51.). Epithelia that specialize in the displacement or the exchange of substances often consist of ciliated cells or brush border cells. The basal cell membrane of brush border cells is often thrown into deep, narrow, parallel folds, oriented at right angles to the cell membrane, which dramatically increase the membrane surface available for exchange processes (Fig. 3.4.3.). Epithelia that have been modified to glandular epithelia consist of membrane-bearing secretory cells. These epithelia will be discussed in a separate chapter.

III.4.1.1. Junctions.

An epithelium's functions necessitate the tight joining

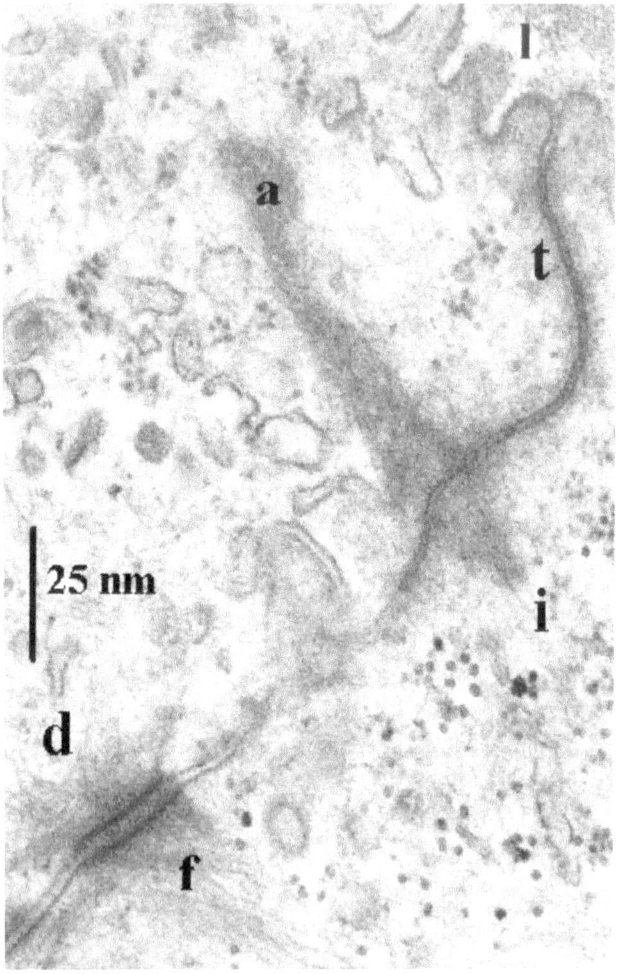

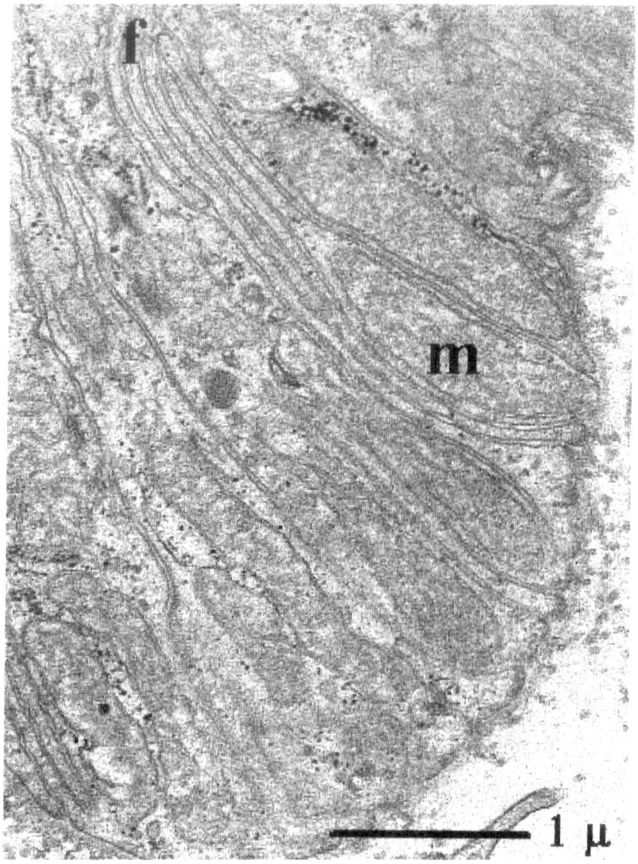

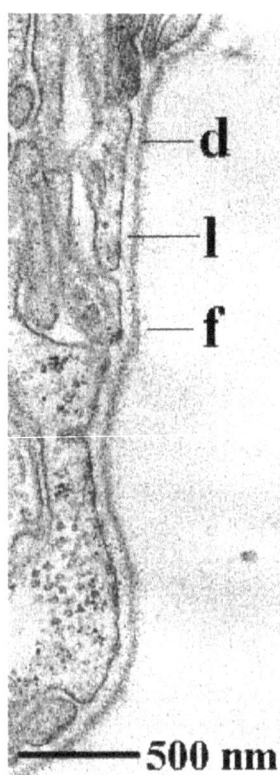

Fig. 3.4.2. (top left) Especially so at their luminal pole, epithelial cells are tightly joined by means of diverse types of junctions, which constitute an entire junctional complex. Topmost is the tight junction or zonula occludens (t), in which the adjoining cell membranes are linked with a dense material that completely fills the intercellular gap. Below this is the intermediate junction or zonula adhaerens (i). In the fibrous lining of the cell membrane's cytosolic face, actin filaments of the terminal web are anchored. The third type of junction is the desmosome or macula adherens (d). In this junction, adjoining cell membranes slightly recede from one another, widening the intercellular gap. The cytosolic face of the membranes is coated with a fibrous material, which anchors the cell's intermediate filaments, the tonofilaments. The intercellular gap contains a layer of dense material, which participates in the joining of both membranes. Intralobular duct, salivary gland, cat, TEM.
Fig. 3.4.3. (top right) In epithelia that participate in ion transport, the basal cell membrane often has deep, narrow folds (f), which greatly increase the membrane surface available for transport processes. The presence of numerous mitochondria (m) indicates that this transport costs energy. Intralobular duct, salivary gland, cat, TEM. **Fig. 3.4.4.** (left) Epithelia rest on a basement membrane. The most conspicuous layer of it, the dense lamina (l), is linked to the epithelial cells by means of fine filaments. The zone occupied by these filaments is the lamina lucida (l). Another kind of filaments (f) course to the adjacent interstitial tissue and will eventually link the dense lamina to its collagen fibrils. They form the lamina fibroreticularis. Choroid plexus, cat, TEM.

of its individual cells, like bricks in a wall. This is done by means of specialized junctions. In a junction, the cell membranes of adjoining cells are interconnected. Several types of junction exist. At the apical pole of prismatic epithelial cells, participating in the formation of simple or pseudostratified epithelia (III.4.1.3.1.-2.), different types of junctions even combine into **junctional complexes** (Fig. 3.4.2.).

The least complex type of junction is the **occluding junction**, also called **zonula occludens** or **tight junction**. In this type of junction, the intercellular space narrows and is filled with dense material, consisting of integral membrane proteins, which traverse and join both cell membranes. Tight junctions lie at the apical pole of epithelial cells, and form a belt, about 300 nanometers wide, which encircles the cell. Tight junctions are called occluding because they occlude the intercellular space, effectively sealing it from the outside world. In this way, passage of substances between the epithelial cells is made impossible. Any transport must occur via the epithelial cells, enabling them to control it. Tight junctions also limit the lateral movements of integral membrane proteins, so that the apical membrane domain can have a different composition, as far as its integral membrane proteins are concerned, from the rest of the cell membrane.

In the **adhering junction**, the intercellular space is filled with fibrous proteins that connect the adjoining cell membranes. The cytosolic faces of the cell membrane sections participating in the junction are coated with dense material, the attachment plaque, in which the ends of the actin microfilaments are anchored. Like the tight junction, the adhering junction forms a continuous belt, the **zonula adhaerens**, about 300 nanometers wide, which encircles the apical pole of the cell, just below the level of the zonula occludens. The actin microfilaments associated with it form a dense mat, or **terminal web**, in the plane determined by the belt and parallel with the apical cell surface. Via the terminal web, the actin microfilament components of the cytoskeleton of adjoining cells are effectively interconnected. This allows tensile forces to be transmitted and spread, contributing to the epithelium's toughness. In addition, the supportive fibers of microvilli and cilia are anchored in the terminal web. The adhering junction occupies a position in between the apical tight junction and the more basally situated desmosomes. Because of this intermediate position, it is called **intermediary junction**.

The third type of junction is the **macula adhaerens** or **desmosome**. Superficially, it somewhat resembles the intermediate junction, but there are some crucial differences between the two. The desmosomes do not form circumcellular belts, as the other junctions do, but are circular patches, with a diameter of about 300 nanometers. Desmosomes are distributed over the lateral cell membranes, the upper limit of their distribution being the intermediate junction. The cell membrane sections participating in this junction recede somewhat, so that the local intercellular space widens, and are coated on the cytosolic face with dense material, the attachment plaque, which is better developed than the one found in the intermediate junction. The attachment plaque anchors the ends of the cytoskeleton's intermediate cytokeratin tonofilaments. Several proteins participate in the anchoring of tonofilaments, among them desmoplakin. In the intercellular space, fibrous proteins connect both adjoining cell membranes, and form a dense band, equidistant from both membranes. Like the intermediate junction, desmosomes effectively link the cytoskeleton of adjoining cells, allowing tensile forces to be transmitted and to spread.

III.4.1.2. Basement membrane.

The basement membrane forms the border between the epithelium and the underlying interstitial tissue. In principle, it is secreted by the lining cells that rest on it. It not only anchors the epithelium to the interstitial tissue, it also functions as a selective permeability barrier. Consequently, not only the epithelium controls the exchange of substances between a body cavity and the underlying tissues, the basement membrane contributes to this control. Basement membranes are also found enveloping muscle and nerve cells, but it is the epithelial basement membranes that reach the highest levels of elaboration.

Ultrastructurally (Fig. 3.4.4.) the basement membrane, or the basement membrane complex, consists of several layers. The most distinctive and most vital layer, in a mechanical sense, is the **lamina densa**, which looks like a dense layer, a few tens of nanometers thick, and running close to and parallel to the basal cell membranes of the epithelium. To this layer, the epithelial cells are anchored and it is in its turn attached to the underlying interstitial tissue. The lamina densa is a dense network of fibrils, made of collagen type IV and a number of other proteins, such as laminin, entactin, and proteoglycans. The narrow space between the dense lamina and the epithelial basal cell membranes is the **lamina lucida**. In this layer, fine **bridging filaments** may be seen, which connect the basal cell membranes with the lamina densa. Integral membrane proteins link the bridging filaments to the cytoskeletal filaments. By means of **anchoring filaments**, made of type VII collagen, the lamina densa is bound to the collagen fibrils of the interstitial tissue. This layer, the **lamina fibroreticularis**, also contains the fibrillary proteins fibronectin and tenascin. In many basement membrane complexes, it is not very distinctive from the underlying interstitial tissue.

III.4.1.3. Epithelium types.

Epithelia are classified on the basis of two criteria: the number of cell layers and the shape of the cells (Fig. 3.4.5.). They range from simple, unilayered epithelia to the highly complex stratified epithelia: the

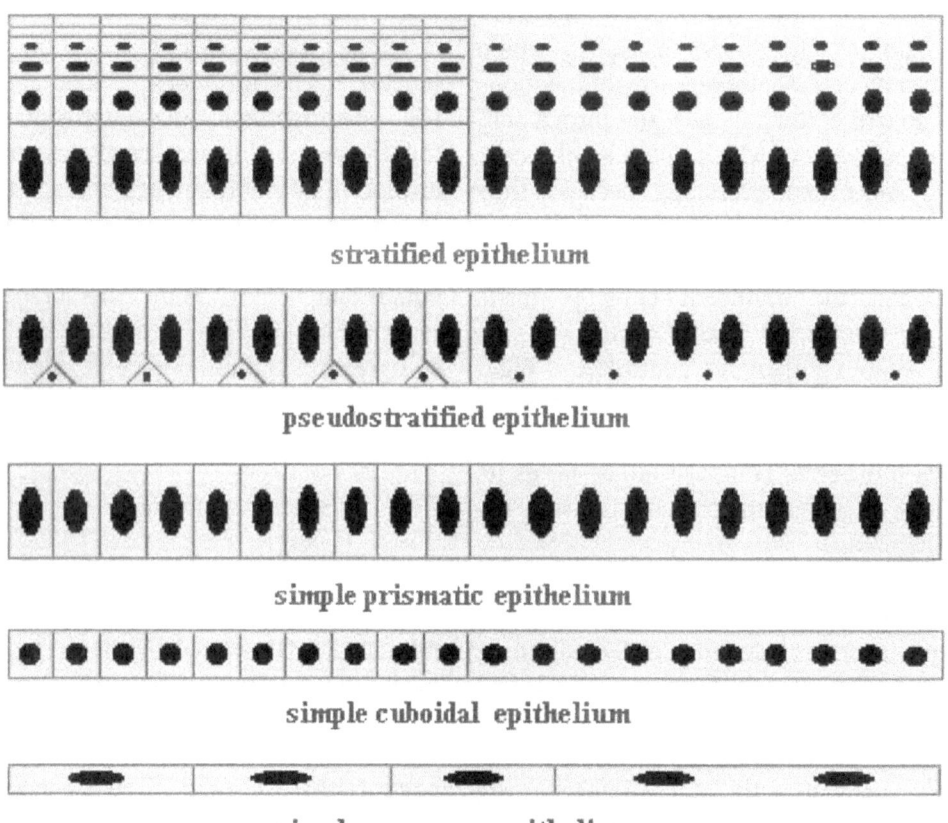

Fig. 3.4.5. There are several types of epithelium. To describe and classify them, 2 criteria are used: the number of cell layers and the shape of the (superficial) cells. Simple epithelia consist of a single layer of cells. Stratified epithelia count 2 or more layers of cells. Pseudostratified epithelia are in fact camouflaged simple epithelia. Regarding cell shape, distinction can be made between squamous, cuboid, and prismatic epithelia.

Malpighian epithelium and the keratinized epithelium.

III.4.1.3.1. Simple epithelium.

An epithelium may consist of a single cell layer. To put it a bit more precisely, every cell of an epithelium may rest on the basement membrane. Such an epithelium is called a **simple epithelium**. In simple epithelia, the shape of the cells may vary from squamous over cuboidal to prismatic. Reference is

then made to a simple squamous, cuboidal, or prismatic (or columnar) epithelium, respectively.

Simple epithelia are found predominantly in the subdiaphragmic segments of the gut, the distal airways and pulmonary alveoli, the kidney excretory ducts, the ducts of glands and reproductive organs, and in the ependymal canal and ventricles of the central nervous system. Squamous and cuboidal epithelia are usually rather passive lining epithelia. They are found in the alveolar parenchyma of the lungs (Fig. 4.14.4.) and in

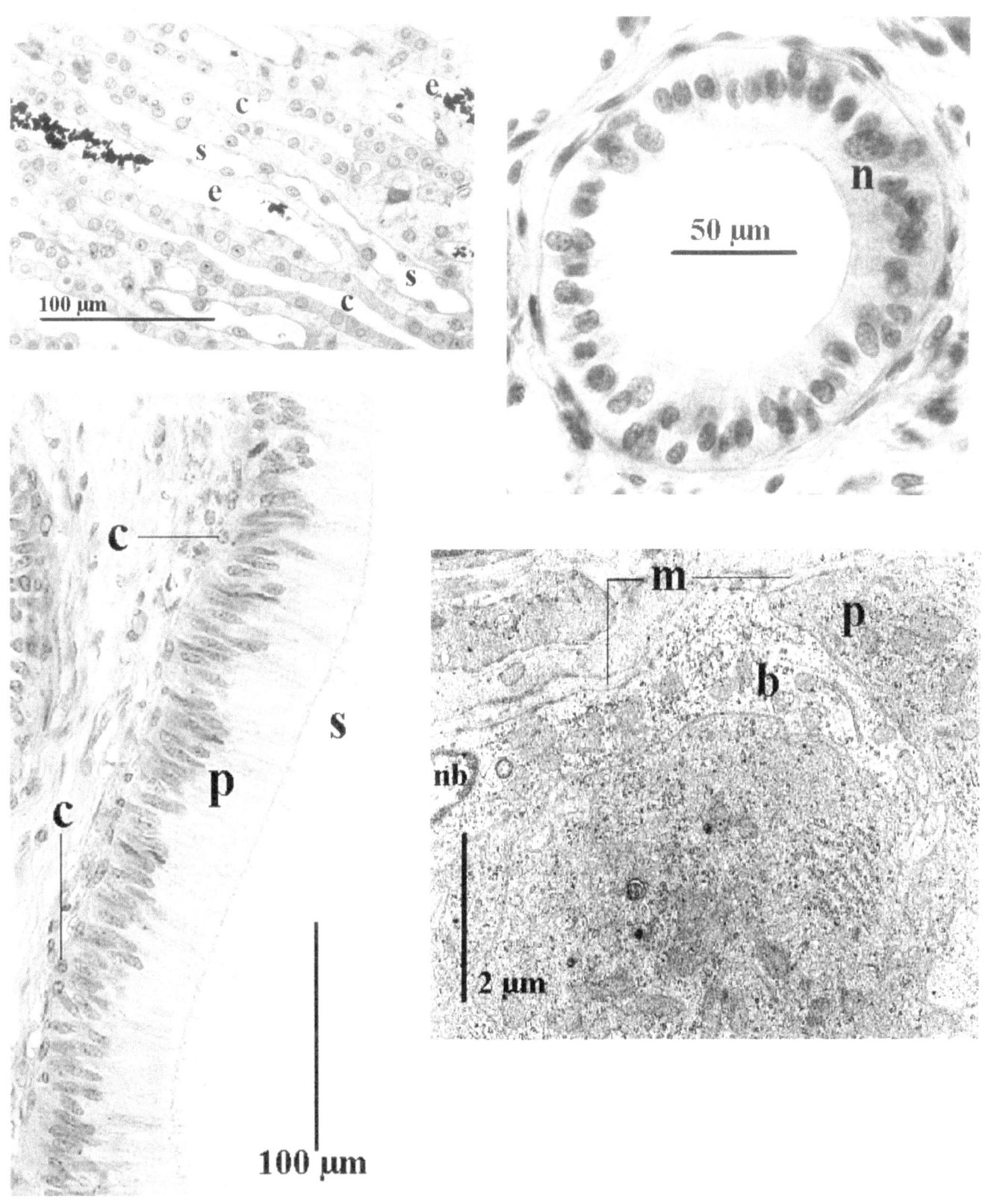

Henle's loops of the kidney (Figs. 3.4.6.-4.8.11.). Simple cuboidal epithelia are found in the renal collecting tubules (Fig. 3.4.6.), and in the ducts of glands and reproductive organs (Fig. 4.10.12.). Simple prismatic (columnar) epithelia often carry cilia or microvilli, show infolding of the basal cell membrane and function in the displacement or exchange of substances. Such epithelia abound in the subdiaphragmic intestine (Fig. 4.15.32.), the renal contorted tubules (Fig. 4.8.4.), the ependyma and choroid plexus of the central nervous system (Fig. 4.4.20.) and the ducts of glands (Fig. 3.4.7.).

Fig. 3.4.6. (top left) Simple epithelia. Squamous epithelium (s), like that of Henle's loop, is made of flattened cells, the nucleus of which bulges into the lumen for lack of room. Such epithelial cells strongly resemble endothelial cells (e), which line blood capillaries (mark the presence of dense erythrocytes). The collecting duct is lined with cuboid epithelium (c). Kidney medulla, cat, 1-micrometer plastic section, toluidin blue. **Fig. 3.4.7.** (top right) Simple prismatic epithelium is composed of a single layer (mark the arrangement of the nuclei, n) of prismatic cells. Intralobular duct, salivary gland, human, HE. **Fig. 3.4.8.** (bottom left) At first sight, pseudostratified epithelium is stratified: beneath a superficial layer of prismatic cells (p), characterized by their slender, elongated nuclei, there is, apparently, a basal layer of cuboid cells with rounded or ellipsoid nuclei (c). This stratification is just an impression, however (see Figure 3.4.9.), and it actually is a simple epithelium. The prismatic cells carry stereocilia (s). Epididymal duct, human, HE. **Fig. 3.4.9.** (bottom right) Ultrastructural observation clearly shows that not just the basal cells (b, nb = nucleus), but the prismatic cells (p) as well, touch the basement membrane (m). According to the definition, this is a simple epithelium. The stratified look in Figure 3.4.8. is a consequence of the different heights of the cells, causing the nuclei to occupy different levels. Epididymal duct, hamster, TEM.

III.4.1.3.2. Pseudostratified epithelium.

A **pseudostratified epithelium** is basically a simple epithelium with cells of unequal height. It consist of low basal cells as well as high prismatic cells. The high prismatic cells are the epithelium's functional cells, which carry out its functions. They do not live indefinitely and have to be replaced regularly. This is achieved by differentiation of basal cells. The high prismatic cells have oval nuclei, oriented with their long axis perpendicular to the basement membrane, while the low basal cells have round nuclei. As a consequence of the different height of both cell types, two rows of nuclei are seen: a lower row of round nuclei and a higher row of oval nuclei. Light optically, when cell membranes cannot be made out, this gives the deceptive impression of a stratified epithelium (Fig. 3.4.8.). In the electron microscope, however, it is clear that both cell types rest on the basement membrane (Fig. 3.4.9.) and, consequently, form a simple epithelium. Thus, pseudostratification can be interpreted as a consequence of a particular mechanism of cell turnover.

A classic example of a pseudostratified epithelium is the respiratory epithelium of the proximal airways (Fig. 4.14.12.). It contains several types of high prismatic functional cells, the most common ones being ciliated cells and goblet cells. Another example of a pseudostratified epithelium is found in the ductus epididymidis. The high prismatic cells carry exceptionally long microvilli, or stereocilia (Fig. 3.4.8.).

III.4.1.3.3. Transitory epithelium.

The exact structure of **transitory epithelium** (Fig. 3.4.10.) is not yet entirely clear, but it is probably a stratified epithelium. Its name implies that its microscopic aspect is transitory, or intermediate, between simple epithelia and stratified epithelia. It has a limited distribution, being found only in the urethers, the urinary bladder, and the proximal urethra.

In transitory epithelium, there are multiple rows of cells. The cells resting on the basement membrane are small, rounded to bluntly pointed, and have little cytoplasm. They are overlaid by successive layers of cells, the apical part of which, carrying the nucleus, is expanded, while the lower part is a narrow process which penetrates the more basal cell layers and, in case of the deeper layers, touches the basement membrane. These are **racket cells**, their shape resembling a tennis racket. The upper layer consists of **superficial cells**, which are the transitory epithelium's functional cells. Racket cells represent successive stages in the differentiation of basal cells to superficial cells. The cytoplasm of the superficial cells, especially so the apical region, contains numerous intermediary filaments and spindle-shaped vesicles (Fig. 3.4.11.). The exposed cell membrane forms irregular infoldings and microvilli. Light optically, the apical cytoplasm appears as a dense band or **crusta**. The cells are joined by means of desmosomes.

The transitory epithelium is thickest in the empty bladder. Here, it may number about ten layers of nuclei. Ultrastructurally, the apical cell membranes of the superficial cells are deeply infolded and particularly rich in vesicles. When the bladder is filled and distended, the racket cells and superficial cells flatten. The number of nuclear layers decreases to about three. The apical membranes of the superficial cells expand by flattening of the folds and incorporation of vesicles. Essentially, transitory epithelium is a passive, impermeable epithelium that is specially adapted to accommodate distension. The cells have the ability to flatten, and the membrane folds and spindle shaped vesicles of the superficial cells represent a membrane reserve that can be consumed as distention advances.

96

III.4.1.3.4. Stratified epithelium.

A **stratified epithelium**, or compound epithelium, numbers at least two but usually several cell layers. Only the basal layer rests on the basement membrane. Stratified epithelia also differ from simple epithelia by the absence of junctional complexes. Usually, their cells are joined by a single type of junctions, the desmosome.

Compound cuboidal or prismatic (columnar) epithelia exist, for instance in the ducts of major glands, but are rare. Usually, they have only 2 layers of cells. They are mostly passive lining epithelia forming the transition between simple prismatic epithelia and stratified epithelia.

The most important stratified epithelia consist largely of squamous cells and have multiple cell layers. Such epithelia arise by cell multiplication in the basal layer, which consists of cuboidal to prismatic cells. The daughter cells form successive layers, according to age. During this apical displacement, the epithelial cells differentiate and flatten. The epithelium may show clearly distinct layers, each corresponding to a successive differentiation stage. The most superficial, squamous cells are the epithelium's functional cells. They are specifically adapted to shield the underlying tissues. Desquamation of the superficial, functional cells is compensated for by continuous supply of fresh cells from below. Differentiation and flattening can be seen as an adaptation to the avascular character of an

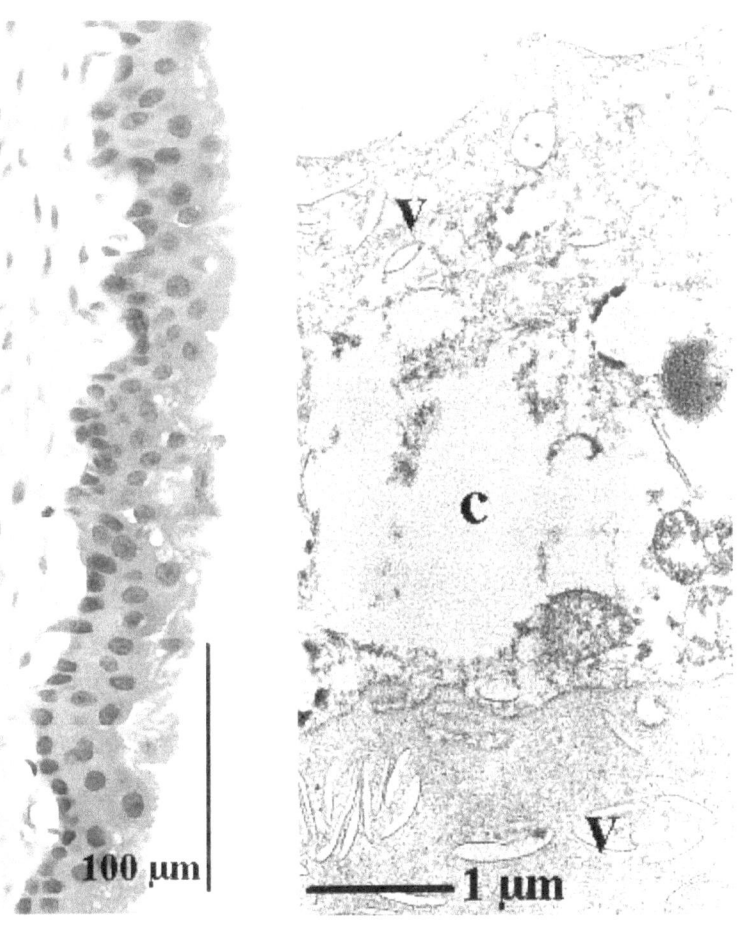

100 μm

1 μm

Fig. 3.4.10. (left) Transitory epithelium is a stratified epithelium. Urine bladder, cat, HE. **Fig. 3.4.11.** (right) The transitory epithelium's superficial cells form a crusta (c). The crusta, as well as the deeper cell layers, contain a large number of membranes in the shape of flattened vesicles (v). When the bladder fills, the epithelium is stretched, and this vesicular membrane is incorporated into the cell membrane. Urine bladder, cat, TEM.

epithelium. The uppermost cells are farthest removed from subepithelial blood vessels and consequently obtain the least food. Since the majority of the cells in multilayered epithelia are squamous, to a variable degree, especially so the functional cells, they are called **stratified squamous epithelia**, although, strictly spoken, this term is not exact. There are two widespread types of stratified squamous epithelia: Malpighian epithelium and keratinized epithelium.

Malpighian epithelium (Fig. 3.4.12.) is found lining body cavities that open into the exterior, such as the mouth and pharynx, the oesophagus, and the rectum. It is primarily a shielding epithelium. Its cells are rich in cytokeratin tonofilaments and they are tightly joined by means of desmosomes. The basal cells are joined to the lamina densa of the basement membrane by hemidesmosomes

Keratinized epithelium (Fig. 3.4.13.) can be regarded as a further differentiation stage of Malpighian epithelium. It is a stratified squamous epithelium, in which the shielding function is developed to extremes. The cytokeratin of the tonofilaments is chemically modified to a very tough protein substance: **keratin**. The cells composing this epithelium are consequently called **keratinocytes** or horn cells. Keratinization is a complicated process, consisting of several steps. Consequently, keratinized epithelium has a distinct layered appearance. Keratinization makes the epithelium impermeable and extremely resistant to mechanical disruption. It is found at the surface of the most exposed body part of all, the skin, where it forms the epidermis.

The basal layer of keratinized epithelium consists of a single row of cuboidal to prismatic keratinocytes, which show multiplication. This is the germ cell layer or **stratum germinativum** (Fig. 3.4.15.). These cells contain numerous tonofilaments, which are anchored in the desmosomes and the **hemidesmosomes** by means of which the keratinocytes are joined to neighbouring cells and the lamina densa of the basement membrane, respectively. The lamina fibroreticularis of the basement membrane is well developed and contains anchoring filaments. The basal cell membrane and the underlying lamina densa often undulate, an adaptation to accommodate more hemidesmomes and to ensure better fixation of the epithelium to the underlying tissue.

The next layer is the prickle cell layer or **stratum spinosum** (Fig. 3.4.16.). It arises from the basal layer by cell multiplication and differentiation. In this layer, flattening sets in. It is built from diamond-shaped cells, oriented with their long axis in the plane of the epithelium. Light optically, they seem to show cross-links, which look like fine parallel filaments, bridging the intercellular spaces. This gives the cells their "spiny" appearance (Fig. 3.4.14.). These so called **Bizzozero bridges** are formed by processes of neighbouring keratinocytes, which are joined at their tips by desmosomes. Their existence may be partially artefactual. During fixation, the keratinocytes may shrink somewhat, causing widening of the intercellular space. Only where desmosomes join them do the cell membranes remain in close proximity, causing the formation of processes.

The keratinocytes of the stratum spinosum differentiate further, giving rise to the next higher cell layer. In this layer, keratinocyte differentiation is already so far advanced that cell multiplication stops. Various phenomena associated with apoptosis appear,

such as pycnotic transformation of the nuclei, which shrink and become heterochromatic. The traditional organelles gradually disappear, probably by autophagocytosis.

The amount of tonofilaments drastically increases, and opaque keratohyalin granules appear, which cause the light optical, basophilic granulation of this layer, the granular layer or **stratum granulosum** (Fig. 3.4.17.). Keratohyalin granules consist of filaggrin, a protein that participates in the aggregation of tonofilaments to bundles. After aggregation, the cytokeratin of the tonofilaments is chemically modified, such as by formation of disulfide cross links, to the much harder and tougher keratin.

On the cytosolic face of the cell membrane, a tough **envelope** is gradually laid down, consisting of the proteins involucrin and loricrin.

Furthermore, secretory vesicles start to accumulate in the cytoplasm. These vesicles, the **keratinosomes**, have a remarkable content: stacks of membranes with a layered aspect, comparable to that of the cell membrane (Fig. 3.4.18.). It is not yet clear how these layered complexes are formed. Eventually, they are liberated by exocytosis (merocrine secretion). These structures are hardly observable after routine treatment with osmium tetroxide. They are much more clearly visible when ruthenium tetroxide is used.

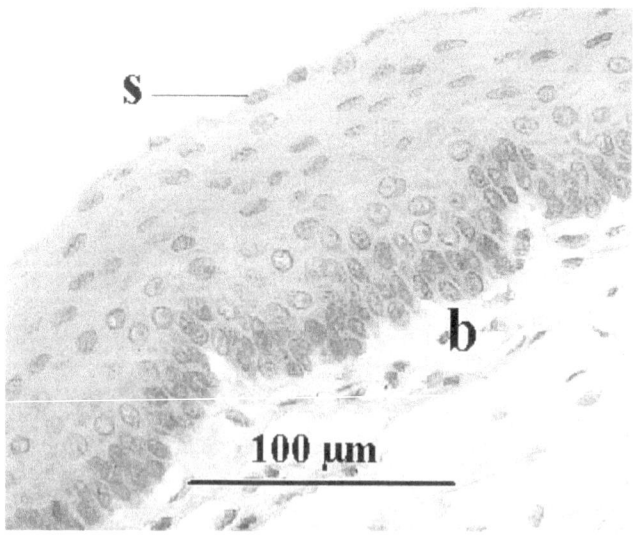

Fig. 3.4.12. Malpighian epithelium is a stratified epithelium with cuboid to prismatic basal cells (b). The superficial cells (s) show a strong tendency to flattening. Malpighian epithelium is only lightly keratinized. Oesophagus, cat, HE.

In a few places, where the keratinized epithelium is extremely thick, the stratum granulosum is succeeded by the stratum lucidum. This layer contains eleidin granules that, like keratohyalin granules, assist in

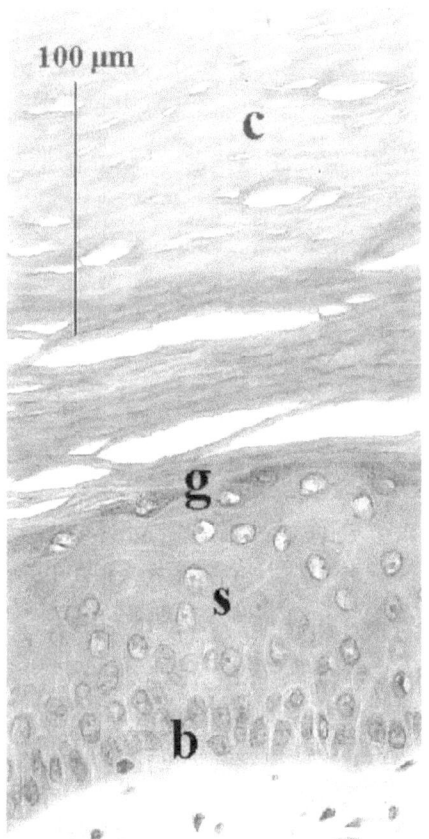 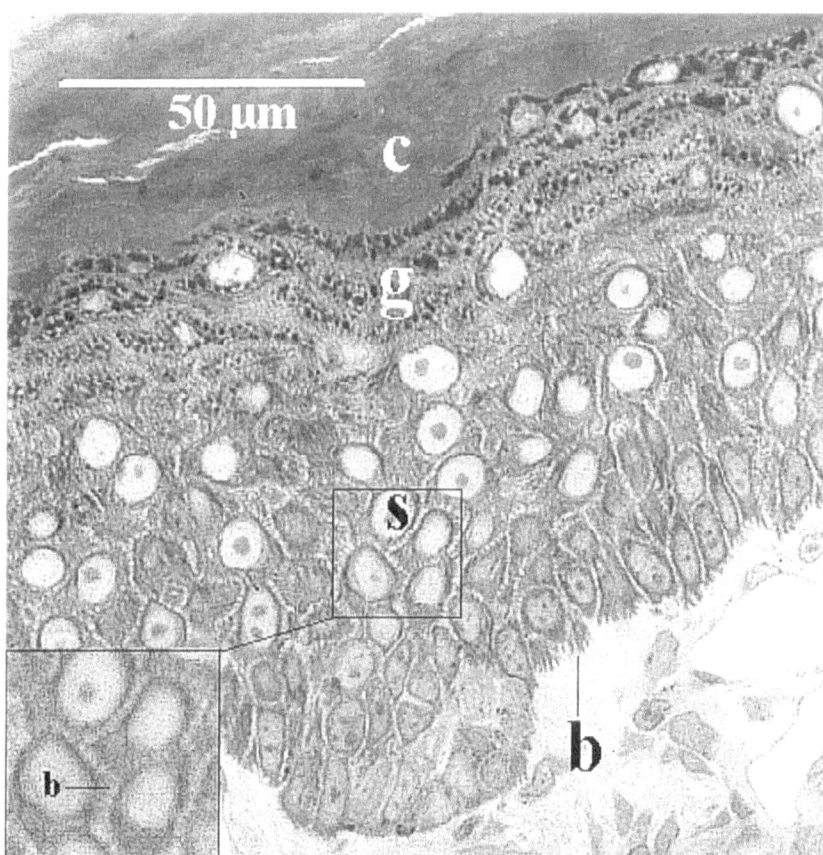

Fig. 3.4.13. (left) The stratified and keratinized epithelium that forms the skin's epidermis is the most complex epithelium. Its functional cells build a keratinized layer, or stratum corneum (c). This layer, which is responsible for the skin's mechanical resistance, does not show any microscopic detail. It is in fact a layer of dead cells, which arises by differentiation out of the deeper, less differentiated layers. Differentiation is a stepwise process, and each step corresponds to a particular layer of the epithelium. The basal layer (b) consists of undifferentiated, prismatic epithelial cells or keratinocytes. Cell multiplication in this layer (it is also called germinative layer or stratum germinativum) allows it to grow thicker. As the cells are moved away from the basal layer, they start to flatten and acquire a rounded nucleus. They form the spiny layer, or stratum spinosum (s, also see Figure 3.4.14.) In the next upper layer, the granular layer or stratum granulosum (g), synthesis of keratin starts, resulting in dark keratohyalin granules. Completion of this keratinization process results in formation of the stratum corneum (c). Foot sole epidermis, human, HE. **Fig. 3.4.14.** (right) The keratinocytes of the basal layer (b) have basal "feet"". The dark pigment visible in this layer is melanin, produced by melanocytes. The spiny layer's keratinocytes (s) seem to be interconnected by short, parallel bridges, Bizzozero's bridges (b, inset). These bridges are in fact cell junctions (Figure 3.4.16.). They give the keratinocytes the spiny aspect from which this layer's name is derived. The granular layer (g) contains dense keratohyalin granules, while the keratinized layer (c) is homogeneously keratinized. Foot sole epidermis, cat, 1-micrometer plastic section, toluidin blue.

aggregating the tonofilaments prior to keratinization.

Usually, the stratum granulosum is directly overlaid with the keratinized layer or **stratum corneum** (Fig. 3.4.19.). In this most superficial layer, the cell nuclei have disappeared completely. The cytoplasm contains nothing but tight bundles of **keratin filaments**. Filaggrin has disappeared. The cell membrane has been replaced by an **envelope**, 3 to 4 times as thick (20 nanometers), consisting of involucrin and loricrin. The desmosomes have been gradually replaced with a layered intercellular **lipid coat**. This coat is made up

of lipid molecules called ceramids, the structure and arrangement of which is similar to the phospholipids of the cell membrane. It is formed by lateral fusion of the layered complexes liberated by exocytosis of keratinosomes (Fig. 3.4.18.). Its layered structure is a consequence, as it is in the cell membrane, of hydrophilic and hydrophobic associations between the ceramid molecules. There is a crucial difference with the cell membrane, however. The lipid coat does not simply consist of bilayers, but of bilayers separated by monolayers. Some ceramids are double headed, others are double tailed. Such ceramids form links between

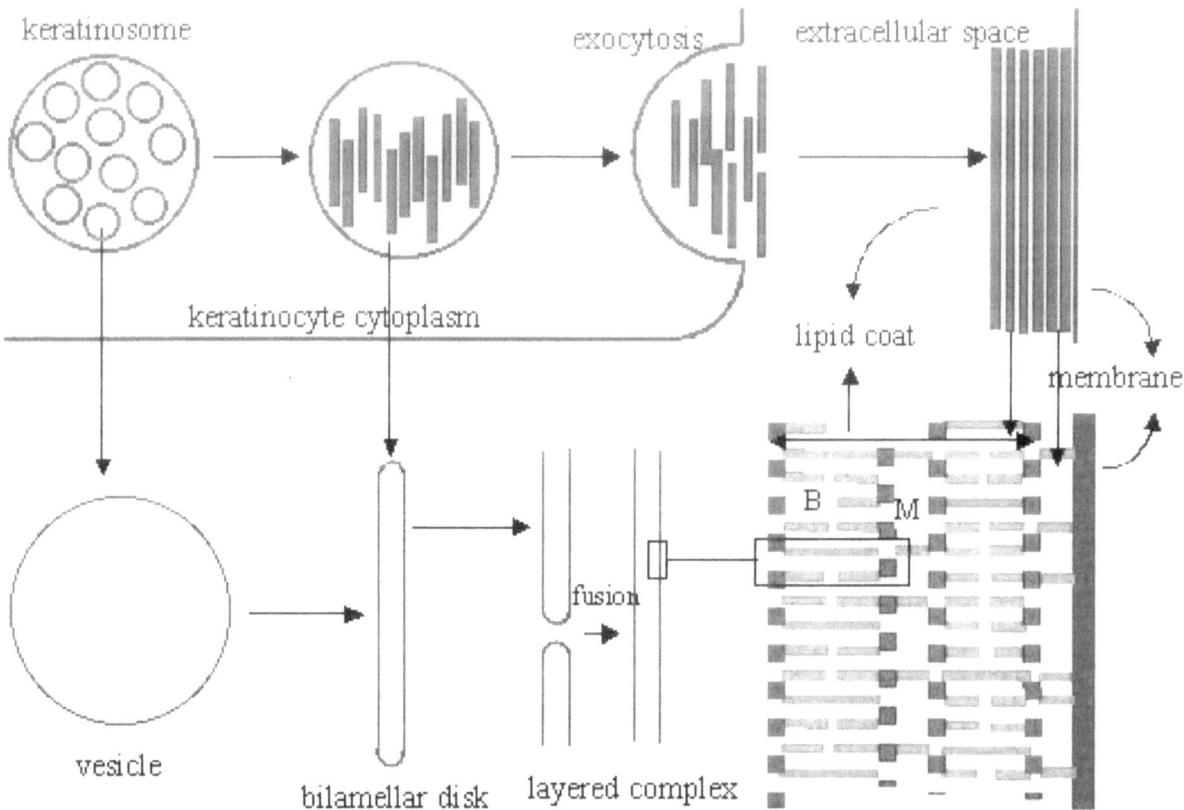

keratinosome   exocytosis   extracellular space

keratinocyte cytoplasm

lipid coat

membrane

B   M

vesicle

fusion

bilamellar disk   layered complex

Fig. 3.4.18. The keratinocytes of the keratinized layer are tightly joined by means of layered lipid complexes that resemble the cell membrane (Fig. 2.2.). These complexes are made of ceramids. Ceramids are lipids that can be thought of as derived from the phospholipids of the cell membrane. Ceramids originally form vesicles inside the keratinosomes. These vesicles flatten to bilamellar disk and eventually fuse, producing layered complexes that leave the cell by exocytosis. In the extracellular space, the layered complexes produced by many cells fuse and build up a lipid layer. This lipid layer is composed of bilayers (b) and monolayers (m). In the bilayers, the ceramid tails interact hydrophobically, as do the phospholipids in the cell membrane. In addition, covalent bonds are formed between ceramid heads, bridging the bilayer, and greatly strengthening it, since covalent bonds are much stronger than hydrophobic bonds. Monolayers are formed where the original bilamellar disks touch. Covalent bonds link them to one another, and to the keratinocyte cell membrane.

hydrophilic and hydrophobic layers, respectively, and contribute to the coherence of the lipid coat. By means of covalent bonds, the ceramid molecules are bound to one another and to the keratinocyte's envelope. This is another essential difference with the phospholipid bilayer of the cell membrane, the cohesion of which is exclusively based on hydrophilic and hydrophobic interactions, and explains its mechanical strength. Thus, the keratinized epithelium's layered structure is a consequence of the gradual differentiation of a tough superficial layer of reinforced cells, the stratum corneum. This layer continuously loses cells by desquamation, which is compensated for by the addition of fresh cells from below. For this reason, an incoherent layer or **stratum disjunctum**, consisting of detaching horn scales, is sometimes distinguished.

III.4.2. Meso- and endothelium including pericytes.

Mesothelium and endothelium are lining tissues of mesodermal origin, which line body cavities that do not open to the exterior world. **Mesothelium** coats the thoracic and abdominal cavities and the organs within them. **Endothelium** lines the inside of blood and lymph vessels, and forms **capillaries**, which pervade the tissues. These lining tissues are much less exposed than epithelia and show less evidence of reinforcement. They control various exchange processes between a luminal space and the underlying tissues. In sharp contrast to epithelia, which show much variation regarding cell shape and number of cell layers, meso- and endothelium are in principle always **simple squamous**. Virtually the only exception are the cuboidal endothelia found in the specialized high

100

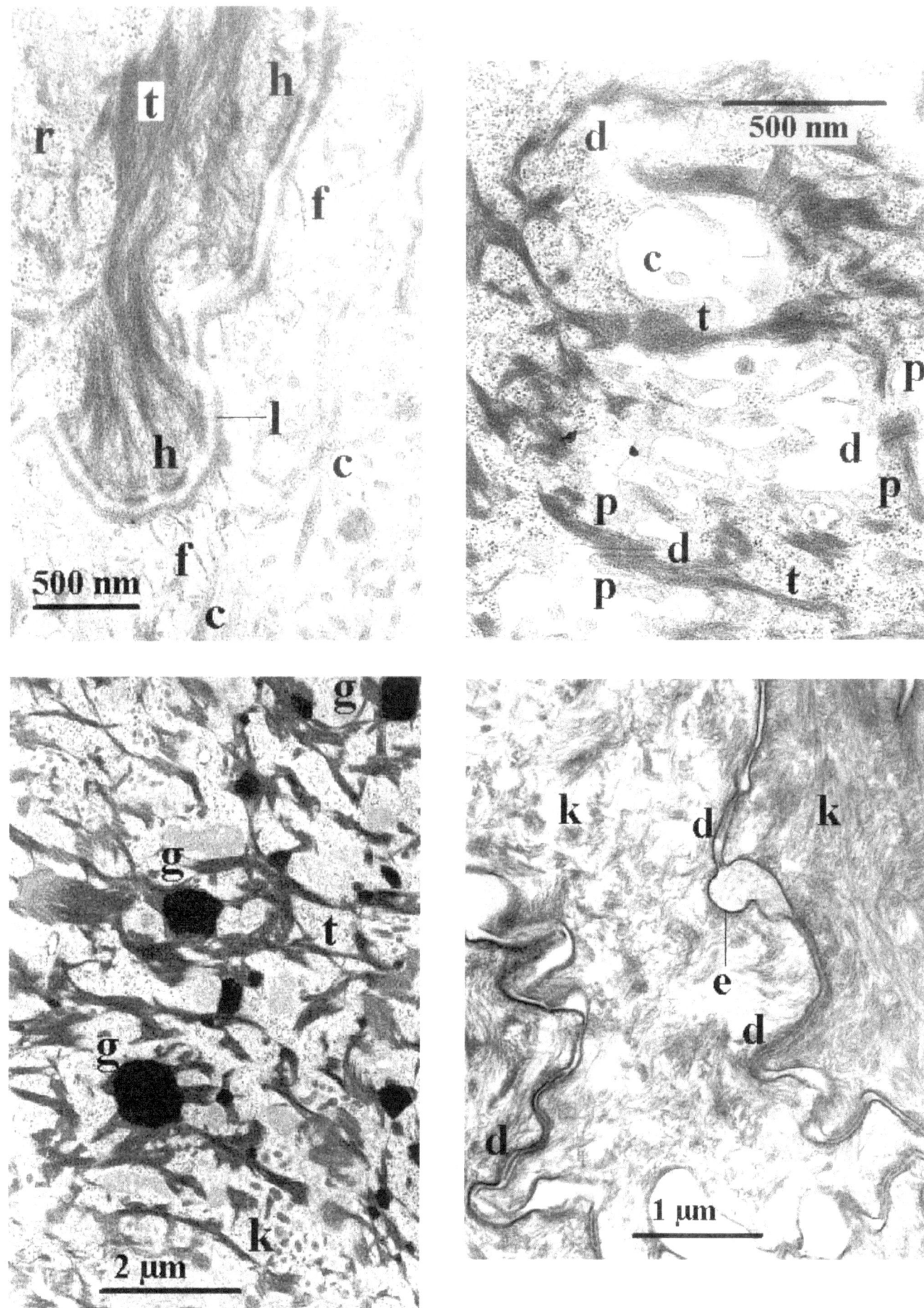

Fig. 3.4.15. (top left) In the keratinocytes of the basal, germinative layer, tonofilaments (t) anchor in a dense proteinaceaous layer on the cytosolic face of the cell membrane. In its turn, this layer is linked to the dense lamina (l) of the basement membrane. This junction looks like one half of a desmosome and is in fact called a hemidesmosome (compare with Figure 3.4.2.). Filaments (f) link the dense lamina to the underlying collagen fibrils (c). The cytoplasm is rich in ribosomes (r), which enable the cells to synthesize keratin. Foot sole epidermis, cat, TEM. **Fig. 3.4.16.** (top right) The keratinocytes of the spiny layer are tightly joined by means of desmosomes (d). The intercellular space is relatively wide. As a result of this, the desmosomes link the tips of 2 processes (p), filled with tonofilaments. These are Bizzozero's bridges (see Figure 3.4.14.). Foot sole epidermis, cat, TEM. **Fig. 3.4.17.** (bottom left) In the granular layer, dense bodies, or keratohyalin granules (g), form on the tonofilaments. This is the first step of the keratinization process. Keratinosomes (k) can also be seen. Foot sole epidermis, cat, TEM. **Fig. 3.4.19.** (bottom right) In the keratinized layer, the tonofilaments have been aggregated into keratin filaments, which completely fill the cell. The cell membrane has been thickened and forms and envelope (e). Remains of desmosomes (d) can be seen. Foot sole epidermis, cat, TEM.

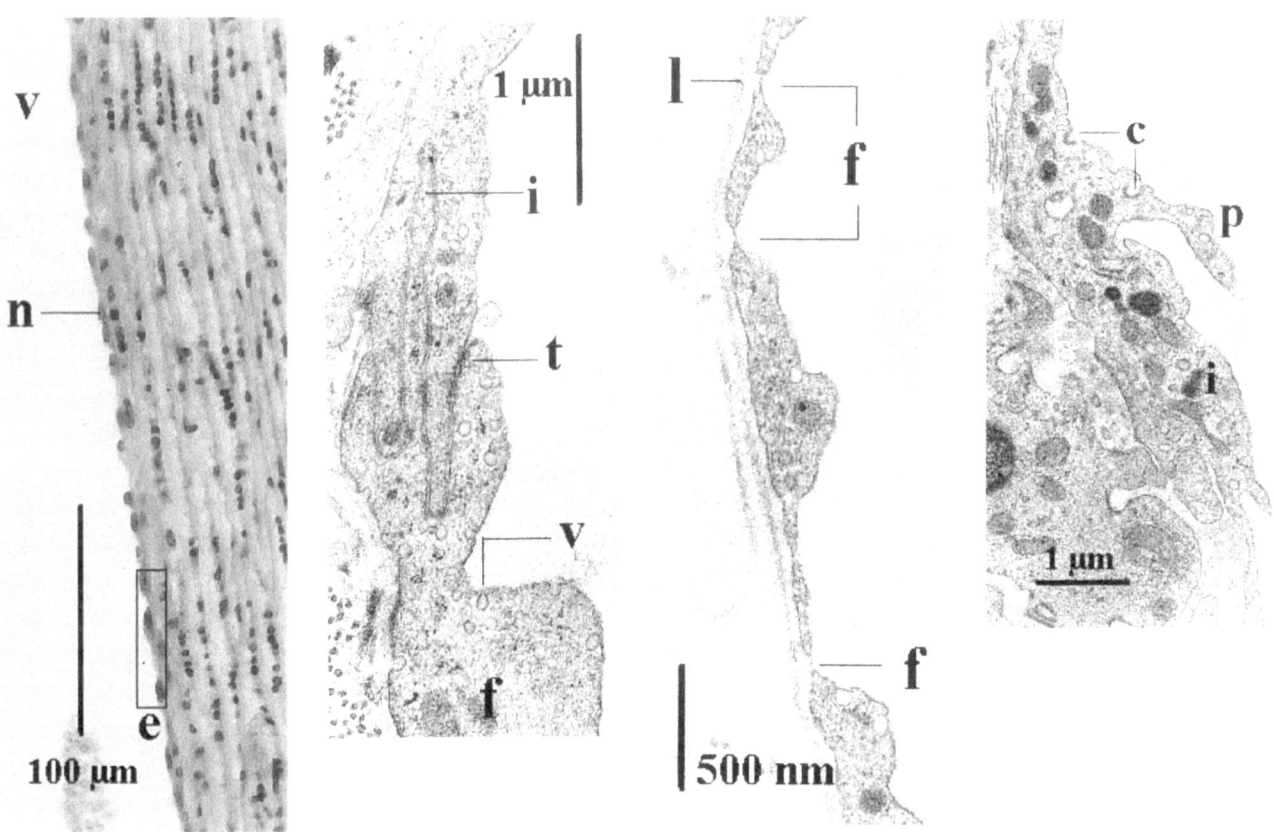

Left to right: **Fig. 3.4.20.** An endothelium (e) lines the lumen of blood vessels (v) and is composed of lining cells which are flattened to such an extent that their cytoplasm can hardly be made out with the light microscope. Consequently, the nuclei, which appear naked, bulge into the lumen for lack of room (n). Aorta, dog, HE. **Fig. 3.4.21.** Adjoining endothelial cells may simply be apposed, but may also interdigitate, like here. The cell membranes are joined by tight junctions (t). Both cell membranes, luminal as well as abluminal, form pinocytotic vesicles (v), which represent a shuttle mechanism. The cytoplasm also contains microfilaments (f). Blood capillary, carotid body, cat, TEM. **Fig. 3.4.22.** Blood capillary endothelial cells often show fenestrations, equipped with a diaphragm (f), which increase their permeability. Fenestrations are the result of local fusion of luminal and abluminal cell membranes. Endothelial cells are linked to the dense lamina (l) of the basement membrane. Blood capillary, choroid plexus, cat, TEM. **Fig. 3.4.23.** Lymph capillary endothelial cells have irregular contours as a consequence of the presence of luminal and abluminal processes (p). The cytoplasmic inclusions (i) represent lysosomal and phagocytosed material. Coated pits (c) can be seen, indicating formation of endosomes. Lymph capillary, small intestinal villus, rabbit, TEM.

endothelial venules of the lymphoid organs and in the splenic sinuses. Endothelial cells are squamous, somewhat elongated cells with an undulating perimeter, oriented with their long axis parallel to the

102

vessel's axis. Usually, endothelial cells are flattened to such an extent that their nucleus, for lack of room, bulges in the vessel's lumen. Their flattened peripheral cytoplasm is often only a fraction of a micrometer thick. The limited resolving power of the light microscope makes it difficult to see. Consequently, with light microscopy, endothelia seem to consist of a row of naked nuclei (Fig. 3.4.20.).

The membranes of adjoining endothelial cells can be simply apposed, but can also overlap or interdigitate. They are joined by means of junctions, predominantly **tight junctions** (Fig. 3.4.21.), although adhering junctions and gap junctions have been observed as well. In addition, they are anchored to the lamina densa of the underlying basement membrane. In all probability, the tight junctions are dynamic: they can reversibly open to allow passage of substances between two endothelial cells. In some specialized capillaries, the endothelial cells are not tightly joined; there may even be spaces between them. Such capillaries, which are typically found in the bone marrow and the lymphoid organs, are called **sinuses**. It goes without saying that such endothelia are highly permeable, they even allow passage of complete cells.

The perinuclear cytoplasm contains some primary organelles and the luminal cell membrane may carry a number of short microvilli. Apart from some microfilaments, the peripheral cytoplasm is dominated by **pinocytotic vesicles** with a diameter of about 70 nanometers (Fig. 3.4.21.). This is especially so in the endothelium which forms the narrowest vessels, the capillaries. The peripheral cell membrane shows numerous caveolae. Their cytosolic face, as in endocytotic profiles, has a dense protein coat that stabilizes the membrane or allows it to change shape. The protein coat does not contain clathrin, however, but caveolin.
Pinocytotic vesicles can be regarded to arise at the luminal cell membrane, by endocytosis, from caveolae. Subsequently, they move to the basal cell membrane, where they undergo exocytosis. This can be demonstrated by the injection of contrast substances in the vessel lumen, which then show up in the interior of the pinocytotic vesicles. The vesicles can be recycled by endocytosis at the basal cell membrane, and shuttle back and forth between both membranes. In this way, various substances may be moved from the vessel's interior to the extracellular spaces of the underlying tissues.
Apart from this dynamic picture of the pinocytotic vesicles, evidence exists that they form rather static connections between the luminal and basal cell membranes. These would consist of more or less

permanent canals, formed by chains of fused vesicles. In this view the caveolae are more or less static structures as well.

Endothelial cells may also contain rod-like vesicles with a dense content, the **Weibel-Palade bodies**. The function of these vesicles is not yet absolutely certain, but they appear to be budding from the Golgi-complex and to undergo exocytosis. They have been demonstrated to contain a number of specific substances, among them factor VIII, also known as von Willebrand's protein, which plays a fundamental role in blood clotting

Endothelial cells that form blood capillaries often show **fenestrations** (Fig. 3.4.22.). These arise by local fusion of luminal and basal cell membranes, forming a diaphragm. The diaphragm contains narrow pores and facilitates the passage of certain substances. The basement membrane crosses the fenestrations uninterruptedly. The dilated, fenestrated capillaries typically found in the endocrine glands, the choroid plexus, and the kidney glomeruli, are called **sinusoidal capillaries**.

Blood capillaries may be associated with **pericytes** or Rouget cells. These cells are completely enveloped by a basement membrane that, at their periphery, joins the endothelial basement membrane. Like endothelial cells, they are flattened, with a bulging nucleus. While the endothelial bulge points towards the capillary center, the pericytal bulge points in the other direction, so that endothelial cells and pericytes look like each other's mirror images. This impression is strengthened further by the presence of numerous caveolae and micropinocytotic vesicles in the pericytes. Pericytes also contain microfilaments. Occasionally, the basement membrane that endothelial cells and pericytes have in common, is interrupted. In these places, cell junctions are formed between the two, especially tight junctions and gap junctions. The extent to which endothelia are covered by pericytes is variable. Presumably, pericytes have contractile properties and can determine the capillary diameter, smooth muscle fibers being absent. In addition, they may have a regulating influence on capillary growth and might influence capillary permeability

The contours of endothelial cells forming lymph capillaries(Fig. 3.4.23.) are not so smooth as those of the blood capillary endothelial cells. They show a number of luminal and abluminal protrusions. The cytoplasm is richer in microfilaments, and apart from micropinocytotic vesicles, they contain lysosomes and phagosomes. These they have in common with macrophages, and it indicates they function in the clearing away of particulate material. Lymph capillary endothelial cells are less tightly joined than those of blood capillaries. The basement membrane is frequently interrupted. In these places, a kind of anchoring filaments may be present. Unlike those associated with the hemidesmosomes of stratified epithelia, these link the cell membrane, not the lamina densa, to the surrounding interstitial tissue. The rather poor coherence of the lymph capillary wall explains its permeability. The task of the lymph capillaries is to recuperate superficial extracellular fluid, which has been lost at the level of the blood capillaries.

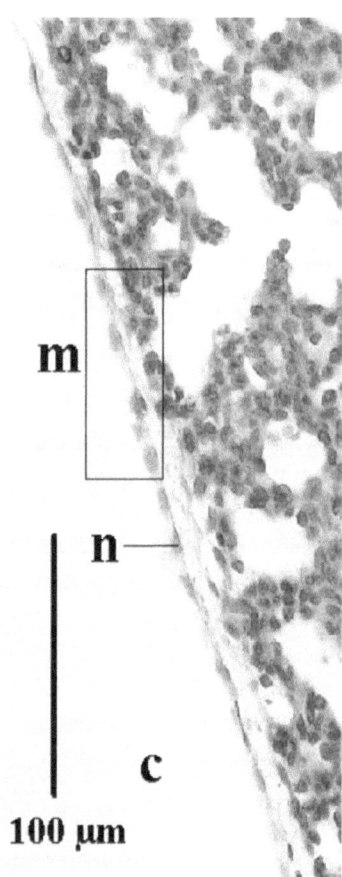

100 μm

Fig. 3.4.24. A mesothelium (m) lines the thoracic and abdominal cavities (c), as well as the organs that lie in them. Usually, they are less extremely flattened than epithelia, and their nuclei (n) form less prominent bulges. Pleura, sheep, HE.

Much of what has been said of endothelial cells is applicable to mesothelial cells. Mesothelial cells are usually less extremely flattened (Fig. 3.4.24.). They are joined by means of tight junctions. They contain microfilaments, pinocytotic vesicles and caveolae.

References.

Allt G., Lawrenson J.G.: Pericytes: cell biology and pathology. Cells Tissues Organs 2001, 169: 1-11.

Anderson R.G.W.: The caveolae membrane system. Annu. Rev. Biochem. 1998, 67: 199-225.

Bundgaard M.: The paracellular pathway in capillary endothelia. Exp. Med. Biol. 1988, 242: 3-8.

Clough G.: Relationships between microvascular permeability and ultrastructure. Prog. Biophys. Molec. Biol. 1991, 55: 47-69.

Downing D.T.: Lipid and protein structures in the permeability barrier of mammalian epidermis. J. Lipid Res. 1992, 33: 301-313.

Eady R.A.J., McGrath J.A., McMillan J.R.: Ultrastructural clues to genetic disorders of skin: the dermal-epidermal junction. J. Invest. Dermatol. 1994, 103: 13S-18S.

Elias P.M.: Stratum corneum architecture, metabolic activity and interactivity with subjacent cell layers. Exp. Dermatol. 1996, 5: 191-201.

Manabe M., O'Guin W.M.: Keratohyalin, trichohyalin and keratohyalin-trichohyalin hybrid granules: an overview. J. Dermatol. 1992, 19: 749-755.

Merker H.J.: Morphology of the basement membrane. Microsc. Res. Tech. 1994, 28: 95-124.

Nehls V., Drenckhahn D.: The versatility of microvascular pericytes: from mesenchyme to smooth muscle? Histochemistry 1993, 99: 1-12.

North A.J., Bardsley W.G., Hyam J., Bornslaeger E.A., Cordingley H.C., Trinnaman B., Hatzfeld M., Green K.J., Magee A.I., Garrod D.R.: Molecular map of the desmosomal plaque. J. Cell Sci. 1999, 112: 4325-4336.

Stevenson B.R., Keon B.H.: The tight junction: morphology to molecules. Annu. Rev. Cell Dev. Biol. 1998, 14: 89-109.

III.5. Glandular tissue.

Glandular tissue is usually derived from epithelium. In fact, glandular tissue, in many cases, is a simple prismatic epithelium that specializes in the synthesis and secretion of bioactive substances: a glandular epithelium. In the simplest case, solitary epithelial cells develop into gland cells, resulting in an epithelium with dispersed gland cells, also known as unicellular glands. Goblet cells (Figs. 4.15.32.-33.) and polarized endocrine cells (Fig. 4.15.40.) may figure as such in the airway and gut epithelia. More frequently, an epithelial cell sheet develops into a continuous glandular epithelium. To form a gland, the epithelium locally proliferates and grows, column-like, into the underlying interstitial tissue. Subsequently, the column becomes hollow, forming a tube. The central hollow, which connects to the outside world, is the lumen. When this continuity with the outside world is maintained during further development, an **exocrine gland** is formed. The lumen serves to evacuate its secretions to the outside world. Exocrine glands largely conserve their epithelial structure. The connection with the overlying epithelium may be lost, resulting in a gland which cannot discharge its secretions into the outside world, but does so instead in the interior, intercellular spaces: an **endocrine gland.** Endocrine glands may greatly modify their original epithelial structure.

GLANDS

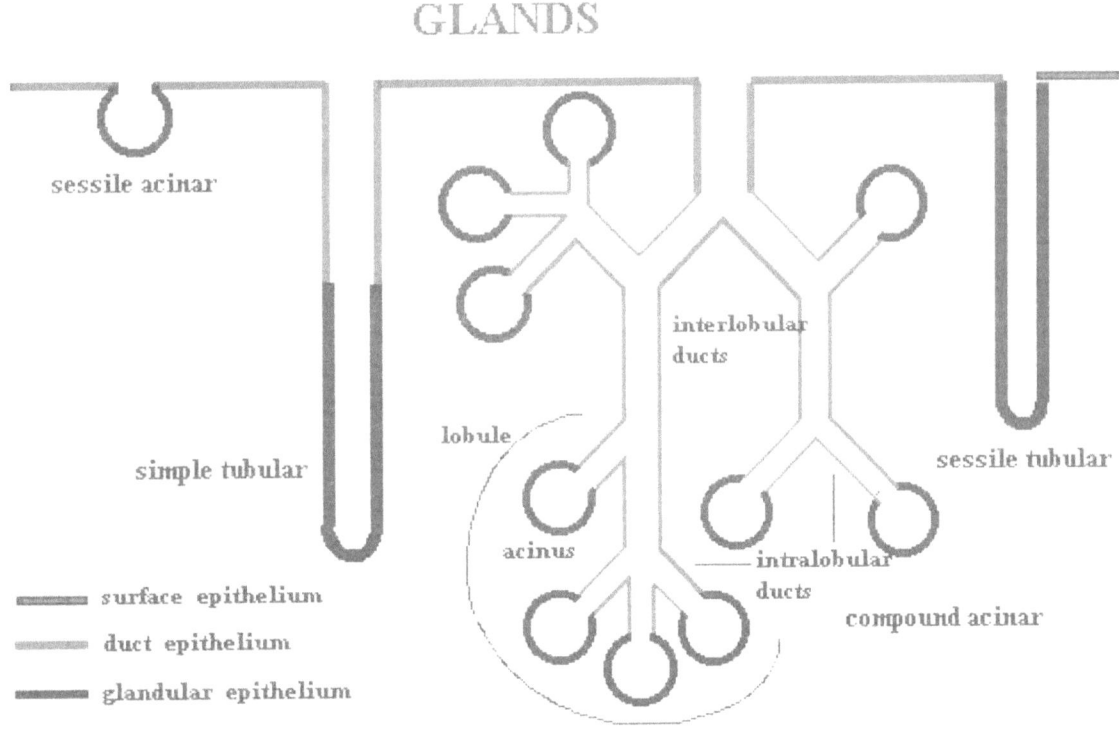

Fig.3.5.1. Types of glands. Glands arise as inpocketings of epithelium into the underlying interstitial tissue. When the resulting gland is globular, it is called an acinar gland, when it is tubular, a tubular gland. In sessile glands, all epithelial cells of the inpocketing develop into gland cells. In more complex glands, only the terminal epithelial cells develop into gland cells, the rest form a duct. Simple glands have an unbranched duct. In compound glands, the duct is branched. Groups of acini (or tubuli, or both) form lobes, surrounded by layers of fibrous connective tissue. The narrow, terminal branches of the ducts, which join the acini or tubuli, are the intralobular ducts. The wider, more central branches of the ducts are the interlobular ducts.

Epithelial cells transform into gland cells by developing characteristics of membrane-bearing cells, such as enzyme-secreting gland cells or peptide hormone-secreting gland cells. This enables them to synthesize and secrete various substances with specific biological effects. Since glandular tissue is directly derived from epithelium, it is to be expected that it retains several of its cytological characteristics. Thus,

105

exocrine gland cells form junctional complexes at their apical pole, and desmosomes. They are linked to the lamina densa of a basement membrane with hemidesmosomes. Their lateral membranes show interdigitations and their basal membranes may be infolded.

III.5.1. Exocrine glands including myoepithelial cells.

The epithelial tube that is the beginning of a gland may continue its development in various ways (Fig. 3.5.1.).

Sometimes, the complete tube develops into a glandular epithelium. Thus, a **sessile gland** is formed. The most obvious examples of these are the endometrial glands (Fig. 4.11.15.), the sebum glands of the skin (Fig. 3.5.2.), Lieberkühn's crypts of the jejunum (Fig. 4.15.32.), and the mucosal glands of the colon and the appendix (Fig. 3.5.3.).

In more complex cases, only the apical cells of the tube develop into gland cells. They form the secretory part of the gland. The epithelium that connects these cells with the overlying epithelium forms the gland's **duct**. Via the duct, the secretory products will be evacuated. In many cases though, the duct is not a passive drain. It can actively regulate the composition of the secretion during its passage, by adding substances to it or absorbing others, and to this end it may develop specific cytological structures. The duct may be unbranched, in which case mention is made of **simple glands**, such as the skin's sweat glands (Fig. 3.5.4.). In addition, the duct may be either straight or coiled. In the most complex glands, the **compound glands**, the duct is branched. To this category belong the largest and most complex glands of the body, such as the salivary glands (Fig. 3.5.5.) and the pancreas (Fig. 4.15.49).

A sessile gland, or the secretory part of a simple or compound gland, may have variable shapes. If it is globular, it is called an **acinus**. If it is tubular, it is called a tubule or **tubulus**. In compound glands, one of both types may dominate, so that mention is made of **acinar glands** (Figs. 3.5.2., 3.5.5.) or **tubular glands** (Figs. 3.5.3.-4., 4.11.15.), respectively. In mixed or tubulo-acinar glands, acini as well as tubules are present in significant numbers. Sessile glands can be acinar, such as the sebum glands, or tubular, such as the endometrial glands. Simple glands, such as the sweat glands, are almost universally tubular. Most compound glands, such as the salivary glands and the pancreas, are acinar or tubulo-acinar.

In many cases, the glandular epithelium is associated with subepithelial **myoepithelial cells** (Fig. 3.5.6.), which have contractile properties and help to evacuate the gland's secretions from the glandular and duct lumen, smooth muscle fibers being absent.

Myoepithelial cells are usually spindle shaped, sometimes star shaped, and form a simple layer, coherent or not, between the glandular epithelium and the basement membrane. Light optically, this may occasionally give the impression of a stratified epithelium. Ultrastructurally, myoepithelial cells closely resemble smooth muscle fibers. They contain microfilament bundles and their cell membrane shows caveolae. They are joined to one another and to the epithelial cells by means of gap junctions and desmosomes, and to the lamina densa of the basement membrane by means of hemidesmosomes.

Myoepithelial cells are most typical in glands associated with the skin and the mouth: the salivary, mammary, sweat and lacrimal glands. They are most numerous in the gland's secretory parts, but may extend to the ducts.

The ducts evacuate the secretory products produced by glands. In glands of the skin and the mouth, the larger part of the duct may be lined by two-layered and stratified epithelia. Otherwise, the ducts are lined by a simple epithelium (Fig. 3.5.5.). In compound glands, the epithelium may differ according to the diameter of the duct branch it lines. In the finest, terminal branches, the epithelium is usually cuboidal, in the more central branches it is prismatic. In this segment of the ducts, the epithelial cells may be brush border cells, with deep infoldings of the basal cell membrane. These characteristics indicate an active participation of these cells in the regulation of the secretion's composition.

III.5.2. Endocrine glands.

Sometimes, the epithelial tube that is the beginning of a gland loses its connection to the overlying epithelium. The deeper, isolated part continues its development to a gland, be it one without a duct. In this way, glands are formed with no connection whatsoever to the outside world. The secretory products are discharged into the intercellular spaces. Such **endocrine glands** only rarely maintain their original epithelial structure. Virtually the only important example of a gland that does that is the thyroid, the endocrine tissue of which is a simple prismatic epithelium lining spherical cavities, and forming follicles (Fig 3.5.7.). Thus, the thyroid contains **follicular tissue**. Usually, endocrine

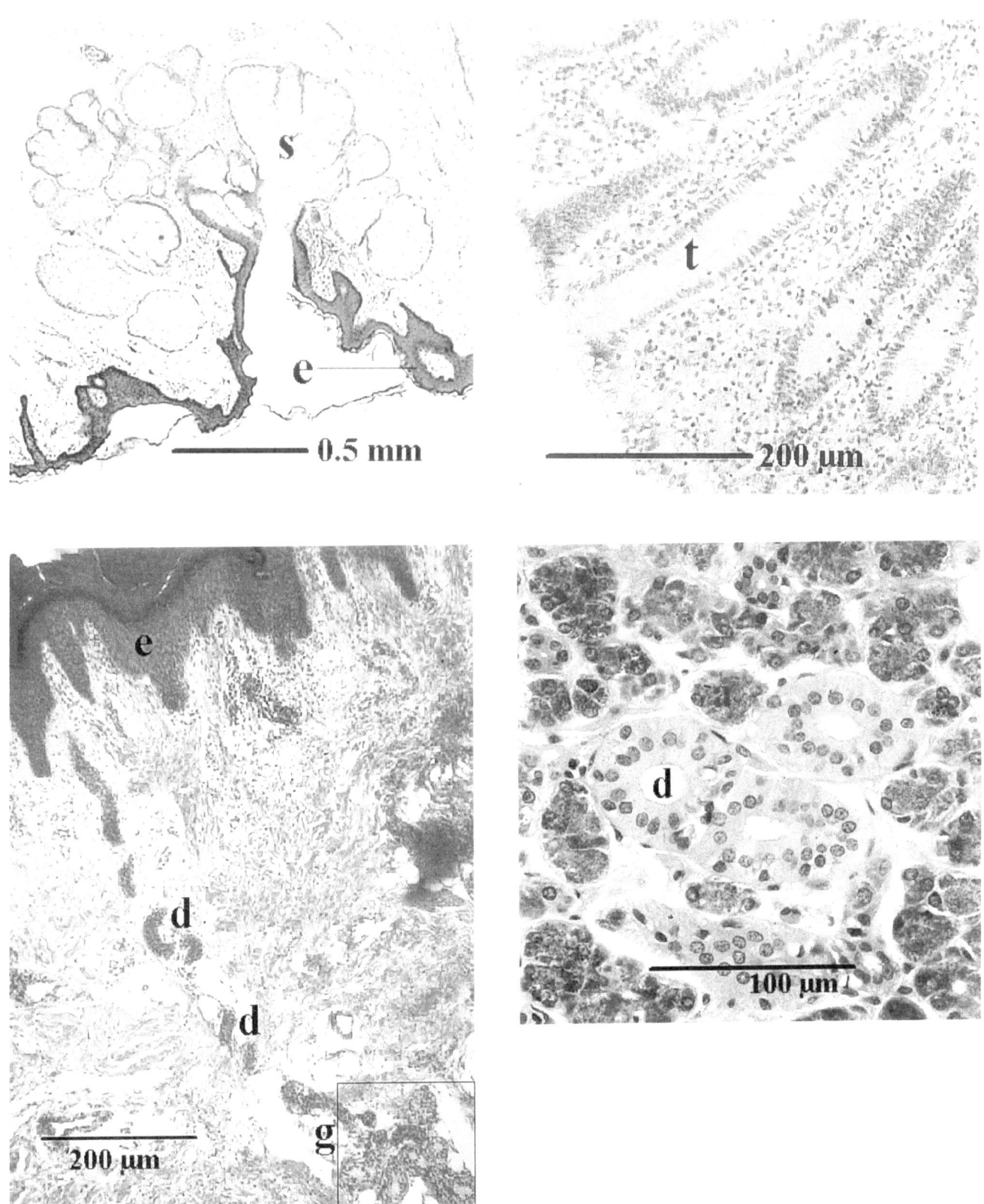

107

Fig. 3.5.2. (top left) Sebaceous glands (s) develop out of inpocketings of the epidermis (e). They are sessile, acinar glands. Nipple, human, HE. **Fig. 3.5.3.** (top right) The mucosal glands of the appendix are sessile, tubular glands (t). Appendix, human, HE. **Fig. 3.5.4.** (bottom left) Sweat glands are simple, tubular glands. The unbranched duct (d) has a straight course, the tubular glandular part (g, rectangle) forms a tight coil. e = epidermis. Skin, human, HE. **Fig. 3.5.5.** (bottom right) Salivary glands are compound, largely acinar, glands. The dark, basophilic acini (a) all show a more or less circular shape in section, which indicates that they are globular structures. In the middle, a few transverse sections of intralobular ducts (d) can be seen. The fact that several of these can be seen in the same section indicates that they are part of a branched system of ducts. Submandibular gland, human, HE.

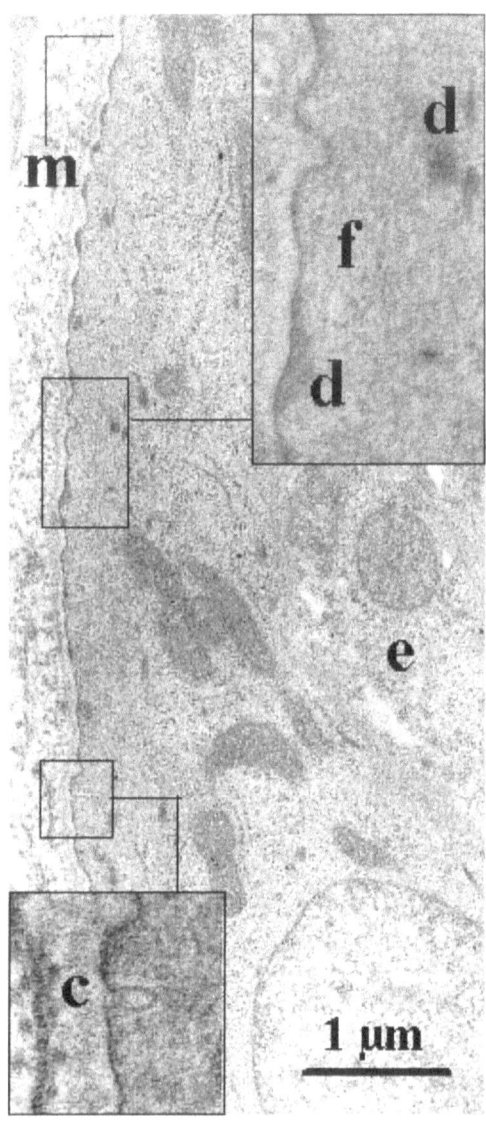

Fig. 3.5.6. Myoepithelial cells are frequently encountered between the basement membrane (m) and the epithelium (e) of glands or ducts. These cells strongly resemble smooth muscle fibers because they contain microfilaments (f), fusiform densities (d) and caveoli (c). Like smooth muscle cells, they are contractile. Sweat gland, cat, TEM.

glandular tissue consists of massive cell cords or trabecules, forming **trabecular tissue** (Fig. 3.5.7.), as is the case in the anterior pituitary gland or adenohypophysis, the parathyroids, and the adrenals. Trabecular tissue does not entirely lose its epithelial

characteristics, though. Cell junctions and a basement membrane are clear reminders that we are dealing with what is, in reality, an epithelium.

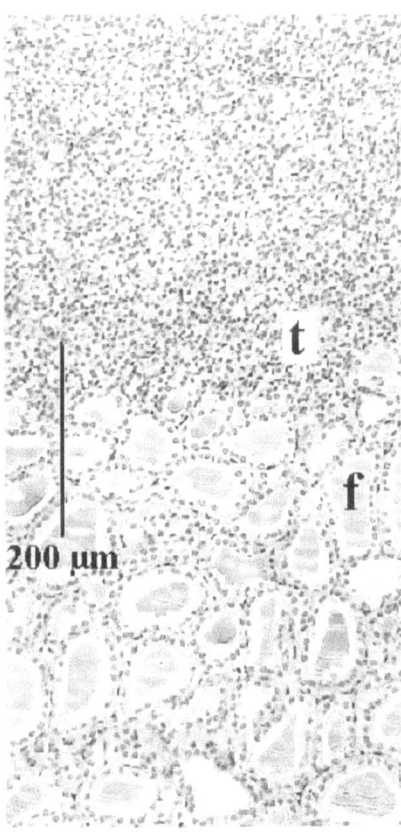

Fig. 3.5.7. Endocrine glandular tissue does not include ducts. In follicular tissue, which is typical of the thyroid gland, the gland cells line cavities or follicles (f). In trabecular tissue, of which the parathyroid gland is an example, the gland cells form massive cell groups or trabecules (t). Thyroid-parathyroid complex, dog, HE.

References.

Redman R.S.: Myoepithelium of salivary glands. Microsc. Res. Techn. 1994, 27: 25-45.

III.6. Nerve tissue.

In several respects, nerve tissue is the most complex tissue. Its constituent cells, the **nerve cells**, may have very complex shapes (II.2.3.). Nerve cells are aggregated into a tissue, but, as we shall see, there are several ways in which nerve cells can be aggregated to form a tissue. Furthermore, in addition to nerve cells, there is a second sharply delineated group of cells that participates in the formation of nerve tissue: **glia cells** (Fig. 3.6.1.). Glia cells, like nerve cells, may have complex shapes (Fig. 3.6.2.). Nerve cells and glia cells may form very complex associations (III.6.1.). Finally, both categories, nerve cells as well as glia cells, can be subdivided into a number of subtypes.

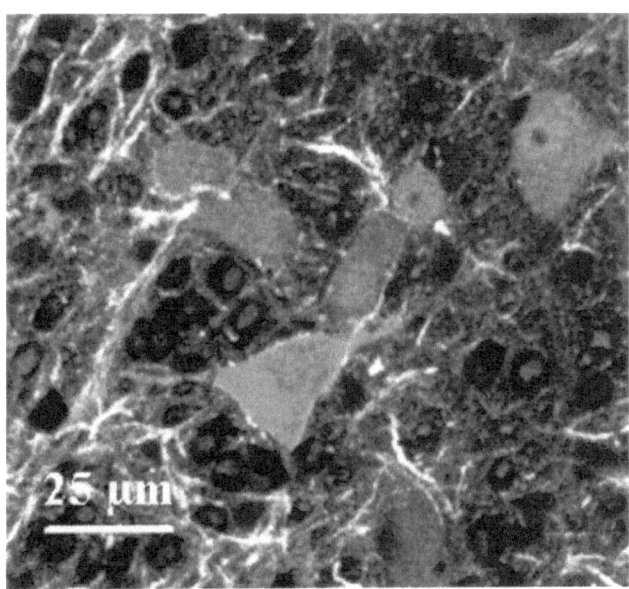 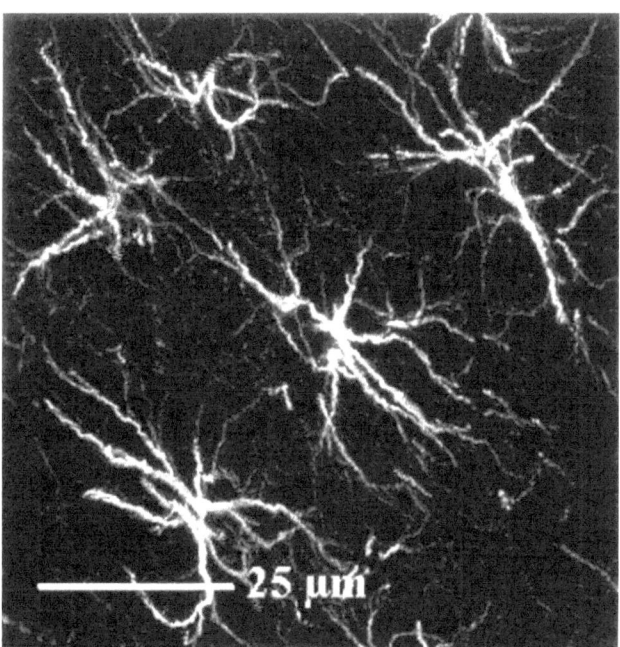

Fig. 3.6.1. (left) Nerve tissue is complex in several respects. Among others, it is composed of 2 sharply divided cell categories: nerve cells and glia cells. In this picture, the nerve cells (n) have been labeled with a fluorochrome, which has been tagged to them by means of an antibody against protein gene product 9.5. Glia cell processes (g) fluoresce with greater intensity, and their fluorochrome has been tagged to them by means of an antibody against glial filbrillary acidic protein. Medulla oblongata, rat, simultaneous recording of two emissions by means of confocal microscopy. **Fig. 3.6.2.** (right) Just like nerve cells, certain types of glia cells, such as astrocytes, have complex shapes due to the presence of processes. Medulla oblongata, rat, TRITC-induced immunofluorescence against glial fibrillary acidic protein, extended depth of focus confocal image.

In nerve tissue, two forms of association between cells are found: bundles and networks. Axons are often grouped in bundles. These bundles conduct action potentials, sometimes over considerable distances. Therefore, this kind of nerve tissue can be called **conductive nerve tissue**. A much more complex form of nerve tissue arises when axon terminals contact the dendrites or perikarya of other nerve cells in order to transmit their action potentials to them. Such contacts between different nerve cells give rise to a network. The point of contact between an axon terminal of one nerve cell and the perikaryon or dendrite of another one is a specialized intercellular junction called a synaptic junction or **synapse**. Synapses are at the basis of the nerve tissue's integrative function (III.6.2.). Because of this, the network variant of nerve tissue can be called **integrative nerve tissue**.

Nerve cells and glia cells have a similar embryonic origin, but diverge early in development. While nerve cells specialize in conduction and transmission of action potentials, glia cells acquire various functions to assist them in these tasks. In conductive nerve tissue, specific types of glia cells associate themselves in a complex way with axons to speed up the conduction of action potentials. In integrative nerve tissue, the association between nerve cells and glia cells is less complex, at least in a morphological sense.

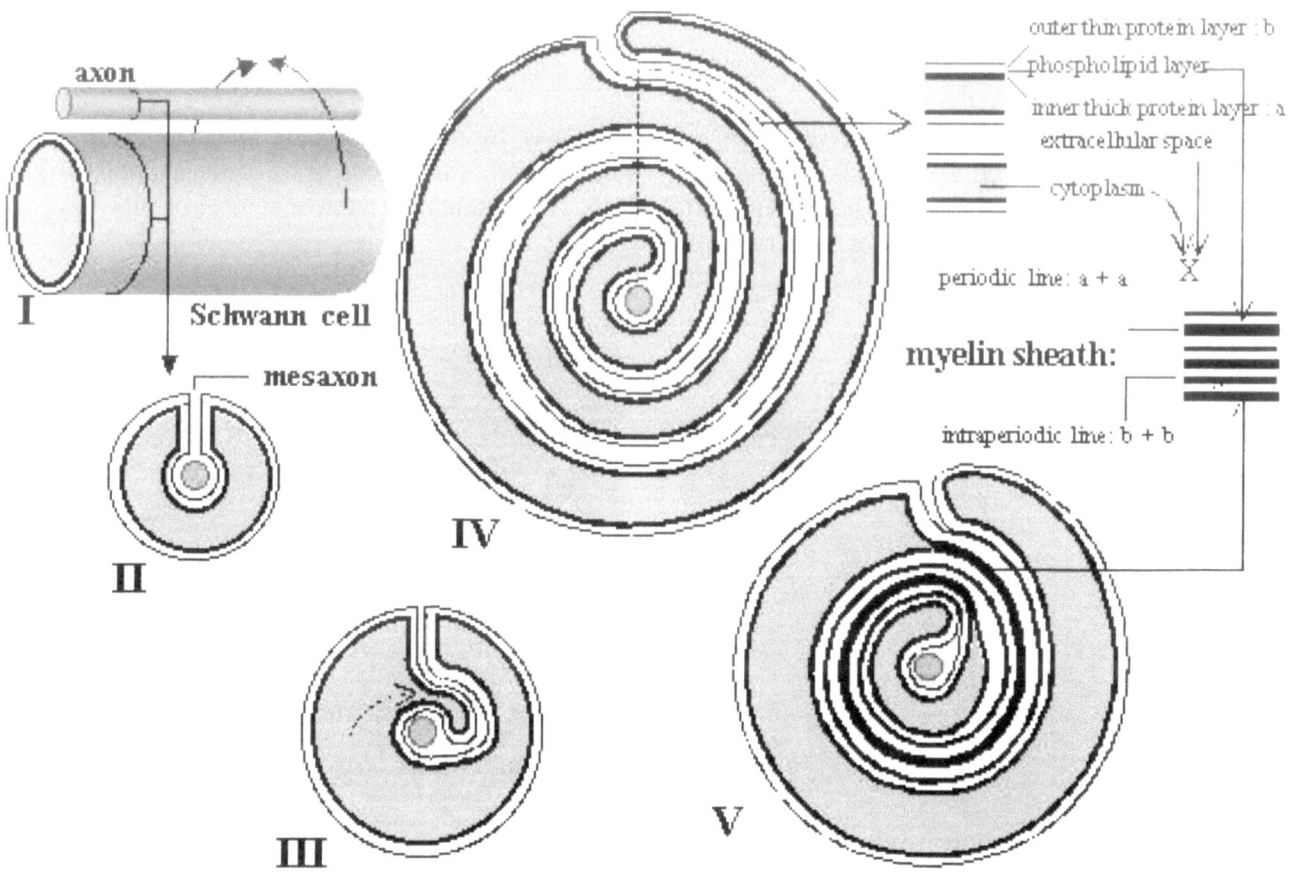

Fig. 3.6.5. Formation of a myelinated nerve fiber. During nervous system development, Schwann cells line up next to an axon (I) and fold around it, so that the axon ends up suspended in a fold of the Schwann cell's membrane, the mesaxon (II). The mesaxon lengthens spirally (III), and the axon is progressively surrounded by a large number of Schwann cell coils (IV). The cytoplasm is extruded from these coils, resulting in fusion of the inner protein layers of the membranes of successive coils. The extracellular space is eliminated by fusion of the outer protein layers of the membranes of successive coils (V). Thus, the resulting myelin sheath is a tight coil of Schwann cell membrane. Axon and Schwann cell not to scale.

III.6.1. Conductive nerve tissue.

Conductive nerve tissue consists of axons, intimately associated with certain types of glia cells: **Schwann cells** and **oligodendrocytes**. In addition, conductive nerve tissue contains less specialized supporting cells, the **fibrillar astrocytes**.

III.6.1.1. Schwann cells.

Schwann cells are exclusively found in the conductive nerve tissue of the peripheral nervous system: the nerves connecting the central nervous system (brain and spinal cord) to the rest of the body. These cells are always found in association with the axon of a nerve cell. Such an association between an axon and a Schwann cell is called a **nerve fiber**. Depending on the complexity of this association, two kinds of nerve fibers can be distinguished: unmyelinated ones and myelinated ones (Fig. 3.6.3.).

Unmyelinated nerve fibers have a relatively simple structure (Fig.3.6.4.). In cross section, they consist of an axon surrounded by a fold of a Schwann cell's cytoplasm. Several axons are accommodated by the same Schwann cell, forming a bundle. The Schwann cell's nucleus occupies the center of the cell, in the center of the axon bundle.

Myelinated nerve fibers have a complex structure and a complex origin (Fig. 3.6.5.).

At some stage during embryonic development, numerous Schwann cells line up next to an axon. The axon deforms the Schwann cells, so that it is suspended in a fold of the Schwann cell's membrane, much like the gut is suspended from the back of the abdominal cavity in a membrane fold, the mesentery. The cell membrane in which the axon is suspended is called the **mesaxon**. In the course of subsequent development, the Schwann cell will wind itself spirally around the axon.

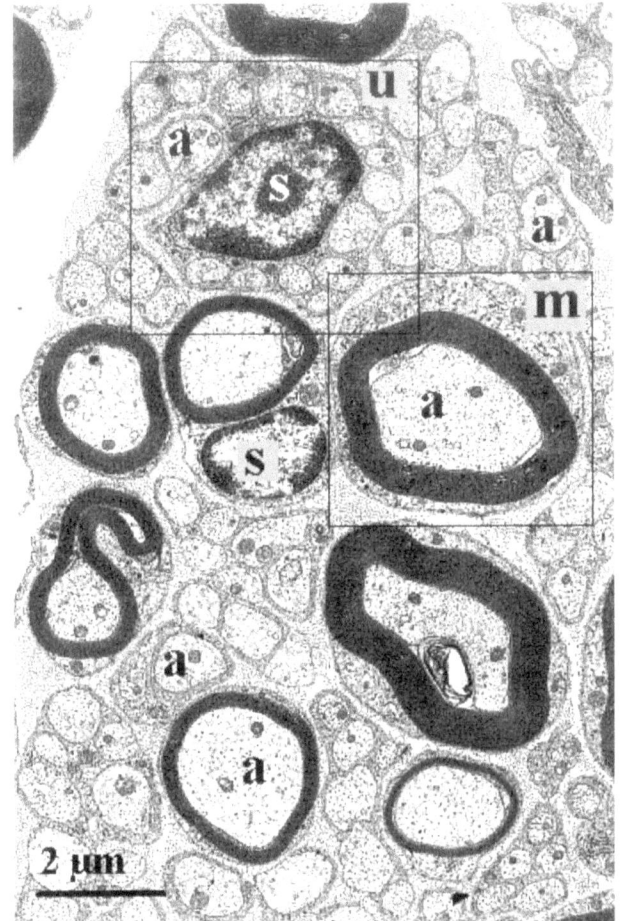

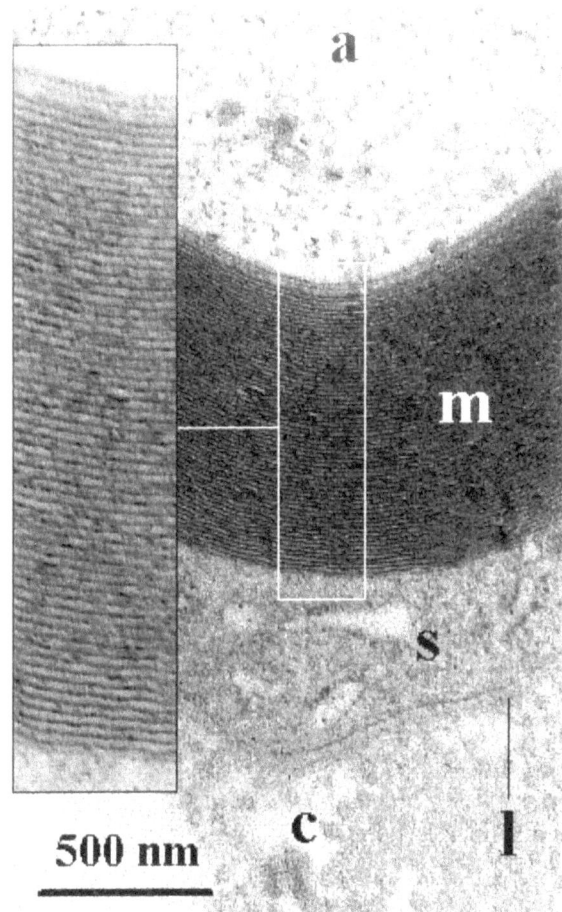

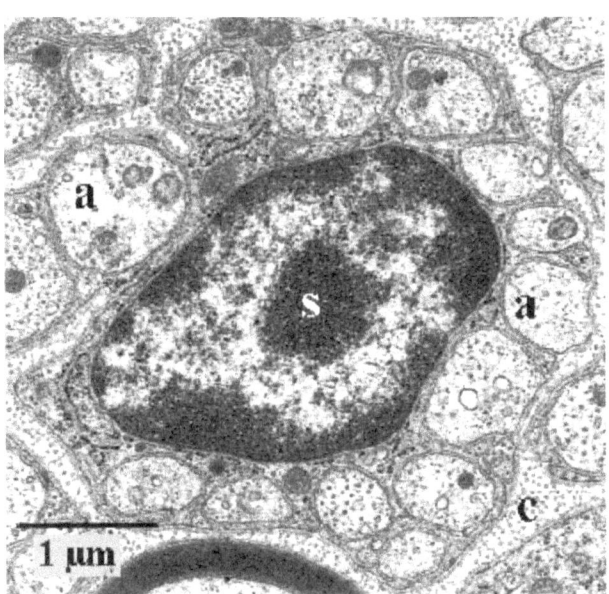

Fig. 3.6.3. (top left) The association between nerve cells and glia cells may very complex. The most complex association is that between axons and Schwann cells (s), which results in the formation of the nerve fibers of the peripheral nervous system. Such nerve fibers can be either unmyelinated (u) or myelinated (m). The second type in particular has a very complex structure. Vagus nerve, rat, TEM. Fig. 3.6.4. (left) A transverse section of a bundle of unmyelinated nerve fibers. The nucleus (n) belongs to a Schwann cell. The Schwann cell's cytoplasm folds and envelops the individual axons (a). c = collagen fibrils. Vagus nerve, rabbit, TEM. Fig. 3.6.6. (above) A transverse section of a myelinated nerve fiber shows the axon (a), the myelin sheath (m) with its characteristic layered structure and the Schwann cell's peripheral cytoplasm (s). Mark the dense lamina (l) of the Schwann cell's basement membrane. c = collagen fibrils. Vagus nerve, rabbit, TEM.

The Schwann cell's membrane has the classical trilaminar structure (II.1.1.). Nevertheless, it is asymmetric. The inner dense protein layer is somewhat thicker than the outer one. As the Schwann cell winds itself around the axon, the outer protein layers of the cell membrane of successive coils touch. Thus, the extracellular space is eliminated. The cytoplasm is extruded from the coils, resulting in the inner protein layers of successive coils touching. The end result is a very compact spiraling of the Schwann cell membrane around the axon, a **myelin sheath**. The relatively thick periodic line is formed by the merging of the inner protein layers of the cell membrane of successive coils. The thinner intraperiodic line is formed by merging of the outer protein layers.

A myelinated nerve fiber thus consists of an axon, wrapped in a myelin sheath (Fig. 3.6.6.). A layer of cytoplasm surrounds the myelin sheath and contains the Schwann cell's nucleus. On the inside of the myelin sheath, touching the axon, another layer of Schwann cell cytoplasm, which has not participated in the formation of the myelin sheath, may be left. The Schwann cell is enveloped by a basement membrane (III.4.1.2.).

The myelin sheath contains proteins but, being derived from cell membrane, is also rich in lipids. During routine preparation for light microscopy, lipid solvents are used and the myelin sheaths appear empty. In the light microscope, transversely sectioned myelinated nerve fibers look like circles, with a dense dot in the center and surrounded by a membrane or neurilemma (Fig. 3.6.7.). Obviously, the neurilemma is not a real cell membrane, which would not be visible in the light microscope. It corresponds to the peripheral cytoplasm of the Schwann cell. The dense central dot is the axon, surrounded with a layer of Schwann cell cytoplasm. Touching the neurilemma, the sausage-shaped Schwann cell nucleus may be seen.

Schwann cells may attain lengths of a millimeter, but remain much too short to myelinate an axon over its entire length, which may be tens of centimeters. To myelinate a complete axon, many tens to hundreds of Schwann cells are necessary. In a longitudinal section of a myelinated nerve fiber, the myelin sheath is seen to be interrupted at more or less regular intervals by transverse "constrictions", the **Ranvier nodes**, which separate successive Schwann cells. The nuclei lie about half way between two nodes. At a node (Fig. 3.6.8.), the exposed part of the axon is narrowed and carries a central swelling. The cytosolic face of the axonal cell membrane is coated with dense material. At both sides of the node, myelinization is incomplete, i.e. the inner protein layers do not touch. Consequently, the Schwann cell membrane forms loops in which cytoplasm is left. The apex of each loop is attached to the axon by means of a tight junction (III.4.1.1.). The inner coils of the Schwann cell are relatively short, and the loops at either end do not reach far. The loops formed by successive, more peripheral coils reach progressively farther along the axon. This is a direct consequence of the trapezium shape of the uncoiled Schwann cell (Fig. 3.6.10.). In this way, a regular row of successive, tightly adhering

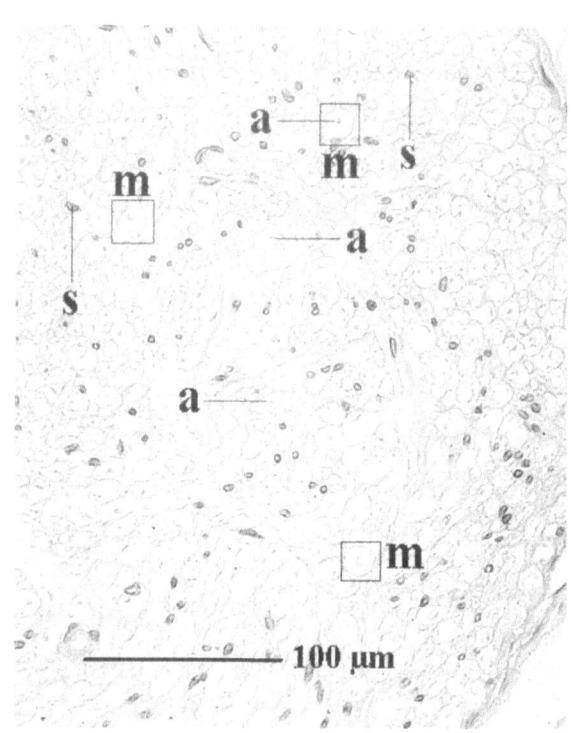

Fig. 3.6.7. Preparation for light microscopy involves the use of lipid solvents. Since myelin sheaths consist of cell membrane and, as a consequence of this, are very rich in lipids, much of them is dissolved. This is why transversely sectioned myelinated nerve fibers (m) look like empty circles under the light microscope. The central dot is the axon (a). The cell nuclei are those of Schwann cells (s) and fibrocytes. Those of Schwann cells are relatively large and euchromatic and may be closely associated with a myelin sheath. Sciatic nerve, human, HE.

loops is formed at either side of the axonal swelling. The last loop forms a number of finger-like protrusions (Fig. 3.6.9.) which interdigitate with the corresponding protrusions of the next Schwann cell, but do not form junctions with them. Thus, unlike the myelinated stretch of the axon, which is sealed off from the extracellular space, the swollen part of it at the Ranvier node remains exposed to it. The basement membrane crosses the nodes uninterrupted.

A longitudinal section of a myelinated nerve fiber also shows a number of interruptions of the myelin sheath that look like slanted lines, the **Schmidt-Lantermann clefts** (Fig. 3.6.11.). These clefts are linear zones where the Schwann cell coils retain cytoplasm and do not participate in the formation of the myelin sheath. The slanted course of these lines is a direct consequence of the trapezium shape of the uncoiled Schwann cell (Fig. 3.6.10.). The function of these clefts remains unclear, but they could make a myelinated fiber more flexible, so that it can adapt to deformation as a consequence of the body's movements. This hypothesis is strengthened by the

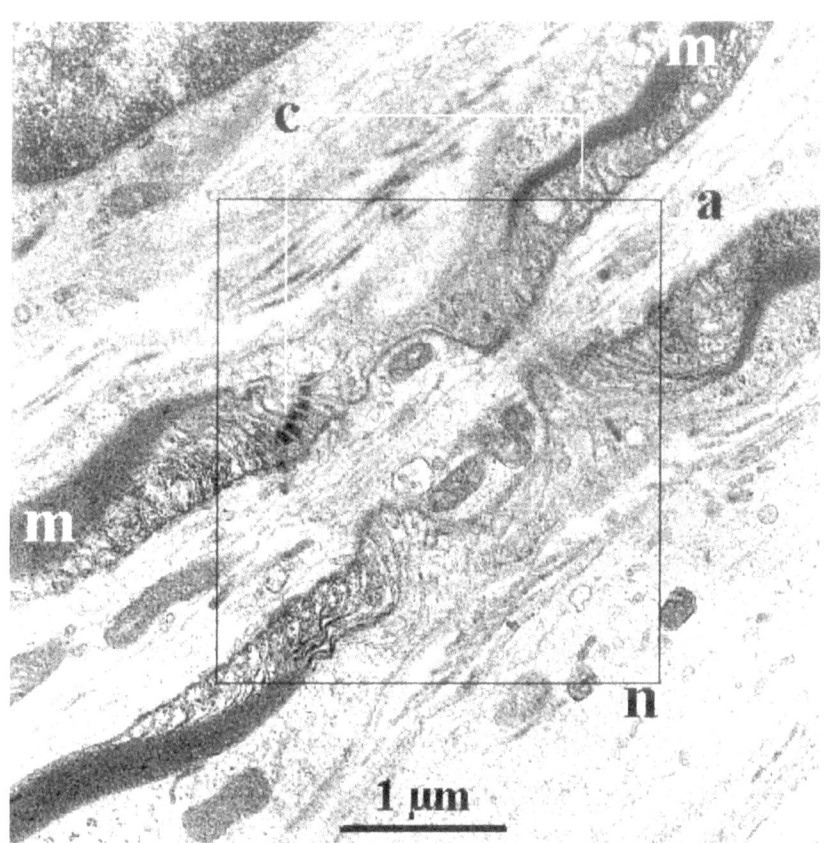

Fig. 3.6.8. Schwann cells are much shorter than the axon they myelinate. Of necessity, the myelin sheath is interrupted at regular intervals by so called Ranvier nodes. A longitudinal section through a Ranvier node shows how an axon (a) initially constricts and, at the actual level of the node, expands again. At both sides of the node, successive coils (c) of the Schwann cell can be observed, as well as part of the myelin sheath (m). Vagus nerve, rabbit, TEM.

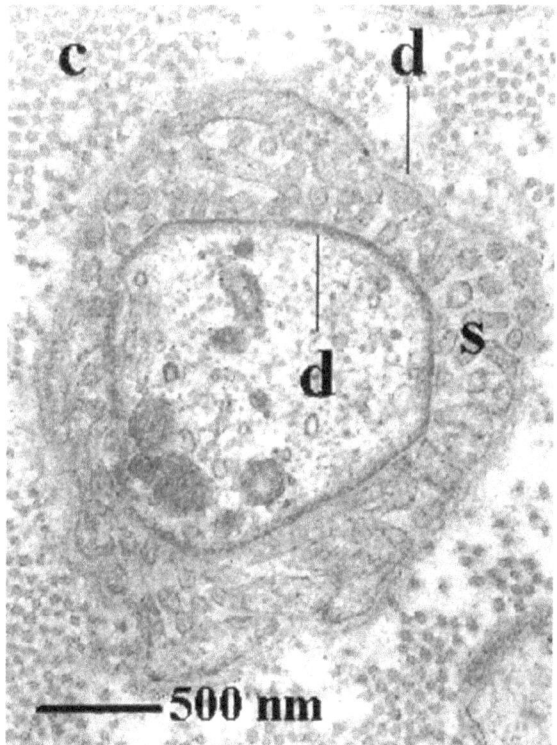

Fig. 3.6.9. A cross section through the middle of a Ranvier node shows how the axon is surrounded by finger-like extensions of the Schwann cell (s). The cytosolic face of the axon's cell membrane is coated with a dense layer (d). Mark the dense lamina (l) of the basement membrane, which crosses the node uninterruptedly. c = collagen fibrils. Vagus nerve, rabbit, TEM.

rarity of Schmidt-Lantermann clefts in the brain where such deformations are, in principle, impossible.

The association of a Schwann cell and an axon is very complex, but of overwhelming physiological

importance. It is clear that myelinated nerve fibers conduct action potentials at much greater velocities than unmyelinated ones. The conduction velocities of unmyelinated fibers are, at most, a few meters per second, while those of myelinated fibers can be ten

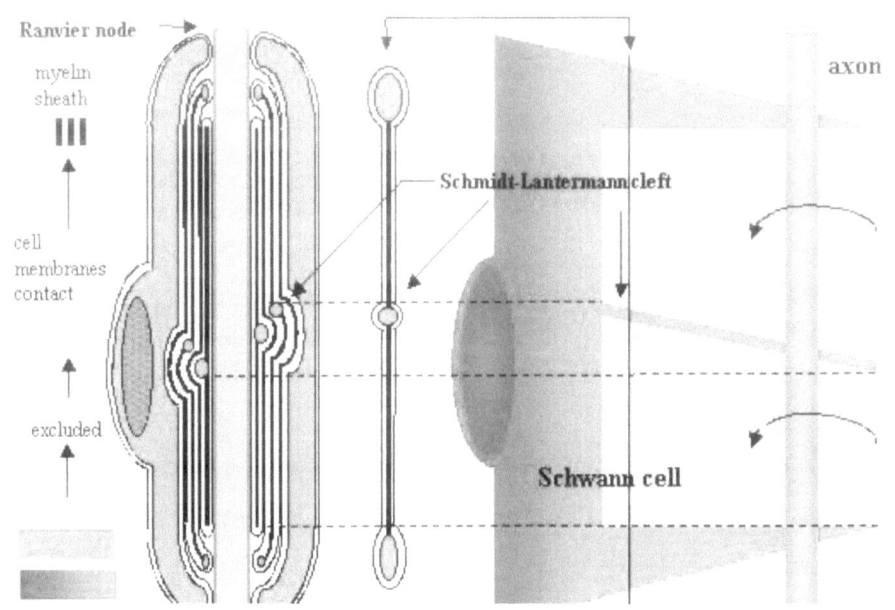

Ranvier node

myelin sheath

‖‖‖

cell membranes contact

excluded

Schmidt-Lantermann cleft

Schwann cell

axon

Fig. 3.6.10. As already shown (Figure 3.6.5.), the Schwann cell's cytoplasm is extruded from its coils during formation of a myelin sheath, resulting in their fusion. However, this drawing of an "uncoiled" Schwann cell shows that local accumulations of cytoplasm are left, resulting in the formation of Schmidt-Lantermann clefts. Other accumulations of cytoplasm are found at the Schwann cell's edges. Because of the slanted course of Schmidt-Lantermann clefts, and the trapezoid shape of the "uncoiled" Schwann cell, longitudinal sections of a myelin sheath will show these clefts as arrow-shaped formations, while successive coils encroach progressively upon the Ranvier node.

times greater. On the scale of the human body, these velocities make conduction of neural signals virtually instantaneous. This considerable difference is determined by the presence or absence of a myelin sheath.

An action potential is able to propagate itself along a membrane by means of a phenomenon referred to as **induction**. A local depolarization creates an electrical field and the membrane pores next to it, being voltage-gated canals, are induced to open. In this way, the action potential spreads and invades successive stretches of membrane. However, lipids are very poor conductors of electricity, so that the myelin sheath will electrically isolate stretches of axon in between the Ranvier nodes. Moreover, it is only at the exposed axonal cell membrane at the nodes that membrane pores are located which determine the distribution of ions at both sides and thus the membrane potential. Consequently, action potentials can only be induced at the nodes. As a result of this, the action potential is not conducted smoothly, as it is in unmyelinated nerve fibers, but "jumps" from one node to the next. This type of conduction is called **saltatory conduction**. Saltatory conduction is not only much faster than smooth conduction, it is also much less energy-consuming. Since the axonal cell membrane

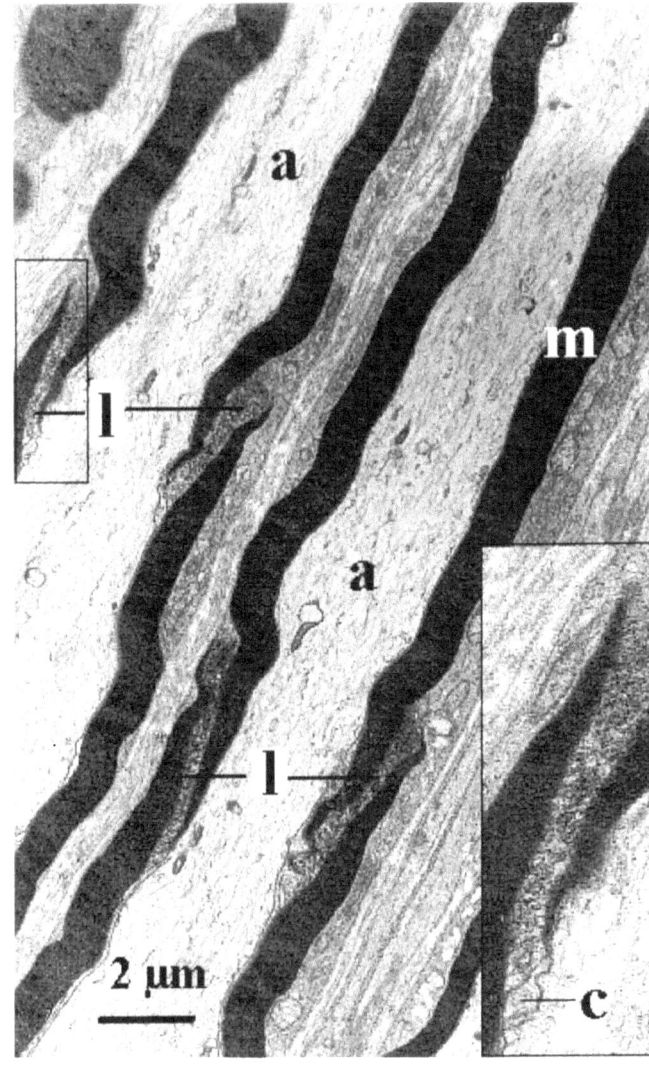

Fig. 3.6.11. In a longitudinal section, Schmidt-Lantermann clefts (l) show up as slanted interruptions (successive coils, c, detach, as it were) of the myelin sheath (m) on both sides of the axon (a). Sciatic nerve, cat, TEM.

depolarizes only locally, few membrane pumps are needed to restore the membrane potential after passage of an action potential.

III.6.1.2. Oligodendrocytes and fibrillar astrocytes.

The oligodendrocyte (Fig. 3.6.12.) is the Schwann cell's counterpart in the central nervous system, where it is an essential part of the conductive nerve tissue and where it myelinates axons. It does not form unmyelinated nerve fibers. The conductive nerve tissue in the central nervous system contains some fibers that are not closely associated with oligodendrocytes. They are either contacted by fibrillar astrocytes or run free in the intercellular spaces.

Oligodendrocytes, as their name implies, are cells with a small number of processes. Only a small amount of cytoplasm is left surrounding the nucleus. Light optically, this gives the impression of a naked nucleus (Fig. 4.4.9.). The nucleus tends to be euchromatic. The processes wind themselves around neighbouring axons and form myelin sheaths, in the same way as the Schwann cells do. Nevertheless, the myelin sheaths formed by oligodendrocytes differ in three respects from those formed by Schwann cells. First, they are not closely associated with the nucleus, which lies in the cell body forming the processes. Therefore, the cytoplasm surrounding the myelin sheath is thinner than that of a Schwann cell. Second, a single oligodendrocyte can myelinate stretches of several axons, since it has several processes. Third, the myelin sheaths of oligodendrocytes lack Schmidt-Lantermann clefts. The Ranvier nodes have the same overall structure as those of the peripheral nervous system. Since there is very little cytoplasm at the periphery of the myelin sheath, however, no interdigitating finger-like extensions are formed. Their place is occupied by the so-called perinodal processes of the fibrillar astrocytes.

In addition to oligodendrocytes, the conductive nerve tissue of the central nervous system contains fibrillar astrocytes (Fig. 3.6.13.), which are not directly involved in the conduction of action potentials, but which support the axons. The nuclei of the fibrillar astrocytes are somewhat less euchromatic than those of the oligodendrocytes. Fibrillar astrocytes carry a number of fairly long and extensively branched processes, supported by bundles of intermediary filaments (Fig. 3.6.14.), which penetrate between the axons of the conductive nerve tissue. They support the myelin sheaths, the naked axons and the endothelial lining of the blood capillaries (III.4.2.). In some places they also support the pia mater (IV.4.8.) and the ependymal cells (IV.4.7.). Around blood capillaries and at the inside of the pia mater, the astrocyte's terminals expand to form end feet and may line up and be joined with tight junctions (III.4.1.1.). Thus, a cohesive lining is formed, light optically visible as a glial limiting membrane.

III.6.2. Integrative nerve tissue.

Integrative nerve tissue contains axon terminals and nerve cell perikarya. Both elements form connections between nerve cells, called **synapses**. In addition, the integrative nervous tissue contains a fairly specific type of glia cell, the **protoplasmic astrocyte**.

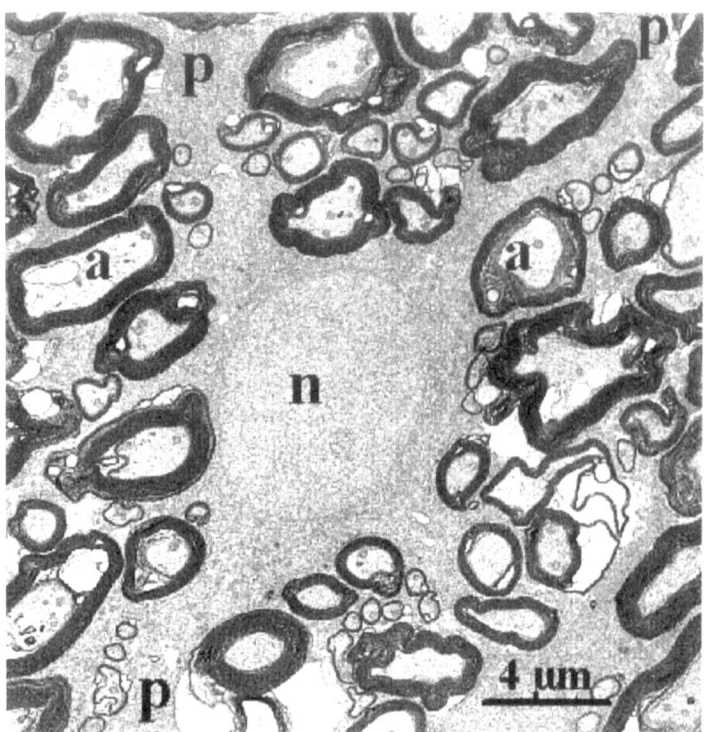

Fig. 3.6.12. Oligodendrocytes form the central nervous system's myelin sheaths. They have a euchromatic nucleus (n), and several processes (p), by means of which they can myelinate several axons (a). Spinal cord, rabbit, TEM.

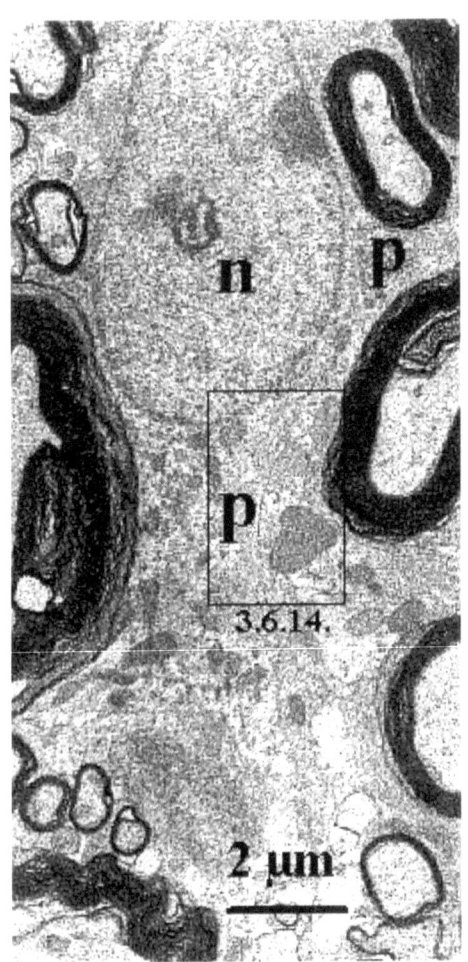

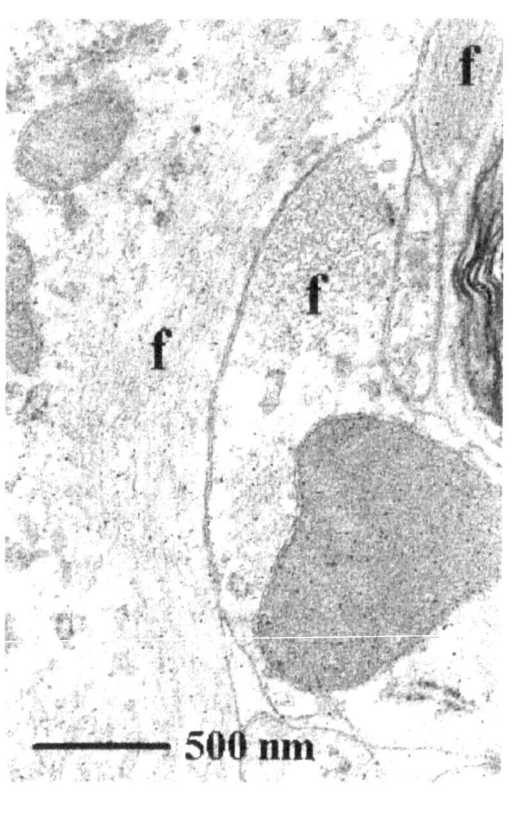

Fig. 3.6.13. (far left) Astrocytes can be regarded as the central nervous system's supporting cells. Fibrillary astrocytes predominate in the conductive tissue of the white matter. Their nucleus (n) is relatively rich in chromatin and they form a number of processes (p), which penetrate between surrounding nerve fibers. Spinal cord, rabbit, TEM. **Fig. 3.6.14.** (left) The cytoplasm of fibrillary astrocytes is rich in intermediary filaments (f), a typical characteristic of reinforced, supporting cell. The fine granulation is artefactual precipitate. Spinal cord, rabbit, TEM.

It is through synapses that nerve cells transmit signals to one another. Interconnected nerve cells form specific circuits that ensure that a stimulus is followed by the correct reaction (Fig. 3.6.15.). A well-known example of this is the quick withdrawal of the hand when it touches a sharp or hot object. This

116

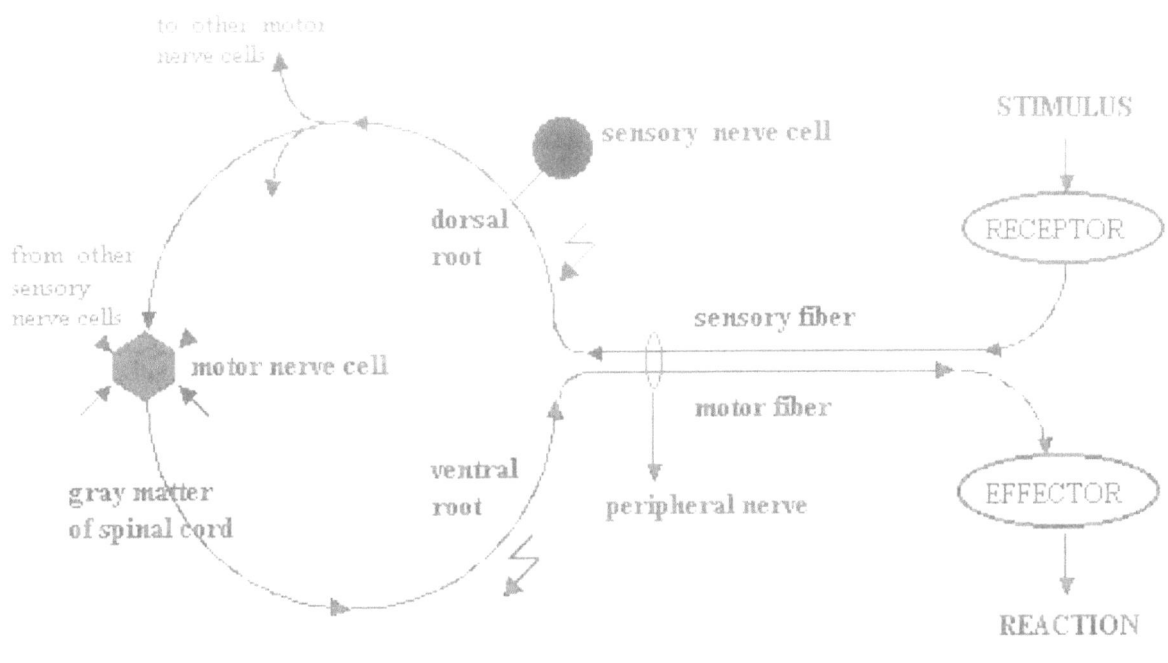

to other motor
nerve cells

sensory nerve cell

STIMULUS

dorsal
root

RECEPTOR

from other
sensory
nerve cells

sensory fiber

motor nerve cell

motor fiber

ventral
root

EFFECTOR

gray matter
of spinal cord

peripheral nerve

REACTION

NEURAL INTEGRATION 1: THE REFLEX ARC

Fig. 3.6.15. In a nutshell, nerve tissue's integrative function ensures that a particular stimulus, picked up by a receptive organ or receptor, is answered by the appropriate reaction of an effector (a muscle fiber or gland cell). This is accomplished by neurally linking the receptor and the effector at the level of the central nervous system, in this case the spinal cord. A stimulus selectively interacts with an appropriate receptor, is converted into an action potential, and conducted to the spinal cord by a sensory nerve fiber. The sensory fiber enters the spinal cord and participates in a synaptic junction with a motor nerve cell. The action potential is transmitted to the motor nerve cell. This nerve cell's axon forms a motor nerve fiber, which leaves the spinal cord. The motor nerve fiber conducts the action potential to an effector, which shows a specific reaction. It looks as though the signal reflects at the level of the spinal cord, entering and returning as it does. This is why this physiological mechanism is called a reflex, and its morphological substrate a reflex arc.

phenomenon, the **reflex**, is the basis of what is called the integrative function of the nervous system. A monosynaptic reflex (Fig. 3.6.15.) is the simplest example of neural integration, but it is rare. Neural integration is almost always more complex (Fig. 3.6.16.) because a given nerve cell will receive signals from several other nerve cells (**convergence**) and in turn, it will transmit a signal to several other nerve cells (**divergence**). Another factor to be taken into account is **summation**. Different stimuli can have opposing effects on the membrane potential. A given nerve cell can be stimulated by some nerve cells, as well as inhibited by others. The membrane of a nerve cell perikaryon may depolarize upon stimulation, but it may also hyperpolarize, when the nerve cell undergoes inhibition. Depolarization decreases the membrane potential, making it more probable that the nerve cell is going to "fire", i.e. to produce an action potential at the axon hillock. Hyperpolarization increases the

membrane potential, reducing the probability of "firing". The perikaryon adds these changes algebraically: the polarity, positive or negative, of the change is taken into account. Only when the sum total depolarization is sufficiently large, and a threshold value is reached, will an action potential arise at the axon hillock. In addition, the magnitude of depolarization determines at what frequency the nerve cell "fires". Nerve cells use frequency modulation to transmit information. Finally, synapses are not static, but dynamic. Repetitive use will give rise to reversible functional and structural changes, which are linked to learning and memory.

III.6.2.1. Synapses.

Synapses (Figs. 3.6.17.-18.) are specialized junctions between two nerve cells that are used to transmit

117

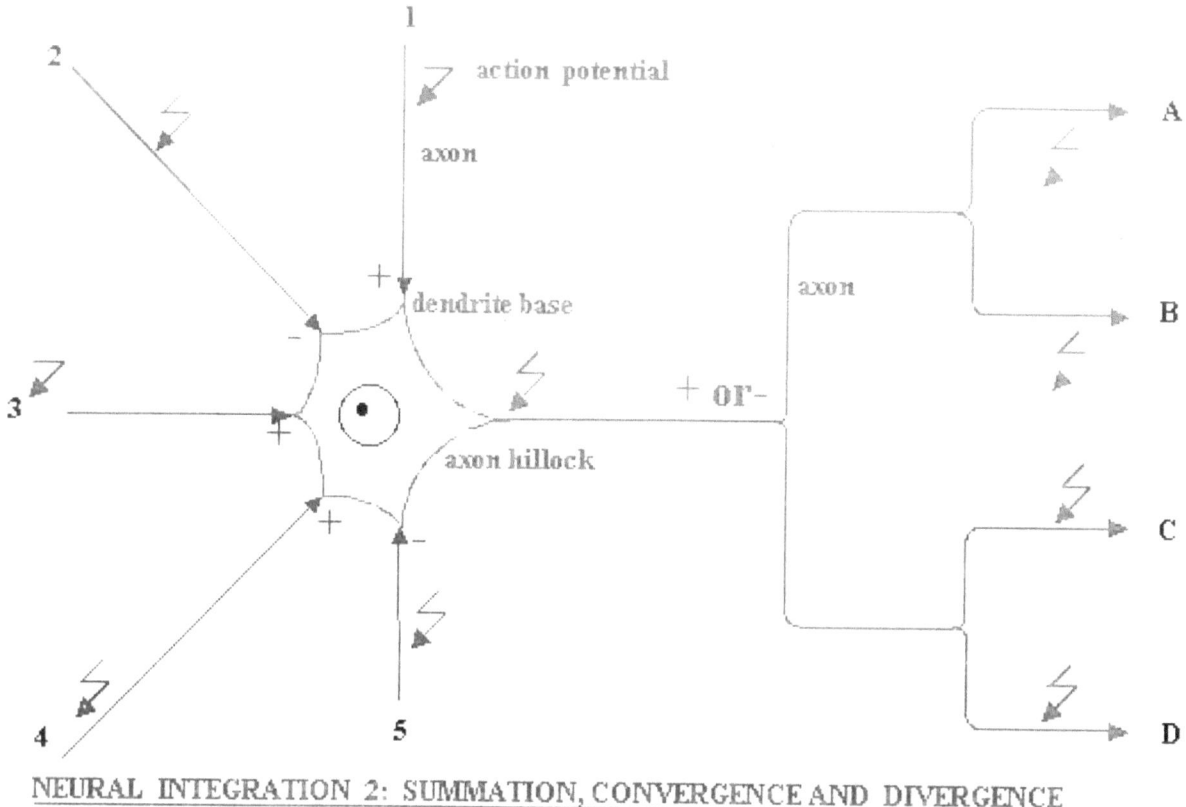

Fig. 3.6.16. Linking the right reactions to particular stimuli through a monosynaptic reflex arc (Figure 3.6.15.), is the simplest example of nerve tissue's integrative function. Usually, the situation is incomparably more complex, although based on the same mechanism, because a nerve cell body is contacted by many nerve fibers (convergence), and in turn sends signals to many other nerve cells (divergence). In addition, a nerve cell body may receive excitatory (+), as well as inhibitory (-), signals. The first depolarize a nerve cell's membrane, enhancing the probability that new action potentials will be induced at the axon hillock, while the second hyperpolarize the cell membrane, lowering this probability. These various stimuli are algebraically added, and when the sum is positive (and sufficiently large), a new action potential arises, excitatory or inhibitory, depending on the type of nerve cell that forms it.

signals from one nerve cell, the **presynaptic nerve cell**, to the other, the **postsynaptic nerve cell**. At the synaptic junction, a narrow intercellular space, referred to as the **synaptic cleft**, and about 20 nanometers wide, extends between both nerve cells.

At a synaptic junction, the presynaptic axon terminal is distended and forms an **end knob** that contains secretory vesicles, the **synaptic vesicles**. Often, the interior face of the presynaptic membrane carries accumulations of a dense material that may appear pyramidal and rest with their bases on the cell membrane. From a top view, seen from the presynaptic axon, these dense bodies are arranged in a hexagonal pattern, called the presynaptic grid. The extent of the free, uncovered membrane patches is similar to the diameter of the synaptic vesicles. The grid's dense bodies may anchor elements of the axonal cytoskeleton to the presynaptic membrane. Upon depolarization of the presynaptic membrane by an

incoming action potential, synaptic vesicles are displaced towards it, probably guided by elements of the axonal cytoskeleton. Between the grid's dense bodies, they dock with the cell membrane and undergo exocytosis, i.e. their contents are emptied, merocrine fashion (II.2.1.1.1.-2., II.2.1.3.), into the synaptic cleft. In the synaptic cleft proper, structural details are occasionally observed. A dense layer can sometimes be seen which runs parallel, but not necessarily equidistant, to the synaptic membranes. A series of filaments that connect the synaptic membranes across the cleft may also be observed. These elements somewhat resemble parts of traditional epithelial cell junctions (III.4.1.1.).

A layer of dense material may coat the postsynaptic membrane's interior face. When present, this layer is always of uniform thickness.

The postsynaptic element is, in principle, a perikaryon or a dendrite. Such synapses are called **axosomatic**

118

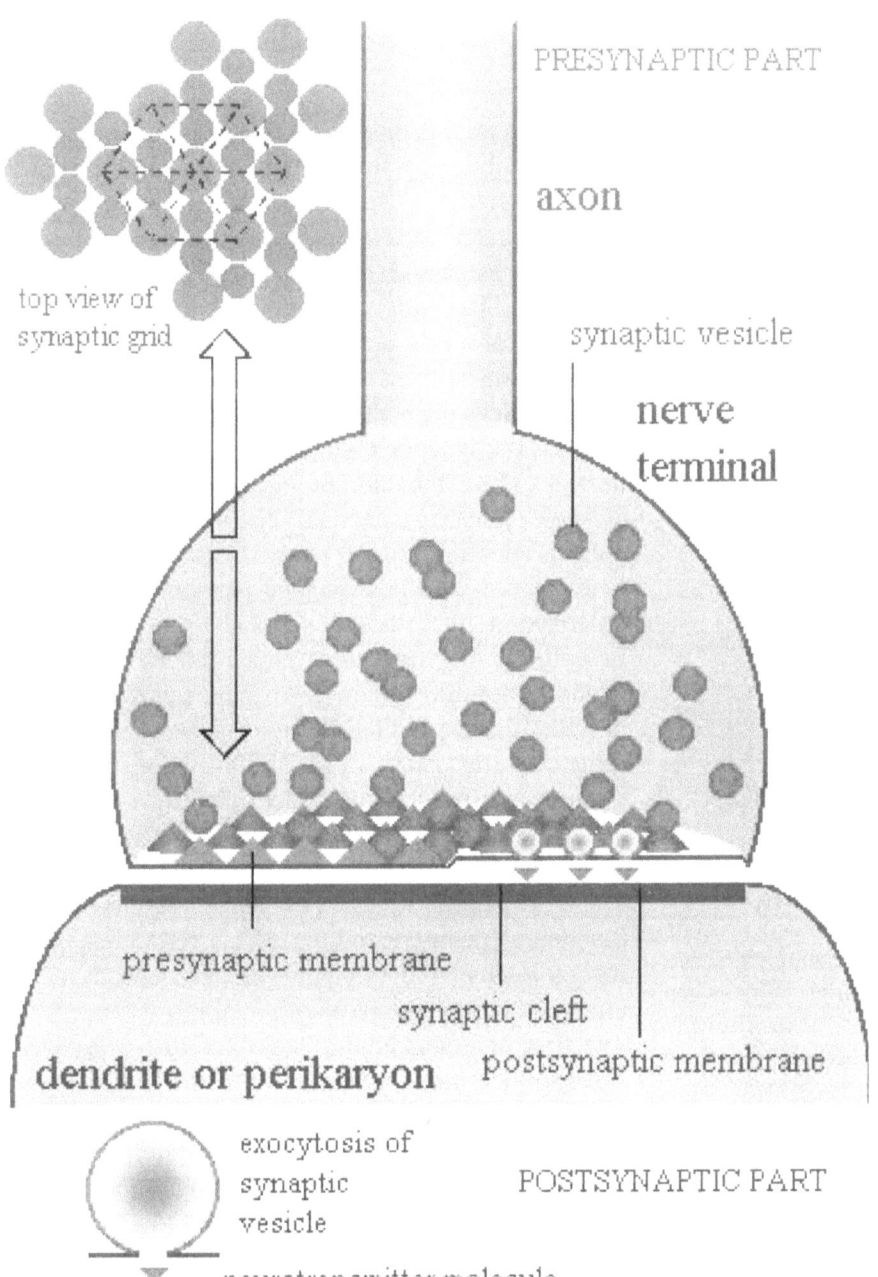

top view of synaptic grid

PRESYNAPTIC PART

axon

synaptic vesicle

nerve terminal

presynaptic membrane

synaptic cleft

postsynaptic membrane

dendrite or perikaryon

POSTSYNAPTIC PART

exocytosis of synaptic vesicle

neurotransmitter molecule

Fig. 3.6.17. A synaptic junction. The axon terminal expands, forming an end knob, which contains synaptic vesicles. The cytosolic face of the end knob's cell membrane, the presynaptic membrane, is studded with pyramidal bodies, arranged (top view, upper left) in a hexagonal pattern. Upon depolarization of the presynaptic membrane by an incoming action potential, the synaptic vesicles dock with the exposed membrane between the pyramidal bodies, and undergo exocytosis. The liberated transmitter molecules enter the synaptic cleft and interact with receptors in the postsynaptic membrane, which is uniformly thickened and belongs (in principle) to a dendrite or a perikaryon, inducing a new action potential.

and **axodendritic**, respectively. In many axodendritic synapses, the dendrite forms a thorny projection: a dendritic spine (Fig. 3.6.18.). In the spine's cytoplasm, a few parallel cisterns of the smooth endoplasmic reticulum are usually present. In some cases, the postsynaptic element may be another axon: an **axoaxonal synapse**. Such synapses are mostly limited to the axon hillock or the axon terminal. While other synapses stimulate the postsynaptic nerve cell, axoaxonal synapses are usually involved in neural inhibition.

Most often, synaptic vesicles are round, with a diameter of about 40 nanometers. Transmission of signals across the synaptic cleft is based on a merocrine secretory mechanism. Upon depolarization of the presynaptic membrane, synaptic vesicles undergo exocytosis. Since the synaptic cleft does not open into the exterior world, nerve cells are in fact endocrine gland cells. The liberated substance is a **neurotransmitter**. Neurotransmitter molecules diffuse across the synaptic cleft and interact with specific receptor molecules or pores in the postsynaptic membrane. As a consequence, the

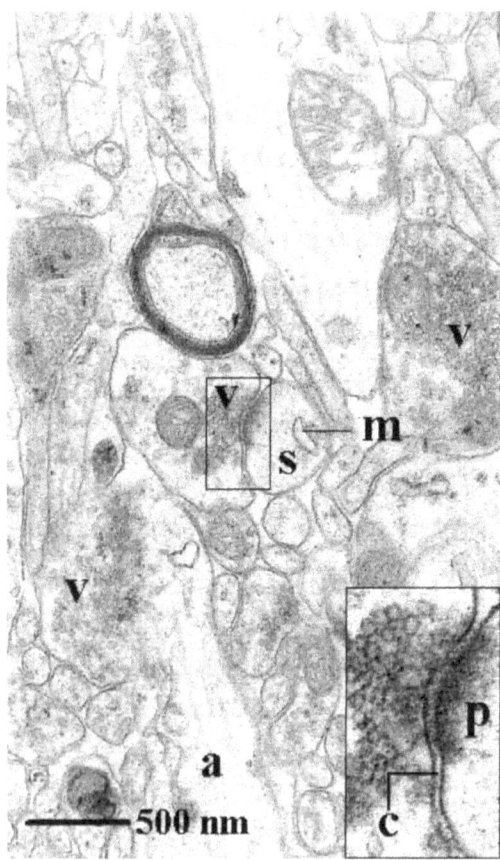

direction only, because only the presynaptic part contains the essential neurotransmitter substance. It can be experimentally demonstrated that nerve fibers are able to conduct action potentials in both senses. In the intact organism, this does not happen, because an action potential is induced at the beginning of the axon (the axon hillock) from where it can only run in a single direction. Once initiated, an action potential cannot spread backwards because, when the action potential has passed, the axon is **refractory** for a brief period (milliseconds), meaning that it is insensitive to induction of a new action potential. Should an action potential arrive from the wrong direction, the synaptic junction lacks the neurotransmitter required to transmit it across the synaptic cleft, and the action potential will decay. Thus, the morphological polarization of the synaptic junction (unequal distribution of vesicles, unequal distribution of dense material at the inner faces of pre- and postsynaptic membranes) confers a polarization in the functional sense as well. Essentially, therefore, the synaptic junction is a switch which either allows current to pass (unidirectionally) or not. It is the biological equivalent of an electronic switch, a transistor. The billions upon billions of synapses in the nervous system are equivalent to the chips in a computer's processor.

Fig. 3.6.18. An axodendritic synaptic junction. An axon (a) forms a terminal expansion or end knob, filled with synaptic vesicles (v). One end knob almost touches a thorny process, or spina (s), of another nerve cell's dendrite. This is the junction's postsynaptic part. The spina characteristically displays a tripartite membrane complex, partially seen here (m). Between end knob and spina is a narrow synaptic cleft. At both sides of the cleft, the cytosolic faces of the membranes are coated with dense material. This is especially prominent at the level of the postsynaptic membrane (p). The presynaptic membrane is rather irregularly thickened. Cerebral cortex, rat, TEM.

membrane's permeability to certain ions is changed. This may lead to either depolarization or hyperpolarization of the postsynaptic membrane. In the first case, the postsynaptic element is stimulated. In the second place, it is inhibited. Because of the crucial intervention of a chemical substance, the transmission of signals between nerve cells is called **chemical neurotransmission**.

Thus, the action potential itself does not cross the synaptic junction. This is to be expected, since an action potential can only be conducted via a membrane, and there is no continuity of membranes at the synaptic junction. The phenomenon of chemical neurotransmission elegantly explains how a signal can cross a synaptic junction. But there is more to it than this: a synaptic junction transmits signals in a single

There are several kinds of chemical substances which function as neurotransmitters. To a certain extent, the morphology of the synaptic vesicles depends on the kind of neurotransmitter they contain.

The first neurotransmitter substance to be discovered was **acetylcholine**. Synapses, or nerve cells, using this substance for neurotransmission are called cholinergic. Synaptic vesicles containing acetylcholine have a diameter of about 40 nanometers and a translucent content. Acetylcholine is produced by choline acetylase. After release, there is reuptake of acetylcholine in the presynaptic end knob, where it is broken down by acetylcholinesterase.

Another well-known neurotransmitter is **noradrenaline**, which is used in adrenergic synapses and nerve cells. Noradrenaline is an amine, derived from the amino acid tyrosine. Its chemical precursor, **dopamine**, is also a neurotransmitter, in dopaminergic synapses. After release and interaction with the postsynaptic membrane, these amines can be broken down in the synaptic cleft by MAO (monoamine oxidase), or they can be taken up in the presynaptic end knob, where they are broken down by COMT (catechol-O-methyl transferase). Another amine with a neurotransmitter function is **serotonin** (5-hydroxytryptamin). Synaptic vesicles containing amines have a diameter of about 40 nanometers and contain a dense core, surrounded by a translucent halo.

They are analogous to the secretory vesicles of amine hormone-secreting gland cells (II.2.1.3.).

From the above, the correlation between transmitter substance and vesicular morphology would appear to be fairly straightforward, but the discovery of many other neurotransmitters has made the situation quite complicated. Some neurotransmitter substances are amino acids, such as **glutamate** and **GABA** (gamma amino butyric acid). GABA is an inhibitory neurotransmitter. It does not depolarize the postsynaptic nerve cell, but hyperpolarizes it, making it less likely that it will generate action potentials. GABA has been linked with translucent, ellipsoid synaptic vesicles. Yet other neurotransmitters are peptides (short strings of amino acids). A few examples of such peptide neurotransmitters, associated with peptidergic synapses, are **VIP** (vasoactive intestinal peptide: it has contractive effects on blood vessels and was first discovered in the gut), **substance P** (P stands for pressure: it enhances blood pressure), and **CGRP** (calcitonin gene related peptide: the gene coding for it is next to that of the hormone calcitonin). As far as is known, peptide neurotransmitters occur in synaptic vesicles with an opaque content and a fairly large diameter of about 120 nanometers. Recently, it was found that **nitrous oxide** (NO) functions as a neurotransmitter in nitrergic synapses. This is a very unusual neurotransmitter in that it is not stored in vesicles, but occurs in soluble form in the cytosol.

At the present time, it is unclear why there are so many neurotransmitter substances. And the picture is further complicated by the phenomenon of colocalization. Many synapses contain more than one kind of neurotransmitter. Synapses may contain two or more kinds of vesicles, each with their own type of neurotransmitter (a common combination is acetylcholine, or an amine, and a peptide), but there are situations in which a single vesicle contains more than one neurotransmitter. Apparently, nerve cells use a very complicated chemical language to talk to each other, and we have only begun to decipher that language.

Relatively simple neurotransmitter molecules (acetylcholine, amines, amino acids) are synthesized locally, in the axonal end knobs by cytosolic enzymes, and concentrated in synaptic vesicles by means of vesicular membrane pumps. The synaptic vesicles are formed by budding from the local smooth endoplasmic reticulum. Upon transmitter release, they are recuperated from the axonal cell membrane and may either be reused directly or recycled via the smooth endoplasmic reticulum. The peptide transmitters are synthesized in the perikaryon's rough endoplasmic reticulum and synaptic vesicles form at the Golgi-complex. They reach the axonal end knob by anterograde transport. Recycling of vesicular membrane is probably via the perikaryon.

Chemical neurotransmission can be manipulated in various ways. Chemical substances that resemble a neurotransmitter to a certain extent may interact with that neurotransmitter's receptors at the postsynaptic membrane, stimulating or inhibiting them. The enzymes that normally break down a neurotransmitter shortly after its release and thus inhibit it, may be unable to handle a "false" neurotransmitter. The results range from excessive, uncontrolled stimulation to total block. These effects may be reversible or permanent. Drugs, anesthetics, and plant, snake and insect toxins are in many cases such "false" transmitters.

III.6.2.2. Cytoplasmic astrocytes.

Associated with integrative nerve tissue are astrocytes, which mainly belong to the cytoplasmic type. Cytoplasmic astrocytes, like nerve cells, have a euchromatic nucleus. It is significantly smaller, however, than a neural nucleus. The cytoplasm forms a number of processes. The perinuclear cytoplasm is somewhat more abundant as in fibrillar astrocytes. Light optically, it cannot be distinguished from the surrounding tissue, which gives the impression of a naked nucleus (Fig. 4.4.9.). The processes are shorter and relatively lacking in filaments as compared to fibrillar astrocytes. At their tips, the processes may be extended to form end feet. The end feet of many astrocytes line nerve cell perikarya and processes and the abluminal face of capillary endothelial cells (III.4.2.). In some places, they line the abluminal face of the ependymal cells (IV.4.7.) and the underside of the pia mater (IV.4.8.). Neighbouring end feet are joined by tight junctions (III.4.1.1.) and form a cohesive layer, particularly around the capillaries and under the pia mater, which may be visible by light microscopy as a glial limiting membrane.

References.

Agnihotri N., Lopez-Garcia J.C., Hawkins R.D., Arancio O.: Morphological changes associated with long-term potentiation. Histol. Histopathol. 1998, 13: 1155-1162.

Dresbach T., Qualmann B., Kessels M.M., Garner C.C., Gundelfinger E.D.: The presynaptic cytomatrix of brain synapses. Cell. Mol. Life Sci. 2001, 58: 94-116.

Harris K.M.: Structure, development and plasticity of dendritic spines. Curr. Opin. Neurobiol. 1999, 9: 343-348.

Hildebrand C;, Remahl S., Persson H., Bjartmar C.: Myelinated nerve fibres in the CNS. Prog. Neurobiol. 1993, 40: 319-384.

Kawai Y.: Ultrastructure of neuronal circuitry in sympathetic ganglia. Microsc. Res. Tech. 1996, 35: 146-156.

Morell P., Norton W.T.: Myelin. Sci. Am. 1980, may, 74-89.

Nakazawa E., Ishikawa H.: Ultrastructural observations of astrocyte end-feet in the rat central nervous system. J. Neurocytol. 1998, 27: 431-440.

Peters A., Palay S.L.: The morphology of synapses. J. Neurocytol. 1996, 25: 687-700.

Smolen A.J.: Morphology of synapses in the autonomic nervous system. J. Electron Microsc. Tech. 1988, 10: 187-204.

Walmsley B., Alvarez F.J., Fyffe R.E.W.: Diversity of structure and function at mammalian central synapses. Trends Neurosci. 1998, 21: 81-88.

IV. ORGANS.

Tissues participate in a structure with a higher level of organization, an **organ**. Organs that closely cooperate form an organ system. A logical sequence in which organs may be discussed suggests itself when the number of tissues they contain, and the complexity of those tissues, is considered. Thus, there are organs in which one type of tissue predominates. These form the first four systems of our classification. In each subsequent system, a tissue predominates which is more complex, according to our discussion of tissues. In the next five, at least two types of tissue predominate. In the last six, several types of tissues are readily apparent, sometimes as much as five or six.

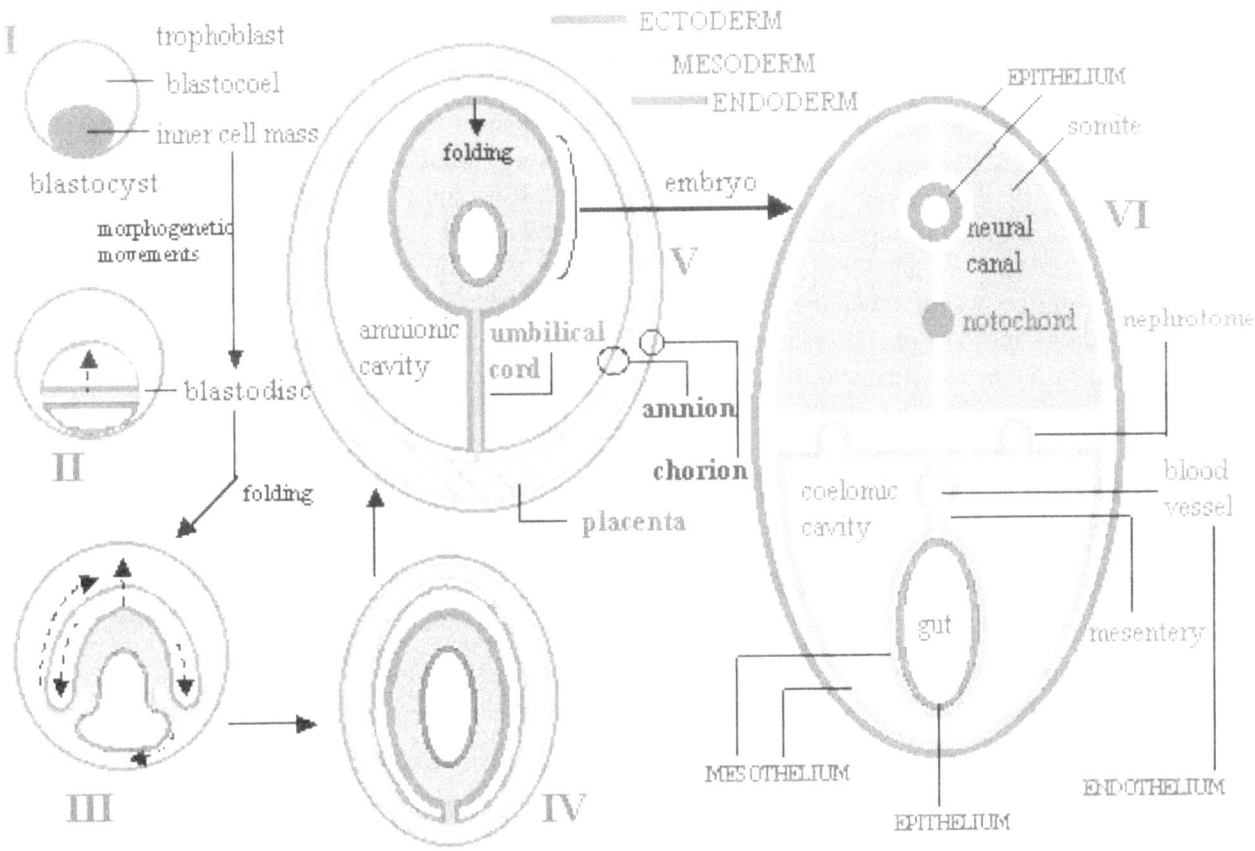

Fig. 4.1. As a result of cell division and multiplication of the fertilized ovum, a blastocyst arises, out of which the embryo and the extraembryonic organs (amnion, chorion, umbilical cord, placenta) will be formed. Morphogenetic migrations of cells result in the formation of 3 germinal layers: ectoderm, mesoderm, endoderm. By subsequent morphogenetic movements, an embryo is formed, and the three germinal layers are manoevered in the right positions, relative to one another, to form the various organs of the body.

Before organs can form, a fertilized ovum or zygote must multiply mitotically, and the daughter cells must engage in morphogenetic migration. Thus, cells that are genetically programmed to form particular tissues will end up in the correct positions, relative to each other, to form organs.

A zygote starts to multiply soon after fertilization. In a few days, it is transformed into a clump of cells, a morula. By the time the morula is ready to be implanted in the wall of the uterus, is has developed a central cavity, and is called a blastula, or blastocyst (Fig. 4.1.). The blastocyst wall, or **trophoblast**, is a simple epithelium. It participates in the formation of an extraembryonic organ, the **chorion**. At one pole of the blastocyst lies an accumulation of cells, the inner cell mass or embryoblast, which will form an embryo, and a number of extra-embryonic organs as well. Through cell migration, the inner cell mass develops a cavity, the equatorial plane of which is occupied by a trilaminar blastodisc. The middle layer is the **mesoderm**. It is bordered by the **ectoderm** and the **endoderm**. The ectoderm spreads over the entire wall of the cavity it borders, the amnionic cavity, and forms the **amnion**, an extra-embryonic organ. In the same way, the endoderm will eventually line the entire cavity it borders, which is the future gut lumen.

The ectoderm and the endoderm will give rise, among them, to most of the later **epithelia** and **glandular tissues**. In addition, the ectoderm will form the **nerve tissue**. The mesoderm will give rise to **lymphoid** and **myeloid tissue**, **interstitial**, **connective**, and **supportive tissues**, **muscle tissue**, **endothelium**, and **mesothelium**. The embryo starts to arch itself, and bulges into the amnionic cavity, which lies at its dorsal side. The connection with the wall of the amnionic cavity progressively narrows, until all that remains is a thin ventral stalk. This stalk is the later **umbilical cord**, yet another extraembryonic organ. Where the umbilical cord joins the chorion, the **placenta** develops.

At the dorsal side of the embryo, the ectoderm folds in, producing a median longitudinal groove, which will later close, forming the neural tube. From the wall of the neural tube, the **nervous system**, including the peripheral nerves and ganglia, as well as the eye's retina and the adrenal medulla, will develop. The rest of the ectoderm forms the epidermis of the **skin**, including its glands and appendages, the thymus, the eye lens, much of the inner ear, the oral and nasal cavities, and the excretory system's distal ducts. The endoderm forms most of the epithelium of the **intestine** and the **respiratory system**, as well as the large glands associated with the gut, the **liver** and the **pancreas**. In addition, it forms a few endocrine glands: the anterior pituitary gland, the thyroid, and the parathyroids. At both sides of the neural tube, the dorsal mesoderm transforms into a series of massive tissue blocks, the somites. These will form much of the **skeleton**, with the bone marrow, and the **skeletal muscles**. The ventral mesoderm, on both sides of the primitive intestine, develops a cavity, the coelomic cavity. At both the dorsal and the ventral side of the intestine, the mesodermal membranes merge into a **mesenterium**. Only the dorsal mesenterium is permanent. This mesoderm will form the visceral muscle tissue, as well as the fibrous tissue, of the intestine and the lungs. In the coelomic wall and mesenterial membranes, the mesoderm develops the **vascular system** and the **lymphoid organs**. The cells lining the blood and lymph vessels lie inside the mesoderm, hence are called endothelium. The coelomic wall is lined with mesothelium, which lies in the middle, i.e. between the inner endothelium and the superficial epithelium. Between the somites and the coelomic space, the mesoderm forms nephrotomes, which give rise to the **kidneys**, and a genital ridge, which gives rise to the **reproductive organs**. The adrenal cortex is also formed in this region.

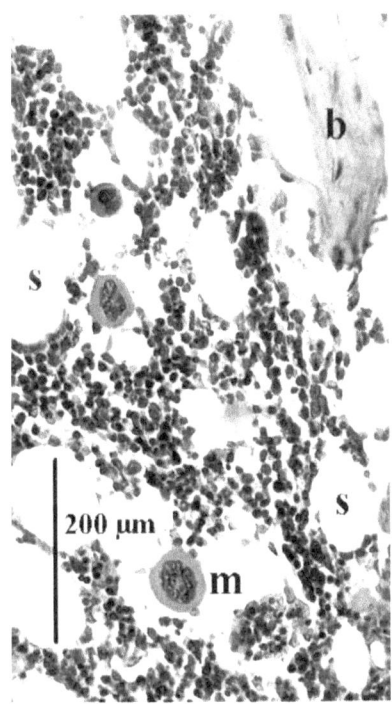

Fig. 4.1.1. Bone marrow consists of masses of hematopoietic cells, resting on (and masking it) a connective tissue reticulum, which also supports thin walled venous sinuses (s). The most conspicuous hematopoietic cells are the megakaryocytes (m). b = bone trabecule. Bone marrow, rat, HE.

IV.1. Lymphoid organs and bone marrow.

The lymphoid organs and bone marrow are predominantly composed of **lymphoid** and **myeloid tissue**, respectively. These tissues are supported mostly by **reticular tissue**, which forms a reticulum. The thymic lymphoid tissue is supported by an analogous reticulum, which has an epithelial (ectodermal) origin. In addition to lymphoid or myeloid tissue, the reticulum supports a dense network of blood or lymph capillaries, made up of **endothelium**, which are often dilated to form sinuses. The endothelium is specially adapted to allow passage of cells. The lymphoid organs and the bone marrow are cellulopoietic organs, i.e. organs that produce cells. To reach the blood or lymph circulation, which some of them will use as a means of transport to their final destination, they have to pass the endothelium. Some cells, in particular lymphocytes, have to go the other way: they have to penetrate from the circulation to the interior of a lymphoid organ. The spleen's mechanism to trap senescent erythrocytes is based on the permeability of its sinus endothelia, which only young erythrocytes can pass.

In the adult organism, myeloid tissue is exclusively found in the interior of certain bones, where it forms the **bone marrow**. Apart from being a blood-forming organ, which produces erythrocytes and thrombocytes, it is also a primary immune organ because, apart from other immune or defender cells, it produces the most important cells of the immune system, the lymphocytes. Lymphoid tissue participates in the formation of other organs, especially the intestine and the airways, but also forms discrete lymphoid organs: the **thymus**, the **lymph nodes**, and the **spleen**. The thymus is, for a number of reasons, different from the other lymphoid organs and lymphoid tissues. As we have seen, its reticulum is derived from ectoderm. Moreover, it houses a specific fraction of the lymphocytes originating in the bone marrow, the T-lymphocytes, which will continue their maturation here. Just like the bone marrow, the thymus is regarded as a primary immune organ, because it only participates in the maturation of lymphocytes, not in their interaction with antigens. The B-lymphocytes of the bone marrow and the T-lymphocytes of the thymus will eventually nest in the peripheral lymphoid tissues and lymphoid organs, where they will contact antigens and become immunologically active. These lymphoid tissues and organs are therefore called secondary. In the lymph nodes, lymphocytes are particularly exposed to antigens via the lymph circulation and in the spleen via the blood circulation.

IV.1.1. Bone marrow.

Microscopically, the bone marrow is dominated by myeloid tissue and dilated blood capillaries or sinuses (Fig. 4.1.1.). The myeloid tissue consists of cell masses mainly formed by the precursor cells of erythrocytes, thrombocytes and granulocytes. It rests on a reticulum or meshwork of fine reticulin fibrils, which also supports the sinus endothelia (Fig. 4.1.2.). Although the distribution of the different types of precursor cells seems random at first, closer inspection reveals certain patterns.

Most easily recognized are the big megakaryocytes. They lie preferentially at the abluminal face of the sinus endothelium. They send finger shaped processes between the endothelial cells into the sinus lumen, where they fragment, forming thrombocytes. Alternatively, the entire megakaryocyte may penetrate into the sinus lumen, and fragment in the circulation, preferably so the pulmonary circulation.

Erythroblasts are found in between the sinuses. They aggregate in groups or nests of about ten cells. In the center of the group, a macrophage is found, which is

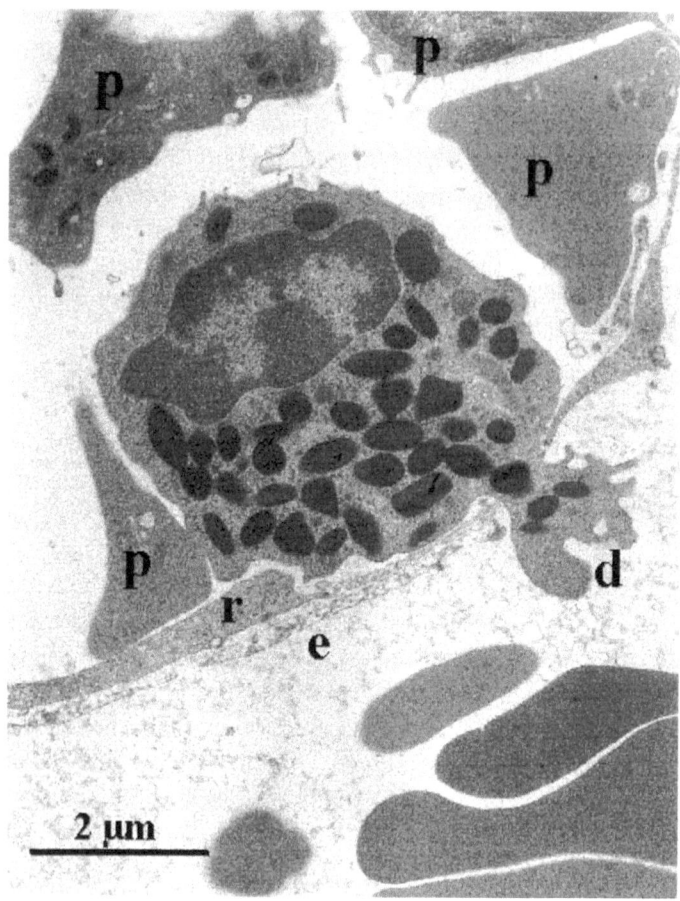

Fig. 4.1.2. Bone marrow's reticulum is made of reticulin fibrils: very thin, diffuse collagen fibrils, synthesized by specialized fibrocytes or reticulocytes (r). Resting on this reticulum, hematopoietic precursor cells (p) are observed. The venous sinuses (mark the erythrocytes) are lined by very thin endothelial cells (e) with wide spaces in between. Mature blood cells, such as an eosinophilic granulocyte, migrate from the reticulum into the venous sinuses by diapedesis (d). Bone marrow, rat, TEM.

derived from a reticulum cell, and which envelops them with its processes (Fig. 3.1.1.). It phagocytoses the nuclei, ejected by the erythroblasts. The enucleated erythrocytes penetrate between the sinus endothelial cells and are liberated in the blood circulation. The bone marrow's macrophages also remove senescent erythrocytes.

The most primitive granulocyte precursors lie farthest from the sinuses and are mainly found near bone tissue or larger blood vessels. As they mature, granulocyte precursors will gradually move closer to the sinuses. Finally, mature granulocytes penetrate between the sinus endothelial cells to the sinus lumen (Fig. 4.1.2.).

Active, blood forming bone marrow is rich in erythrocytes and therefore has a red color: red marrow. With age, reticulum cells progressively transform into white adipose tissue, and blood formation decreases. This inactive marrow has a yellowish color caused by the presence of fat: yellow marrow. In the neonate, red marrow is found in virtually every bone of the skeleton. It occupies the central marrow cavity, as well as the spongy bone surrounding it, of the long bones, and the spongy bone in the other bones. The amount of red marrow decreases with age as it is progressively replaced with yellow marrow. In the adult, red marrow only remains in the flat bones of the skull roof, as well as

in the ribs, the breastbone, the pelvis, the collarbones and the vertebrae.

IV.1.2. Thymus.

The thymus lies in the upper thoracic cavity, occupying the space between the heart and the lungs. It is different from the other lymphoid organs, not only because of its function, but also because of its origin. The thymus is maximally developed in the younger organism and involutes as the organism ages. Embryologically, the thymus is largely derived from the epithelium of the third gill pouch. Both ectodermal and endodermal contributions to this epithelium are likely. Left and right thymus germs later merge ventrally. The epithelium grows into a spongy cell mass or **reticulum**. This reticulum is analogous to that of other lymphoid organs, but is in fact an epithelium. Septa, originating from the surrounding dense fibrous tissue partition the reticulum into lobes and blood vessels penetrate it. During the later stages of embryonic development, the reticulum is colonized by primitive lymphoid cells from the bone marrow. Since the reticulum's mazes are narrowest in the center, most lymphoid cells cannot penetrate that far and nest themselves at the periphery. This results in the typical histological

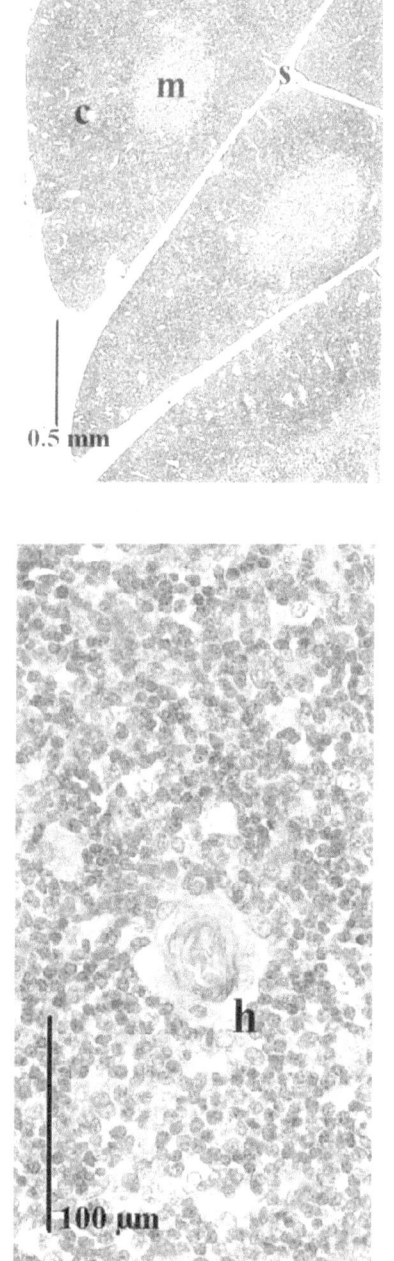

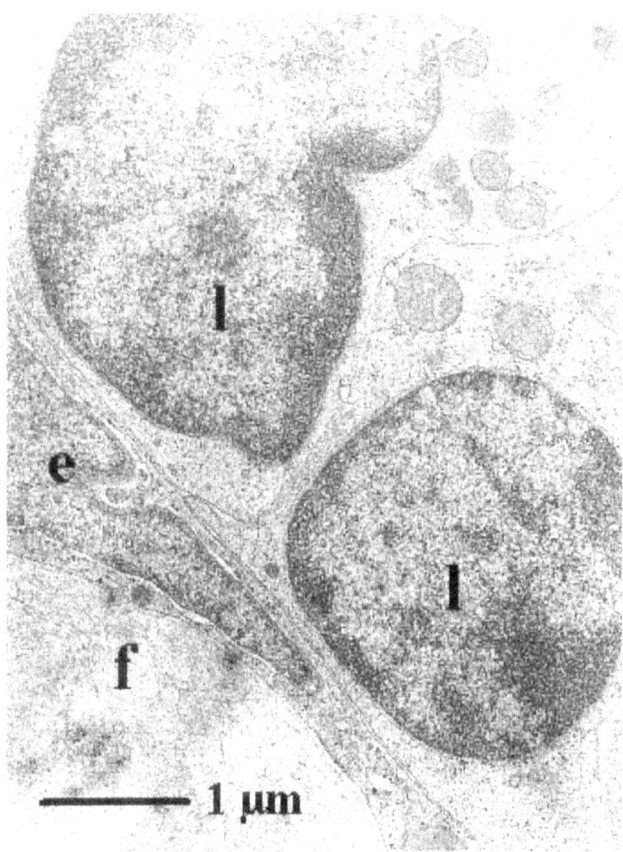

structure of the thymus: a lobed organ, partitioned by fibrous tissue septa, which displays a lymphocyte-rich, dark basophilic **cortex** and a lymphocyte-poor, pale **medulla** (Fig. 4.1.3.).

Ultrastructurally, the reticulum (Fig. 4.1.4.) retains several characteristics that betray its epithelial nature. The reticular cells are interconnected by desmosomes and contain bundles of cytokeratin tonofilaments. Their epithelial character also explains why little extracellular matrix is formed. The reticulum is best developed in the cortex. Developing T-lymphocytes are closely associated with reticular cells, often called **thymic nurse cells**, and often lie deeply embedded in the reticular cell cytoplasm. They may

be distinguished from one another by the character of their nuclei. Reticular cells tend to have larger, euchromatic nuclei, while lymphocytes have small, heterochromatic nuclei. The cell membranes of both cells may interdigitate. Smaller reticular cells line the fibrous tissue septa and the outer perimeter of the blood vessels, and are found in the medulla. In the central medulla of a thymic lobe, **Hassal's bodies** (Fig. 4.1.5.) are frequently found. These are eosinophilic, layered aggregates, formed by squamous reticular cells. Their cytoplasm shows evidence of incipient keratinization, judging from the presence of keratohyalin granules. Apoptosis in the center of Hassal's bodies may be related with the absence of blood vessels. The exact significance of these bodies is unknown.

The lymphoid cells or lymphocytes trapped in the reticular mazes of the cortex are thymus dependent lymphocytes or T-lymphocytes. In the course of their development, they gradually move towards the medulla. Ripening of T-lymphocytes involves the development of specific membrane receptors, complementary to antigens to which the body may eventually be exposed. The thymus can be viewed as an organ that eliminates, from a very large population of developing T-lymphocytes, those which would react to the body's own substances, because their receptor happens to be complementary to one of them. This development may involve controlled exposure of the developing T-lymphocytes to the body's own substances. Such lymphocytes as react to them will be induced to die by apoptosis and are engulfed by macrophages. The others will be allowed to enter the blood circulation at the cortico-medullary junction and eventually nest in the secondary lymphoid tissues and lymphoid organs, where they will be responsible for the cellular aspects of the immune response (III.1.5.). Essentially, the thymus's function is the formation of a circulating T-lymphocyte store, sufficient for life, from which suitable lymphocytes will be selected to respond to an immune challenge.

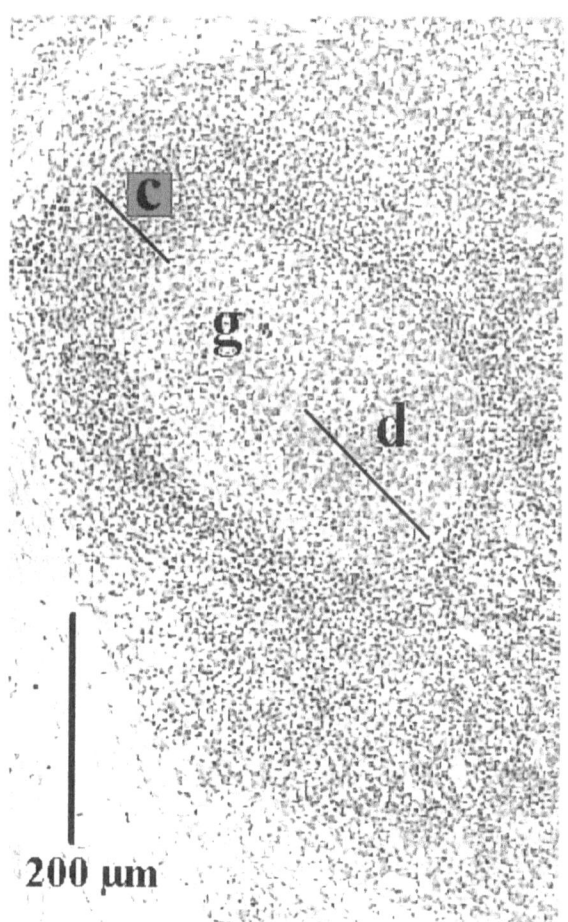
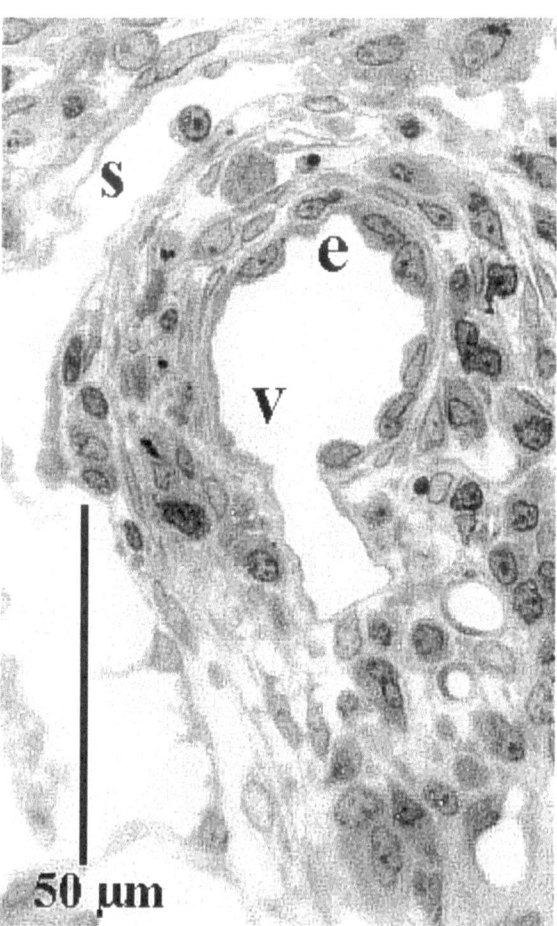

Fig. 4.1.10. (left) A cortical lymph follicle is subdivided in a dark corona (c) or mantle zone, and a paler reaction center or germinative center (g), which in turn displays an eccentric dark zone (d). Mark the "shift" of the germinative center in the direction of the medulla, to the lower right. Also, the corona is thickest in the opposite direction, towards the capsule. The corona contains the as yet unstimulated B-lymphocytes. Antigenically stimulated B-lymphocytes, the so-called centroblasts, undergo clonal expansion in the dark zone, followed by lymphoblastic transformation to so-called centrocytes in the germinative center. Lymphoblastic transformation is the first step towards development of plasma cells. The nuclei become euchromatic and they get separated by increasing volumes of cytoplasm, which explains the pale aspect of the germinative center. Lymph node, human, HE. **Fig. 4.1.11.** (right) A high endothelial venule (v). The endothelial cells (e) are much higher than in other endothelia. s = lymph sinus. Lymph node, rabbit, 1-micrometer plastic section, toluidin blue.

128

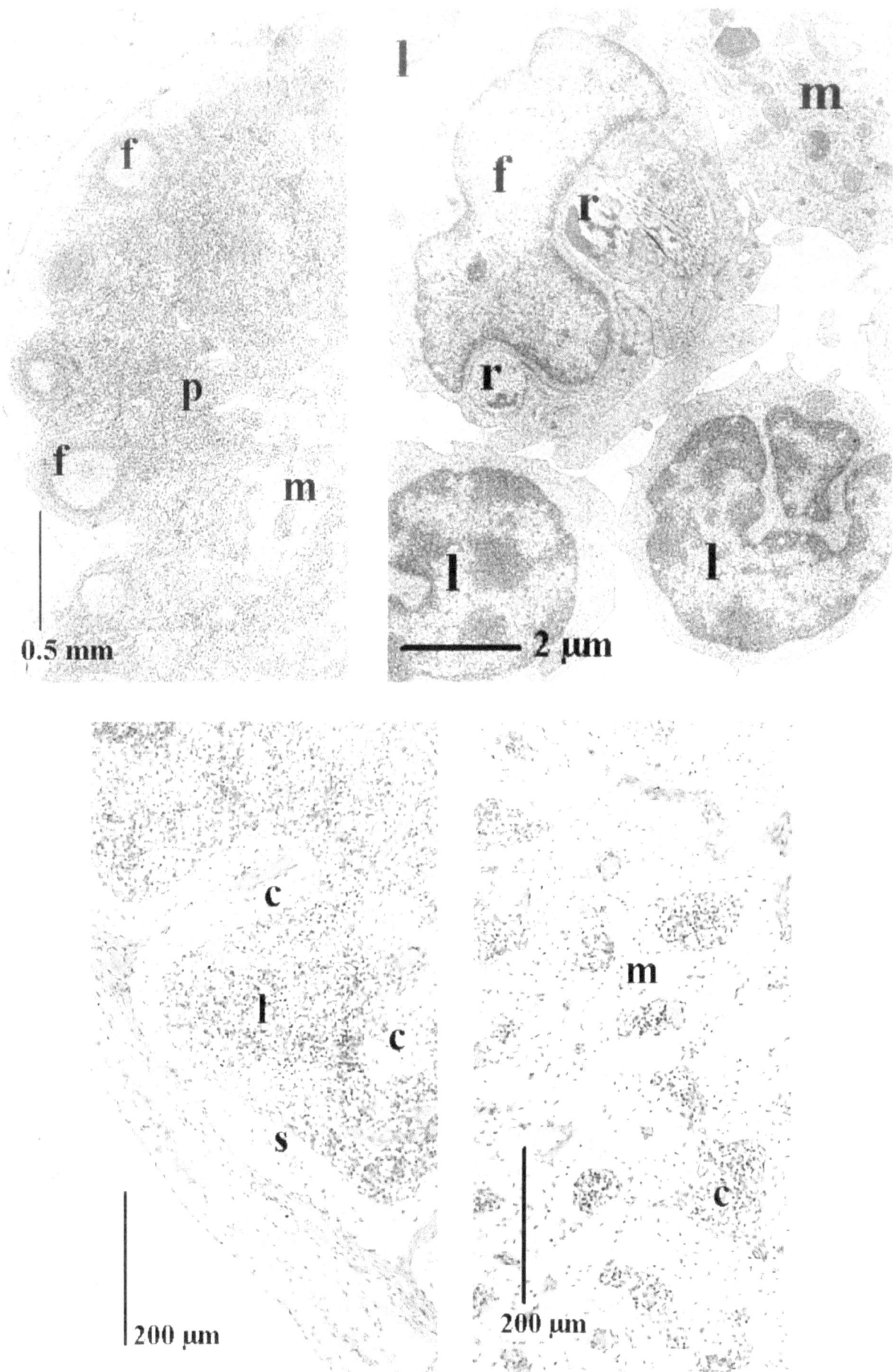

Fig. 4.1.6. (top left) A lymph node has a peripheral cortex, in which the lymphoid tissue aggregates into follicles (f). At deeper levels lies a paracortex (p), where the lymphoid tissue is more uniformly distributed, followed by a central medulla (m), containing little lymphoid tissue. Lymph node, human, HE. **Fig. 4.1.7.** (top right) Reticulin fibrils (r) and reticulum cells (specialized fibrocytes, f) form a reticulum, which supports lymphocytes (l), and macrophages (m). Macrophages assume the role of antigen presenting cells. Lymph node, rabbit, TEM. **Fig. 4.1.8.** (bottom left) Beneath the lymph node's fibrous connective tissue capsule lies a subcapsular sinus (s), in which lymph circulates. Via the septa, radiating from the capsule, branches of the subcapsular sinus, the cortical sinuses (c), penetrate into the lymph node. l = lymphoid tissue. Lymph node, human, HE. **Fig. 4.1.9.** (bottom right) The lymph node's medulla contains a labyrinthine medullary sinus (m). The lymphoid tissue is aggregated into medullary cords (c). Lymph node, human, HE.

From puberty onwards, the thymus will start to involute. In growing measure, white adipose tissue replaces fibrous tissue. Lymphocyte stores are depleted, causing collapse of the reticulum. Finally, all that remains is an inert mass of fibro-adipose tissue.

IV.1.3. Lymph nodes.

Lymph nodes (Fig. 4.1.6.) are globular or kidney-shaped accumulations of lymphoid tissue, a few millimeters in diameter, which are widely distributed in the interstitial tissues and along the lymph vascular system.

Lymph nodes are enveloped with a fibrous tissue capsule from which septa penetrate the node. During embryonic development, the reticulum's mazes (Fig. 4.1.7.) fill with lymphocytes. Most of these nest at the periphery, giving rise to a cell-rich, basophilic **cortex**. The central **medulla** is much poorer in lymphoid cells, with the exception of a number of **medullary cords**. In the peripheral cortex, lymphocytes form ellipsoid aggregations, the **lymph follicles**. In the deeper levels of the cortex, bordering the medulla, lymphocytes are distributed more evenly and form a **paracortex**. At the lymph node's convex side, several afferent lymph capillaries, carrying lymph to the node, penetrate the capsule, discharging lymph into a **subcapsular sinus** (Fig. 4.1.8.). The lymph carries antigens and antigen presenting cells. The subcapsular sinus is confluent with a number of **cortical sinuses**, which follow the course of the septa and drain into a number of relatively wide **medullary sinuses** (Fig. 4.1.9.). At the concave side of the lymph node, the medullary sinuses drain into a single or a few efferent lymph capillaries, carrying lymph away from the node. The endothelial wall of the sinuses is extremely permeable, allowing lymph to circulate in the reticular mazes and cells to pass from the lymph into the reticulum or vice versa.

In the lymph follicles (Fig. 4.1.10.) of the peripheral cortex, the most common type of lymphocytes are B-lymphocytes from the bone marrow. They enter the lymph node via specialized capillaries, the **high endothelial venules**, which are situated in the paracortex (Fig. 4.1.11.). These capillaries have an unusual cuboidal to prismatic endothelium. When an antigen is in circulation, B-lymphocytes are stimulated by helper T-cells that have been activated by this antigen. As a consequence of this, they undergo mutation, followed by proliferation or clonal expansion. Mutation generates multiple types of B-lymphocytes, some of which will react to different aspects of the antigen. By clonal expansion, multiple copies of each B-lymphocyte type will be generated. Only those B-lymphocytes which react to the antigen will be selected and undergo lymphoblastic transformation. Those that do not will die by apoptosis and are removed by macrophages. Lymphoblastic transformation involves growing more cytoplasm, causing the small, heterochromatic cell nuclei to disperse. A direct consequence of lymphoblastic transformation is that the lymph follicles develop a clearer **germinal center**, while not activated B-lymphocytes form a dark peripheral **corona** or mantle zone (Fig. 4.1.10.). The germinal center is often shifted in the direction of the medulla, thus occupying an eccentric position. Clonal expansion takes place at the "basal" pole of the germinal center, pointing towards the medulla, which remains darker. The proliferating B-lymphocytes of this **dark zone** are called centroblasts. The non-proliferating B-lymphocytes of the germinal center's clear zone are called centrocytes. Activated B-lymphocytes start to migrate to the medulla and leave the lymph node via the efferent capillaries. The efferent capillaries carry them to the blood circulation, form where they can enter the tissues. During this trip, they will transform to plasma cells. B-memory cells do not undergo lymphoblastic transformation and stay behind in the corona.

The paracortex is dominated by T-lymphocytes from the thymus, which have likewise penetrated into the lymph node via the high endothelial venules. The cortical sinuses partition the paracortex into a number of cords, with a high endothelial venule in their center. When T-lymphocytes are activated by antigens, they undergo clonal expansion and differentiate. Cytotoxic cells leave the node via the efferent capillaries. T-helper cells migrate to the peripheral cortex to activate B-lymphocytes. Memory T-cells stay behind. Clonal expansion may cause hypertrophy of the paracortex.

The medullary cords contain mainly B-lymphocytes and their descendants, the plasma cells, as well as macrophages.

Essentially, the lymph node is and organ which, in a controlled and regulated fashion, brings antigens in contact with specific populations of T- and B-lymphocytes. Antigens do not enter the lymph node in free circulation, however. They are processed by **antigen presenting cells**, which incorporate them in their cell membrane. These cells may reside inside or outside the lymph nodes. In the second case, antigen-presenting cells will carry antigens to the lymph nodes. We have already met two kinds of antigen-presenting cell: T-lymphocytes and macrophages. There is a third kind of antigen presenting cell: **dendritic cells**. Dendritic cells may have some resemblance to macrophages, and the difference between the two is not always apparent. A useful distinction seems to be their method of endocytosis. While macrophages are fairly indiscriminate, engulfing large particles, dendritic cells, when they are phagocytic at all, sample antigenic material in a more sophisticated way, by pinocytosis and receptor-mediated endocytosis. Both cell types develop processes, but those of dendritic cells may be quite extensive and complicated. They have large, euchromatic nuclei. The cytoplasm of dendritic cells is poorer in organelles than that of macrophages. Proliferating B-lymphocytes are selected, and tested

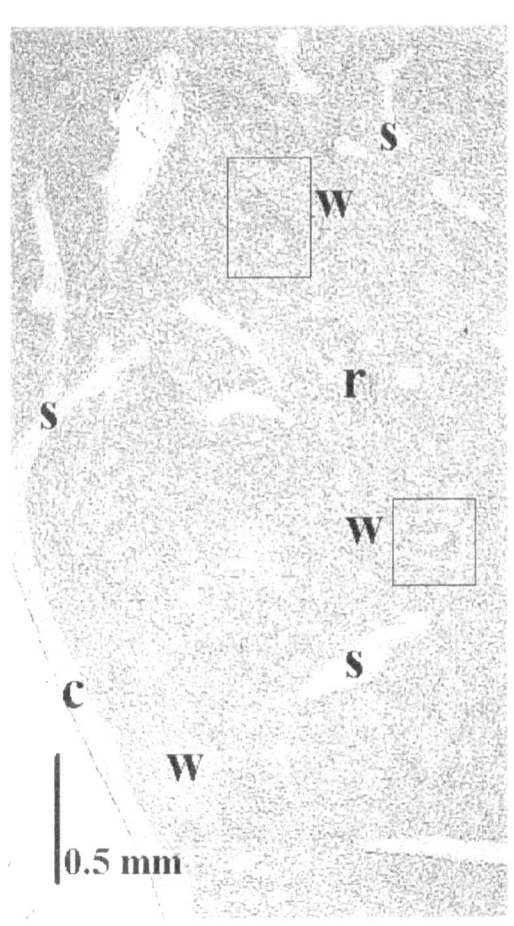
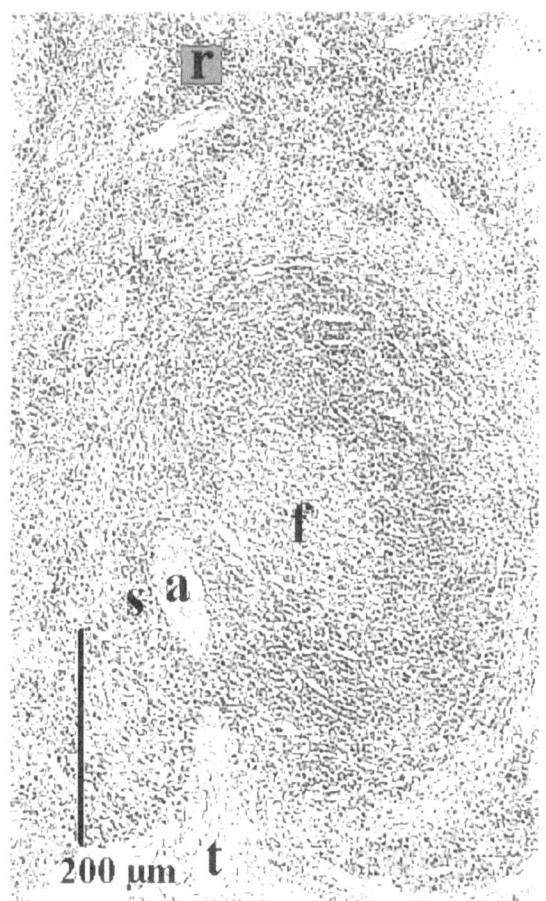

Fig. 4.1.12. (left) The spleen is surrounded by a capsule (c), which forms septa (s). Through these, trabecular vessels penetrate into the organ. The red pulp (r) derives its color from blood, which circulates in large venous sinuses. Where venous sinuses are lacking, lymphoid tissue is apparent, the white pulp (w). Spleen, cat, HE. **Fig. 4.1.13.** (right) Lymphoid tissue is most evident in the white pulp, where venous sinuses are lacking. The white pulp's lymphoid tissue envelops branches of the trabecular arteries (t), the central arteries (a). Thus, a periarterial lymphoid sheath (s) is formed, wherein lymph follicles (f), containing a germinative center, develop. r = red pulp. Spleen, goat, HE.

for their reaction with the antigen they present, by **follicular dendritic cells**, which are permanent residents of lymph node follicles and probably descend from reticular cells. Follicular dendritic cells form slender, extensive processes with a filiform or beaded appearance, which penetrate between the lymphocytes and are joined to one another by desmosome-like junctions, forming a three-dimensional network. They do not phagocytose, but carry antigens on the outside of their cell membrane.

T-lymphocytes are stimulated by a number of dendritic cell types, most of which probably descend from precursors in the myeloid tissue and only migrate to the lymph nodes when they have sampled antigen. These cells originally reside in the peripheral interstitial tissues and epithelia, (Langerhans's cells) or in the circulatory fluids (veiled cells). In the paracortical zones, they develop into **interdigitating cells**.

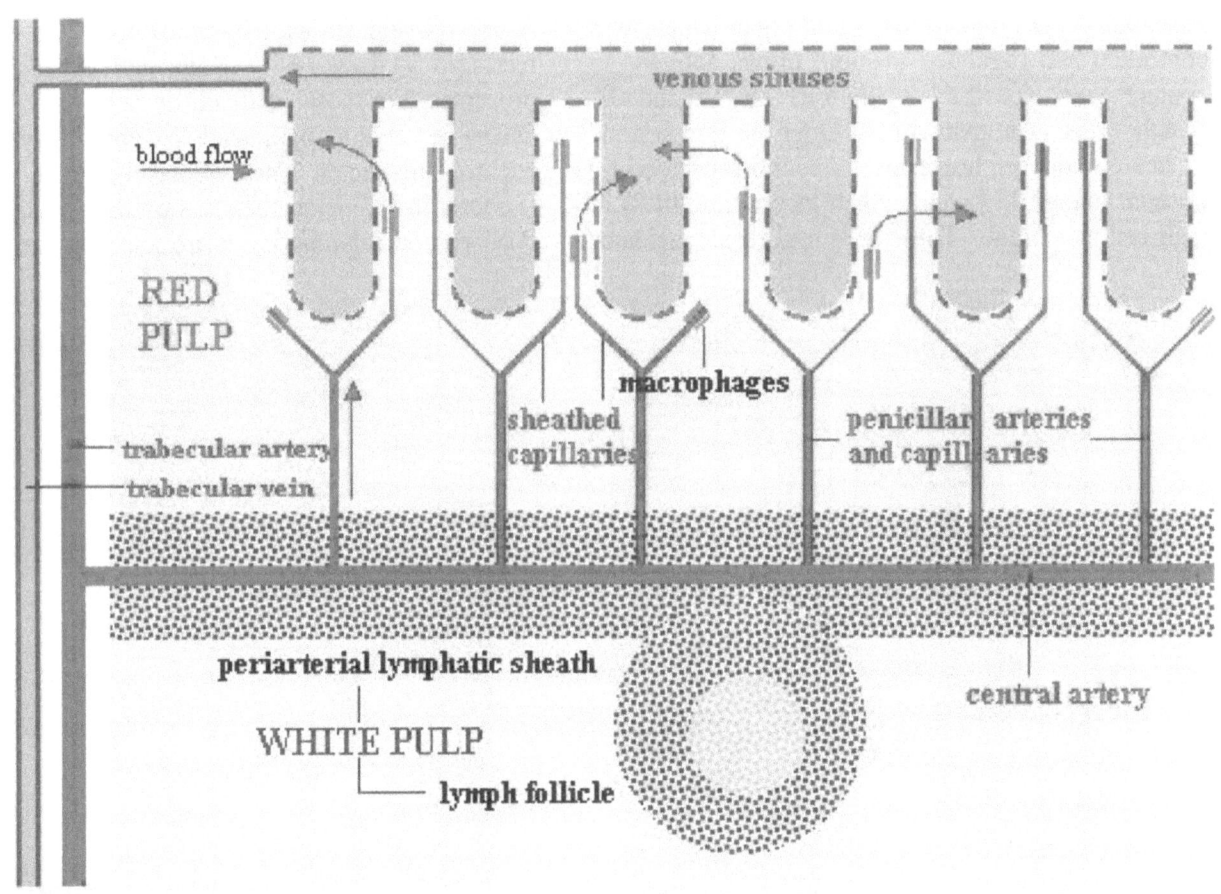

Fig. 4.1.14. The splenic blood circulation is unusual and plays an essential part in the selection and trapping of senescent erythrocytes, which will subsequently be degraded. The central arteries branch into penicillar arteries, which in their turn form capillaries. The terminal capillaries become sheathed by macrophages, and are called sheathed capillaries. These capillaries open into the extracellular space. Here, blood leaves the vascular tract. The spleen has an open circulation. Only young, healthy and sufficiently plastic erythrocytes can reenter the circulation, by insinuating themselves between the endothelial cells lining the venous sinuses. Senescent erythrocytes can no longer do this and are trapped.

IV.1.4. Spleen.

The spleen is a relatively large lymphoid organ that lies in the left upper abdominal cavity. In fact, it is an organ with a double function. On the one hand, it has an immunological function. On the other hand, it can be conceived of as a filter that removes senescent or damaged erythrocytes from the circulation and degrades them. Consequently, the spleen is a lymphoid organ with an exceptionally rich blood supply. Unique to the spleen, some of this blood even circulates extravascular.

Microscopic observation (Fig. 4.1.12.) reveals the spleen to be filled to overflowing with erythrocytes. They give a large part of the splenic tissue a red color: the **red pulp**. In the red pulp, concentrations of lymphoid tissue are distributed, collectively called

132

the **white pulp**. The spleen has a dense fibrous tissue capsule, which sends septa into the spleen's interior. Through these septa, trabecular arteries enter the spleen and trabecular veins leave it. In young individuals, this capsule also contains some visceral muscle tissue. Oxygen shortage may lead to contraction of the splenic capsule, so that erythrocytes are literally pressed out to replenish the circulating erythrocyte stock, increasing the blood's oxygen carrying capacity.

The white pulp occurs in two forms. One form envelopes the arterioles, which are branches of the trabecular arteries and penetrate the red pulp. It forms a **periarteriolar lymphatic sheath** (Fig. 4.1.13.). Associated with this sheath is the second form of white pulp: the occasional, eccentrically situated **lymph follicle**. These sheathed arterioles are also called the **central arterioles**. The splenic reticulum is arranged in concentric layers around the central arteriole and is stocked with T-lymphocytes and interdigitating cells. The lymph follicles are populated mainly by B-lymphocytes and follicular dendritic cells. Antigen presenting cells penetrate the white pulp from the red pulp. Activated T- and B-lymphocytes and plasma cells migrate to the red pulp, where they penetrate between the endothelial cells of the venous sinuses to reach the blood circulation.

The red pulp contains large venous sinuses (Fig. 4.1.14.), surrounded with reticulum that is stocked with erythrocytes: **Bilroth's cords**. The central arteriole gives rise to side branches which course radially, leave the white pulp and split up in a number of fine branches or penicilli. These form capillaries, which get enveloped by a cellular sheath consisting of macrophages, the **sheathed capillaries**. These macrophages engulf antigens, carried by the blood. The sheathed capillaries empty in the reticulum of the red pulp. This means that the spleen has an open circulation, i.e. that blood circulates outside the vessels. Eventually, erythrocytes re-enter the blood circulation at the level of the venous sinuses. The sinus endothelium has a particular structure (Fig. 4.1.15.). The endothelial cells are distinctly elongated, spindle shaped, and oriented with their long axis parallel to the sinus axis. In cross sections, they are cuboidal. Their cell basis contains dense bundles of microfilaments, running parallel with the basement membrane. Individual endothelial cells show almost no junctions with other endothelial cells. The basement membrane is discontinuous and shows large gaps. The incomplete basement membrane and the slits between the endothelial cells allow erythrocytes to cross the sinus endothelium.

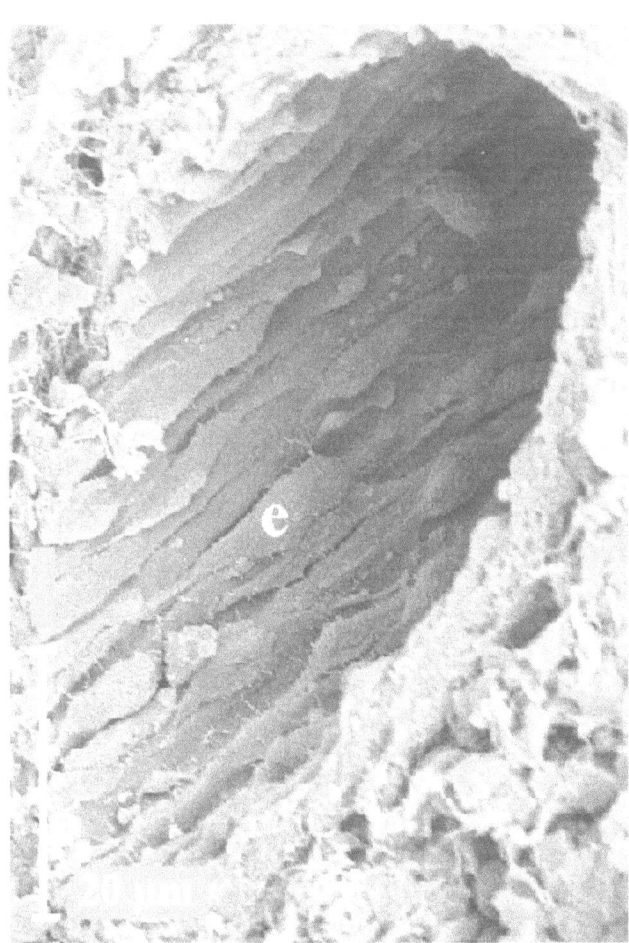

Fig. 4.1.15. The endothelial cells (e) lining the venous sinuses are elongated and lie parallel to the longitudinal axis of the sinuses. They are not flattened, but rather domed, bulging into the lumen. Spleen, rabbit, SEM.

Erythrocytes only manage to do this, however, when they are plastic enough to insinuate themselves in the reticular mazes and the intercellular slits of the sinus endothelium. Senescent erythrocytes do not succeed in this and are trapped, whereupon they are engulfed by macrophages. The sinuses are drained by the trabecular veins.

References.

Alam R.: A brief review of the immune system. Allergy Immunol. 1998, 25: 727-738.

Bodey B., Kaiser H.E.: Development of Hassall's bodies of the thymus in humans and other vertebrates (especially mammals) under physiological and pathological conditions: immunocytochemical, electronmicroscopic and in vitro observations. In Vivo 1997, 11: 61-86.

Brelinska R., Warchol J.B.: Thymic nurse cells: their functional ultrastructure. Microsc. Res. Tech. 1997, 38: 250-266.

Chadburn A.: The spleen: anatomy and anatomical funcion. Semin. Hematol. 2000, 37 suppl. 1: 13-21.

Cyster J.G.: Chemokines and cell migration in secondary lymphoid organs. Science 1999, 286: 2098-2101.

Fu Y.X., Chaplin D.D.: Development and maturation of secondary lymphoid tissues. Annu. Rev. Immunol. 1999, 17: 399-433.

Gretz J.E., Anderson A.O., Shaw S.: Cords, channels, corridors and conduits: critical architectural elements facilitating cell interactions in the lymph node cortex. Immunol. Rev. 1997, 156: 11-24.

Imai Y., Yamakawa M.: Morphology, function and pathology of follicular dendritic cells. Pathol. Int. 1996, 46: 807-833.

Kendall M.D.: Functional anatomy of the thymic microenvironment. J. Anat. 1991, 177: 1-29.

Lichtman M.A.: The ultrastructure of the hemopoietic environment of the marrow: a review. Exp. Hematol. 1981, 9: 391-410.

Lindhout E., de Groot C.: Follicular dendritic cells and apoptosis: life and death in the germinal centre. Histochem. J. 1995, 27: 167-183.

Liu Y.J., Grouard G., de Bouteiller O., Banchereau J.: Follicular dendritic cells and germinal centers. Int. Rev. Cytol. 1996, 166: 139-179.

Reid C.D.L.: The biology and clinical applications of dendritic cells. Transfusion Med. 1998, 8: 77-86.

Stockwin L.H., McGonagle D., Martin I.G., Blair G.E.: Dendritic cells: immunological sentinels with a central role in health and disease. Immunol. Cell Biol. 2000, 78: 91-102.

Von Gaudecker B.: Functional histology of the thymus. Anat. Embryol. 1991, 183: 1-15.

Wilkins B.S.: Histology of normal hematopoiesis: bone marrow histology I. J. Clin. Pathol. 1992, 45: 645-649.

IV.2. Skeleton.

The skeleton consists of **connective** and **supportive tissues**, predominantly so the highly specialized **cartilage** and **bone**. Both tissues form the parts of the skeleton, the bones. These roughly come in two varieties that can be distinguished according to their embryological development: the relatively simple **mesenchymal bones** and the complex **enchondral bones**. Dense fibrous connective tissue and a few rarer tissue types also participate in the formation of the skeleton, mainly in the specialized places of contact between bones: **joints** and **intervertebral disks**.

IV.2.1. Mesenchymal bones.

During embryological development, mesenchymal bones are formed out of primitive mesenchymal tissue. Anatomically, the best known of these are the flat bones that make up the skull roof. In general, mesenchymal bones, also called intramembranous bones, lie superficially, cannot move relative to one another and serve to shield weak, underlying organs.

Where mesenchymal bones will form, primitive mesenchymal cells differentiate to osteoblasts. The osteoblasts deposit fibrous bone and transform to walled-in osteocytes. Meanwhile, the surrounding mesenchymal tissue develops into dense fibrous tissue: the bone membrane or **periost**. In the periost's deeper layers, undifferentiated mesenchymal cells form a **cambium** or osteogenic layer. They differentiate to osteoblasts, which deposit lamellar compact bone in the form of circumferential lamellae, which envelop the central mass of fibrous bone. Thus, these lamellae are formed by mesenchymal bone formation under the periost: **subperiosteal growth**. In effect, this process deposits successive layers of new bone on older bone, which makes the bone grow in a fashion that is analogous to cartilage's appositional growth. Eventually, the fibrous bone is degraded and replaced, from the center outwards, by lamellar spongy bone. In the mazes of the spongy bone, bone marrow forms out of mesenchymal tissue.

A mature mesenchymal, flat bone thus consists of a central mass of spongy bone with bone marrow, enveloped by circumferential lamellae of compact bone (Fig. 4.2.1.). Flat bones grow by continued subperiosteal bone formation. While new layers of compact bone are added at the surface, the deeper layers are degraded by osteoclasts and replaced with

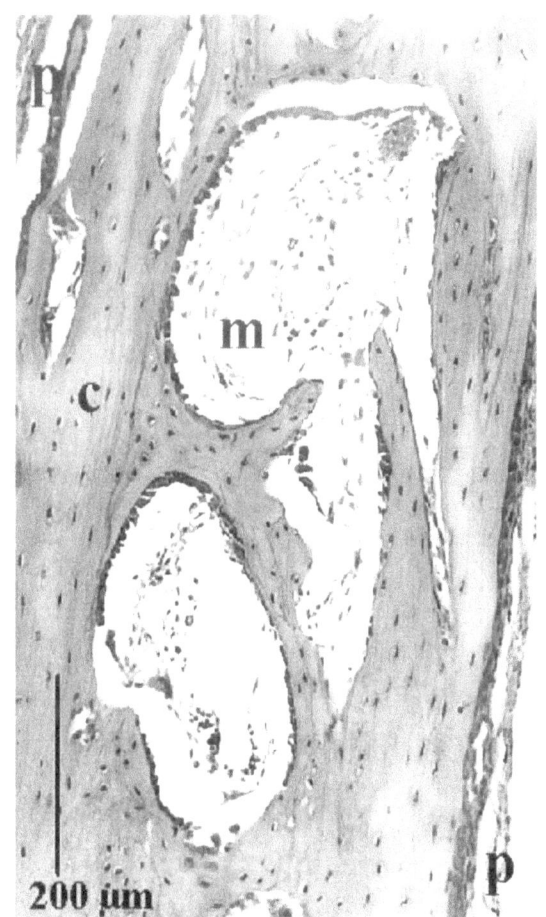

Fig. 4.2.1. Mesenchymal bones consist of a superficial layer of compact bone (c) in the shape of circumferential lamellae, and a central core of spongy bone with bone marrow (m). The bone is lined with periosteum (p). Cranial bone, rat, HE.

spongy bone. As a result of this, and without reckoning with remodeling processes, the dimensions of the whole bone and the central spongy bone mass increase, while the thickness of the circumferential lamellar layer remains relatively constant.

IV.2.2. Enchondral bones.

Enchondral bones have a much more complex history of formation and a much more complicated structure then do mesenchymal bones. Anatomically, they are a diverse lot. The **long bones** are those of the arms and legs: humerus, radius, ulna, femur, tibia, and fibula. The **short bones** are those of the hands and feet: the carpals and metacarpals, and the tarsals and metatarsals, respectively. From a histological point of view, these can be regarded as scaled down and simplified long bones. The bones forming the base of the hands and feet, the bones of the shoulder and hip girdles, and those of the rib cage are also enchondral

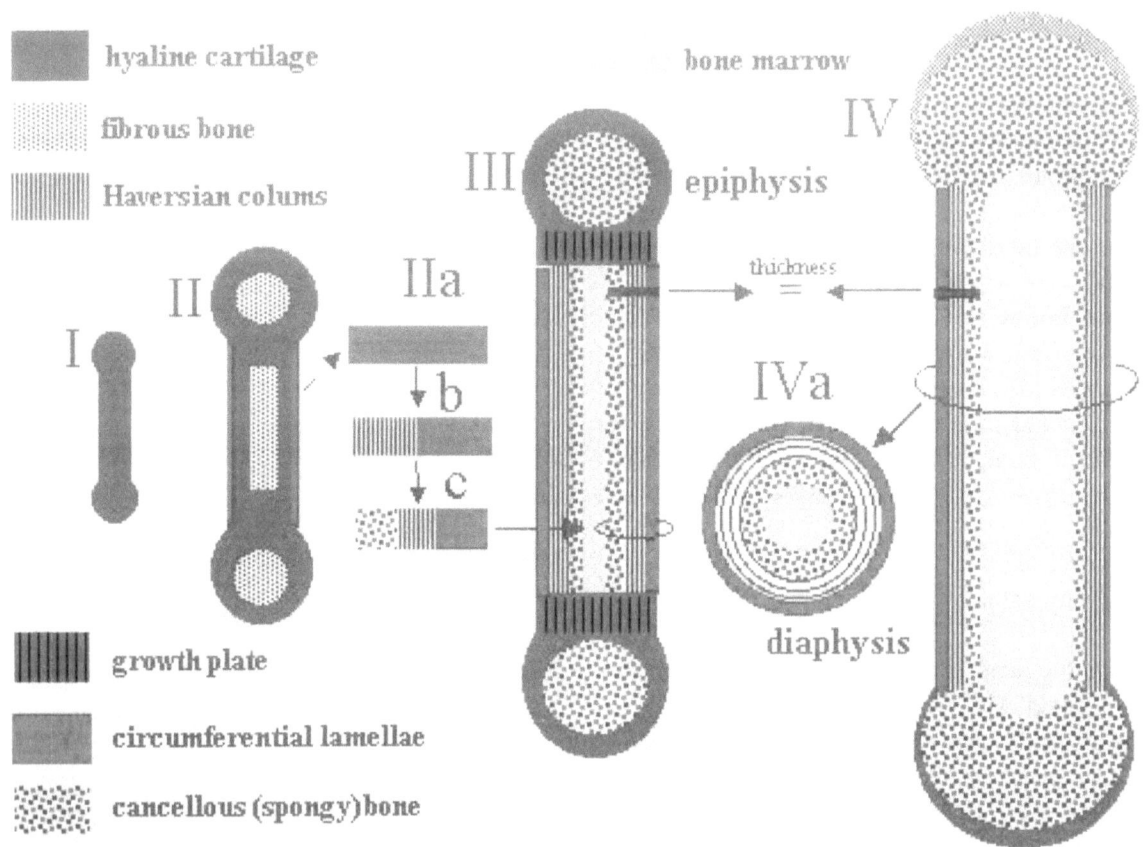

Fig. 4.2.2. Long bones are enchondral bones: they arise from fetal precursor bones, entirely made of hyaline cartilage, and enveloped with perichondrium (I). In the center of the epiphyses and the diaphysis, cartilage calcifies, is degraded, and replaced with fibrous bone. Subsequently, this fibrous bone is degraded from the center outwards, resulting in the formation of a marrow cavity. At the level of the diaphysis, the perichondrium is converted into a periosteum. Instead of cartilage, lamellar bone is now deposited, in the shape of circumferential lamellae (II). While the periosteum continually adds new lamellae at the periphery, the deepest ones are consecutively degraded, and replaced with compact lamellar bone, in the shape of Haversian columns. In their turn, these are degraded, the deepest ones first, and replaced with spongy bone (IIa and III). Degradation of the deepest spongy bone widens the marrow cavity, while the thickness of the diaphyseal wall tends to remain constant. This mechanism, subperiosteal bone formation (II, III), allows diametrial growth of the diaphysis. Analogously, the fibrous bone of the epiphysis is degraded, and replaced with spongy bone. At the epiphyseal rim, a layer of cartilage is preserved, but the perichondrium is lost. Thus, articular cartilage is formed. In the young individual, 2 layers of cartilage are preserved, separating the epiphyses from the diaphysis: the growth plates (III). These enable longitudinal growth of the diaphysis. Bone lengthening stops when the growth plates are finally eliminated (V).

bones. The most complex enchondral bones are the **vertebrae**. Some bones, especially those of the face and the jaws, have a mixed origin, partly mesenchymal, partly enchondral.

Enchondral bones are not formed directly, but arise from fetal precursor "bones" made of hyaline cartilage. These precursors, by a complicated process of ossification, degradation, and replacement, are transformed to bones: enchondral bone formation. Enchondral bone formation is not only a mechanism by which bone is formed, it is also a mechanism by which bone grows. In general, bones grow in length by enchondral growth. Bones can also grow in thickness: this is by subperiosteal growth, which is

independent of cartilage. Thus, the term enchondral does not exactly describe this type of bone. Enchondral bones generally lie rather deep, may be able to move relative to one another because they are often connected via mobile joints, and serve primarily in the support of the body and the attachment of muscles.

IV.2.2.1. Long bones.

Long bones derive their name from their elongated shape. They consist of a relatively narrow, cylindrical shaft or **diaphysis**, which expands at both ends to form an **epiphysis**, which may have a fairly complex shape. The epiphyses carry the articular faces of the bone, and often offer insertion places to the muscles.

The formation of a long bone begins in the diaphysis of its cartilage precursor (Fig. 4.2.2.). For a while, this precursor has been growing, both appositionally and interstitially. At a certain moment, mesenchymal cells in the perichondrium enveloping the diaphysis no longer differentiate to chondroblasts, but to osteoblasts. Technically, the perichondrium is now a **periost**. This periost deposits, by subperiosteal bone formation, a number of **circumferential lamellae**

around the fetal diaphysis. Interstitial growth in the cartilage stops, the chondroblasts hypertrophy and the matrix is calcified. These phenomena are the onset of cartilage degeneration and ultimate degradation. Blood vessels penetrate into the calcified cartilage, allowing access to macrophages, which degrade the calcified matrix. Mesenchymal cells in the walls of the ingrowing blood vessels transform into osteoblasts, which deposit **fibrous bone** on the remnants of the calcified cartilage matrix left over by the macrophages. Eventually, this fibrous bone will be degraded, and a central diaphyseal **marrow cavity** will be formed.

Meanwhile, the periost has been depositing a number

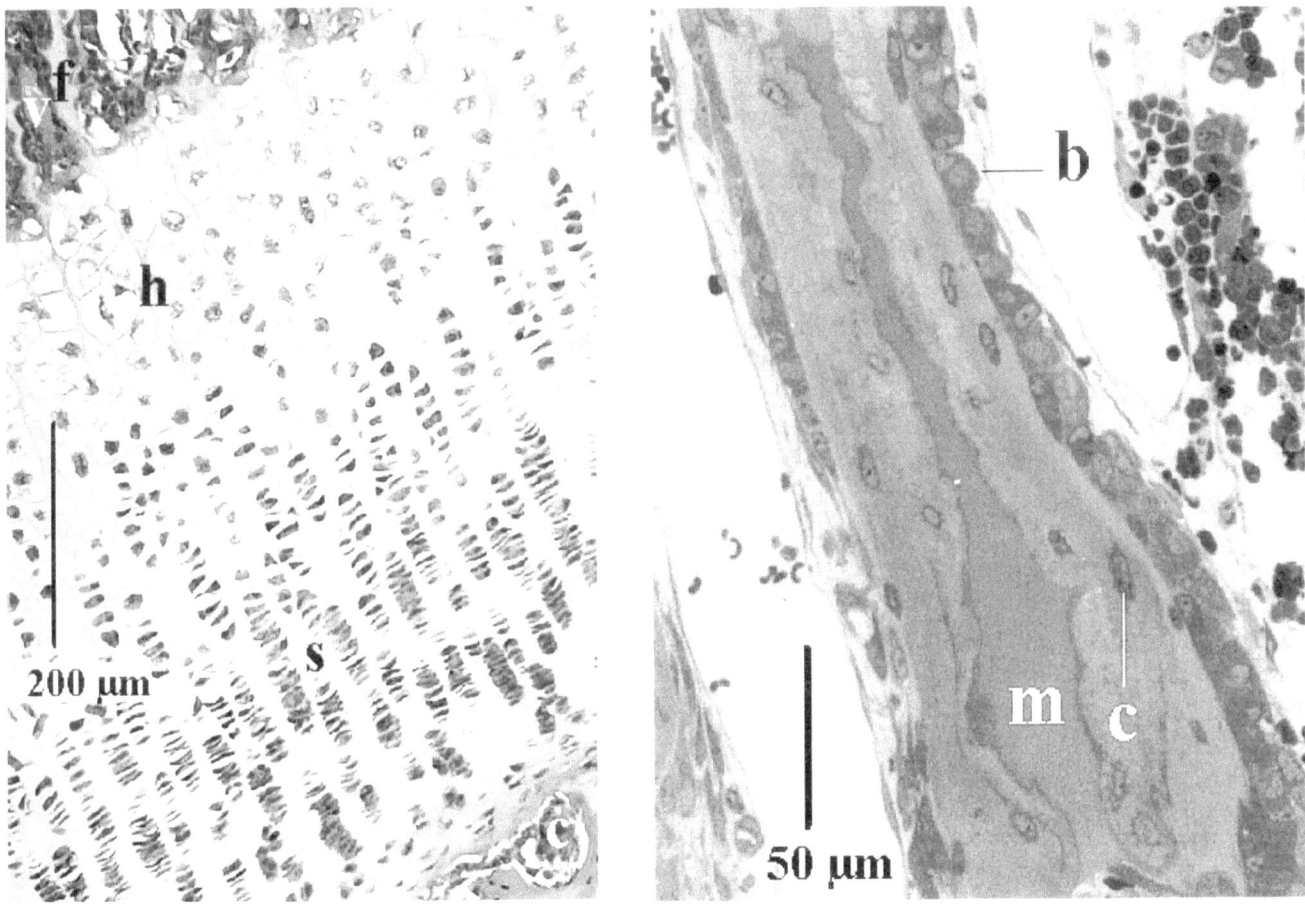

Fig. 4.2.3. (left) The cartilaginous growth plate of a long bone enables longitudinal growth because of its peculiar mechanism of interstitial growth: axial growth. While the chondrocytes multiply, they maintain a constant orientation of their metaphase plane: at right angles to the bone's long axis. Thus, successive cell generations form long rows of cells, parallel to the bone's long axis. These rows of flattened chondrocytes, looking like stacks of coins, occupy the most distinctive layer of the growth plate, the serial zone (s). Continuing cell multiplication in the serial zone thickens the growth plate and consequently lengthens the whole bone. The oldest cartilage, which lies closest to the diaphysis, has now played its part and no longer serves any purpose. The chondrocytes will die by apoptosis, and it will be degraded and replaced with bone. Before the chondrocytes die, they become hypertrophic (h). From the diaphysis, blood vessels (v) penetrate into the spaces formerly occupied by chondrocytes. The cartilage matrix is degraded, and osteoblasts deposit fibrous bone (f) on what remains of it. c = cancellous (spongy) bone of the epiphysis. Long bone, rabbit, HE. **Fig. 4.2.4.** (right) A fibrous bone trabecule. In its center, calcified cartilage matrix (m) still shows. Around it, fibrous bone has been deposited by osteoblasts (b), which get walled in, in the process, and convert into osteocytes (c). Ileum, rabbit, 1-micrometer plastic section, toluidin blue.

of circumferential lamellae. The oldest, deepest lamellae are gradually degraded. Osteoblasts then deposit lamellar bone, and the deeper circumferential lamellae are replaced with lamellae that are arranged concentrically around blood vessels that run parallel to the diaphyseal axis. In this way, **osteons** or **Haversian columns** are formed. The central blood vessels are interconnected via transverse canals of Volkmann. The osteons in particular are responsible for the bone's strength and are suited to the accommodation of longitudinal tensile and compressive forces. While new osteons are formed at the periphery, under the expanding layer of circumferential lamellae, the older, deeper osteons are degraded by osteoclasts. Osteoblasts then deposit new lamellar bone, this time in the shape of cancellous or **spongy bone** containing bone marrow. While the spongy bone layer is added to peripherally, its deeper layers are degraded, causing expansion of the marrow cavity (Fig. 4.2.2.).

In a somewhat later stage, cartilage degeneration, characterized by chondroblast hypertrophy and matrix calcification, starts at the centers of the fetal epiphyses. Upon vascularization, calcified cartilage is degraded by macrophages and replaced by a mass of fibrous bone. Subsequently, the fibrous bone is degraded and replaced with spongy bone containing bone marrow. While the spongy bone mass grows, the perichondrium deposits additional cartilage at the epiphyseal surface. Locally, the perichondrium disappears, giving rise to a smooth articular surface. This part of the epiphyseal cartilage is the **articular cartilage**. At its exposed surface, the collagen fibrils form a much denser network than deeper down and they run parallel to the surface. Another specialized layer of cartilage is preserved at the junction between diaphysis and epiphysis, the epiphyseal plate or **growth plate**, which will play an essential role during longitudinal growth of the bone (Fig. 4.2.2.).

The **longitudinal growth** of a long bone begins in the growth plate. In the growth plate (Fig. 4.2.3.), interstitial growth takes place, be it of a special kind. During normal interstitial growth, the orientation of the mitotic spindle will vary randomly in the course of successive chondroblast mitoses. Not so in the growth plate. Here, the orientation of the mitotic spindle is fixed: parallel to the longitudinal axis of the bone. Consequently, the daughter cells of multiplying chondroblasts line up, forming an axis parallel to the bone's longitudinal axis. This particular variant of interstitial growth is called **axial growth**. In this way, the growth plate forms a transverse zone containing a number of parallel, longitudinal rows of flattened chondroblasts, which

look like stacks of coins. This part of the growth plate is the **serial zone**. Continued axial growth in the serial zone lengthens the growth plate and consequently the entire bone. The growth plate cartilage has now played its part and will gradually be replaced with bone. When axial growth has moved them to a certain distance from the epiphysis, the chondroblasts stop multiplying. They begin to hypertrophy and later the cartilage matrix calcifies. Thus, a **hypertrophic zone** is formed, followed by a **provisional calcification zone** (provisional, because the calcified cartilage is not maintained: it will be degraded and replaced by another type of calcified tissue, bone). The chondroblast's degeneration involves some aspects of apoptosis, such as nuclear shrinkage. Cell death may be speeded up by matrix calcification, since this hampers diffusion of oxygen and food substances. From the marrow cavity, blood vessels grow into the calcified area of the growth plate. They prefer the way of least resistance: the rows of dead chondrocytes. They bring along macrophages, which degrade the calcified matrix, and mesenchymal cells, which transform into osteoblasts and deposit fibrous bone on the leftover matrix fragments (Fig. 4.2.4.). Thus, between the diaphysis and the growth plate, a layer of fibrous bone is formed. It borders the marrow cavity and the diaphyseal spongy bone, but does not contain bone marrow. In its center, it is degraded, causing lengthening of the marrow cavity. At its periphery, it will be replaced with lamellar bone and incorporated into the diaphysis.

When a bone reaches its adult dimensions, the chondroblasts of the growth plate stop multiplying and they all hypertrophy, whereupon the entire growth plate calcifies and is degraded. A fully-grown bone also lacks fibrous bone tissue. The spongy bone of the diaphysis has fused with that of the epiphyses, but the marrow cavity is limited to the diaphysis.

A long bone's **diametric growth** occurs by subperiosteal bone formation. The cambium layer's (Fig. 4.2.5.) mesenchymal cells transform to osteoblasts, which deposit circumferential lamellae. While new lamellae are added superficially, the deeper, older, ones are degraded by osteoclasts. Local mesenchyme cells differentiate to osteoblasts, which deposit concentric layers of lamellar bone around longitudinal blood vessels: osteons or Haversian columns. In their turn, the deeper osteons are degraded and replaced by spongy bone. The deeper spongy bone is degraded, widening the marrow cavity.

Thus, in a cross section of a growing, as well as a

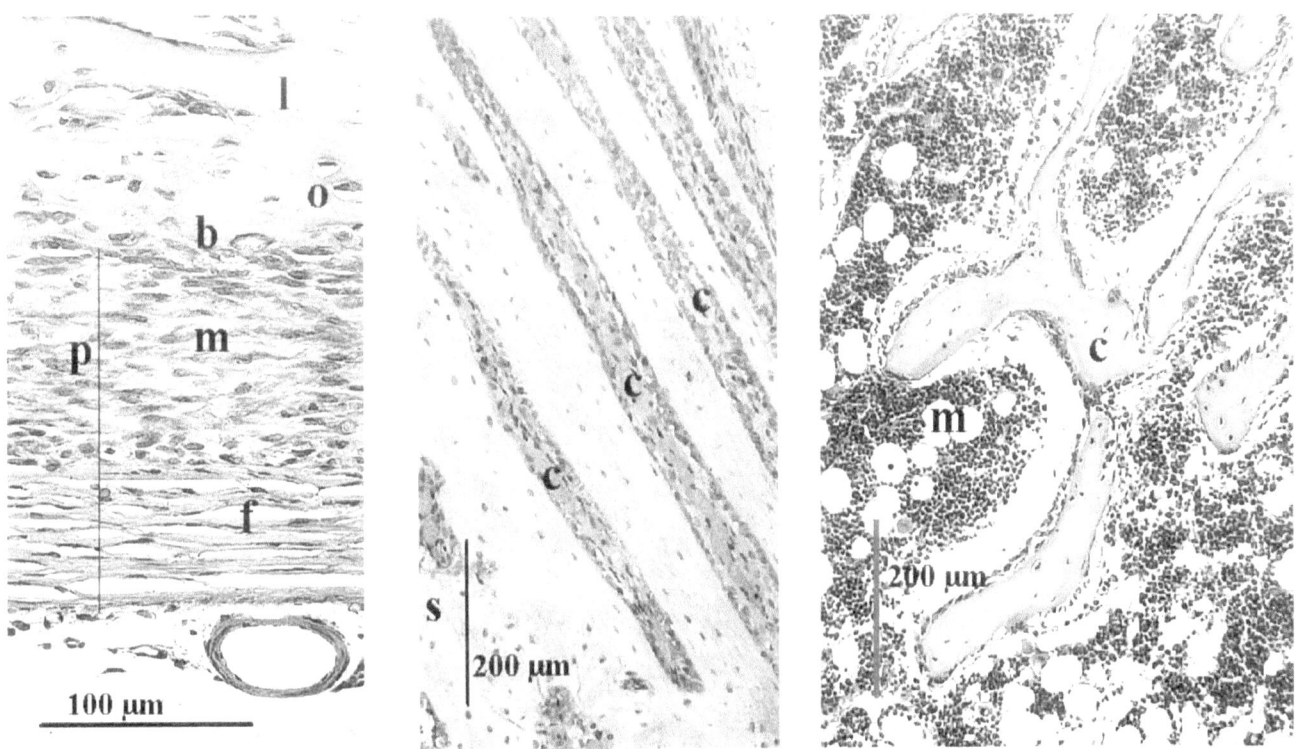

Left to right: **Fig. 4.2.5.** The periost (p) or bone membrane consists of a layer of primitive mesenchymal tissue (m), covered with a layer of dense fibrous tissue (f). Mesenchymal tissue (mark the numerous, closely packed cells, which indicates that there is little matrix) represents the osteogenic layer or cambium. The deeper cells can differentiate into osteoblasts (b), which synthesize lamellar bone (l), and end up as walled in osteocytes (o). This mechanism, subperiosteal bone formation, adds new circumferential lamellae to existing bone and allows diametrial growth of the diaphysis. Long bone, rabbit, HE. **Fig. 4.2.6.** Central to the circumferential lamellae lies a layer of compact bone, the lamellae of which are arranged in concentric cylinders, which lie parallel to the bone's long axis: osteons or Haversian columns. The hollow axis of each column is a Haversian canal (c), lined with osteoblasts, and containing a blood vessel. Mark the orange color of the erythrocytes. Towards the diaphyseal center lies spongy, or cancellous, bone (s). Humerus, rabbit, HE. **Fig. 4.2.7.** Central to the level occupied by Haversian columns, the bone lamellae form a labyrinth, cancellous bone (c). Its cavities are filled with bone marrow (m). Humerus, rabbit, HE.

mature, diaphysis, the following concentric layers, starting at the surface, are encountered: periosteum (Fig. 4.2.5.), compact bone in the shape of circumferential lamellae, a layer of compact bone forming osteons or Haversian columns (Fig. 4.2.6.), a layer of spongy bone containing bone marrow (Fig. 4.2.7.), and a marrow cavity. The absolute thickness of the diaphyseal wall does not greatly increase during diametric growth, while the marrow cavity and of the whole diaphysis continually expand, causing the relative thickness of the diaphyseal wall to decrease.

During growth of a long bone, there is proportional **epiphyseal growth**. Initially, the epiphysis is still largely cartilage. The deeper layers of the peripheral cartilage, which grows interstitially and, except for the articular cartilage, subperichondrially, calcify and degenerate and are replaced with fibrous bone. In its turn, the fibrous bone is degraded and replaced with lamellar spongy bone, which contains bone marrow. Thus, the central mass of spongy bone expands by enchondral bone formation. Between the articular cartilage and the growth plate, the perichondrium is eventually transformed into a periosteum, whereupon subperiosteal growth adds new layers of compact lamellar bone, which make the epiphysis expand. The deeper layers are gradually degraded and replaced with spongy bone.

During growth of a long bone, **remodeling** is necessary, and for a number of reasons. In the long run, as the organism gradually reaches its adult size and proportions, the shape of the bones may have to be adapted to changing load patterns. In the short run, on the contrary, the shape of the bone has to be conserved. Longitudinal bone growth would inevitably lead to changes in shape because the basis of the epiphysis, where the growth plate and the fibrous bone layer are situated, is wider than the diaphysis. This would lead to widening of both the diaphysis and its marrow cavity during longitudinal growth, independently of the diametric growth of the diaphysis. In reality, the epiphysis is connected to the diaphysis through a conical connecting part, the **metaphysis**. Essentially, remodellation during longitudinal growth involves the conservation of the metaphyseal shape. This is obtained by selective degradation of bone at the edge of the cone basis, followed by deposition of new bone at the inside, at the periphery of the marrow cavity. This bone is deposited by locally differentiated osteoblasts, which may be covered with interstitial tissue, forming an **endosteum**, which is analogous to the periosteum. The relative shares of the various bone tissue types making up the wall of the metaphysis are conserved by the mechanisms already discussed under diametric growth.

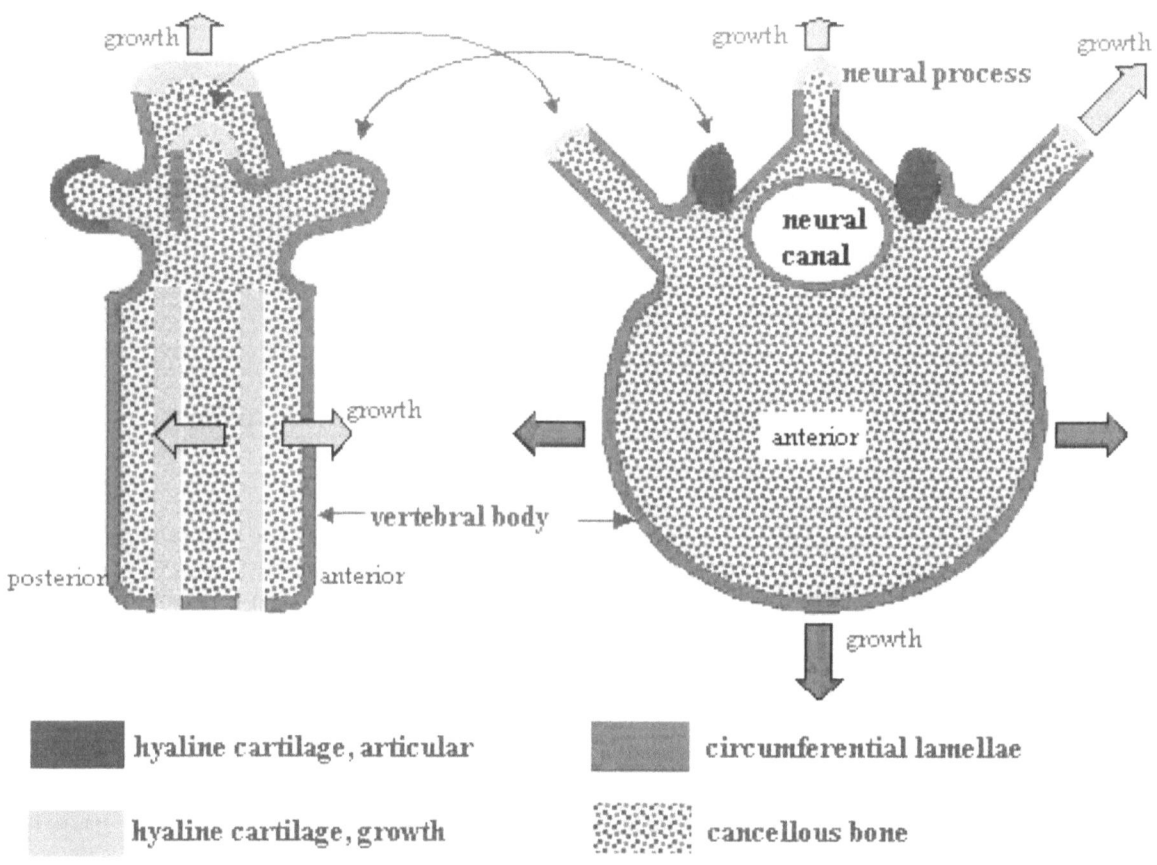

Fig. 4.2.8. A vertebra consists of a vertebral body and a number of processes. Some of these form articular surfaces with adjoining vertebrae, while others serve to attach muscles and tendons. Inside the neural canal runs the spinal cord. The vertebral body is made of spongy bone, enveloped with circumferential lamellae, and grows in girth by means of subperiosteal bone formation (dark arrows). A growing vertebral body also contains 2 transverse cartilaginous growth plates, and grows in length by means of enchondral bone formation (light arrows). The processes grow stouter by subperiosteal growth, and lengthwise by enchondral growth, originating in a terminal growth plate. In those processes that serve in articulation, this growth plate develops into a layer of articular cartilage. In the other processes, it is eventually completely replaced with bone.

IV.2.2.2. Vertebrae.

The vertebrae envelop the spinal cord and protect it. In addition, they have an essential supporting function: they make up the vertebral column, which constitutes the skeleton's axis. They also serve as insertion points to muscles.

During embryological development, the neural tube is supported by a notochord (Fig. 4.1.). At regular interspaces along the notochord, concentric nuclei of cartilage develop, which are the precursors of the **vertebral bodies**. At the dorsal side of the prospective vertebral bodies, additional cartilaginous precursors form in the shape of plates, to the left and right of the neural tube. They fuse with one another on the dorsal midline, resulting in the formation of a **neural arch**. Their basis fuses with the vertebral body, resulting in the formation of a **neural canal**, which completely encloses the neural tube or primitive spinal cord. Where vertebral bodies and neural arch join, processes, or **zygapophyses**, develop, allowing the vertebrae to articulate with one another. Other processes, the **neural processes**, offer insertion points to muscles and ligaments.

The cartilaginous vertebrae initially grow interstitially and subperichondrially. Eventually, in the center of the vertebral bodies and in the neural arches, enchondral bone formation starts. Cartilage hypertrophies, calcifies, is degraded, and is replaced with bone. Initially, this is fibrous bone, which is subsequently degraded and replaced with lamellar spongy bone containing bone marrow.

Some time after initiation of enchondral bone formation, the perichondrium is transformed to a periosteum. By subperiosteal bone formation, lamellar bone is deposited in the shape of circumferential lamellae.

Vertebrae grow by enchondral, as well as subperiosteal, growth (Fig. 4.2.8.). The vertebral body is a cylinder that expands diametrially by subperiosteal growth. The cylinder's length increases by means of enchondral growth. Enchondral bone formation in the vertebral body does not entirely transform it into bone: a transverse layer of cartilage is maintained at both its ends, forming two growth plates which enable the vertebral body to lengthen. Another layer of cartilage is maintained which joins the neural arch to the vertebral body. This layer functions as a growth plate, which allows the neural arch to expand. Finally, growth plates are situated at the tips of the zygapophyses and the neural processes, enabling them to lengthen. The growth plates of the neural processes will eventually be replaced with bone. Those of the zygapophyses may be conserved as articular cartilage.

Vertebrae form articulating joints through the zygapophyses. In addition to this, they are interconnected through ligaments, which transform a series of vertebrae into a vertebral column. Most of these ligaments consist of dense fibrous and ordered connective tissue. A notable exception is the ligamentum flavum, which consists of elastic tissue.

It runs on the inside of the neural canal and facilitates stretching of the vertebral column after bending.

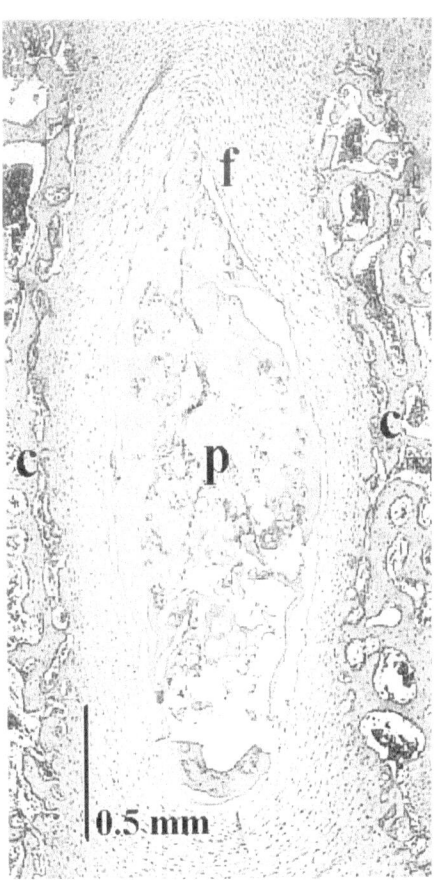

Fig. 4.2.9. An intervertebral disk contains a nucleus pulposus (p), a specialized form of interstitial tissue with a largely fluid matrix, which serves as a buffer. It is enveloped and contained by a layer of fibrous cartilage, the annulus fibrosus (f). c = spongy bone of 2 successive vertebral bodies. Spine, rat, HE.

IV.2.3. Intervertebral disks.

Intervertebral disks (Fig. 4.2.9.) form shock-absorbing cushions between the bodies of adjoining vertebrae. Their inside is hollow and filled with a viscous fluid. This **nucleus pulposus** is enveloped with concentric layers of fibrous cartilage, the **annulus fibrosus**. The nucleus pulposus is an unusual type of interstitial tissue. Its matrix is fluid, since it contains only ground substance and no fibrils. The shock-absorbing characteristics of the intervertebral disks are explained by the fact that fluid is incompressible. This fluid is secreted by clusters of physaliphorous cells, which are distributed throughout the nucleus pulposus. These cells are remnants of the embryonic notochord.

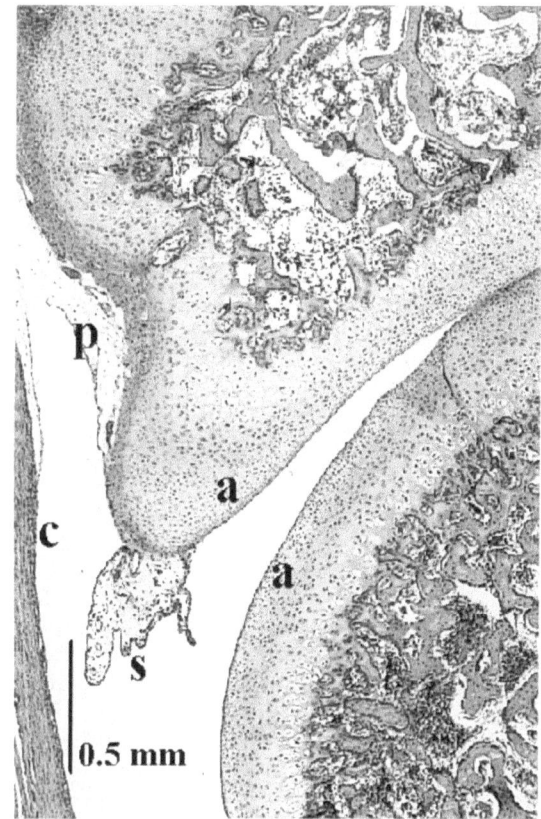

fact specialized matrix-secreting cells. The give away is the possession of processes and the abundant rough endoplasmic reticulum. Similar synovial cells line the inside of the joint capsule. They only secrete ground substance, no fibrils, and into the synovial space. Here, the ground substance is mixed with derivatives of the blood plasma and forms the lubricating synovial fluid. It also allows diffusion of oxygen as well as food and waste molecules between the synovial capillaries and the avascular articular cartilage. Other synovial lining cells are macrophages with antigen-presenting properties.

References.

Behrsin J.F., Briggs C.A.: Ligaments of the lumbar spine: a review. Surg. Radiol. Anat. 1988, 10: 211-219.

Iwanaga T., Shikichi M., Kitamura H., Yanase H., Nozawa-Inoue K.: Morphology and functional roles of synoviocytes in the joint. Arch. Histol. Cytol. 2000, 63: 17-31.

Fig. 4.2.10. Bones may articulate relative to one another in a joint. The smooth articular faces are made of hyaline cartilage, lacking a perichondrial coat, the articular cartilage (a). Perichondrium (p) is present outside the actual articular surfaces. The joint is encapsulated with dense fibrous tissue, the joint capsule (c). Inside the capsule is a synovial cavity, filled with a lubricating fluid. This is produced by the synovium (s), an interstitial tissue mass pervaded with blood vessels, and lined with specialized matrix-secreting cells, the synovial cells. Heel joint, rabbit, HE.

IV.2.4. Joints.

Joints allow movement or articulation of two bones relative to one another. The cartilaginous articular surfaces proper, where both bones actually touch, are enclosed in a synovial space, which is filled with a lubricating fluid and lined with a dense fibrous joint capsule. This capsule also ensures that both bones are held in close apposition. Within the synovial space, a specialized structure made up of interstitial tissue is found, the **synovium** (Fig. 4.2.10.). Its deeper parts are richly vascularized, its surface may form complicated folds that are lined by one or more layers of **synovial cells**. These superficially resemble an epithelium, called the synovial membrane. Their apical membrane forms microvilli and microplicae. They may even form a rudimentary basement membrane and, in addition to gap junctions, desmosomes. However, most of these cells are in

142

IV.3. Muscular system.

The muscular system fixes the skeleton in certain positions and can move the individual bones relative to one another. It is predominantly made up of **skeletal muscle tissue**. To form **muscles**, individual muscle fibers are joined into bundles by means of fibrous tissue sheaths. Dense fibrous **connective tissue** also forms the **tendons** that join the muscles to the skeleton. Although it is not very conspicuous, **nerve tissue** is a vital component of the muscular system. Each individual skeletal muscle fiber is contacted by a motor nerve fiber that forms a specialized end knob or **motor end plate**. Both muscles and tendons are in contact with the terminals of sensory nerve fibers which, in the muscles, participate in the formation of complex sensory organs, the **muscle spindles**.

IV.3.1. Muscles.

Fundamentally, a muscle is a collection of muscle fibers, arranged according to a particular pattern, which are joined by fibrous tissue sheaths (Fig. 4.3.1.). An individual muscle fiber is enveloped by a thin layer of fibrous tissue, the **endomysium**. Several fibers form a bundle, enveloped by a thicker fibrous tissue layer, the **perimysium**. The whole muscle, consisting of multiple bundles, is enveloped by a thick and densely fibrous connective tissue layer, the **epimysium** or fascia. In all these fibrous tissue layers, blood vessels and nerve fibers run.

At both ends of the muscle, the long, cylindrical muscle fibers are attached to a tendon via a specialized **myotendinous junction** (Fig. 4.3.2.). At such a junction, the muscle fiber membrane shows a number of finger-like processes and its inner face is coated with a dense proteinaceous layer, the internal lamina. The internal lamina consists of specialized proteins that bind the actin microfilaments of the terminal I-band. Therefore, it is the equivalent of a Z-membrane. Transmembrane proteins join the internal lamina to the lamina densa of the enveloping basement membrane, which in its turn is connected to the collagen fibrils of the tendon. During muscle fiber contraction, this arrangement allows for efficient transmission of force from the actin microfilaments to the collagen fibrils.

Muscle fibers may be shorter than the muscle in which they occur, and yet not be joined to other fibers, but to fibrous tissue. Such fibers may be fusiform, with tapered ends. They are usually anchored, via their basal lamina, to the collagen

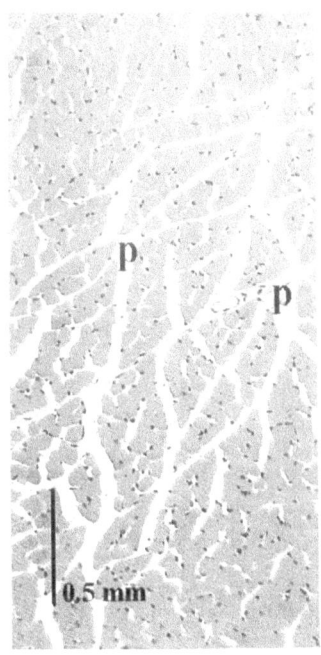

Fig. 4.3.1. A skeletal muscle consists of parallel bundles of skeletal muscle fibers, sheathed with fibrous connective tissue. Individual fibers are sheathed with a very thin connective tissue layer, the endomysium. A bundle of several fibers is sheathed by a thicker layer of connective tissue, the perimysium (p). A large number of such bundles, i. e. an entire muscle, is sheathed by a connective tissue fascia or epimysium. Gluteus muscle, transverse section, rabbit, HE.

fibrils of the endo- and perimysia. Other fibers are cylindrical, and are anchored to **tendinous intersections**, which are transverse bands of dense ordered fibrous tissue, similar to tendons. In this case, a muscle not only consists of parallel fibers, but of serial ones also. Contrary to tendons, tendinous intersections are symmetrical: both faces show muscle fiber insertions, with a structure similar to myotendinous junctions.

IV.3.2. Tendons.

Tendons, which bind skeletal muscles to bones, consist of **dense ordered fibrous tissue** (Fig. 4.3.3.), in which the collagen fibrils run parallel to the tendon's longitudinal axis. The collagen fibrils are arranged into bundles, sheathed with a thin layer of loose fibrous tissue, the **peritendineum internum**. The whole tendon is enveloped with a thicker layer of fibrous tissue, the **peritendineum externum**. Frequently, the peritendineum externum is lined with mesothelium, forming a serosa or **epitenon**. The surrounding tissues form a sheath, lined with a corresponding serosa, the **peritenon**. Between both

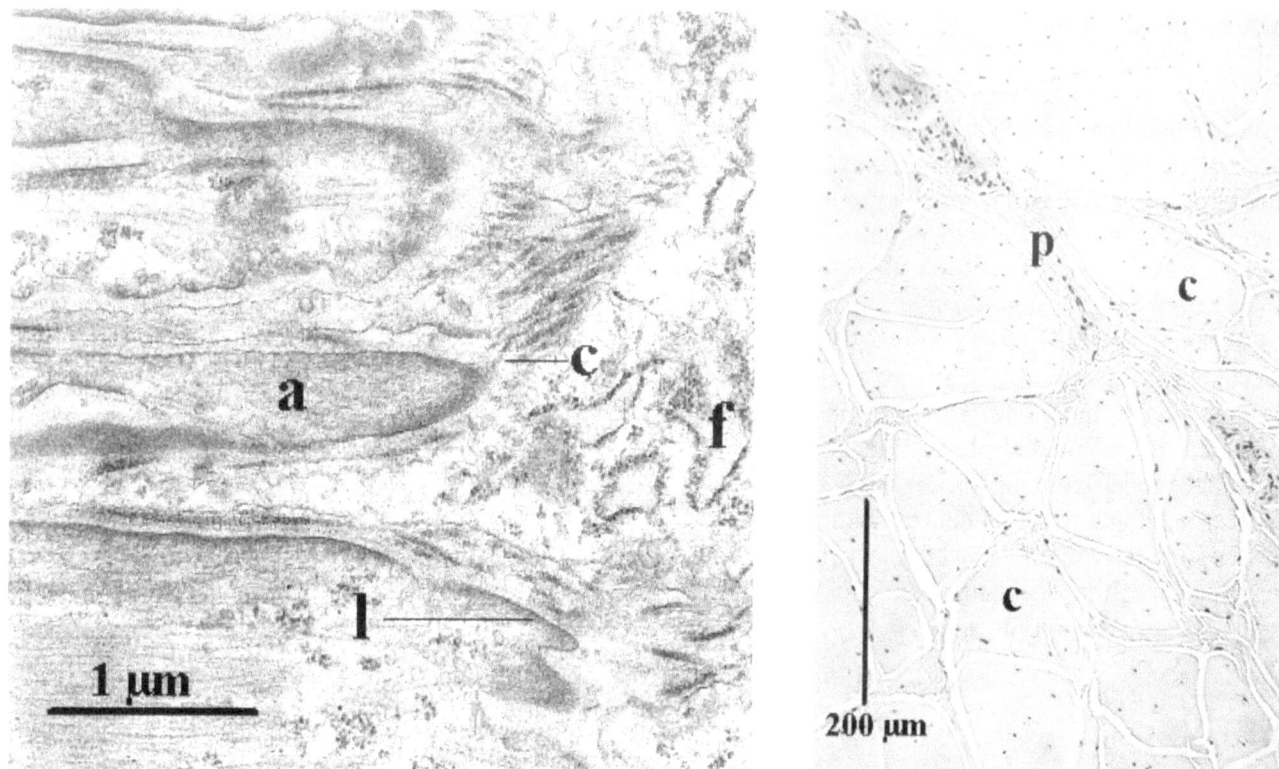

Fig. 4.3.2. (left) Tendons are anchored to muscle fibers by means of specialized myotendinous junctions. The muscle fiber terminal participating in such a junction develops a number of finger-like processes. The cytosolic face of the cell membrane is coated with a dense internal lamina (l), which anchors both the actin microfilaments (a) of the myofibrils and the collagen fibrils (c) of the tendon. Below, the cytoplasm of a fibrocyte (f) shows. Skeletal muscle, hamster, TEM. **Fig. 4.3.3.** (right) A tendon consists of a large number of parallel bundles of collagen fibers (c), i.e. ordered dense fibrous tissue. Several of these are sheathed with a thin layer of loose fibrous tissue, the peritendineum internum (p). Finger tendon, human, HE.

is a narrow space and both serosae facilitate the tendon's movements relative to the surrounding tissues.

At one end, a tendon is attached to a muscle by a myotendinous junction. At the opposite end, it is anchored to a bone by **Sharpey's fibers**. These are the tendon's own collagen fibrils, which are embedded in the peripheral bone tissue. The attachment site of a tendon to a bone may be reinforced with fibrous cartilage.

IV.3.3. Motor end plates.

Muscles are connected to the spinal cord by means of motor nerves. Bundles of myelinated motor nerve fibers run in the perimysium. Each individual muscle fiber is contacted by a single motor nerve fiber terminal. This is a relatively long, flattened end knob, which indents the muscle fiber: the **motor end plate** (Fig. 4.3.4.). The free surface of the motor end plate is covered with a few flattened Schwann cells,

which do not form myelin. The basement membrane of the Schwann cells merges with that of the muscle fiber. The part of the muscle fiber that accommodates the motor end plate is the sole plate.

The motor end plate contains numerous cholinergic synaptic vesicles and forms a synaptic junction with the sole plate. This myoneural junction differs on a number of points from the synaptic junctions found in nerve tissue, however. To begin with, the cytosolic faces of the pre- and postsynaptic membranes (those of the motor end plate and the sole plate, respectively) are largely clear of dense coats. At most, the motor end plate membrane carries a number of local densifications, or active zones, towards which the synaptic vesicles tend to converge. The active zones have the shape of ribbons, which run parallel to the long axis of the motor end plate. Secondly, the pre- and postsynaptic membranes do not run entirely parallel, because the sole plate forms a number of deep and narrow furrows, which may be bifurcated. These furrows lie perpendicular to the superficial cell membrane and together constitute a

144

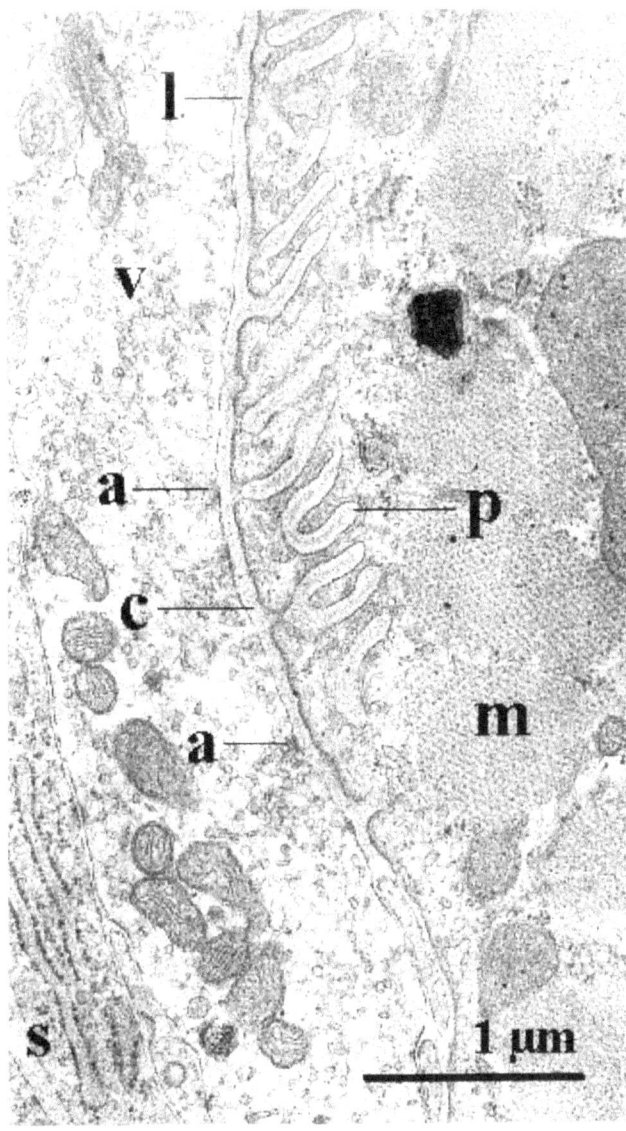

IV.3.4. Muscle spindles.

Muscle spindles are receptor organs that lie in the perimysia of various muscles (Fig. 4.3.5.). They consist of a bundle of parallel, specialized muscle fibers, called **intrafusal fibers** to distinguish them from the ordinary muscle fibers, the extrafusal fibers. A muscle spindle lies parallel to the neighbouring extrafusal fibers and is itself constituted of about ten intrafusal fibers. Intrafusal fibers not only are much thinner (diameter: 5 to 10 micrometers) and shorter (length: up to a few millimeters) than extrafusal ones, they also have a deviating microscopic structure. The biggest difference of all is that the intrafusal fibers receive a dense sensory innervation.

A muscle spindle is enveloped with a fibrous capsule, in which blood vessels and nerve fibers run. The intrafusal fibers lying close to the spindle axis have a dilated center, caused by the accumulation of cell nuclei. This nuclear bag (Fig. 4.3.6.) gives its name to the axial intrafusal fibers: **nuclear bag fibers**. At both sides of the nuclear bag, the intrafusal fiber narrows and its nuclei form an axial row: a nuclear chain. Both the nuclear bag and the nuclear chain zones conserve only remains of the myofibrils, and there is no cross striation. The terminals of the nuclear bag fibers show, except for their diminutive diameter, the normal microscopic structure of a skeletal muscle fiber, with peripheral nuclei and a well developed transverse striation. At the periphery of the muscle spindle lie intrafusal fibers which are shorter than the axial nuclear bag fibers and do not contain a nuclear bag. They show a single, continuous nuclear chain and are called **nuclear chain fibers**. In contrast to nuclear bag fibers, their nuclear chain zone conserves a peripheral cross striation.

Sensory nerve fibers (Fig. 4.3.6.) contact both types of intrafusal fibers at the level of the nuclear bags and nuclear chains. At the nuclear bag level, intrafusal fibers are encircled by snake-like, spirally wound nerve terminals. The nuclear chain zones are contacted by branched terminals resembling bird feet. Both types of nerve terminals indent the intrafusal fibers and are loaded with mitochondria. The intrafusal muscle fiber ends, the structure of which is identical to that of extrafusal fibers, are contacted by motor nerve fibers, forming motor end plates.

Muscle spindles are mechanoreceptors that are sensitive to deformation by stretching. Skeletal muscle fibers continually maintain a tonus to fix the skeleton in certain positions. If this tonus is insufficient, a skeletal muscle is stretched by the

Fig. 4.3.4. The terminal of a motor nerve fiber, loaded with clear synaptic vesicles (v), forms a motor end plate, which is the presynaptic part of a synaptic junction with a skeletal muscle fiber. In a few places, the cytosolic face of its cell membrane carries a dense material, the active zones (a). The dense lamina of the basement membrane continues into the synaptic cleft (c). The postsynaptic muscle fiber's membrane is the sole plate (p). It is slightly thickened and forms tubular, branched inpocketings, also containing dense lamina. s = Schwann cell cytoplasm, mi = mitochondria, my = myofibrils. Skeletal muscle, rabbit, TEM.

kind of secondary synaptic cleft, at the bottom of the primary synaptic cleft. They greatly expand the available postsynaptic membrane surface for incorporation of receptor molecules. In both synaptic cleft divisions, a narrow dense layer runs parallel and equidistant to the pre- and postsynaptic membranes. Upon leaving the junction, it merges with the lamina densa of the basement membrane.

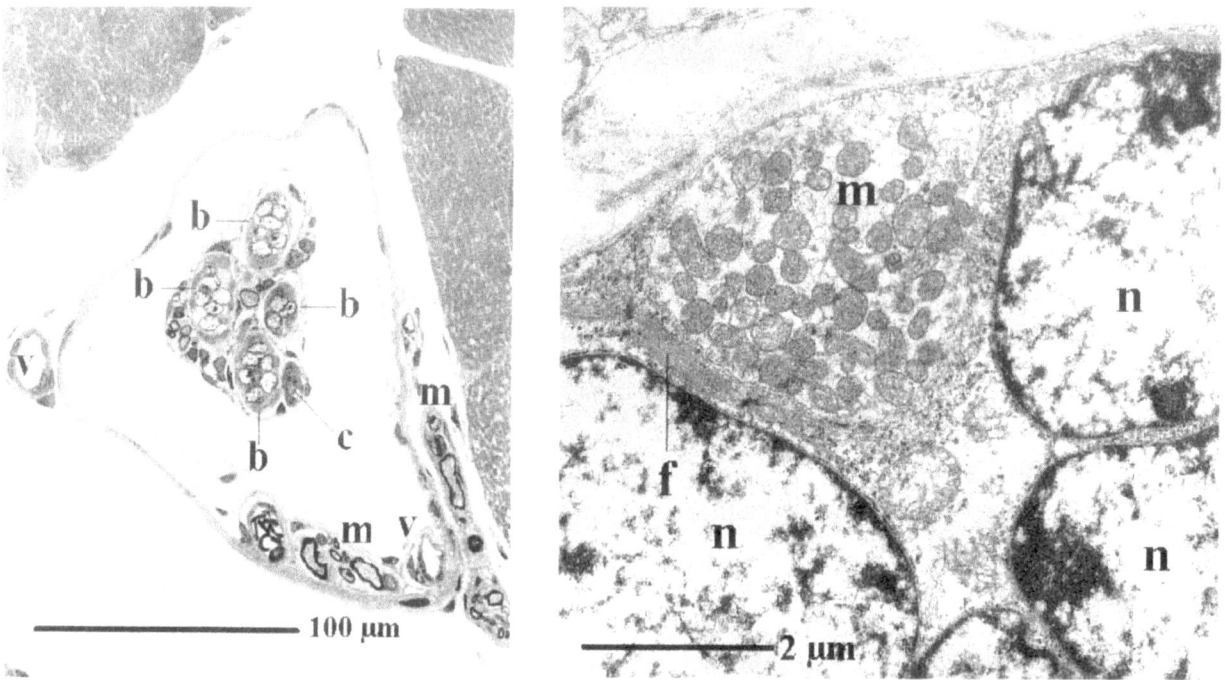

Fig. 4.3.5. (left) A transverse section of a muscle spindle. It is surrounded by a capsule, carrying blood vessels (v) and myelinated nerve fibers (m). In the center is a bundle of intrafusal fibers (compare their dimensions with those of the extrafusal fibers at the upper left and to the right). Except for a single nuclear chain fiber with a central nucleus (c), 4 nuclear bag fibers show, characterized by an accumulation of nuclei (b). Neck muscle, rabbit, 1-micrometer plastic section, toluidin blue. **Fig. 4.3.6.** (right) A nuclear bag fiber, with numerous cell nuclei (n), is contacted by the end knob of a sensory nerve fiber, loaded with mitochondria (m). The nuclear bag fiber's cytoplasm contains traces of myofibrils (f). Neck muscle, rabbit, TEM.

weight of the body or a part of it. Since muscle spindles run parallel to the skeletal muscle fibers, they are stretched as well. This deformation of the intrafusal fibers causes deformation of the sensory nerve terminals and induces action potentials running along the sensory nerve fibers to the spinal cord. In the gray matter of the spinal cord, these fibers synapse with motor nerves, which form fibers innervating the extrafusal fibers of the same muscle. Through a reflex mechanism, stretching of intrafusal muscle fibers will result in compensatory contraction and increased tonus of extrafusal fibers. In this way, muscle spindles ensure that the length and, indirectly, the tonus of a skeletal muscle are maintained between narrow values.

The motor innervation of the intrafusal fiber terminals has several functions. The nuclear bag and nuclear chain zones of the intrafusal fibers have elastic properties and will shorten upon compensatory contraction of the extrafusal fibers, so that their stimulation stops. In contrast, the terminals, similar to extrafusal fibers, can be passively stretched, but not shortened. They can only shorten by shifting of the myofilaments, and the only way to do that is by neural stimulation of the fiber. In addition, some muscles can sustain different lengths, according to the particular position they have to fix. When muscles have to shorten to accommodate themselves to another position, the motor fibers innervating the intrafusal fibers can cause these to shorten accordingly. Finally, contraction of the intrafusal fiber ends may stretch the central zones, increasing the muscle spindle's sensitivity.

References.

Benjamin M., Ralphs J.R.: Tendons and ligaments - an overview. Histol. Histopathol. 1997, 12: 1135-1144.

Hijikata T., Ishikawa H.: Functional morphology of serially linked skeletal muscle fibers. Acta Anat. 1997, 159: 99-107.

Trotter J.A.: Functional morphology of force transmission in skeletal muscle. Acta Anat. 1993, 146: 205-222.

IV. Nervous system.

During embryonic development, the nervous system develops from the neural tube. Before the neural groove closes to form a tube, groups of cells separate from the edges of the groove, the neural crest. While the neural tube forms the central nervous system, the neural crest gives rise to the ganglia of the peripheral nervous system and an endocrine gland, the adrenal medulla. The brain originates as an expansion of the cranial end of the neural tube. The original expansion is constricted in a few places, producing a number of brain vesicles. These give rise to the main subparts of the brain, such as the cerebrum and the cerebellum. The rest of the neural tube does not expand but becomes the spinal cord. Brain and spinal cord constitute the central nervous system. The peripheral nervous system consists of cranial and spinal nerves, connecting the brain and the spinal cord, respectively, to the rest of the body.

The wall of the newly formed neural tube is a simple prismatic epithelium, the neuroepithelium, which rests on a peripheral basement membrane. Later on,

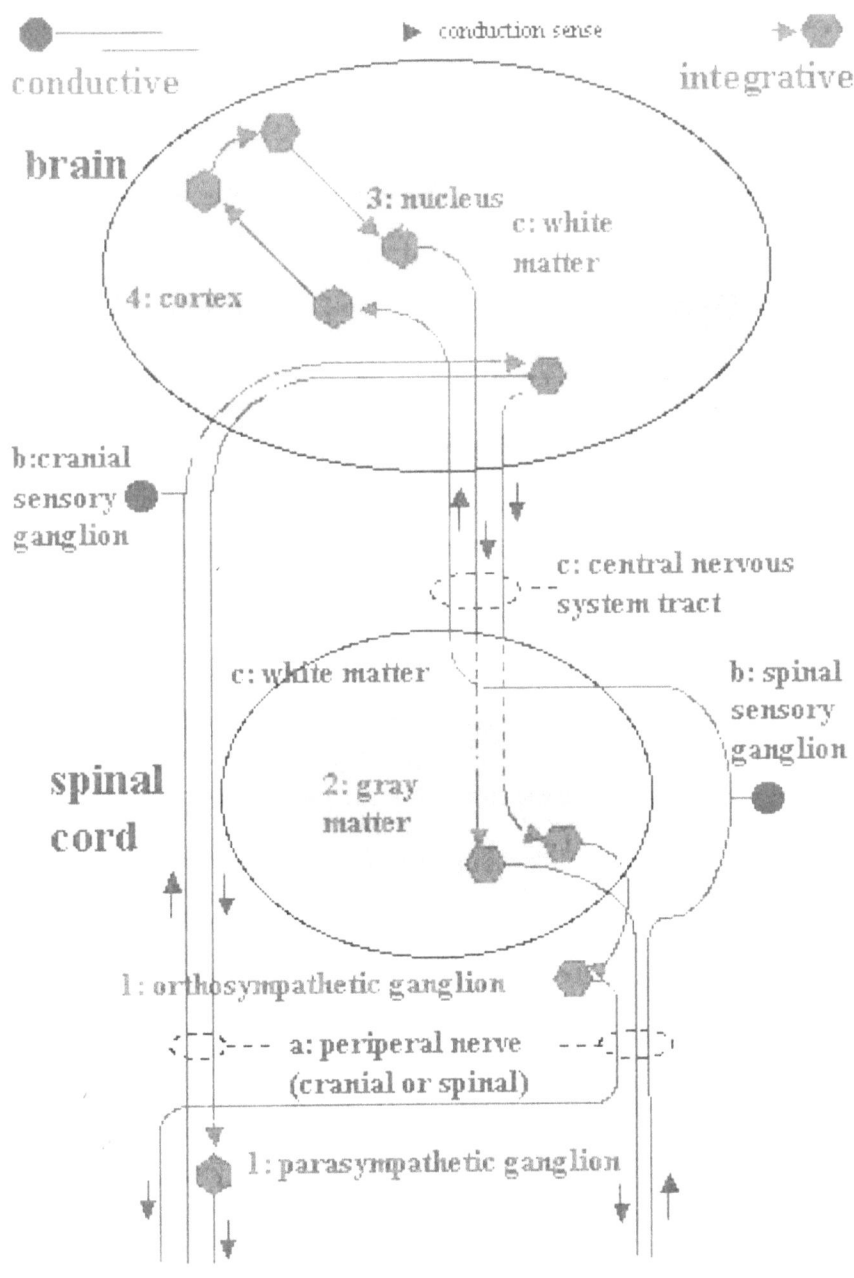

NERVOUS TISSUE

Fig. 4.4.1. The nervous system is dominated by nervous tissue, which occurs in two forms: conductive and integrative. Conductive tissue is composed of nerve fibers, the function of which is to conduct action potentials. This tissue is found in spinal and cranial peripheral nerves (a) and sensory ganglia (b), and in the white matter of the brain and the spinal cord (c). Integrative tissue is composed of nerve cell perikarya with their dendrites, carrying synaptic junctions with axon terminals of other nerve cells. In this tissue, action potentials are transmitted from one nerve cell to the next. It is organized to various degrees of complexity. In its simplest form, it is found in the ortho-and parasympathic motor ganglia (1). Increasingly complex integrative tissue is found in the spinal cord's gray column (2), the brain nuclei (3), and the brain cortex (4).

cell multiplication gives the neuroepithelium a stratified character. The neuroepithelial cells develop and differentiate into nerve cells and glia cells. The nerve cells grow axons that contact target cells in both the central and peripheral nervous systems. The most central layer of neuroepithelial cells, lining the tube's lumen, is not greatly involved in this transformation and largely retains its original epithelial character. These are the ependymal cells. In a few places, the neuroepithelium retains its simple character throughout embryonic development, giving rise to choroid plexus cells.

The dominant tissue type which forms the nervous system is, of course, **nerve tissue**. It occurs in two forms: conductive nerve tissue and integrative nerve tissue (III.6.1.-2., Fig. 4.4.1.).

Conductive nerve tissue consists of bundles of nerve fibers, which conduct action potentials from one part of the nervous system to another, sometimes over considerable distances, up to tens of centimeters.

Integrative nerve tissue consists of perikarya and dendrites of nerve cells, and axon terminals that contact them to form synaptic junctions. In the integrative nerve tissue, action potentials are transmitted from one nerve cell to another, the nerve cells forming networks or circuits, often quite complicated ones.

In addition to nerve tissue, the nervous system contains, to a lesser extent, other kinds of tissue, such as glandular tissue, epithelium, endothelium, and fibrous tissue.

Occasionally, nerve cells are found which do not discharge their transmitters near the dendrites of other nerve cells, but in stead into the general intercellular space and from there into the blood. In effect, these neurotransmitters have become hormones. Technically, the nerve cells producing them are hormone-secreting gland cells. Morphologically, they are indistinguishable from typical nerve cells. Such **neurosecretory cells** form two endocrine glands, closely associated with the brain: the **pineal gland** and the **neurohypophysis**.

The **ependyma** and the **choroid plexi** are made up of neuroepithelial cells that have hardly, if at all, participated in the transformation of the neuroepithelium from simple to stratified. Consequently, they still form an **epithelium**, lining the interior spaces of the central nervous system, the spinal canal and the brain's ventricles, which stem from the embryonic neural canal. Since they are not nerve cells, but do descend from the neuroepithelium, they can be regarded as glia cells. They are primarily involved in the production and circulation of the

cerebrospinal fluid, which fills the spinal canal and the ventricles and bathes the surrounding nerve tissue.

In the peripheral nervous system, bundles of nerve fibers are enveloped by sheaths of **fibrous tissue**. The central nervous system contains little fibrous tissue and consequently has a weak consistency. It is enveloped, on the other hand, by three concentric fibrous tissue sheaths, the **meninges**.

The **endothelium** forming the central nervous system's capillaries is specifically adapted to make it relatively impermeable to larger molecules. Thus, a blood-brain barrier is formed, which helps to maintain the chemical composition of the cerebrospinal fluid.

Microglia were initially regarded as yet another category of glia cells, derived from the neuroepithelium. Later, they turned out to be entirely different kinds of cells altogether. They are defender cells, replacing the lymphoid tissue, which is completely absent in the central nervous system.

IV.4.1. Conductive nerve tissue.

In the peripheral nervous system, conductive nerve tissue forms the **nerves**. Nerves contain sensory nerve fibers as well as motor nerve fibers. The morphologies of both are absolutely identical. Their only difference lies in the direction in which they conduct action potentials. Sensory nerve fibers conduct action potentials towards the central nervous system, while motor nerve fibers conduct action potentials away from the central nervous system. The axons of the sensory nerve fibers originate from perikarya that do not receive synaptic input. They accumulate at certain places along the nerves: the **sensory ganglia**. In the central nervous system, conductive nerve tissue forms the **white matter**. In the spinal cord, the white matter is found at the periphery. In the central nervous system, on the other hand, it occupies a central position. White matter derives its color from the high number of myelinated nerve fibers.

IV.4.1.1. Nerves.

The peripheral nervous system consists of 12 pairs of cranial nerves, connected to the brain, and about 30 pairs of spinal nerves, connected to the spinal cord. The cranial nerves contain motor nerve fibers, sensory nerve fibers, or a mixture of both. The spinal nerves always contain both motor and sensory nerve fibers. Inside the vertebral canal, they split, forming

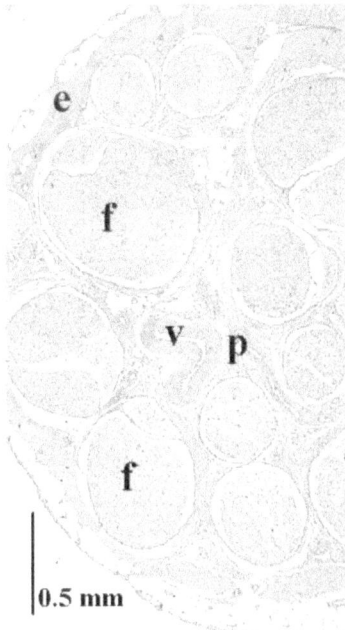

Fig. 4.4.2. A transverse section of a peripheral nerve shows several bundles of nerve fibers (f, detail: Figure 3.6.7.), sheathed in a layer of fibrous connective tissue, the perineurium (p). The nerve itself is sheathed in a thicker layer of connective and adipose tissue, the epineurium (e). The epineurium forms septa, which carry blood vessels, the vasa nervorum (v). Sciatic nerve, human, HE.

a dorsal root and a ventral root. By way of the dorsal root, the sensory fibers of the nerve enter the spinal cord. Motor fibers, on the other hand, leave the spinal cord by way of the ventral root and continue down the spinal nerve. On entering the spinal cord, sensory nerve fibers synapse with motor nerve cells of the gray matter or run up the spinal cord towards the brain, to synapse with brain nerve cells. Interneurons may be intercalated between the sensory nerve fibers and the motor or brain nerve cells. The connection between an incoming sensory fiber and an outgoing motor one is the simplest example of a reflex arc, ensuring that a certain stimulus will be followed by the correct response.

A peripheral nerve (Fig. 4.4.2.) is a collection of **nerve fibers**, subdivided into bundles by sheaths of **fibrous tissue**. Each individual nerve fiber, myelinated (by Schwann cells) or not, is ensheathed by a very thin layer of fibrous tissue, the **endoneurium**. A bundle of nerve fibers, containing hundreds of fibers, is ensheathed by a thicker layer of loose fibrous tissue, the **perineurium**. The perineurium may contain layers of flattened cells, the perineural cells, which are assumed to be analogous to the mesothelial cells covering the arachnoidea, the

middle of the three meninges (IV.4.5.). The entire nerve, containing several bundles of nerve fibers, is ensheathed by a layer of dense fibrous tissue, the **epineurium**. The epineurium is a direct continuation of the dura mater, the outer meninge. The perineurium and the deeper layers of the epineurium contain blood vessels, the **vasa nervorum**.

IV.4.1.2. Sensory ganglia.

The sensory ganglia are collections of perikarya of the nerve cells that form the sensory fibers of the peripheral nerves.
The dorsal root of each spinal nerve carries a sensory ganglion. Therefore, it is also called a **dorsal** or a **spinal ganglion**. The perikarya it contains are always those of pseudounipolar nerve cells. In addition, sensory ganglia are located on some, but not all, cranial nerves. Most often, they also contain the perikarya of pseudounipolar nerve cells. The only exceptions are the sensory ganglia carried by the cranial nerves that are connected to the organs of hearing and balance. They contain the perikarya of bipolar nerve cells.

Sensory ganglia (Fig. 4.4.3.) are encapsulated by a relatively thick layer of dense fibrous connective tissue, which is continuous with the dura mater of the central nervous system and the epineuria of the spinal nerves. Their interior contains little fibrous tissue.
The perikarya of the pseudounipolar or bipolar nerve cells are not evenly distributed. They are found in greatest number at the periphery of the ganglia, where they form a cortex. In the center, they form a few longitudinal cords. Between the cords run numerous myelinated and unmyelinated nerve fibers, originating at the surrounding perikarya. The perikarya have no synaptic contacts whatsoever.
The perikarya are lined by a single layer of squamous or cuboidal glia cells, the satellite cells. Satellite cells have little cytoplasm, contain mostly primary organelles, and form processes that run parallel to the surface of the perikaryon and interdigitate with those of neighbouring satellite cells. The boundary between nerve cells and satellite cells is irregular, since both form spikes that indent the other's surface. These spikes may deceptively resemble axonal end knobs. Satellite cells are joined by means of desmosomes (III.4.1.1.). Their abneural surface is coated with a basement membrane. They may form a thin myelin sheath at the level of the perikarya of bipolar nerve cells. For this reason, they are regarded as analogous to Schwann cells.

149

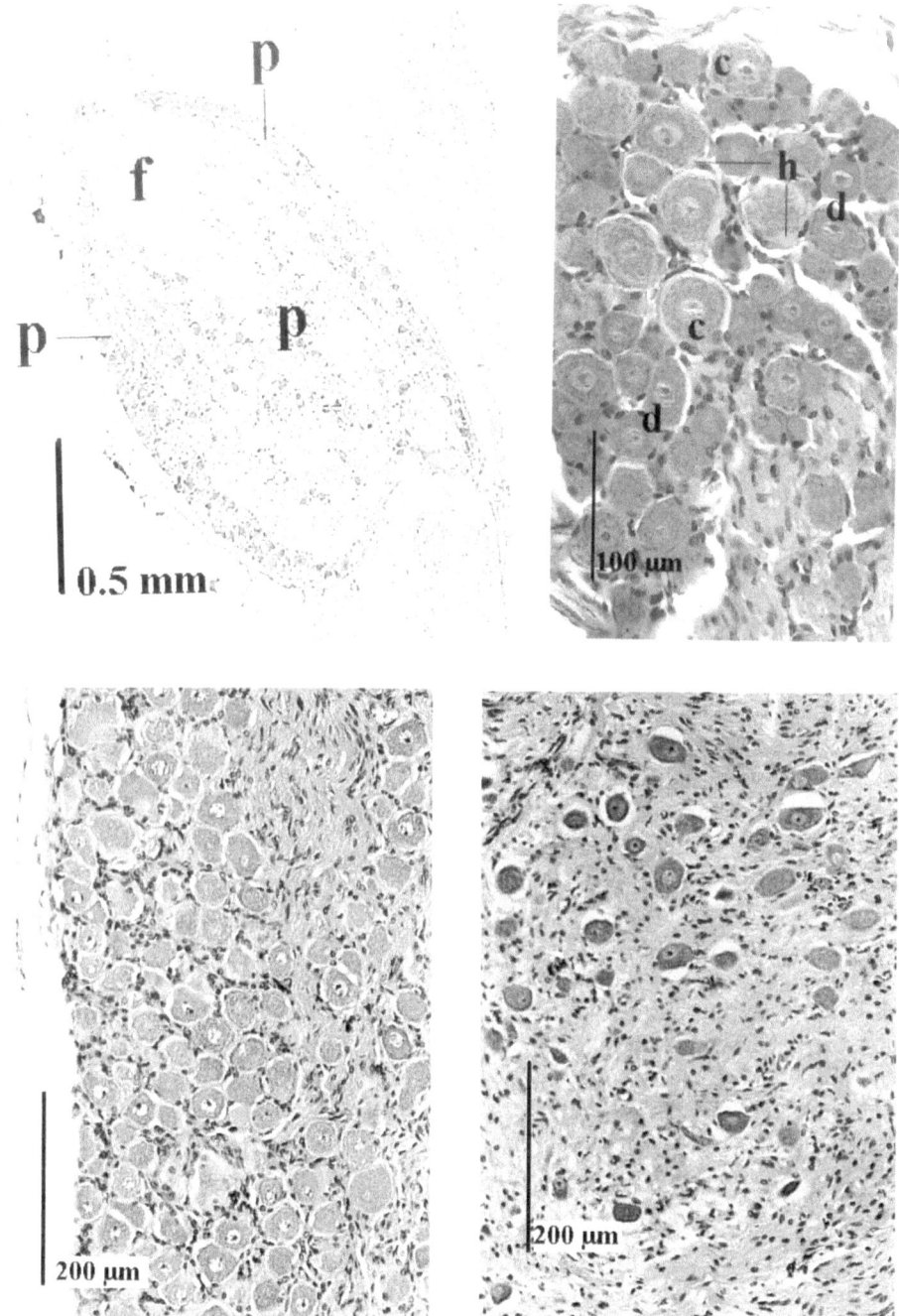

Fig. 4.4.3. (top left) A sensory ganglion contains the perikarya (p) of pseudounipolar (sometimes bipolar) nerve cells. These perikarya form a peripheral cortex, as well as a number of more centrally running cords. This arrangement leaves ample room for the passage of bundles of sensory nerve fibers (f). Spinal ganglion, sheep, HE. **Fig. 4.4.4.** (top right) The pseudounipolar sensory nerve cells of spinal ganglia belong to 2 types: large clear ones, with coarsely granular Nissl substance (c), and small dark ones, with finely granular Nissl substance (d). Mark the axon hillocks (h). Spinal ganglion, rat, HE. **Fig. 4.4.5.** (bottom left) In cranial sensory ganglia, the pseudounipolar nerve cell perikarya have a more homogeneous look, especially regarding size. Nodose ganglion, goat, HE. **Fig. 4.4.6.** (bottom right) The perikarya of multipolar motor nerve cells, occupying a motor ganglion, are smaller and more homogeneously distributed (compare with Figure 4.4.5.). Superior cervical ganglion, sheep, HE.

In spinal ganglia, two kinds of perikarya or ganglion cells can often be distinguished (Fig. 4.4.4.). Some of the perikarya are relatively large, with diameters of 100 micrometers or more. The Nissl substance is coarsely granular, with the granules widely spaced, giving the perikaryon a pale appearance. Other perikarya are smaller and contain a finely granular, homogeneous Nissl substance, making them appear darker. The large, pale ganglion cells probably form myelinated nerve fibers that constitute the sensory innervation of the skin and the muscles. The small, dark ganglion cells, on the other hand, are thought to form mostly unmyelinated nerve fibers and supply the sensory innervation of the entrails. The perikarya of cranial sensory ganglia (Fig. 4.4.5.) have a much more uniform look.

IV.4.1.3. White matter.

Apart from glia cells, most of which are oligodendrocytes and fibrillar astrocytes, white matter contains myelinated (by oligodendrocytes, Fig. 4.4.9.) nerve fibers. The glia cell bodies are scattered between the nerve fibers. Since they contain little perinuclear cytoplasm, their nuclei appear naked by light microscopy.

In the spinal cord, the white matter occupies the periphery (Fig. 4.4.8.). This peripheral layer of white matter is very thin at the spinal cord's sacral levels, progressively thickening nearer to the brain. As the spinal cord approaches the brain, more and more nerve fibers join it, connecting it with ever more body parts. At the cervical level, the white matter reaches its maximum thickness. Every nerve fiber running between the brain and the trunk or limbs has to pass this point. The white matter of the spinal cord is at the outside of the original neural tube and is coated with a basement membrane. Under the basement membrane is a continuous layer of astrocytic end feet: the glial limiting membrane.
The nerve fibers of the spinal cord are arranged in discrete longitudinal bundles, called fascicles or tracts. Some of these contain "ascending" fibers that conduct action potentials, generated in receptor organs, to the brain. Others are collections of "descending" fibers, which conduct action potentials from the brain to the spinal cord's motor nerve cells. The best example of such fascicles is found in the dorsal column, the area of white matter delimited by the dorsal horns of the gray matter. This area is occupied by two fascicles, both containing ascending nerve fibers from the spinal ganglia: the **fasciculus cuneatus** and the **fasciculus gracilis**.

In most of the brain, but not everywhere, the white matter occupies a central position. It occasionally forms conspicuous formations. A spectacular example is the **corpus callosum**, a collection of nerve fibers forming a bridge between the two hemispheres of the cerebrum.

IV.4.2. Integrative nerve tissue.

Like conductive nerve tissue, integrative nerve tissue assumes a number of aspects. The peripheral nerves carry expansions, caused by the accumulation of perikarya giving rise to axons of motor nerve fibers: **motor ganglia**. Inside these ganglia, motor nerve cells receive synaptic input from nerve fibers originating in the central nervous system. In the central nervous system, integrative nerve tissue forms **gray matter**. In the spinal cord, gray matter occupies a central position. In the brain, it is found both in central and peripheral positions. **Brain nuclei** are accumulations of gray matter in the centrally located white matter. At the brain's periphery, gray matter forms a **cortex**. Apart from glia cells, mostly protoplasmic astrocytes, the gray matter contains nerve cell perikarya and their dendrites and axon terminals forming synaptic junctions with these (Fig. 4.4.9.). In contrast to the nerve cells, the astrocytes contain little perinuclear cytoplasm, giving the impression, by light microscopy, of naked nuclei. Essentially every nerve cell encountered in the gray substance is a multipolar one. The absence of myelin explains the relatively dark coloration of gray matter.

IV.4.2.1. Motor ganglia.

Motor ganglia are found in association with spinal, as well as with a number of cranial, nerves. The perikarya they contain are always those of multipolar nerve cells. They are postsynaptic nerve cells, i.e. they are innervated by presynaptic nerve fibers, originating at nerve cells in the brain or the spinal cord. Thus, the distance from the central nervous system to a peripheral organ is covered by two successive nerve fibers. The presynaptic one is usually myelinated, the postsynaptic one usually not.

In a functional sense, motor ganglia come in two varieties. Some of them are associated with the peripheral nerves originating at the cervical, thoracic, and lumbar segments of the spinal cord. These are the **orthosympathetic ganglia**. Most of these, the **paravertebral ganglia**, lie close to the spinal cord. Consequently, the presynaptic fibers that enter them are short. The postsynaptic fibers are long and innervate the body wall and limbs. A few others, the

prevertebral ganglia, lie at greater distances from the spinal cord, and the presynaptic fibers associated with them are relatively long. The postsynaptic fibers leaving them are short and innervate the viscera. The **parasympathetic ganglia** are associated with cranial nerves. Here, the greatest discrepancy in length between pre- and postsynaptic fibers is found. Parasympathetic ganglia are usually intramural, i.e. they lie in the peripheral organs. Consequently, their presynaptic fibers are very long, their postsynaptic ones very short. In the sacral regions of the spinal cord, the distinction between ortho- and parasympathetic ganglia and nerves becomes unsharp. Motor ganglia have no close connection to higher nerve centers and we are usually not aware of the actions of the nerve fibers associated with them. They are part of what is called the autonomic nervous system. In general terms, the actions of orthosympathetic, or simply sympathetic, nerves prepare the body for action, among others by increasing the respiratory rate and heart rhythm, and by inhibiting the peristaltic action of the intestine. Their effects allow the body to generate short, intense bursts of energy. Parasympathetic nerves do the opposite, and are generally active during time periods of rest. In general, sympathetic postsynaptic nerve fibers use noradrenaline as their neurotransmitter, while parasympathetic postsynaptic nerve fibers use acetylcholine.

Intramural parasympathetic ganglia will not be discussed here, because they do not form separate organs. Orthosympathetic ganglia have a capsule of dense fibrous connective tissue, confluent with the epineurium of the nerve with which they are associated. The deeper layers of the capsule may contain a few layers of flattened perineural cells, equivalent to the mesothelial cells covering the arachnoidea (IV.4.5.). The multipolar nerve cells or ganglion cells of motor ganglia are relatively small and are evenly distributed in a tangle of myelinated and unmyelinated nerve fibers (Fig. 4.4.6.). It is not uncommon to come across binuclear ganglion cells or ganglion cells with an eccentric nucleus. The satellite cell cover of the ganglion cells, coated with a basement membrane, is not as cohesive as it is in sensory ganglia. It is interrupted to allow passage of presynaptic nerve fibers, synapsing with the ganglion cells. These are generally cholinergic (Fig. 4.4.7.).

Apart from ordinary nerve cells, orthosympathetic ganglia may contain a smaller, relatively rare kind of cells (Fig. 4.4.7.). Their cytoplasm is loaded with dense vesicles storing an amine, dopamine. A particular property of amines is that they form complexes with formaldehyde, which can be induced to fluoresce, the color of this fluorescence depending specifically on the amine. This characteristic gives the cells their name: **SIF-cells** (Small Intensely Fluorescent). Their nuclei are smaller and denser than those of the nerve cells. They receive synaptic input from the same presynaptic nerve fibers that contact the nerve cells. In turn, they form synaptic junctions with the nerve cells in which they are the presynaptic element. Therefore, they are regarded as dopaminergic interneurons between the presynaptic fibers and the ganglion cells. SIF-cells may also be closely associated with fenestrated blood capillaries, making it likely that they secrete dopamine into the blood. In that case, they would function as endocrine gland cells.

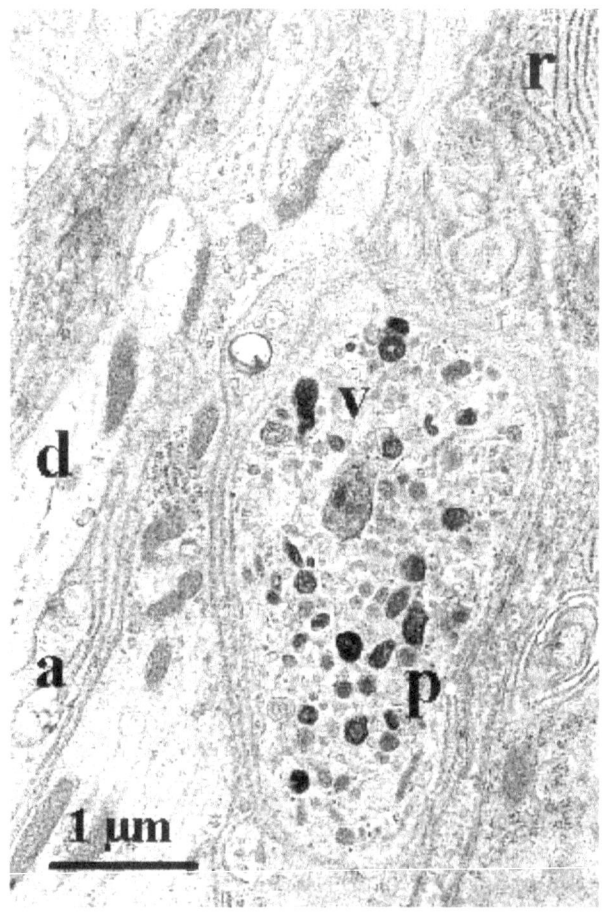

Fig. 4.4.7. In some motor ganglia, SIF-cells are encountered in addition to motor nerve cells. SIF-cells contain adrenergic synaptic vesicles (v). In this particular image, they also contain material in various degrees of digestion. Mark the presence of synaptic junctions between axons (a) of presynaptic nerves from the spinal cord and dendrites of the local, ganglionic nerve cells (d), which contain rough endoplasmic reticulum (r). Their synaptic vesicles are cholinergic. Superior cervical ganglion, rabbit, TEM.

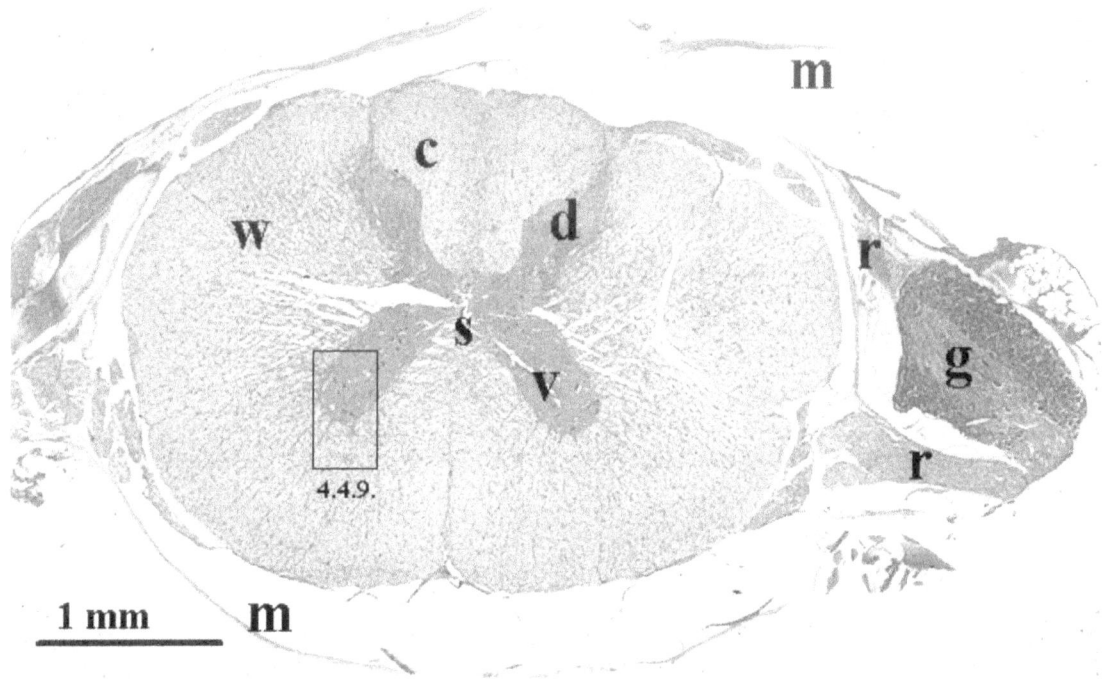

Fig. 4.4.8. A transverse section of the spinal cord shows a peripheral band of white matter (w) and a central, butterfly-shaped zone of gray matter. The white matter encompasses, among others, the dorsal columns (c). Grey matter forms the gray column, which has 2 dorsal (d), as well as 2 ventral (v), horns. The dorsal horns reach the spinal cord's periphery, the ventral ones are surrounded by white matter. In the gray column's center is the spinal canal (s). Peripheral nerves connect to the spinal cord by means of dorsal and ventral (r) roots. The dorsal root carries a spinal ganglion (g). Remains of the dura mater (m) can be seen. Cervical spinal cord, rat, HE.

IV.4.2.2. Gray matter of the spinal cord.

Gray matter forms the central axis of the spinal cord (Fig. 4.4.8.). In cross section, it has the shape of a fat letter H or a butterfly, displaying two **dorsal horns** and two **ventral horns**. Usually, the ventral horns are wider than the dorsal ones. The ventral horns never reach the spinal cord's periphery, always remaining separated from it by a broad band of white matter. The dorsal horns form a thin process, which extends to the edge of the spinal cord. In some segments of the spinal cord, the gray matter forms less prominent **lateral horns**. The relative size of the gray matter is maximal at the lower cervical and the lumbar levels of the spinal cord. Here, the motor nerve cells that innervate the limbs are concentrated.

The most striking nerve cells of the spinal cord's gray matter are the **somatic motor nerve cells** of the ventral horns (Figs. 4.4.9.-10.). They are the largest nerve cells to be found in the spinal cord. Their perikarya and dendrites display numerous synaptic junctions, formed by sensory fibers from the peripheral nervous system and descending fibers from the brain. The somatic motor nerve cells give rise to motor fibers, which leave the spinal cord by

way of the ventral roots and form synaptic junctions with skeletal muscle fibers (IV.3.3.).

The lateral horns are occupied by the relatively small perikarya of the nerve cells that send presynaptic fibers to the motor ganglia of the peripheral nervous system.

In the dorsal horns, various types of small multipolar nerve cells are found, which are more or less arranged in layers according to type. Some of these are contacted by incoming sensory nerve fibers and form ascending fibers to the brain. Others are interneurons, which receive synaptic input from incoming sensory fibers and form synaptic junctions with somatic motor nerve cells. Alternatively, they may connect descending fibers from the brain with somatic motor nerve cells. The dorsal third of the dorsal horns, the substantia gelatinosa, is relatively poor in nerve cells, due to the entrance of numerous sensory fibers.

IV.4.2.3. Brain nuclei.

Brain nuclei are accumulations of gray matter in the brain's white matter. Only a few of the most important or striking ones will be mentioned.

153

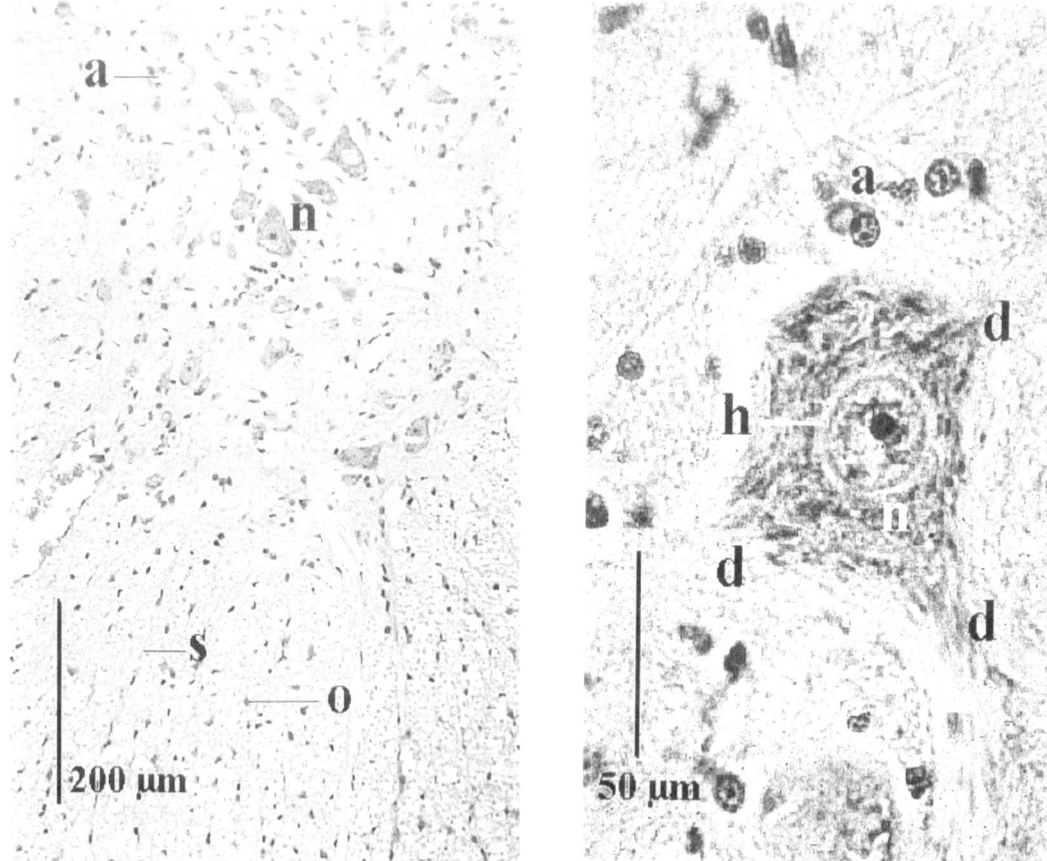

Fig. 4.4.9. (left) The gray column's ventral horn contains the perikarya of multipolar motor nerve cells (n), the axon of which forms a nerve fiber that leaves the spinal cord through the ventral root. The "naked" nuclei between these nerve cells belong to glia cells, predominantly protoplasmic astrocytes (a). The white matter is composed of large numbers of myelinated nerve fibers (compare with Figure 3.6.7.). Between these fibers lie the nuclei of oligodendrocytes and fibrillar astrocytes (o). The "septa" (s) are not made of connective tissue, but of astrocyte cytoplasm. Cervical spinal cord, rat, HE.

Fig. 4.4.10. (right) The perikaryon of a multipolar motor nerve cell of the spinal gray column's ventral horns has a polygonal shape because of the presence of multiple processes, the bases of which lie in the section plane. The central nucleus is fairly large, rounded, euchromatic, and contains a prominent nucleolus. It is surrounded by a clear, granule-free halo (h). This is the region occupied by Golgi-complexes. The cytoplasm is rich in basophilic Nissl substance (n). Since the Nissl substance penetrates into the bases of the processes, these are dendrites (d). The perikaryon lies in a tangle of nerve and glia cell processes, wherein the nuclei of astrocytes (a) are seen. Spinal cord, human, HE.

The **cuneate** and **gracile nuclei** are in the brain stem, the cranial prolongation of the spinal cord. The sensory nerve fibers that have ascended in the fasciculus cuneatus and the fasciculus gracilis of the spinal cord terminate on the perikarya of these nuclei, which are accumulations of nerve cells. Another distinctive brain stem nucleus is the **olivary nucleus**, which sends "climbing" fibers to the cerebellum. In histological sections, it has an undulated appearance.

The cerebellum has several nuclei (Fig. 4.4.11.). The largest one is the **dentate nucleus**, which derives its name from its cogged or crenellated appearance in sections.

In the mesencephalon, one of several nuclei to be found is the **substantia nigra**, which contains dopaminergic nerve cells. These also produce melanin, a dark pigment, which explains the name given to this nucleus. Melanin is a polymer of DOPA, the precursor molecule of dopamine. Nerve fibers from the substantia nigra form inhibitory synapses in the corpus striatum of the cerebrum, and they use dopamine as a neurotransmitter. Parkinson's disease, a severe motor disorder, is caused by degeneration of these nerve cells.

The most important nucleus of the diencephalon is the **thalamus**, which is actually a collection of brain nuclei. Almost every ascending tract to the cerebrum passes via the thalamus. The thalamic nerve cells give rise to fibers that ascend to the cerebrum. Ventral to the thalamus, in the floor of the third brain

154

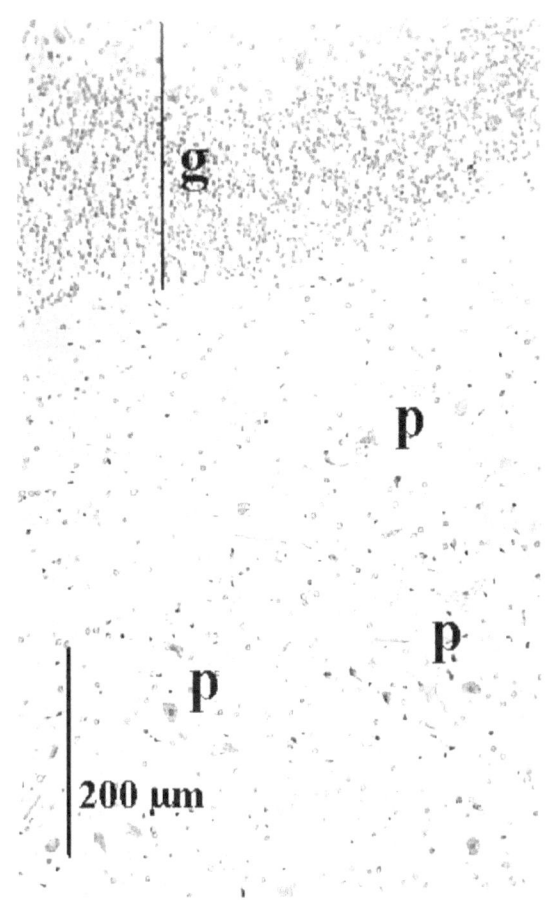

Fig. 4.4.11. A brain nucleus is an accumulation of nerve cell perikarya (p) in the white matter. g = gray matter (cerebellar cortex). Cerebellum, rat, HE.

ventricle, is the **hypothalamus**, which contains neurosecretory cells and functions to regulate the anterior pituitary gland.

In the white matter of the cerebral hemispheres, on both sides of the lateral ventricles, is an extensive formation of gray matter, crossed by bundles of nerve fibers, which give it a striped appearance. This is called the **corpus striatum**. The corpus striatum consists of subparts, including the caudate nucleus, the globus pallidus and the putamen. The caudate nucleus is elongated, extends along the lateral ventricle and thickens to form the amygdala. The corpus striatum receives nerve fibers from the cerebral cortex, the thalamus and the substantia nigra. It also sends fibers, mostly to the thalamus.

IV.4.2.4. Cerebellar cortex.

The cortex of the cerebellum is not smooth, but forms a fairly regular pattern of transverse (to the body's axis) folds or folia (Fig. 4.4.12.). In comparison to a smooth cortex, these folds enlarge the cortical surface, creating additional room for neural perikarya and synapses.

The cerebellar cortex is composed of several types of multipolar nerve cells, which are arranged in three distinctive layers, according to type (Fig. 4.4.13.). The largest nerve cells of the cerebellum are the **Purkinje cells**. They form a simple layer in the middle of the cortex. The **molecular layer** lies at the surface of the cerebellar cortex. It only contains a few nerve cell perikarya: those of molecular nerve cells and basket cells. The molecular nerve cells are relatively small and lie close to the surface. The basket cells are somewhat bigger and lie deeper. Their name is derived from their intensively branched axon, with which they surround the perikaryon of a Purkinje cell, resulting in the image of a Purkinje cell resting in a basket. The molecular layer is almost entirely occupied by axon terminals and dendritic trees, forming synaptic junctions. The deepest cortical layer, which rests on the white matter, is the **granular layer**. It contains, almost exclusively, granular nerve cells.

The perikarya of **Purkinje cells** (Fig. 4.4.14.) are shaped like tear drops pointing to the molecular layer. The point is the base of the dendritic tree. The rounded part of the perikaryon has a diameter of about 20 micrometers. The dendritic tree is very extensive. Its branches lie in a single plane, which extends far into the molecular layer, perpendicular to the axis of the local cortical fold. The dendrites are thickly set with spines. They receive the axon terminals of granular nerve cells and climbing fibers. The axon is very thin. It originates on the side of the perikaryon opposite the base of the dendritic tree, and follows a straight course into the granular layer. The axons of the Purkinje cells form the only nerve fibers that leave the cerebellar cortex. They will form inhibitory synapses in the cerebellar nuclei.

Molecular nerve cells and basket cells are inhibitory interneurons. Both receive synaptic input from granular nerve cells. Basket cell axonal end knobs form axodendritic, axosomatic and axo-axonal synapses with Purkinje cells. The axodendritic synapses do not involve the dendritic spines. The end knobs are filled with translucent, ellipsoid synaptic vesicles. Molecular nerve cells form axodendritic synapses with Purkinje cells.

Granular nerve cells are very small, having a diameter of only about 6 micrometers. They do not have a large amount of cytoplasm and their nuclei are heterochromatic. Consequently, granular nerve cells deceptively look like glia cells (Figs. 4.4.13., 4.4.14.). Granular nerve cells send their axon to the molecular layer, where it splits in two, forming a letter T. Both branches run in opposite directions, perpendicular to the plane of the Purkinje dendrites. These are the **horizontal fibers** (Fig. 4.4.15.). They form compact bundles, almost completely free of glia cells. The granular nerve cells are excitatory interneurons, i.e. they connect incoming fibers, such as the mossy fibers, to the cortical nerve cells and stimulate these. The axon terminals of the horizontal fibers contain globular, translucent synaptic vesicles and form synaptic junctions with the dendritic spines of the Purkinje cells (Fig. 4.4.16.), and with the other cortical nerve cells.

Ascending fibers from outside the cerebellum, the mossy fibers and the climbing fibers, penetrate the cortex. Both are excitatory. **Mossy fibers** only reach the granular layer. Their terminals, loaded with translucent synaptic vesicles, synapse with the dendrites of the granular nerve cells. A mossy fiber axonal end knob is large, and is indented by large numbers of granular cell dendrites (Fig. 4.4.17.). These complexes, the glomeruli, are so large that they can be observed by light microscopy. They appear like nucleus-free zones in the granular layer (Figs. 4.4.13.-14.). **Climbing fibers** reach into the molecular layer. Their end knobs, loaded with translucent synaptic vesicles, form synaptic junctions with the dendritic spines of the Purkinje cells.

IV.4.2.5. Cerebral cortex.

The cortex of the cerebrum is the highest "level" of the entire nervous system. It is not smooth, but shows a complex pattern of folds (gyri) and grooves (sulci). These folds and grooves have the same function as the cerebellum's folia. They increase the cortex's surface, thereby creating additional room for nerve cells. The cerebral cortex comprises areas where sensory signals arrive by way of ascending nerve fibers: the sensory cortex. Sight, hearing, smell and tactile senses each have their own discrete areas of projection in the sensory cortex. Signals leave the motor cortex for the body by way of descending fibers. An important part of the cortex is the association cortex, where signals are exchanged between cortical areas.

The cerebral cortex is composed of a number of multipolar nerve cell types. The most important ones are the **pyramidal nerve cells** and the granular or **stellate nerve cells**. The cerebral cortex has a layered structure because these nerve cells are aggregated according to type. These layers are not as sharply delineated, however, as those of the cerebellar cortex. Globally, six layers can be distinguished, the upper one containing very few nerve cells: the **molecular layer**. As it is in the cerebellum, this layer is largely made up of axons and dendritic trees, which form synaptic junctions. The molecular layer is followed by an **external granular layer** with stellate cells and small pyramidal nerve cells, a **pyramidal layer** with intermediary pyramidal nerve cells, an **inner granular layer** with stellate cells, a **ganglion layer** with large pyramidal nerve cells, and a **multiform layer** with a varied population of nerve cells. This layered structure shows local variations. The sensory cortex, where many ascending fibers enter the cortex, appears granular because of the paucity of pyramidal nerve cells, making the stellate cells more apparent. The motor cortex, on the other hand, is agranular because of the relatively small number of stellate cells.

Ascending fibers reach the cerebral cortex mainly from the thalamus, passing via the corpus striatum. They are particularly numerous in the sensory cortex, and tend to terminate at the upper cortical levels. Their terminals form synaptic junctions with the dendrites of pyramidal nerve cells, either directly or via interneurons, the most important of which are the stellate cells. The pyramidal nerve cells also come into mutual synaptic contact, either directly or via interneurons. They are the only nerve cells of the cerebral cortex that give rise to nerve fibers which will leave the cortex. Such descending fibers are primarily associated with the motor cortex.

Thus, the most important cerebral nerve cells are the **pyramidal nerve cells**, which derive their name from the characteristic shape of their perikaryon (Figs. 2.52., 4.4.18.). The perikaryon's top points at the cortical surface. Its base is slightly convex. In the center of it, the axon originates, and runs straight in the direction of the white matter underneath the cortex. On the way, it forms collaterals, i.e. branches that run perpendicular to it. From the top and from the edge of the basis, dendrites emerge. The apical dendrite is unusually long. It runs straight at the cortical surface, mirroring the axon on the other side, and only forms branches at its terminal. The most superficially situated pyramidal nerve cells have short apical dendrites and long axons. The reverse applies to the deeper nerve cells.
The pyramidal nerve cell's dendrites are set with spines, which are the postsynaptic part of excitatory synaptic junctions. The axonal end knobs forming

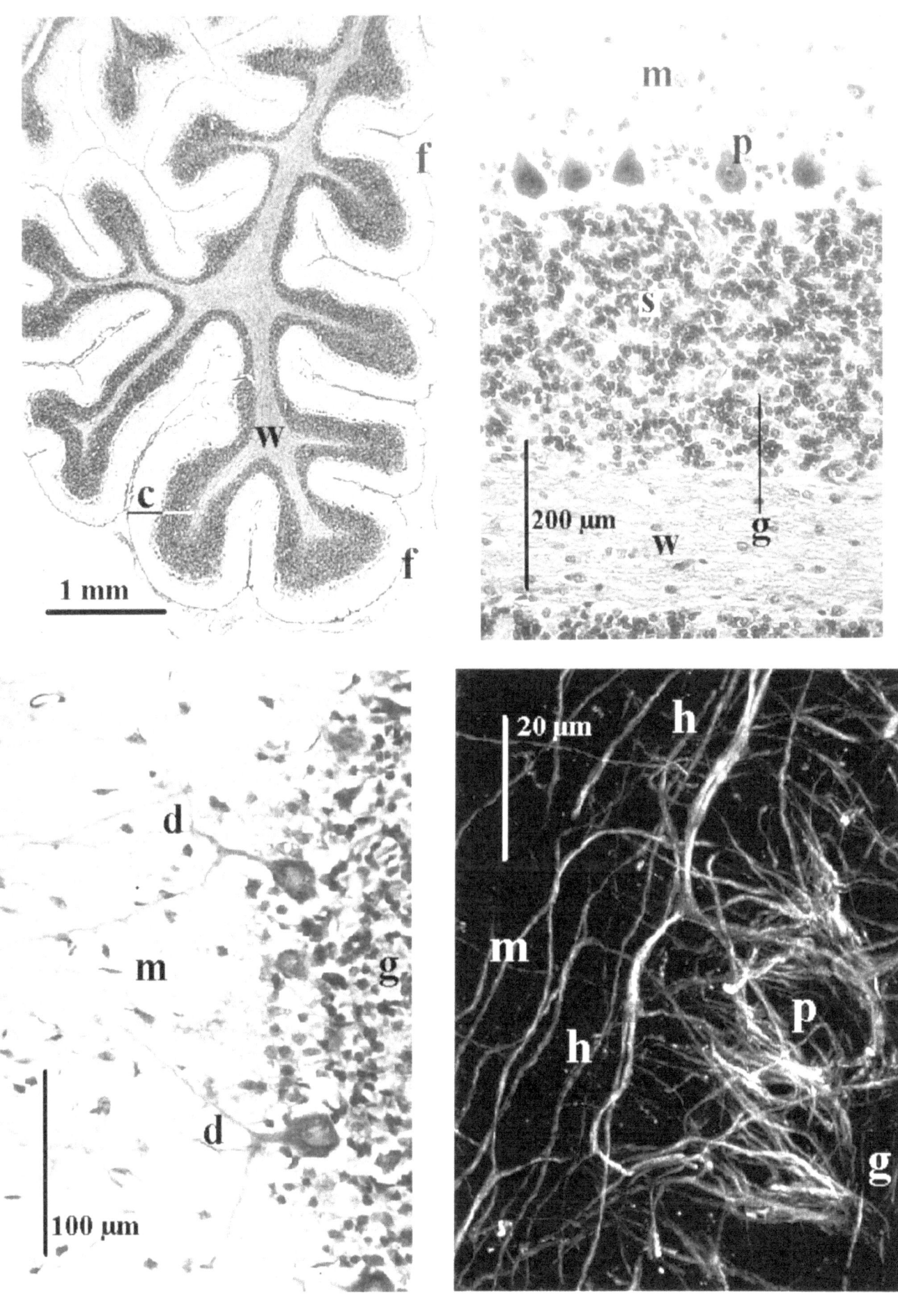

Fig. 4.4.12. (top left) The cerebellum has a layered cortex (c), which forms folds, or folia (f). In sections, this results in a dendroid, branched pattern, the arbor vitae (tree of life). The white matter (w) lies centrally. Cerebellum, rat, Klüver-Barrera. **Fig. 4.4.13.** (top right) The cerebellar cortex has three layers. The topmost one is the poorly staining molecular layer (m). It contains very few nerve cell perikarya. The deepest layer, which rests on the white matter, is the granular layer. It is rich in granular, or stellate, nerve cells (s). These nerve cells have a deceptive resemblance to glia cells because of their dense nuclei and scant cytoplasm. This layer also contains numerous glomeruli (g). It rests on the white matter (w). Sandwiched between both layers are the Purkinje cells (p). These are very conspicuous because they are the cerebellum's largest nerve cells and because they are arranged in a single row. Cerebellum, rat, Klüver-Barrera. **Fig. 4.4.14.** (bottom left) The Purkinje cells of the cerebellar cortex have a perikaryon shaped like a raindrop, pointing with its tip towards the molecular layer (m). This shape is caused by the presence of only 2, opposite, processes (compare with a more typical multipolar nerve cell, Figure 4.4.10.). The axon, which is very thin and cannot be seen here, originates at the blunt side of the perikaryon and runs towards the granular layer (g). At the opposite, pointed, side of the perikaryon, the stem of the extended dendritic tree (d) originates. The dendritic branches lie in a plane that, in this image, coincides with the plane of section. Cerebellum, cat, Klüver-Barrera. **Fig. 4.4.15.** (bottom right) In this image, the perikarya of the Purkinje cells (p) are not visible, but the spaces they occupy are delimited by the axons coming in (among others) from the molecular layer (m). Other axons originate in the granular layer (g), cross the Purkinje cell level and enter the molecular layer. There, they split into 2 branches, forming a letter T. These branches lie parallel to the surface of the cerebellar cortex, which is why they are called horizontal fibers (h). Cerebellum, rat, immunofluorescent visualization of neurofilament protein, extended depth of focus confocal image.

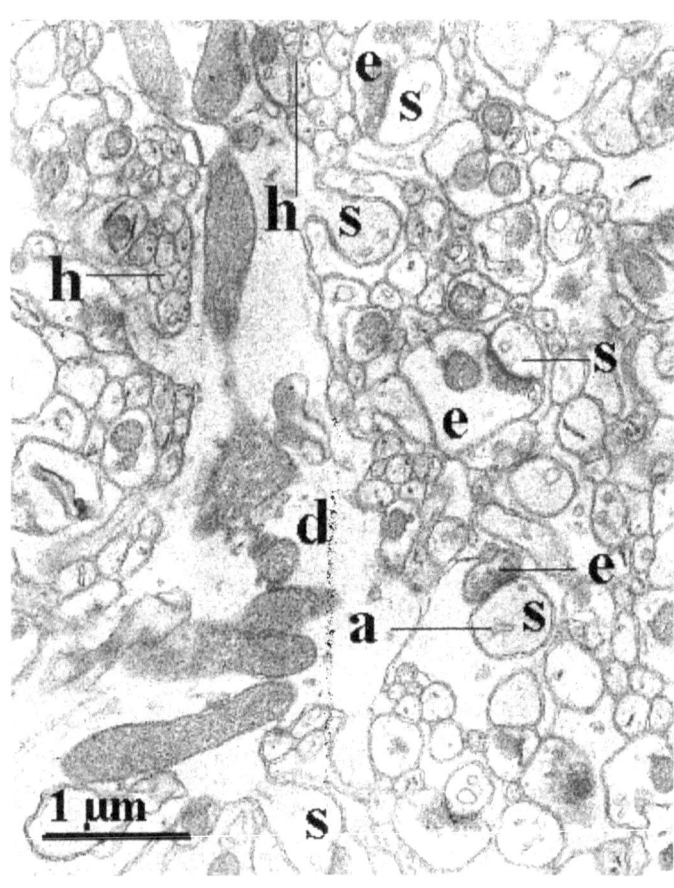

1 µm

Fig. 4.4.16. The molecular layer of the cerebellar cortex largely consists of the very thin, parallel axons of granular nerve cells, the horizontal fibers (h). These axons form synaptic junctions with the dendrites of Purkinje cells (d). In this image, the section plane is perpendicular to the horizontal fibers, which are cut transversely, and parallel to the plane of the Purkinje cell dendritic trees. The actual synaptic junctions are formed between a distended axonal end knob (e) of a horizontal fiber, filled with synaptic vesicles, and a Purkinje cell dendritic spine (s). Cerebellum, rat, TEM.

the presynaptic part of these junctions are filled with round synaptic vesicles and belong to other pyramidal nerve cells, subcortical ascending fibers and excitatory interneurons, particularly stellate cells. At the dendrites, the perikaryon and the axon, synaptic junctions are also formed without spines. Such junctions are much less frequent. When present, the axonal end knobs contain ellipsoid synaptic vesicles and use GABA (III.6.2.1.2.) as a neurotransmitter. These end knobs belong to inhibitory interneurons. The cortical nerve cells frequently use glutamate or aspartate as neurotransmitters.

The other nerve cell types of the cerebral cortex are interneurons. They form various and sometimes very

158

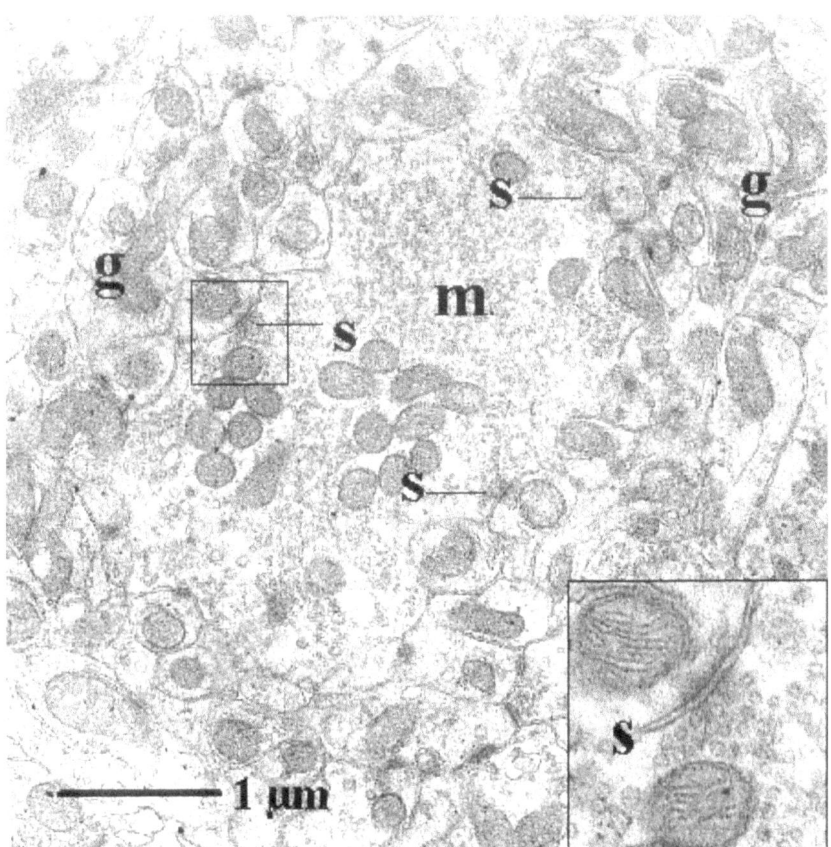

Fig. 4.4.17. A glomerulus of the granular layer of the cerebellum corresponds to the bulky end knob of a so-called mossy fiber (m), filled with mitochondria and large numbers of synaptic vesicles, which forms a large number of synaptic junctions (s) with dendrites of granular nerve cells (d). One synapse is shown enlarged at the lower right corner. Cerebellum, rat, TEM.

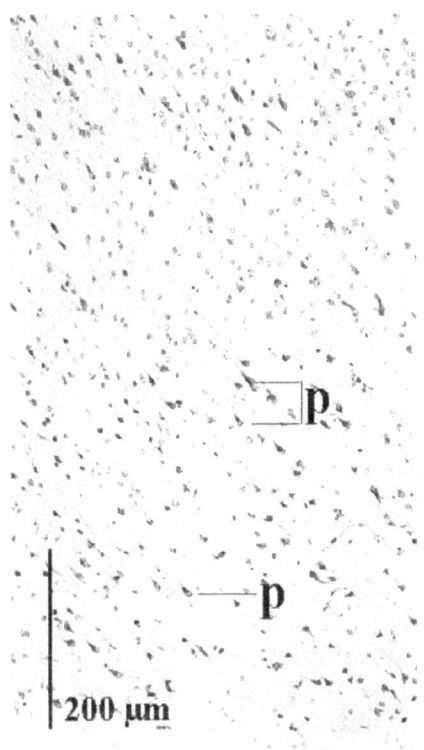

Fig. 4.4.18. The cerebral cortex, except for its superficial molecular layer, is composed of multiple layers of pyramidal nerve cells (p) and stellate cells (granular nerve cells). These layers are much less distinct than those of the cerebellar cortex. Cerebrum, human, HE.

complex connections, mainly between ascending fibers and pyramidal nerve cells and between the pyramidal nerve cells themselves. With the exception of the stellate cells, their dendrites do not carry spines. The **stellate cells** are small interneurons with scarce cytoplasm and a heterochromatic nucleus. They look similar to glia cells and are equivalent to the granular nerve cells of the cerebellum. Stellate cells are the most important excitatory interneurons of the cerebral cortex. More rare, inhibitory, types of interneuron are, among others, the fusiform cells, the horizontal cells, and the Martinotti cells.

The above description applies to the **neocortex**, which is, from an evolutionary point of view, the most recent part of the brain. It is well developed in mammals only. Almost the entire surface of the cerebral hemispheres is neocortex. At the ventral and medial sides of the cerebral hemispheres, however, a few patches of less complex cortex are tucked away, which have a much longer evolutionary history than the neocortex.

The **olfactory cortex** receives sensory nerve fibers from the olfactory bulbs. These are virtually the only sensory fibers not to reach the cortex by way of the

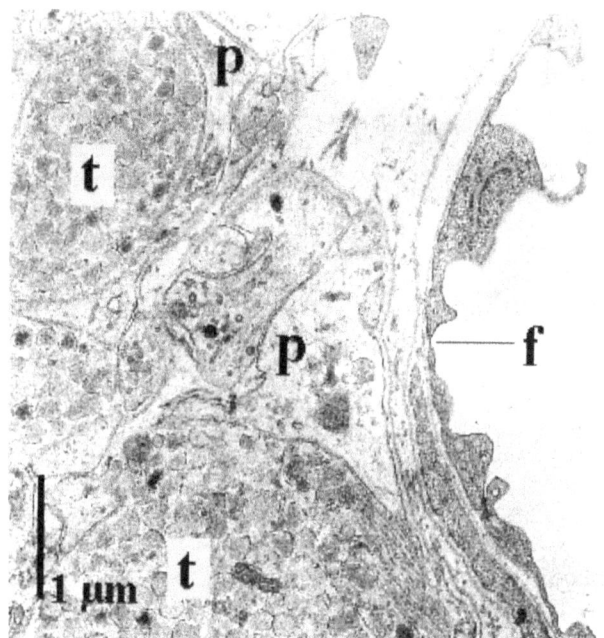

IV.4.3. Pineal gland and neurohypophysis.

The **pineal gland** is a dorsal appendage of the brain, a few millimeters long. Its stalk is hollow and this space is continuous with the third brain ventricle. The actual glandular tissue is at the top of the organ. It is composed of pinealocytes and astrocytes.

Pinealocytes are the pineal gland's neurosecretory cells. They are multipolar cells, forming processes containing dense vesicles. Some of these processes do not contact postsynaptic nerve cells, but rather fenestrated capillaries, similar to the sinusoidal capillaries of endocrine glands (IV.7.). Other processes form synaptic junctions in which they are presynaptic to nerve cells. In this case, their terminals often display a synaptic rod surrounded by translucent vesicles. Synapses like these are uncommon, but are typical for the rod and cone photoreceptor cells of the retina (Fig. 4.12.25.) and the cochlear and vestibular hair cells. Apparently, pinealocytes are receptor cells, transmitting signals to nerve fibers that leave the pineal gland. In addition to this, pinealocytes appear to receive orthosympathetic, adrenergic nerve fibers from outside the pineal gland. The pineal gland is best developed before puberty, and involutes at later age. In the ageing gland, extracellular, calcified granules may appear.

The hormone produced by the pineal gland is **melatonin**, a derivative of serotonin. The name melatonin is derived from an observation in amphibia, where melatonin acts on the skin's pigment cells, the melanocytes (IV.9.1.1.). It induces aggregation of their pigment granules, causing bleaching of the skin. In higher vertebrates, the main function of melatonin seems to be to contribute to the regulation of the sleep-awake cycle. The concentration of melatonin fluctuates during each 24-hour cycle under the influence of changing light intensities. This points at a connection between the retina and the pinealocytes. Although pinealocytes, like the retinal photoreceptors, form synaptic end knobs with rods, it is unlikely that they are directly influenced by light. In full daylight, the concentration of melatonin is minimal. With decreasing light intensity, higher concentrations of melatonin have a sleep-inducing effect. Before the onset of puberty, the pineal gland also appears to inhibit, via the hypothalamus, the gonadotroph cells of the pituitary gland.

The **neurohypophysis** is a ventral appendage of the brain. It is composed of bundles of unmyelinated nerve fibers, which originate in the hypothalamic nuclei. The hypothalamic nerve cells are

Fig. 4.4.19. The neurohypophysis contains the terminals (t) of neurosecretory nerve fibers, originating in the hypothalamus, enveloped by the filamentous processes of the local glia cells, the pituicytes (p). These terminals are filled with neurosecretory vesicles. They approach a fenestrated capillary (c), where the liberated hormones will enter the blood circulation. Neurohypophysis, cat, TEM.

thalamus. The olfactory cortex has only three layers: a molecular layer at the surface, followed by a pyramidal layer and a polymorphous layer.

The **olfactory bulbs** are two elongated masses of white matter, coated with a cortex. At the surface of this cortex, where a molecular layer is found, axons from the olfactory mucosa of the nose enter. They form synaptic junctions with the dendrites of tufted cells and mitral cells. The dendritic tree of a mitral cell is extensive, and gives rise to a nucleus-free zone, a glomerulus. The mitral glomeruli are arranged in a simple layer. Underneath the glomeruli, an external plexiform layer is found, containing nerve fibers and perikarya of tufted cells. In turn, this is followed by a layer with perikarya of mitral cells. Mitral cells somewhat resemble pyramidal nerve cells. The mitral cell perikarya rest on an internal plexiform layer, rich in nerve fibers, and a granular layer. The underlying white substance contains fibers that run to the olfactory cortex.

The **hippocampus** derives its name from its characteristic shape, which is that of a sea horse. It is implicated in the regulation of memory and emotional behavior. The hippocampal cortex is trilaminar, i.e. a superficial molecular layer is followed by a pyramidal layer and a polymorphous layer.

morphologically similar to normal nerve cells, but do not form synapses. They discharge their secretory product into the blood stream, which makes them neurosecretory cells. The top of the neurohypophysis is closely associated with a classical endocrine gland, the anterior pituitary gland (IV.7.1.). The neurohypophysis itself is also called the posterior pituitary gland.

The neurohypophysis contains numerous fenestrated, sinusoidal capillaries (IV.7.), surrounded by the axonal end knobs of hypothalamic neurosecretory cells (Fig. 4.4.19.). The end knobs are filled with dense vesicles containing hormone, the neurosecretory vesicles. Dilated end knobs, or end knob aggregates, are visible light optically as intensely staining **Herring bodies**. The glia cells are modified astrocytes, called **pituicytes**.

The neurohypophyseal hormones are peptides, which are synthesized in the nerve cell perikarya of the hypothalamus and are displaced by anterograde axoplasmic transport to the axonal end knobs. By way of the local sinusoidal capillaries, into which they are discharged, they reach the corticotroph, thyrotroph and gonadotroph endocrine cells of the pituitary gland and stimulate them to secrete their own hormones. Thus, the endocrine activities of the pituitary gland are regulated by the neurohypophysis. Because of this close association, both organs, in spite of their very different microscopic structure, can be regarded as a single entity, the hypophysis. In addition, the neurohypophysis produces hormones that interact with other organs. The **antidiuretic hormone** stimulates absorption of water from the lumen of the collecting tubules of the kidneys (IV.8.1.2.). Hypothalamic nerve cells release it upon stimulation by water loss, which leads to a decreased volume of extracellular fluid and a higher salt concentration. **Oxytocin** stimulates smooth muscle cells and myoepithelial cells (III.5.1.) to contract, particularly those of the milk glands, helping the expulsion of milk. The nipples are mechanically stimulated during breast-feeding, and sensory nerve fibers convey this signal to the hypothalamic nerve cells by way of the brain stem.

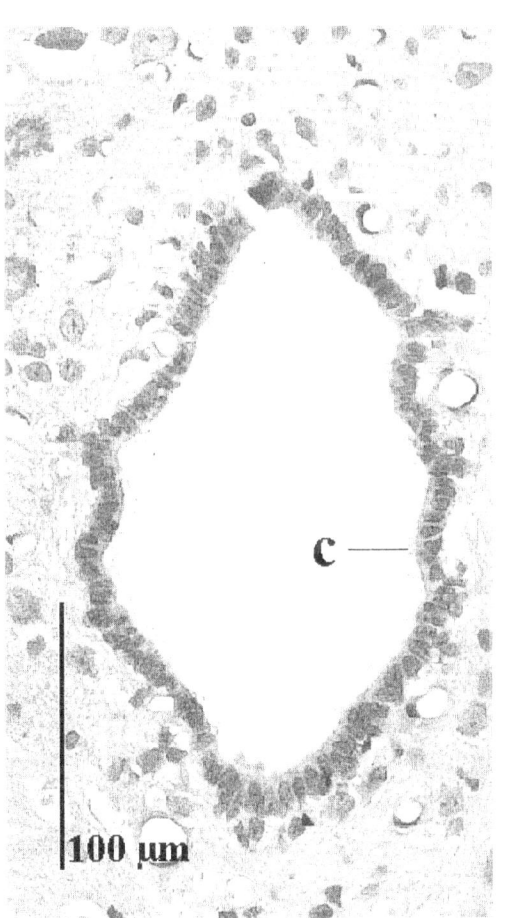
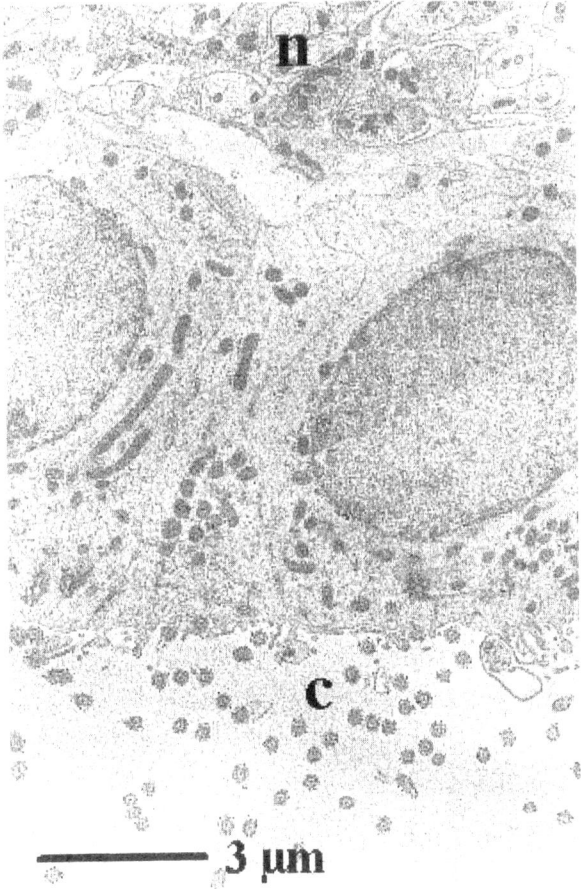

Fig. 4.4.20. (left) The spinal canal's lumen is lined with a simple prismatic epithelium (mark the single row of nuclei), composed of ependyma cells, whose cilia (c) can be made out. Spinal cord, rat, HE. **Fig. 4.4.21.** (right) Ependyma cells are typical ciliated cells. Their cilia (c) extend into the lumen of the spinal canal. Spinal cord, rat, TEM.

IV.4.4. Ependyma and choroid plexi.

The brain contains four relatively wide cavities with a complex shape, the **ventricles** - two lateral ones in the cerebral hemispheres, and a third and fourth one in more caudal parts of the brain. The fourth ventricle narrows to form the **spinal canal**, which runs the length of the spinal cord.

The ventricles and the spinal canal are lined with a simple cuboidal to prismatic "epithelium", or ependyma, made up of **ependyma cells** (Fig. 4.4.20.). Ependyma cells are ciliated cells (Fig. 4.4.21.). Like typical epithelial cells, they are joined by apical junctional complexes (III.4.1.1.). In contrast to typical epithelial cells, they may form a basal process that extends into the underlying fibrous tissue, and the basement membrane on which they rest is, at most, poorly developed. Their bases may be contacted by astrocyte end feet. By the beating of their cilia, they propel the cerebrospinal fluid filling the ventricles and the spinal canal.

In a few places in the roof of the third and fourth ventricles and in the walls of the lateral ventricles, the brain's original neuroepithelium is still present in another form: choroid plexus cells. The fibrous tissue on which these cells rest is continuous with the pia mater, the innermost of the three meninges. It is rich in blood vessels, and forms a number of complex folds, the choroid plexus (Fig. 4.4.22.), which are lined with a simple layer of choroid plexus cells and penetrate deep into the ventricular space. **Choroid plexus cells** (Fig. 4.4.23.) carry an apical brush border, composed of microvilli. They contain numerous mitochondria and their basal cell membrane forms deep, narrow folds. They usually rest on a well-developed basement membrane. The underlying capillaries are fenestrated. Choroid plexus cells are secretory brush border cells. They extract certain components from the blood plasma and secrete them into the ventricles: mostly ions and low molecular weight organic molecules. Thus, they contribute to the formation of cerebrospinal fluid. The basal cell membrane's folds, as well as the apical microvilli, increase the available membrane area, creating room for membrane pumps, needed for these transport processes. By way of the fourth ventricle, cerebrospinal fluid drains to the subarachnoidal space.

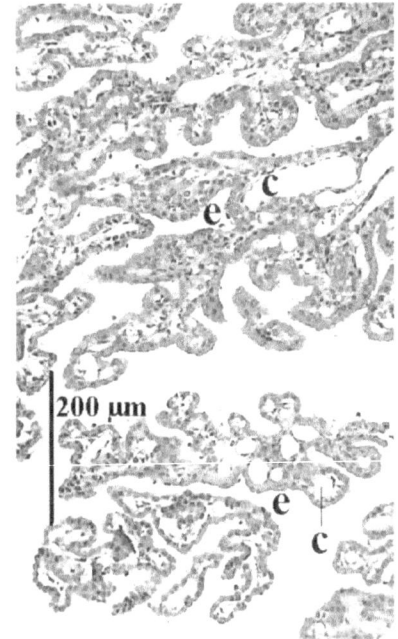
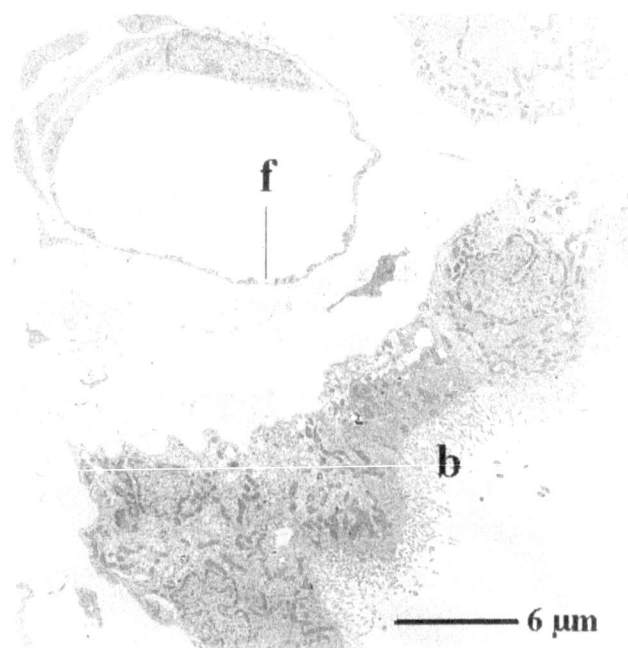

Fig. 4.4.22. (left) In a few places, the ependyma cells lining the ventricles contact the pia mater, because no nervous tissue develops here. Thus, a choroid plexus is formed. The epithelium (e) develops a large number of deep, branched folds, thereby considerably increasing its surface. The ependyma cells of this epithelium change into choroid plexus cells. The interstitial tissue, derived from the pia mater, contains large numbers of capillaries (c). Cerebrum, cat, HE.
Fig. 4.4.23. (right) Choroid plexus cells are equipped with a brush border (b). The underlying capillaries (c) are fenestrated. Cerebrum, cat, TEM.

IV.4.5. Meninges.

The outermost of the three concentric fibrous tissue sheaths, or meninges (Fig. 4.4.24.), encapsulating the central nervous system, is the **dura mater**. The dura mater, or dura, is composed of dense fibrous connective tissue. The dura mater of the spinal cord is separated from the vertebrae by an epidural space, filled with loose fibrous tissue and a venous plexus. The dura mater of the brain merges with the periosteum of the skull. Locally, the dura contains venous sinuses. It is separated from the underlying arachnoid by a subdural space.

The **arachnoid** is a thin, avascular layer of loose fibrous tissue, somewhat resembling a cobweb, hence its name. Locally, it forms cell masses, the arachnoid villi, which penetrate into the venous sinuses of the dura. Cerebrospinal fluid, which drains from the fourth ventricle to the subarachnoid space, is discharged into the venous blood by way of these villi. Between the arachnoid and the pia mater is a wide subarachnoid space, bridged by fibrous tissue strands that carry blood vessels.

The **pia mater** is the innermost of the meninges. The pia of the brain accurately follows the contours of the cortical folds. It is a relatively thin layer, composed of loose fibrous tissue, rich in blood vessels. It is separated from the underlying nervous tissue by a basement membrane and a glial limiting membrane.

The subdural and subarachnoid spaces are lined with mesothelial cells.

IV.4.6. Blood brain barrier.

Blood vessels penetrate the central nervous system from the pia mater. Initially, they are coated with fibrous tissue, but the capillaries traversing the nervous tissue are only coated with a glial limiting membrane, a layer of glia end feet, joined by tight junctions (III.4.1.1.). The capillary endothelial cells (III.4.2.) rest on a relatively thick (20 to 50 nanometers) basement membrane. They are joined by tight junctions, do not show many pinocytotic vesicles, and are unfenestrated. All this indicates that the central nervous system's capillaries are relatively impermeable. In fact, it can be demonstrated that even fairly small molecules, particularly lipids, do not easily penetrate from the blood to the cerebrospinal fluid. Thus, there exists a blood brain barrier that serves to protect the delicate nerve cells from potentially drastic changes in the chemical composition of the cerebrospinal fluid that bathes them. These specific characteristics of the capillaries, which are vital to the existence of the

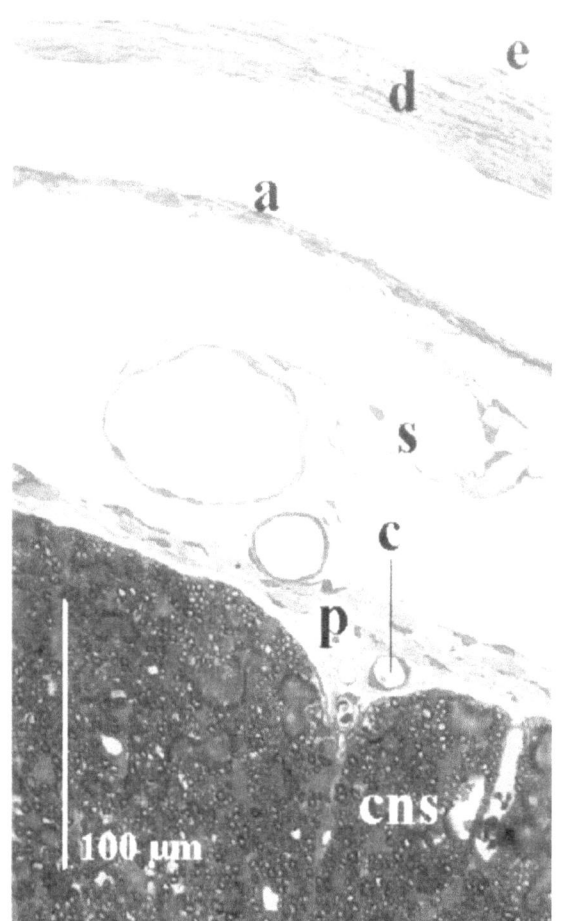

Fig. 4.4.24. The central nervous system is shielded by 3 concentric fibrous tissue sheaths, the meninges. The outer dura mater, or dura, is made of dense fibrous tissue (d). At the level of the spine (here) it is separated from the surrounding bone by an epidural space (e). It is separated from the flimsy arachnoid (a) by a subdural space. Fibrous tissue strands (s) connect the arachnoid to the pia mater, or pia (p). The pia, which rests on the central nervous system's surface (cns), is composed of loose fibrous tissue, and carries numerous capillaries (c). Spinal cord, rabbit, 1-micrometer plastic section, toluidin blue.

barrier, are induced during development by the surrounding glia cells.

IV.4.7. Microglia.

Microglia are not really glia cells since they do not descend from the neural ectoderm. Rather, they have a mesodermal origin. They may be derived from pericytes (III.4.2.), which have penetrated the capillary basement membrane.

The cytological structure of these cells, at least in the resting stage, somewhat resembles that of astrocytes. They are relatively small and carry branched processes. Microglia are the most important defender cells of the central nervous system. Like macrophages, they are involved in phagocytosis and antigen presentation. Upon infection or tissue damage, they are transformed to macrophage-like cells, with shorter, less strongly branched processes. These changes are reversible, unless the central nervous tissue is so badly damaged that nerve cells die, in which case they are permanently transformed.

References.

DeFelipe J., Farinas I.: The pyramidal neuron of the cerebral cortex: morphological and chemical characteristics af the synaptic inputs. Prog. Neurobiol. 1992, 39: 563-607.

Goldstein G.W., Betz A.L.: The blood-brain barrier. Sci. Am. 1986, september: 70-79.

Janzer R.C.: The blood-brain barrier: cellular basis. J. Inherit. Metab. Dis. 1993, 16: 639-647.

Matthews M.R.: Small, intensely fluorescent cells and the paraneuron concept. J. Electr. Microsc. Tech. 1989, 12: 408-416.

Nieuwenhuys R.: The neocortex. An overview of its evolutionary development, structural organization and synaptology. Anat. Embryol. 1994, 190: 307-337.

Spector R., Johanson C.E.: The mammalian choroid plexus. Sci. Am. 1989, november: 48-55.

Streit W.J., Graeber M.B.: Microglia: a pictorial. Prog. Histochem. Cytochem. 1996, 31: 1-90.

Streit W.J., Kincaid-Colton C.A.: The brain's immune system. Sci. Am. 1995, november, 38-43.

IV.5. Vascular system.

The vascular system is a closed system of intensively branched tubes, the blood and lymph vessels, in which blood and lymph, respectively, circulate.

Blood vessels form tubes that conduct blood to the organs of the body, the **arteries,** and tubes that conduct blood away from them, the **veins**. The propulsive force necessary for blood circulation is provided by a pump, the **heart**, from which the arteries radiate and toward which the veins return. Arteries as well as veins are conductive and distributive blood vessels and have a relatively thick, impermeable wall. On their way to the organs, arteries frequently bifurcate, and grow thinner accordingly. When the arteries enter the tissues of a peripheral organ, they split up in a large number of extremely thin walled vessels, the capillaries, which pervade the organ. Blood capillaries only consist of an endothelium (III.4.2.). These vessels not only conduct blood but, in addition, allow exchange of substances between the blood inside them and the surrounding tissues. The capillary beds of the organs are drained by veins, of very small diameter at first, which merge into ever-larger veins and ultimately reach the heart.

Lymph vessels conduct lymph from the peripheral organs to the heart. At the blood capillary level, fluid enters the intercellular spaces, and is lost form the blood vascular space. This fluid is drained from the tissues by lymph capillaries. Lymph capillaries too have an extremely thin and permeable wall, made up of endothelium. Lymph capillaries are drained by larger and larger lymph vessels, which eventually open into the venous part of the blood vascular tract, close to the heart, returning the tissue fluid to the blood stream. Lymph capillaries end blindly and the lymph vascular system, contrary to the blood vascular tract, is made up exclusively of return vessels.

Apart from the ubiquitous interstitial and connective tissues, the vascular system is predominantly made up of **endothelium** and **muscle tissue**.

Endothelium lines the vessel's internal space or lumen and rests on a thin layer of loose fibrous tissue. Both layers form the internal coat or **tunica intima**. Most often, the endothelial cells are unfenestrated and interconnected through tight junctions. They rest on a continuous basement membrane. Occasionally, they form a basal process that contacts a deeper smooth muscle fiber. In this myoendothelial junction, both basement membranes fuse. The microscopic characteristics of this

endothelium, in contrast to the capillary endothelium, indicate a low permeability, illustrating the purely conductive function of the larger blood vessels.

The muscle tissue, mostly smooth muscle tissue, consists of circular and helicoidal fibers, and makes up the intermediate vessel coat or **tunica media**. In addition to smooth muscle fibers, the tunica media contains varying amounts of collagen fibers, elastic fibers and fenestrated elastic membranes. These are synthesized by the smooth muscle fibers.

Finally, the tunica media is coated with an external vessel coat or **tunica adventitia**, consisting of loose fibrous tissue, which gradually merges with the surrounding tissues. In the largest blood vessels, which lie in the body cavities, the tunica adventitia is coated with mesothelium.

In principle, elastic membranes separate the tunica intima from the tunica media and the tunica media from the tunica adventitia: the **elastica interna** and the **elastica externa**, respectively. They are almost exclusively limited to the arteries, however, and an elastica externa is only found in the larger arteries. The wall of the larger blood vessels is supplied with blood by smaller blood vessels, the vasa vasorum. In addition, the blood vessel wall contains nerve fibers, the nervi vasorum. Locally, sensory nerve fibers are found which participate in specialized receptor organs: the arterial **chemo-** and **baroreceptors**.

IV.5.1. Heart.

The heart is a pump, but a compound one: it consists of a right heart and a left heart, separated from one another by a septum, and each half has a relatively weak atrium and a strongly muscular ventricle. Via the pulmonary arteries, the right ventricle pumps blood to the lungs, where it is loaded with oxygen. The oxygenated blood is conducted back to the heart by the pulmonary veins and enters the left atrium. This is the small or pulmonary circulation, which exclusively involves the lungs. The left atrium pumps blood into the left ventricle, which in turn pumps it into the large circulation, comprising the rest of the body. Deoxygenated blood returns through the vena cava, and enters the right atrium. The atria are separated from their ventricles by a valve, which prevents reflux of blood upon relaxation of the atrium. Additional valves are situated at the points of entry or exit of the blood vessels.

The heart wall is constructed from the same elements as the blood vessels, but with different names. The heart lumen and consists of endothelium, resting on a

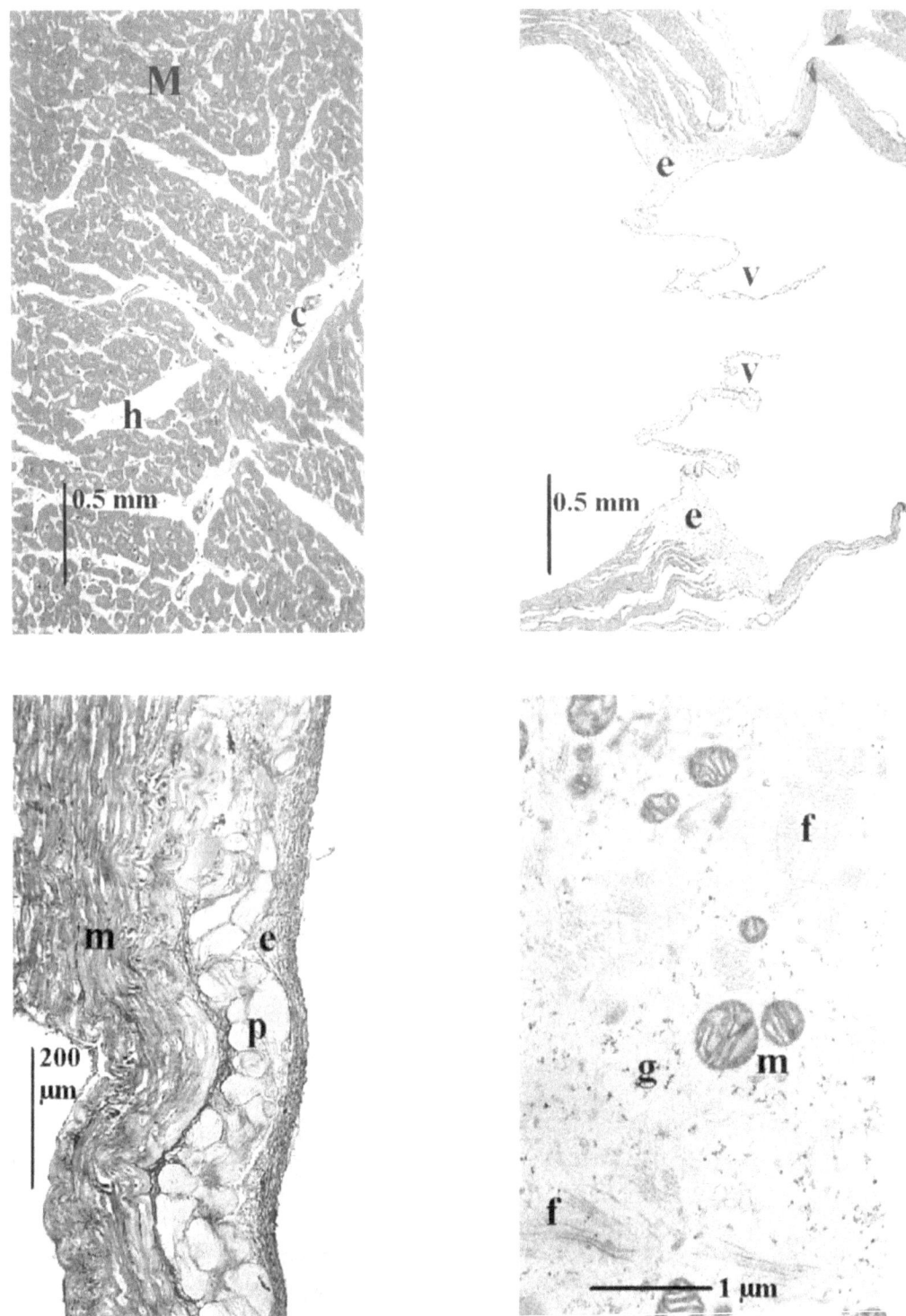

Fig. 4.5.1. (top left) Most of the cardiac wall is a thick layer of cardiac muscle tissue, the myocard (m). The cardiac muscle fibers are arranged in bundles, separated from one another by interstitial tissue, Henle's clefts (h), containing the coronary vessels (c). Heart, human, Masson stain. **Fig. 4.5.2.** (top right) An atrioventricular valve (v) is derived from endocard (e) and thus consists of a core of loose fibrous tissue, lined with endothelium. Heart, cat, HE. **Fig. 4.5.3.** (bottom left) The myocard's inside is coated with endocard (e): a fibrous tissue layer lined with endothelium. In the deeper layers of the endocard, the subendocard, strongly modified cardiac fibers are found: Purkinje fibers (p). These are larger than ordinary myocardiac fibers (m) and, as a consequence of their lack of myofibrils, their cytoplasm is much paler. They are unable to contract, but serve as natural pacemakers and conductors of contractile stimuli. Heart, human, Masson stain. **Fig. 4.5.4.** (bottom right) A Purkinje cell's cytoplasm contains only traces of myofibrils (f) and only small numbers of mitochondria (m). Glycogen granules (g) represent an energy store. Heart, rabbit, TEM.

thin layer of loose fibrous tissue. The endocard forms the cardiac **valves** (Fig. 4.5.2.). Apart from endothelium and loose fibrous tissue, these valves are reinforced with a central layer of denser fibrous tissue. The thickest layer of the cardiac wall is the tunica media or **myocard**, which consists of a cardiac muscle tissue (Fig. 4.5.1.). The spaces between individual fibers, Henle's spaces, are filled with loose fibrous tissue, in which the vasa vasorum of the heart, the coronary vessels, run. Locally, denser fibrous tissue is found in the myocard, serving as a cardiac skeleton on which the cardiac muscles fibers insert. Elastic fibers are scarce. The tunica adventitia or **epicard** is a thin layer of loose fibrous tissue, lined with mesothelium. The same mesothelium lines the pericardial space and, with the underlying loose fibrous tissue, forms the pericard.

In the endocard, bundles of physiologically specialized cardiac muscle fibers are found, which play an essential role in the mechanism of cardiac contraction and make up the so called cardiac pacemaker and conduction system. Rhythmic depolarizations occur spontaneously in the heart's pacemaker, the sino-atrial node, which is situated at the junction of the largest veins with the atria. The rhythm with which the pacemaker depolarizes can be modulated neurally: it is the only example of cardiac muscle fibers that have a motor innervation. Thanks to the electric coupling, through the gap junctions of the intercalated disks, of subsequent conduction system fibers, a depolarization wave is initiated which runs to the atrio-ventricular node, at the junction of atrium and ventricle. The atrio-ventricular node is normally dominated by the sino-atrial node, but when this influence is removed, it also shows pacemaker activity, be it at a slower rhythm. The atrio-ventricular node gives rise to bundles of Hiss, which course through the interventricular septum and radiate in the ventricular endocard. Starting in the bundles of Hiss, the physiological specialization of the cardiac muscle fibers is combined with a morphological specialization: they form Purkinje fibers. The Purkinje fibers transmit the rhythmic depolarizations, or contraction stimuli, of the sino-atrial node to the myocard, resulting in contraction of the ventricles at a rhythm imposed by the sino-atrial node.
Purkinje fibers (Figs. 4.5.3.-4.) are bigger than normal cardiac fibers and do not form clear processes. Their nucleus is pycnotic and often situated eccentrically. Remains of myofibrils and cross striation are seen here and there at the periphery. The triad system is not well developed. Consequently, Purkinje fibers are not equipped for contraction. Their center is loaded with glycogen, which dissolves and is flushed during preparation, giving them a translucent appearance. They contain small numbers of mitochondria. All this points to a largely anaerobe metabolism based on glycolysis, a clear contrast with the contractile muscle fibers of the myocard. Purkinje fibers are joined to one another and to the myocardial fibers by means of intercalated disks.

Locally, the atria contain cardiac muscle fibers that, apart from a contractile apparatus, contain dense vesicles with a diameter of up to 300 nanometers, especially in the perinuclear zone. These vesicles contain hormones that regulate blood pressure. These specialized cardiac muscle fibers are called **myoendocrine cells**.

IV.5.2. Arteries.

Arteries are characterized by a relatively thick wall and, consequently, a relatively narrow lumen. This is caused by the strong development of the media. The tunica media shows variable amounts of smooth muscle tissue.

In the largest arteries, such as the aorta, the tunica media contains massive amounts of undulating elastic membranes (Fig. 4.5.6.). These are the **elastic arteries**. Smaller amounts of elastic membranes occur in the tunica intima and tunica adventitia, blurring the boundaries between these layers (Fig. 4.5.5.). Elasticas cannot clearly be discerned. The yellowish color of the elastic arteries is a consequence of their elevated content of elastic tissue.
Elastic arteries are exclusively conductive. Their function is to lead the blood from the heart to the main subdivisions of the body: head, trunk, and limbs. Because of their elastic wall, their diameter can change according to pressure. During systole, when the heart pumps blood into an elastic artery, the wall is stretched. The artery reverts to its original diameter during diastole. This contributes to the conversion of a pulsing blood flow to a smooth one.

Elastic arteries are followed by narrower **muscular arteries**, which contain less elastic tissue, so that the reddish color of the smooth muscle fibers is more apparent. In the larger muscular arteries, the tunica media is bordered on both sides by an undulating elastica. Subsequent generations of muscular arteries decrease in diameter, and the tunica media progressively thins. The elastica externa is lost

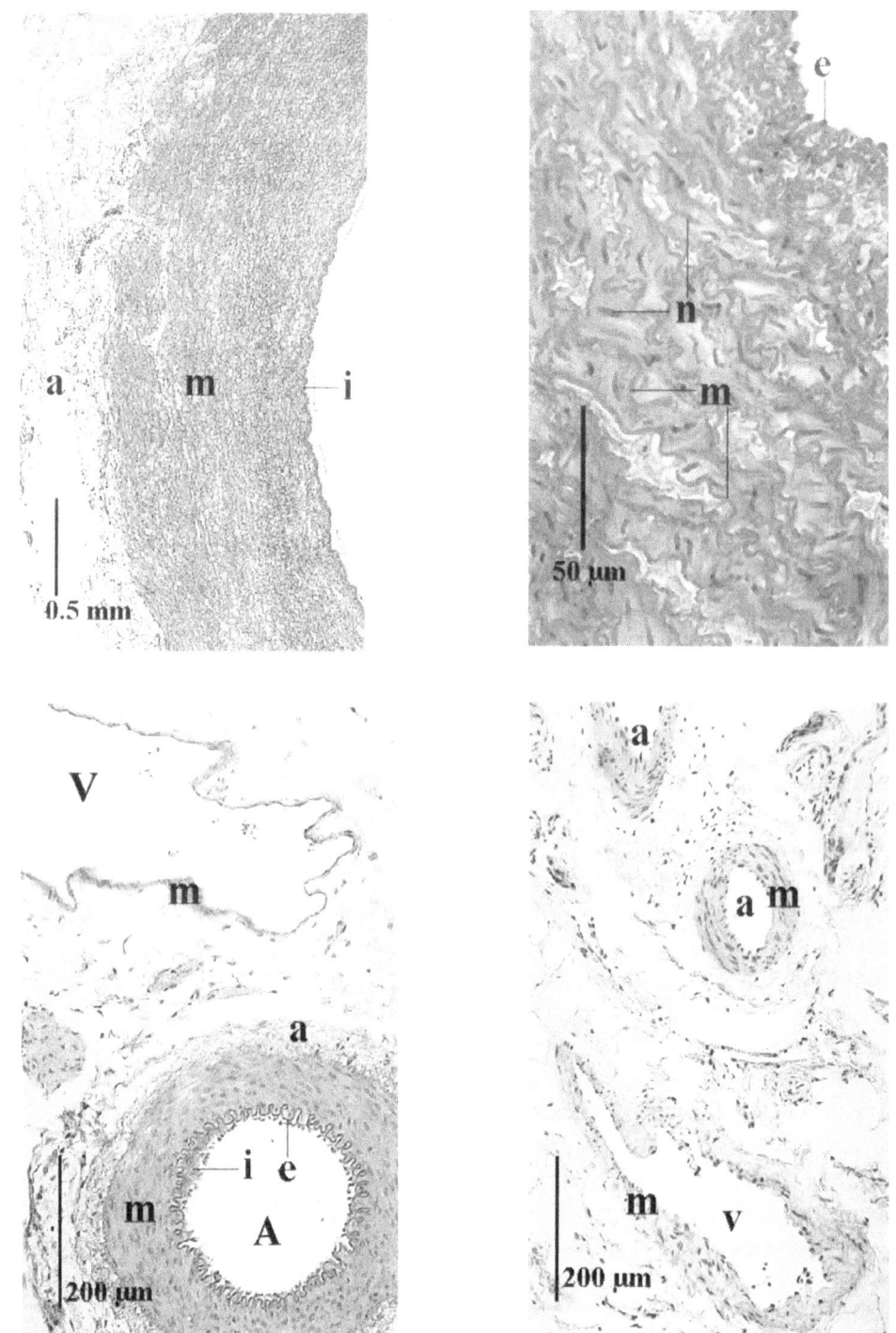

Fig. 4.5.5. (top left) The wall of an elastic artery is composed of three concentric layers. A thin tunica intima, or intima (i), consisting of an endothelium lining a layer of loose fibrous tissue, borders the arterial lumen. The thick middle layer is the tunica media, or media (m). It is composed of visceral muscle tissue and large numbers of elastic membranes. At the outside of the media is a thick layer of loose fibrous tissue, the tunica adventitia, or adventitia (a). Aorta, dog, HE. **Fig. 4.5.6.** (top right) A stronger magnification of Figure 4.5.5. shows the bulging nuclei of the endothelial cells of the intima (e). The media contains wavy elastic membranes (m). The nuclei (n) between them belong mostly to smooth muscle fibers. Aorta, dog, HE. **Fig. 4.5.7.** (bottom left) The media (m) of a muscular artery (A) contains relatively little elastic membrane and consists largely of visceral muscle tissue. The intima (i) is separated from the media by an undulating elastic membrane, the internal elastica (e). The adventitia (a) merges with the surrounding fibrous tissue. At the same level as these arteries, veins (V) are encountered. They have a larger lumen and a thinner wall than the corresponding arteries. The media (m) is very thin. Kidney hilar interstitial tissue, rabbit, HE. **Fig. 4.5.8.** (bottom right) Arterioles (a) are the narrowest segments of the arterial system. They lack an internal elastica. The corresponding venous elements, or venules (v), have relatively wider lumina and thinner walls. m = media. Tendon interstitial tissue, human, HE.

168

relatively early and most muscular arteries only show an elastica interna (Fig. 4.5.7.). The smallest muscular arteries, not visible through the naked eye, have lost the elastica interna as well. These are the **arterioles** (Fig. 4.5.8.). In the smallest arterioles, a cross section of the tunica media shows only a few smooth muscle fibers. In the transition to a capillary, these are lost, so that the capillary wall is in fact a tunica intima.

Muscular arteries are distributive. Subsequent generations distribute arterial blood to ever-smaller regions of the body. As long as they retain a tunica media, they are contractile. The degree of contraction is neurally determined and defines the amount of blood a certain region receives. The smallest arterioles can be regarded as precapillary sphincters that determine how much blood enters the capillary beds.

IV.5.3. Veins.

Veins have a relatively wide lumen and a thin wall (Fig. 4.5.7.). This is a consequence of the tunica media's minor development. In contrast, the tunica adventitia is relatively thick. Veins, especially those of the lower limbs, contain valves. These are protrusions of the intima: they consist of loose fibrous tissue, lined with endothelium. The smallest veins, only visible through a microscope, are called **venules** (Fig. 4.5.8.). They arise from capillaries that acquire a tunica media. The somewhat larger veins have an elastica interna. The largest have an elastica externa as well.

The venous blood pressure is substantially lower than the arterial blood pressure, because arterial blood has been distributed over so many capillaries. The low blood pressure and the large diameter account for the low speed of venous blood flow, much lower than in the corresponding artery. The valves prevent blood from flowing back. The thin venous wall expands easily. Therefore, the veins constitute a blood reservoir, which may contain several times more blood than the arteries.

IV.5.4. Lymph vessels.

Lymph vessels resemble thin walled veins and also contain valves (Fig. 4.5.9.). In microscopic slides, they may be distinguished from blood vessels by the fact that they do not carry erythrocytes.

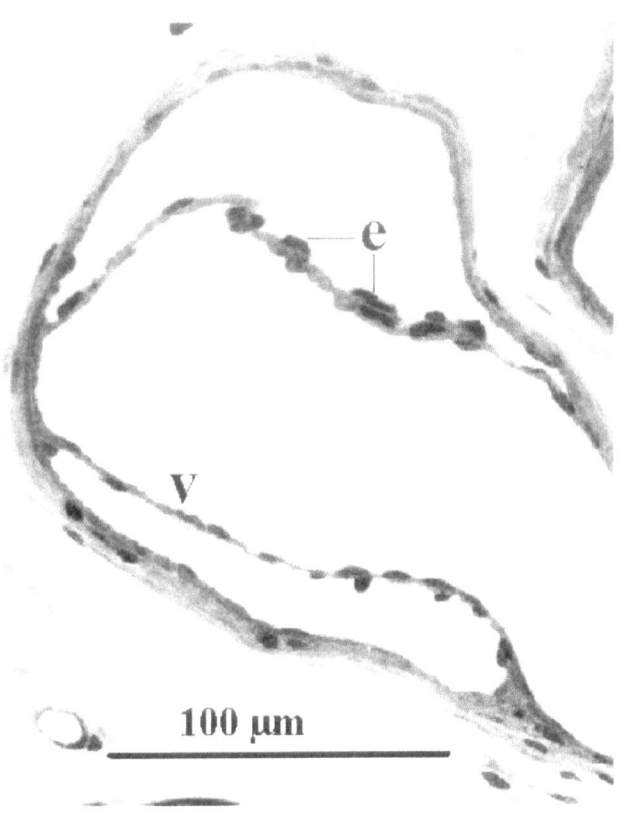

Fig. 4.5.9. Typical in lymph capillaries is the presence of valves, formed by the intima. A valve (v) has a loose fibrous tissue core, lined with endothelium (e). Tongue interstitial tissue, rat, 1-micrometer plastic section, toluidin blue.

IV.5.5. Arterial chemoreceptors and baroreceptors.

In a few places, sensory nerve fibers are closely associated with arteries and may give rise to veritable receptor organs. Distinction can be made between chemoreceptors, which monitor the chemical composition of the blood plasma, and baroreceptors, which monitor blood pressure.

Because of their anatomical location, the **arterial chemoreceptors** are also known as **carotid** and **aortic bodies**. The left and right carotid bodies are located in the neck region, closely associated with the bifurcation of the common carotid artery into an internal and an external carotid artery (Fig. 4.5.10.). Aortic bodies are found in variable numbers in the upper thoracic cavity, in close association with the aortic arch. Smaller aggregations of chemoreceptive tissue are found in various places along the abdominal arteries.

Carotid and aortic bodies are minute organs, but have a profound physiological significance. As chemoreceptors, they are stimulated by decrease of the arterial oxygen tension. They receive a rich blood supply from the artery they are associated with.

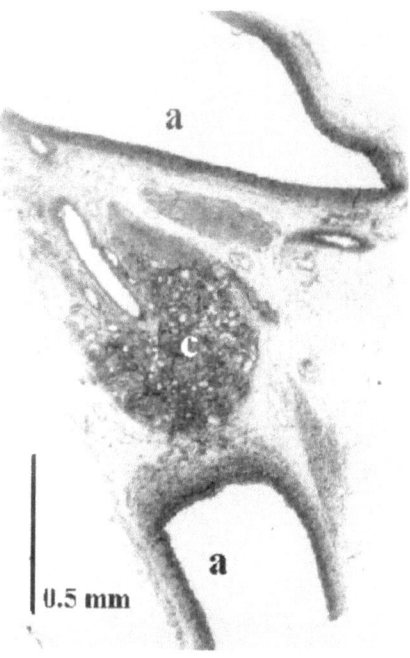

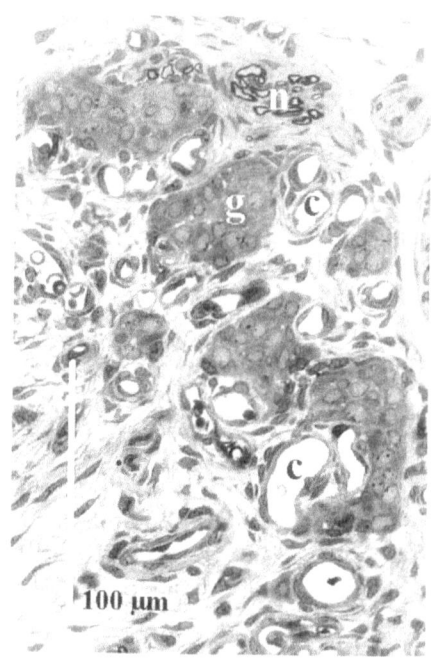

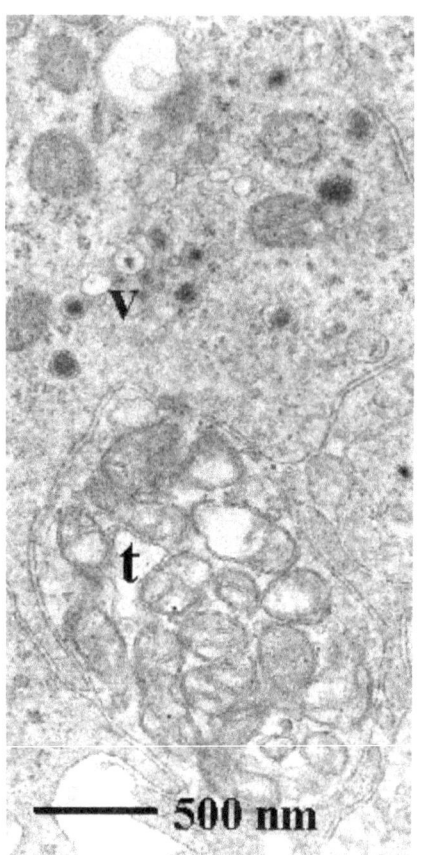

Fig. 4.5.10. (top left) The carotid body (c) is a chemoreceptor organ that is found where the common carotid artery bifurcates in an internal and an external artery (a). Carotid bifurcation, rabbit, 1-micrometer plastic section, toluidin blue. **Fig. 4.5.11.** (above) The carotid body is composed of gland-like lobes or glomeruli (g) of chemoreceptive glomus cells. Numerous capillaries (c) running in the fibrous connective tissue septa indicate that the carotid body has an abundant arterial blood supply. Mark the presence of myelinated sensory nerve fibers (n). Carotid body, rabbit, 1-micrometer plastic section, toluidin blue. **Fig. 4.5.12.** (left) The carotid body's chemoreceptive glomus cells contain dense vesicles (v) and have the cytological structure of endocrine, amine- or peptide hormone-secreting cells. Closely associated with glomus cells are the terminals (t), loaded with mitochondria, of sensory nerve fibers. Carotid body, rabbit, TEM.

Sensory nerve fibers of the cranial glossopharyngeal and vagal nerves, respectively, connect them to the brain stem. Here, they synapse with, among others, motor neurons innervating the respiratory muscles of the thoracic cage. If the arterial oxygen tension drops beneath a critical level, these chemoreceptors, through a reflex mechanism (Fig. 3.6.15.), stimulate the respiratory muscles. The respiratory rhythm increases, and normal arterial oxygen tension is restored. Thus, the arterial chemoreceptors contribute to the maintenance of blood gas levels between narrow limits and insure that the body receives sufficient oxygen. This explains their strategic position along the aorta, which supplies most of the body with oxygenated blood, and along the carotid artery, which conducts oxygenated blood to the brain.

Arterial chemoreceptors consist of globular aggregations of chemoreceptive cells or **glomus cells** and flattened supportive cells, separated from one another by fibrous tissue septa (Fig. 4.5.11.). In these septa and between the glomus cells, numerous capillaries and nerve fibers are seen.

The supporting cells envelop glomus cell groups and mainly contain primary organelles. The glomus cells have the structure of endocrine, amine hormone-secreting cells (Fig. 4.5.12.). They form synaptic junctions (III.6.2.1.) with the terminals of sensory nerve fibers, which are loaded with mitochondria. The presynaptic element is the glomus cell. Its dense granular vesicles function as synaptic vesicles and the inner face of the cell membrane is irregularly thickened. On the other side of the intercellular space or synaptic junction, the inner face of the neural cell membrane carries a corresponding, homogeneously thick, dense layer, and there are no vesicles in proximity. Thus, the nerve terminal is the postsynaptic element. The glomus cell membrane carries receptor molecules that are stimulated by low oxygen concentrations. When the arterial oxygen tension decreases below a border level, the glomus cell depolarizes and its dense vesicles undergo exocytosis, releasing neurotransmitter. The sensory nerve terminals are depolarized and action potentials are generated, which run towards the central nervous system. The exact nature of the neurotransmitter(s) involved is still debated. Many suitable substances have been located in the glomus cells, among them the amine dopamine and several peptides.

The story of glomus cell-nerve terminal interactions does not end here, however. In addition to the synapses just discussed, which can be termed **afferent synapses**, and often next to them, another type of synapse has been described. The polarity of these synapses is reversed. The sensory nerve terminal contains local accumulations of translucent synaptic vesicles and the inner face of its membrane is irregularly thickened. Thus, it is the presynaptic element. The inner face of the glomus cell membrane carries a corresponding, homogeneously thick, dense layer and it is the postsynaptic element. These synapses enable the sensory nerve terminal to influence the glomus cell: they are **efferent synapses**. Probably, both types of synapses make up a local regulatory mechanism that regulates glomus cell activity. When the glomus cell is stimulated, it depolarizes the sensory nerve terminal through the afferent synapses. As already discussed, this may give rise to action potentials in the nerve fibers to the brain stem. In addition, depolarization of the nerve terminal activates the efferent synapses, which may inhibit the secretory activity of the glomus cell. Thus, this regulatory mechanism contains an afferent limb and an efferent limb, as a reflex does. Unlike a true reflex, which passes by way of the central nervous system (Fig. 3.6.15.), this mechanism is limited to the peripheral nerve terminal. It is termed an **axon reflex**.

The **arterial baroreceptors** are mechanoreceptors, associated with the internal carotid artery. Immediately after the common carotid artery bifurcation, this vessel expands and forms a thin-walled sinus. In the tunica media of this carotid sinus, smooth muscle fibers are scarce, but collagen and elastic fibrils are abundant. In the tunica media and the tunica adventitia, numerous sensory nerve fibers are found, which locally expand to form nerve terminals, loaded with mitochondria.

Baroreceptors are sensitive to deformation and are stimulated when the sinus wall is stretched, as it is by increasing blood pressure. Blood pressure can be restored to normal levels by relaxation of the vessel walls, decreasing of the cardiac contraction frequency, or decreasing of the blood's volume by increased urine production.

References.

Forssmann W.G., Nokihara K., Gagelmann M., Hock D., Feller S., Schulz-Knappe P., Herbst F.: The heart is the center of a new endocrine, paracrine, and neuroendocrine system. Arch. Histol. Cytol. 1989, 52: S293-S315.

Gonzalez C., Almaraz L., Obeso A., Rigual R.: Carotid body chemoreceptors: from natural stimuli to sensory discharges. Physiol. Rev. 1994, 74: 829-898.

Kimani, J.K.: Elastin and mechanoreceptor mechanisms with special reference to the mammalian carotid sinus. Ciba Found. Symp. 1995, 192: 215-236.

Thornell L.E., Eriksson A.: Filament systems in the Purkinje fibers of the heart. Am. J. Physiol. 1981, 241: H291-H305.

Verna A.: Ultrastructure of the carotid body in the mammals. Int. Rev. Cytol. 1979, 60: 271-330.

IV.6. Extra-embryonic organs.

Extra-embryonic organs are those that arise from parts of the blastocyst that do not participate in the formation of the embryo proper (Fig. 4.1.). They contribute to nourishing the embryo during its development inside the uterus. They are predominantly formed of **epithelium** and **endothelium**.

IV.6.1. Amnion.

The amnion is a membrane that lines the space surrounding the embryo and is derived from extra-embryonic ectoderm. Histologically, it is a mucosa, consisting of an epithelium that rests on a fibrous tissue lamina propria. The apices of the epithelial cells point towards the embryo. The deeper layers of the lamina propria merge with the chorion. The epithelium is simple cuboidal to prismatic. The epithelial cells carry numerous apical, slightly irregular microvilli. The basal cell membrane forms protrusions. The cytoplasm is loaded with glycogen granules. Secondary organelles are scarce. The cells form typical junctions, especially tight junctions and desmosomes.

The amnion epithelial cells absorb certain components of the blood plasma and secrete them in the amniotic space, creating amniotic fluid. In addition, they regulate this fluid's composition and volume.

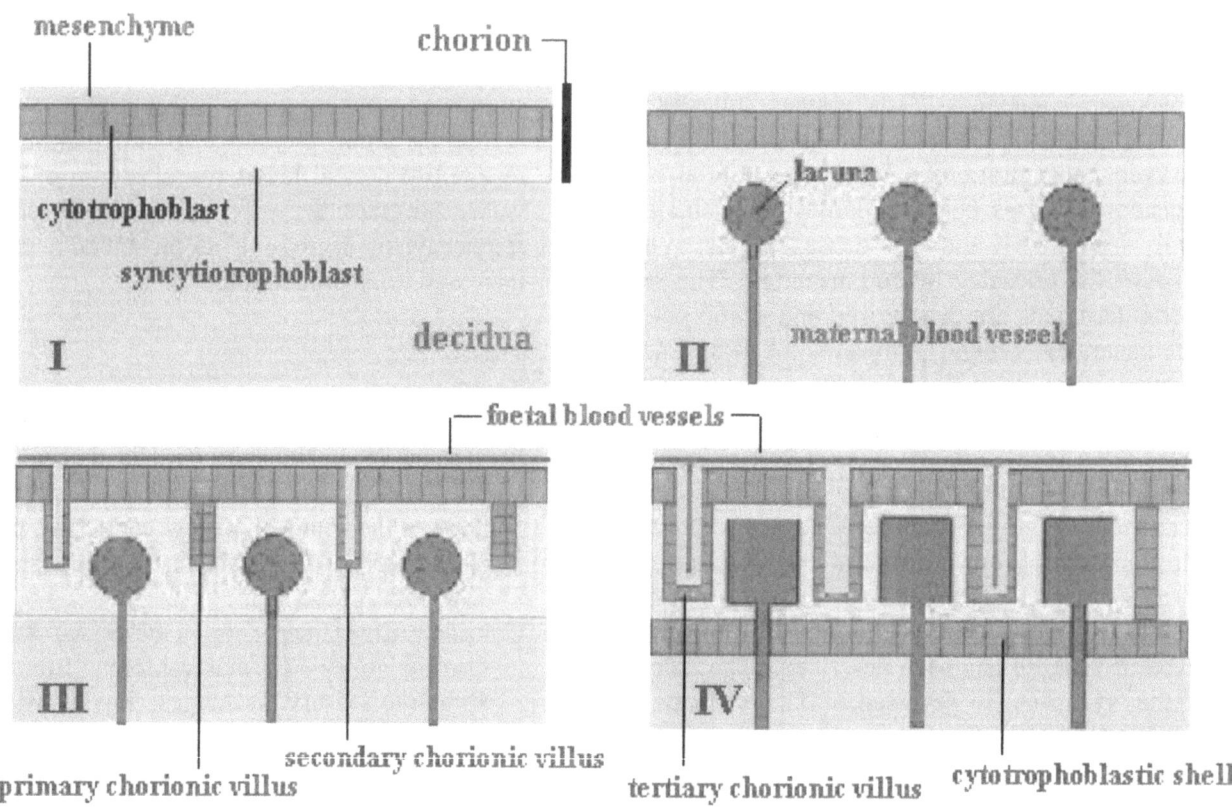

Fig. 4.6.1. Chorionic epithelium is stratified, consisting as it does of a deeper cytotrophoblast and a superficial syncytiotrophoblast. The syncytiotrophoblast contacts the decidua, i.e. the uterine epithelium (I). It locally degrades the decidua, so that cavities appear, filled with maternal blood, the lacunae (II). The cytotrophoblast develops villi (III). Primary villi are made exclusively of epithelium, while in secondary villi an interstitial tissue core appears. When blood vessels penetrate this core, a tertiary villus is formed (IV). The cytotrophoblast spreads over the deeper, intact decidua and forms a cytotrophoblastic plate.

172

IV.6.2. Chorion and placenta.

The chorion is a mucosa, which envelops the amnion. Both have a common lamina propria. The chorion's epithelium faces the decidua, the specialized region of the endometrium (IV.11.3.2.) that allows blastocyst implantation. Locally, the chorion contacts and penetrates the decidua and forms a **placenta** (Fig. 4.6.1.). The placenta ensures intensive contact between the maternal blood and the blood of the developing embryo. Through the placenta, the embryo takes up food molecules and oxygen from the maternal blood and gets rid of waste molecules and carbon dioxide.

The chorion is lined with a stratified epithelium, derived from the trophoblast. Its basal layers consist of individual cells and form the **cytotrophoblast**. The superficial layers form a syncytium, the **syncytiotrophoblast**. Along its entire surface, the chorion develops protrusions, the chorionic **villi**, which penetrate the decidua. At a particular spot, the development of the villi is carried to greater extremes, and a placenta is formed. A chorionic villus originally consists of cytotrophoblast, covered with syncytiotrophoblast. In this stage, the villus is called a primary villus. The primary villus is invaded by the underlying chorionic interstitial tissue, which forms a central core. In this way, a primary villus is transformed into a secondary one. Eventually, the interstitial tissue core is invaded by capillaries, and a tertiary villus is formed (Fig. 4.6.2.). Meanwhile, the villi acquire a more complicated, dendritic shape by the formation of branches, which greatly increase the extent of the villus-decidua interface, facilitating the exchange of substances between mother and embryo. While it grows into the decidua, the trophoblast degrades the endometrial epithelium. In a later stage, it degrades the decidual tissue. Eventually, even the walls of the endometrial blood vessels are degraded. The end result is that the chorionic villi of the placenta bathe in maternal blood, which circulates in extravascular, intervillous spaces. A placenta having a structure like this is called a hemochoreal placenta. From the tips of the villi, the chorionic epithelium spreads over the intact, non-degraded, surface of the decidua and merges into a **basal plate**.

The syncytiotrophoblast of a fully developed villus shows distinct signs of differentiation. The apical cell membrane forms irregular microvilli and shows endocytosis, which indicates the existence of intensive transport of low molecular weight and high molecular weight substances, respectively. The apical cytoplasm is loaded with vesicles, part of which are secretory

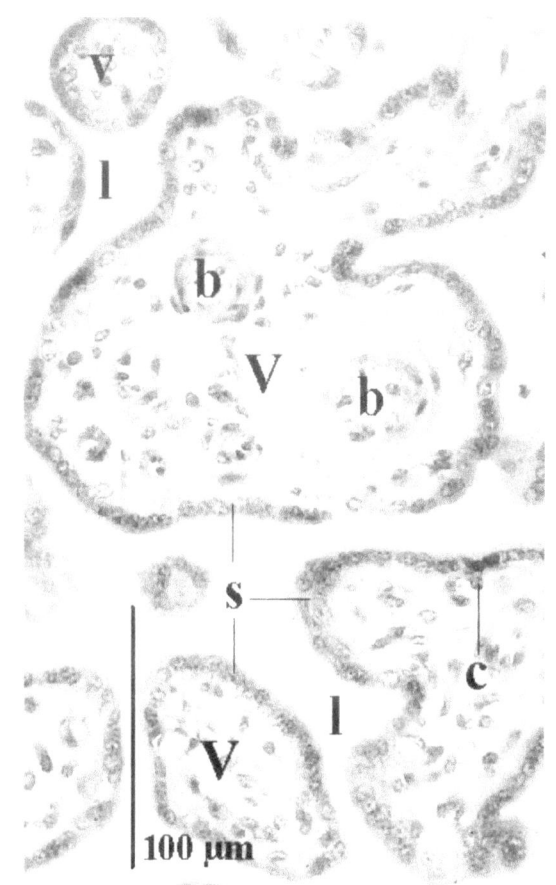

Fig. 4.6.2. Placental villi (v) are lined with syncytiotrophoblast (s). The cytotrophoblast (c) has been reduced to individual epithelial cells. The villous interstitial tissue contains blood vessels (b), indicating that these villi are tertiary. Maternal blood circulates in the lacunae (l). Placenta, human, HE.

vesicles, part of which belong to the smooth endoplasmic reticulum. The basal cytoplasm is basophilic and contains a well-developed rough endoplasmic reticulum, indicating protein production. Some of these proteins are enzymes, needed to degrade the decidua during implantation of the trophoblast, others are hormones, such as human chorion gonadotrophin. Steroid droplets and mitochondria with tubular cristae are encountered as well, indicating steroid hormone synthesis.

The underlying cytotrophoblast contains relatively undifferentiated cells. These show mitosis and thus supply cells, which will participate to the syncytiotrophoblast. Initially, the cytotrophoblast has a coherent epithelial structure, but as the villi develop, its coherence is gradually lost. Eventually, all that remains of the cytotrophoblast is a rather small number of isolated cells.

The underlying interstitial tissue contains macrophages (Hofbauer's cells). The capillaries are of the permeable, sinusoidal, type. As the villi develop, they become more numerous and more closely associated with the chorionic epithelium, thus moving closer to the maternal blood. The interstitial tissue is invaded with cytotrophoblast cells, which secrete **matrix-type fibrinoid**. This eosinophilic material is heterogeneous: it is a mosaic of patches showing similarities, in structure as well as in composition, to either basement membrane or ground substance.

The basal plate joins the placenta to the intact decidua. It consists, as do the villi, of cytotrophoblast and syncytiotrophoblast. The latter lines the intervillous spaces. The former rests on the interstitial tissue, which appears to be "glued" to the underlying decidua by **fibrin-type fibrinoid**. This is composed of fibrils with the characteristic 24-nanometer period transverse striations of fibrin and, in contrast to matrix-type fibrinoid, is completely free of cells. It originates from the blood and is analogous to a blood clot.

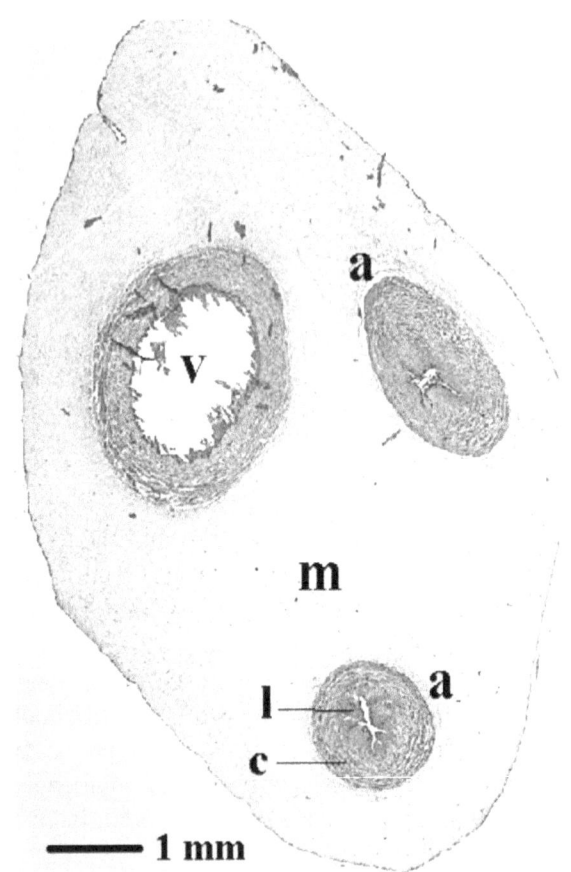

—— 1 mm

Fig. 4.6.3. The umbilical cord contains 3 blood vessels, sheathed in mucous tissue (m), which is lined with amnionic epithelium. The thick-walled vessels are arteries (a), the single thin-walled one is a vein (v). These vessels do not have a standard structure. The media is double: its inner layer is longitudinal (l), its outer layer circular (c). In addition, there is no typical adventitia of loose fibrous tissue, as the media directly contacts the mucous tissue. Umbilical cord, human, HE.

IV.6.3. Umbilical cord.

The umbilical cord (Fig. 4.6.3.) arises from the embryonic stem that connects the embryo with the amnion. Consequently, it is covered with epithelium, derived from the same extra-embryonic ectoderm that also lines the amniotic cavity. The umbilical cord's interior contains blood vessels and interstitial tissue. The interstitial tissue is mucous tissue, called **Wharton's jelly**, which confers a certain rigidity to the umbilical cord and prevents nicking of the cord and twisting of the blood vessels. Three blood vessels course in the umbilical cord's interior: two arteries and a single vein. The arteries are of the muscular type and conduct deoxygenated blood from the embryo to the placenta. The vein conducts oxygenated blood to the embryo. As in blood vessels elsewhere, the umbilical arteries have a relatively thick wall and narrow lumen, while the umbilical vein has a thin wall and wide lumen. In other respects, these vessels deviate form other blood vessels. They have a double-layered tunica media. In its inner layer, the smooth muscle fibers have a circular or spiral arrangement, while in its outer layer the fibers run longitudinally. There are no distinct elastics. A typical tunica adventitia, consisting of loose fibrous interstitial tissue, is absent. The tunica media rests directly on the mucous tissue of Wharton's jelly.

References.

Jones C.J.P., Fox H.: Ultrastructure of the normal human placenta. Electron Microsc. Rev. 1991, 4: 129-178.

Jones C.J.P., Jauniaux E.: Ultrastructure of the materno-embryonic interface in the first trimester of pregnancy. Micron 1995, 26: 145-173.

Kaufmann P., Huppertz B., Frank H.G.: The fibrinoids of the human placenta: origin, composition and functional relevance. Ann. Anat. 1996, 178: 485-501.

Novak R.F.: A brief review of the anatomy , histology, and ultrastructure of the full term placenta. Arch. Pathol. Lab. Med. 1991, 115: 654-659.

IV.7. Endocrine system.

The endocrine system contains a number of endocrine glands consisting of **glandular tissue** and **endothelium**, which forms numerous blood capillaries. The glandular tissue produces hormones, which enter the blood circulation. Typically, the capillaries are dilated and fenestrated, which increases their permeability. This is essential, considering that the hormones have to pass the endothelium of the capillary wall to enter the circulation. Such capillaries are called **sinusoidal capillaries**. Glandular tissue and endothelium are enveloped in and supported by loose fibrous interstitial tissue. The whole gland is enveloped in denser fibrous connective tissue, which may form thin and incomplete septa. Usually, endocrine glands show much less septal fibrous tissue than do exocrine glands. This may be explained by the absence of ducts in endocrine glands. Most endocrine glands have an ecto- or endodermal origin.

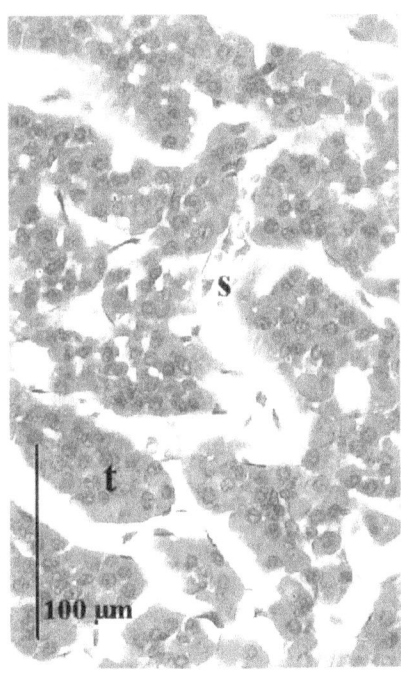

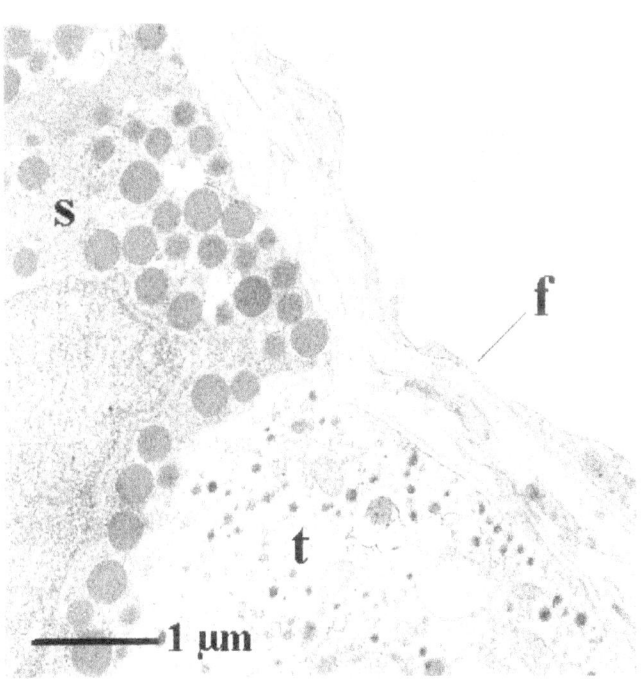

Fig. 4.7.1. (left) The anterior pituitary gland's endocrine tissue is arranged in trabecules (t), interspersed with numerous, expanded capillaries, the sinusoidal capillaries (s). Anterior pituitary gland, rabbit, HE. **Fig. 4.7.2.** (right) The anterior pituitary contains several types of organotroph cells, two of which can be seen here. The cell containing large secretory vesicles is a somatotroph (s), which secretes somatotroph hormone. The cell containing small secretory vesicles is a thyrotroph (t), which secretes thyroid-stimulating hormone. Both cells lie near a sinusoidal capillary, which shows fenestrations (f). Anterior pituitary, cat, TEM.

IV.7.1. Anterior pituitary gland.

The anterior pituitary gland arises as an invagination, known by embryologists as Rathke's pouch, of the ectoderm of the palate. Later, this pouch will close and separate from the ectoderm. It envelops the top of a corresponding invagination of the epithelium forming the floor of the primitive brain. Thus, the anterior pituitary gland becomes a brain appendage, the stem that connects it to the brain developing into the neurohypophysis. The anterior pituitary gland is also called the **adenohypophysis**. Both form the hypophysis proper, or pituitary gland. In man and most mammals, only the terminal part, the **pars distalis**, of the anterior pituitary gland has endocrine activity. The human anterior pituitary has a volume of somewhat less than 1 cubic centimeter and most of it is pars distalis. A minor part of the anterior pituitary forms a sheath that partly envelops the neurohypophyseal stem: the pars tuberalis. The pars intermedia of the anterior pituitary is a thin layer of tissue between the pars distalis and the tip of the neurohypophysis.

The reason why the anterior pituitary should be so closely associated with the brain is well known: the hormone productions of its various organotroph cell types are controlled by other hormones, produced by specialized neurons or neuroendocrine cells. The most important of these form the hypothalamic nuclei. Their axons form the hypothalamo-hypophyseal tractus and course in the neurohypophysis (IV.4.3.). They terminate next to sinusoidal capillary networks that drain to the anterior pituitary via portal veins. Their hormones are peptides, which are synthesized in the perikarya, reach the terminals by axoplasmic transport and are secreted through exocytosis. The exact nature of the hormonal influence of the hypothalamus on the anterior pituitary depends on the cell type. Somatotrophs and mammotrophs undergo stimulation as well as inhibition. The other organotroph cell types: thyreotrophs, corticotrophs and gonadotrophs, only undergo inhibition. The target organs of these cells are themselves endocrine glands, the hormonal secretions of which inhibit the hypothalamus. Thus, these organotroph cells, their target organs, and the hypothalamus, are part of a feedback loop.

The pars distalis has, except for a few follicles, a trabecular structure (Fig. 4.7.1.). The trabecules intermingle with a dense network of sinusoidal capillaries.

The anterior pituitary contains about 5 cell types with endocrine activity, the **organotroph cells**, named after the target organ that they influence through their hormonal secretion. These cell types have diameters of 10 to 15 micrometers, the somatotrophs and mammotrophs being somewhat smaller than the other cell types. They display the typical cytological characteristics of symmetrical, peptide hormone-secreting gland cells (II.2.1.1.2.). They differ from each other mainly in the numbers and dimensions of their secretory vesicles (Fig. 4.7.2.). In general, the secretory vesicles are rounded or polygonal and have an opaque content which fills the vesicle completely, so that no submembranous halo shows. Some organotrophs, i.e. the somatotrophs, the lactotrophs, and the corticotrophs, secrete pure peptide hormones and have a well-developed rough endoplasmic reticulum. Others, such as the thyreotrophs and gonadotrophs, secrete glycopeptide hormones and, in addition to rough endoplasmic reticulum, their Golgi-complex is relatively well developed. These characteristics may change during the secretory cycle or according to the physiological parameters of the body.

In addition to hormonally active organotroph cells, the pars distalis contains smaller and less well developed **folliculo-stellate cells**. These cells do not contain secretory vesicles. They form processes, with which they envelop the organotroph cells. Occasionally, they may form follicles. They are joined to one another and to the organotroph cells by means of desmosomes. Probably, they are not a homogeneous cell category. Some of them may be resting or inactive organotroph cells. Others probably regulate the activities of the organotroph cells.

Somatotroph cells secrete the somatotroph hormone or growth hormone. This is one of the hormones that stimulate metabolism. In the growing organism, it stimulates the longitudinal growth of the bones by inducing mitosis in the chondrocytes of the growth plates. Somatotrophs are mainly located in the posterio-lateral parts of the pars distalis and may occur in large numbers, accounting for almost half the total volume of the pars distalis. They contain numerous secretory vesicles with a diameter of somewhat more than 300 nanometers.

Mammotroph or **lactotroph cells** secrete prolactin, or lactotroph hormone, which stimulates growth of the milk glands and production of milk. They are evidently present in greatest numbers at the end of pregnancy and during lactation. They are preferably located in the lateral parts of the pars distalis and may account for 20 percent or more of its total volume. Their secretory vesicles are relatively scarce and their diameters may attain values of 900 nanometers, making them the largest vesicles found in any organotroph cell type. In times of inactivity, lysosomes appear, by means of which the cells engage in autophagocytosis, clearing their superfluous vesicles and even parts of other organelles. This intracellular elimination of secretory product has been described in a number of endocrine cell types and is referred to as **crinophagocytosis**.

Corticotroph cells secrete adrenocorticotroph hormone, which induces the zona fasciculata of the adrenal cortex to produce its own steroid hormones. They represent some 20 percent of the volume of the pars distalis and are mainly found in its anterio-central part. This is the only organotroph cell type with a deeply indented nucleus. The secretory vesicles are scarce to fairly numerous, with diameters of about 200 nanometers. These cells frequently contain lipid droplets.

Thyrotroph cells secrete thyrotroph hormone, which incites the thyroid follicles to thyroid hormone production. They represent about 5 percent of the volume of the pars distalis and have the same anterio-central distribution as the corticotrophs. It is the only organotroph cell type which is distinctly elongated, instead of rounded. The secretory vesicles are scarce to fairly numerous and have diameters of somewhat less than 150 nanometers, the smallest secretory vesicles of any organotroph cell type.

Gonadotroph cells stimulate the development of gametes and the production of hormones by the endocrine cells of the reproductive organs. They represent about 5 percent of the volume of the pars distalis and are distributed mainly in its lateral parts. Their secretory vesicles are numerous and have diameters of somewhat less than 300 nanometers. The rough endoplasmic reticulum shows dilated cisterns. Lipid droplets and lysosomes may be present. It is the only organotroph cell type that secretes two hormones. One of these is follicle-stimulating hormone. In the female, this hormone induces ripening of ovarian follicles and oocytes, and induces the follicles to secrete estrogen. In the male, this hormone stimulates spermatogenesis. The other hormone is called, in the female, luteinizing hormone. It stimulates the development of the corpus luteum and its secretion of progesterone. In the male, this hormone is the interstitial cell-stimulating hormone, which incites the interstitial cells of the testes, the Leydig cells, to secrete testosterone.

IV.7.2. Thyroid gland.

The thyroid gland lies on the ventral side of the larynx. In the embryo, the thyroid is formed as a ventral gland-like invagination of the pharyngeal endoderm. This invagination separates from the endoderm and migrates caudally, where it comes to rest on the ventral side of the larynx. It forms two lateral lobes, which remain connected through a narrow isthmus. The isthmus may carry a triangular cranial projection, the pyramid, which is a leftover of the embryonic thyroid's "duct".

The thyroid is the only endocrine gland of any significance in the human body that has a follicular structure (Fig. 4.7.3.). The glandular tissue does not form solid cords, but hollow **follicles**. Originally, these follicles were tubular invaginations of epithelium, which were pinched off. Their epithelial structure has been carefully preserved. The largest follicles have diameters of a few hundred micrometers. Their wall is a simple cuboidal to prismatic epithelium, formed by gland cells, the **thyreocytes** (Fig. 4.7.4.). At first sight, it may be confusing to notice that the thyreocytes, which form an endocrine tissue, should have the cytological structure of polarized, exocrine, enzyme-secreting gland cells. This deviating structure is explained by the fact that the synthesis proper of thyroid hormone occurs extracellulary, in the follicular lumen. The thyreocytes in fact only supply the raw materials that are necessary to synthesize thyroid hormone, and they secrete them, merocrine fashion, at their apical pole, which borders the follicular lumen. These raw materials form a viscous mass, the **colloid**, which fills the follicular lumen. In fact, the only reason why thyreocytes can be regarded as endocrine cells at all, is that they, in the end, secrete a hormone into the circulation. To be able to do this, they must phagocytose and enzymatically degrade colloid to liberate hormone. Consequently, in a certain stage of

their life cycle, the thyreocytes show characteristics of macrophages: apical phagosomes and lysosomes. As a consequence of colloid absorption, peripheral spaces called resorption vacuoles appear in the colloid. The liberated hormone is secreted, merocrine fashion, at the basal cell pole, in close proximity to sinusoidal capillaries. In summary, thyreocytes are complex, doubly polarized cells: they absorb raw materials at their basal pole and secrete them at their apical pole, while finished hormone travels in the opposite direction.

The thyroid follicles produce the thyroid hormone or thyroxin. This is not a pure hormone, however, but a mixture of several closely related hormonally active substances. They are derived from an amino acid, tyrosine, which is iodated and subjected to condensation reactions. The follicular thyreocytes take up tyrosine and iodium ions and secrete them, by means of membrane pumps, into the follicular lumen. The thyreocyte's apex carries microvilli, probably to accommodate large numbers of membrane pumps. In addition, the thyreocytes synthesize a glycoprotein, thyroglobulin, which they secrete, merocrine fashion, in the follicular lumen. In the colloid, the negatively charged iodium ions are oxidized to neutral iodium by a peroxidase, which is also synthesized by the thyreocytes. Neutral iodium atoms are bound to tyrosine molecules, which condensate and form complexes with thyroglobulin. Thyreocytes engulf these complexes by means of pseudopodia and phagocytose them. Thyroglobulin is enzymatically degraded, and variously iodated and condensed tyrosine molecules, forming thyroxin, are secreted at the basal cell pole.

In periods of prolonged stress, such as cold, thyroxin stimulates mitochondrial oxidative phosphorylation: the production of ATP with the energy obtained from breakdown of glucose and fatty acids. Thus, thyroxin stimulates the basal body metabolism. It is self evident that insufficient production of thyroxin leads to metabolic disorders, which may cause impaired development. As part of a regulatory mechanism, thyroxin inhibits the hypothalamus, causing inhibition of the hypophyseal thyrotroph cells. If insufficient iodium is supplied to the body in the food, insufficient thyroxin is produced. Consequently, the thyroid is unable to inhibit the hypothalamus. The hypothalamus will continue to stimulate the hypophyseal thyrotrophs, which will, in turn, stimulate the thyroid follicles. This may lead to thyroid hypertrophy, or goiter.

On closer inspection, the thyroid contains a second type of endocrine cell. In the loose fibrous interstitial

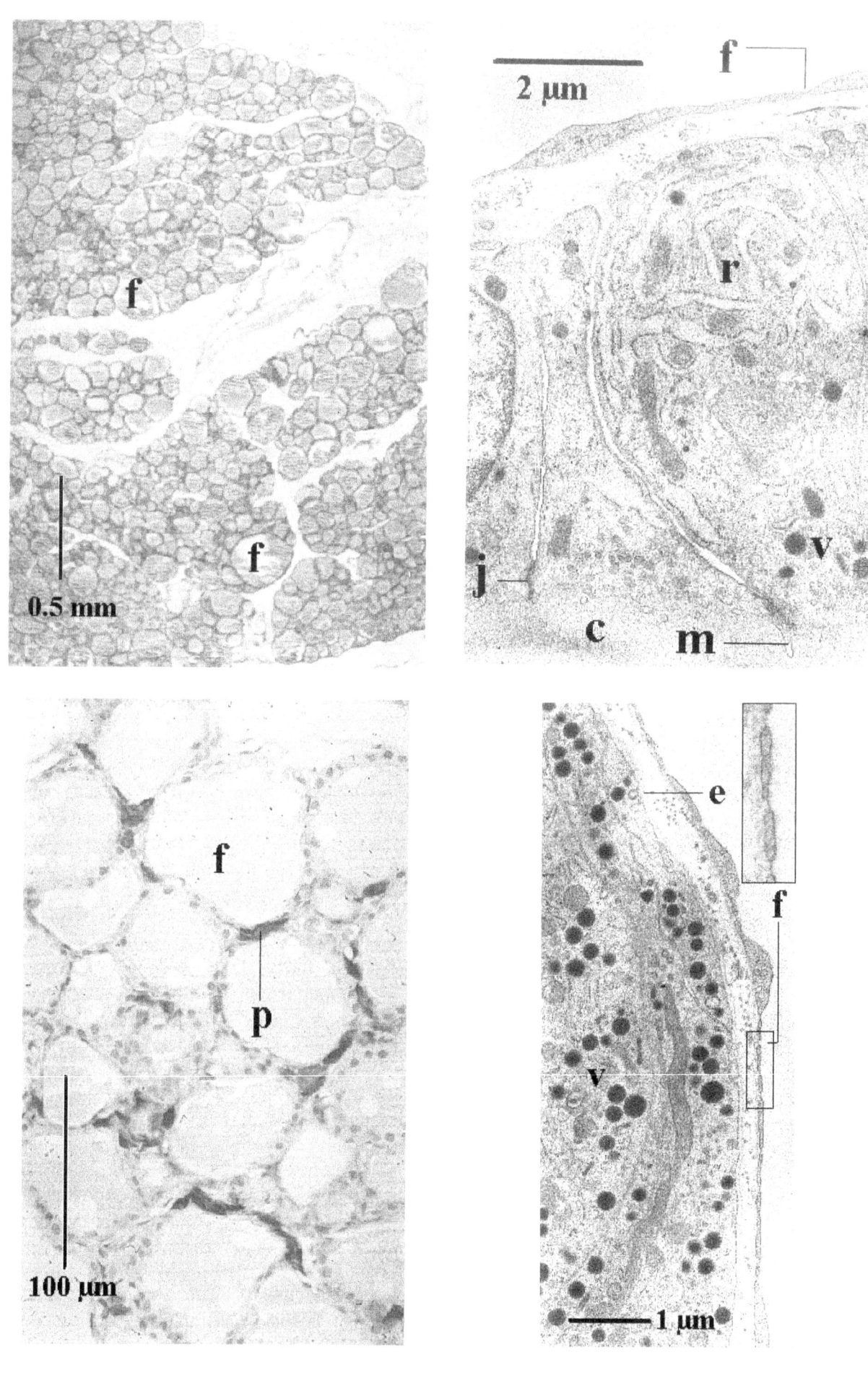

Fig. 4.7.3. (top left) The thyroid gland contains fibrous tissue septa, which divide the glandular tissue into lobes, composed of follicles (f). The follicular wall is a simple cuboidal or prismatic epithelium, composed of thyreocytes. The follicular lumen is filled with colloid. Thyroid gland, dog, HE. Fig. 4.7.4. (top right) The follicular wall is a simple epithelium of thyreocytes, which are joined by means of apical junctional complexes (j), and carry a few short microvilli (m). The colloid (c) is a homogeneous fluid. The thyreocytes contain abundant rough endoplasmic reticulum (r) and dense secretory vesicles (v). Remarkably, the vesicles do not distribute evenly along the cell's perimeter, as they do in other endocrine cells, but concentrate at the cell apex, as they would do in exocrine gland cells. A fenestrated capillary (f) comes in close proximity of the thyreocytes. Thyroid, cat, TEM. Fig. 4.7.5. (bottom left) In the interstitial tissue separating the follicles (f), and invading the follicular epithelium, numerous parafollicular cells are observed (p). Thyroid, dog, immune reaction to calcitonin, visualized with peroxidase. Fig. 4.7.6. (bottom right) Parafollicular cells are loaded, at their periphery, with secretory vesicles (v), the contents of which can be liberated by exocytosis (e) near a fenestrated (f), sinusoidal capillary. Thyroid, cat, TEM.

tissue that envelops the follicles, clusters of **parafollicular cells** (Fig. 4.7.5.) are found. These cells also occur in the follicular walls, but never contact the lumen. They have the typical cytological structure of peptide hormone-secreting gland cells (II.2.1.1.2.). They contain numerous secretory vesicles with diameters between 100 and 200 nanometers (Fig. 4.7.6.)

The parafollicular cells produce the hormone calcitonin. Calcitonin is released when the calcium concentration of the blood increases and reaches a critical level. It inhibits the osteoclasts of the bone tissue (III.2.4.5.). Since calcium loss, mainly via the urine, is no longer compensated by osteoclastic activity, blood calcium levels drop. This inhibits calcitonin release. Thus, calcitonin works antagonistically to parathormone. In contrast to the thyreocytes, the parafollicular cells are not under hypothalamic and hypophyseal control.

In summary, the thyroid is in fact a multiple gland. Its active components, follicles and parafollicular cells, both have their characteristic cytological structure and function. The reasons for this close association of what amounts to two endocrine glands are not as clear as they are in the anterior pituitary. Probably, one component has some regulatory influence on the other.

IV.7.3. Parathyroid glands.

The parathyroid glands derive their name from their close association with the thyroid. Usually, there are four of them, a cranial pair and a caudal pair, and they lie dorsal of the thyroid lobes. They are minute organs, only a few millimeters in diameter. During embryological development, they are formed from the endoderm of the fourth gill pouch.

Like other endocrine glands, the parathyroids (Fig. 4.7.7.) do not have prominent septa, but with

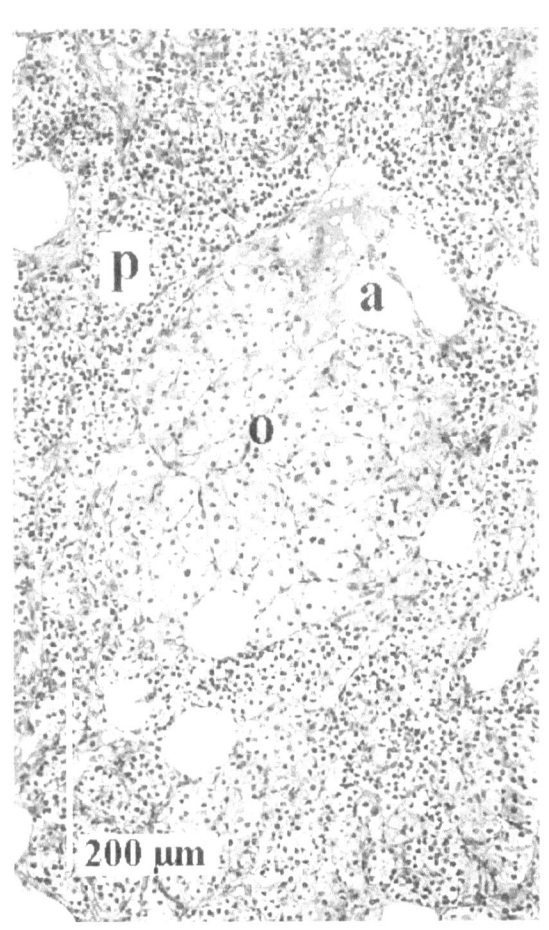

Fig. 4.7.7. Apart from principal cells (p), which are its active endocrine cells, the parathyroid contains additional cell types, such as oxyphilic cells (o). Oxyphilic cells lie in groups, are clearly larger than principal cells, and have a granular, eosinophilic (or oxyphilic) cytoplasm. A few white adipocytes (a) are also seen. Parathyroid, human, HE.

increasing age, the development of adipose tissue makes them more conspicuous. The glandular tissue is made up of three cell types.

The most numerous cells are the **principal cells**, which show the characteristic cytological structure of peptide hormone-secreting cells. They contain only small numbers of secretory vesicles, with diameters of about 300 nanometers. They also contain variable amounts

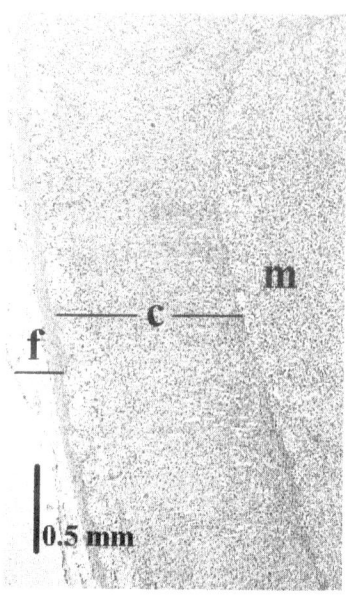

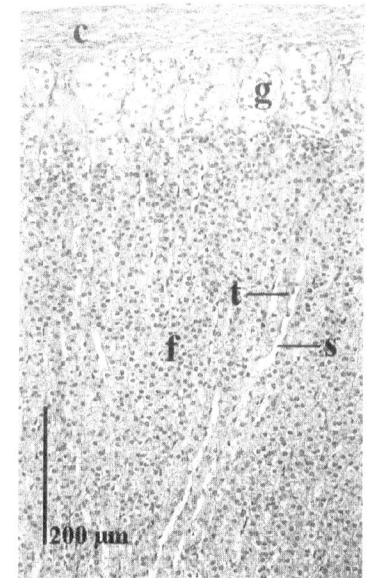

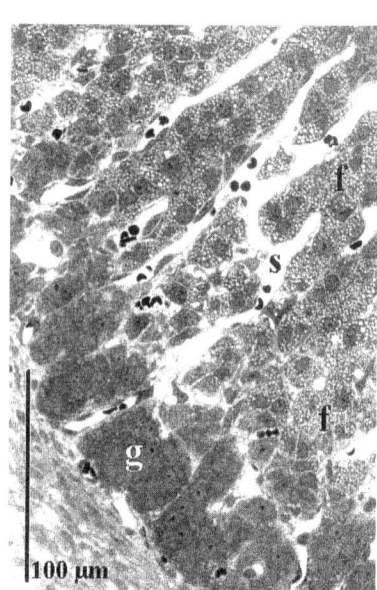

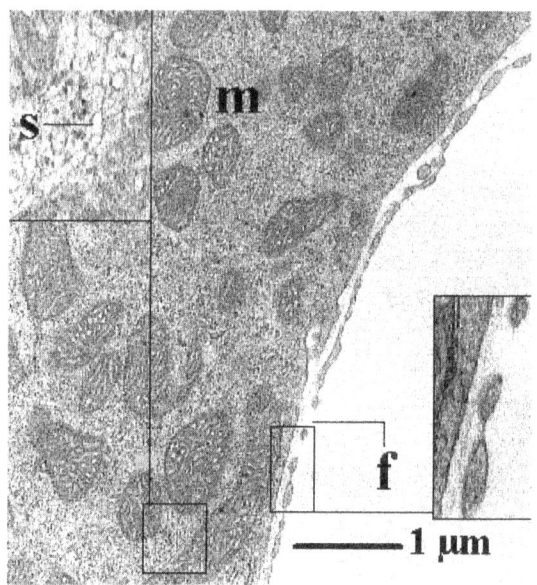

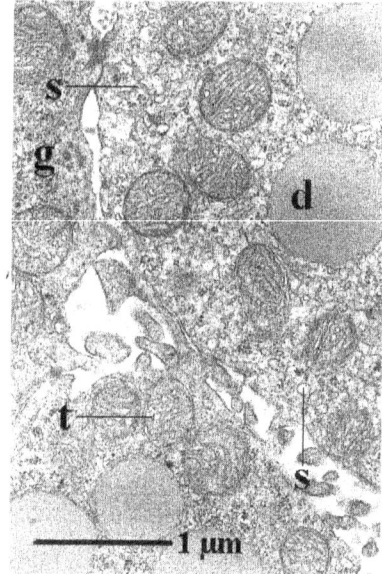

Fig. 4.7.8. (top left) The adrenal gland is subdivided in a cortex (c) and a medulla (m). The organ is embedded in a capsule of fibrous and adipose tissue (f), but does not contain septa. Adrenal gland, dog, HE. **Fig. 4.7.9.** (top right) The adrenal cortex is further subdivided into 3 layers, the 2 most important of which can be seen here. Beneath the capsule (c) is the zona glomerulosa (g), in which the endocrine cells are arranged in rounded, globular trabecules. Next is the zona fasciculata (f), the trabecules of which are narrow, elongated, fascicle-like (t). These trabecules are about 2 cells wide, run parallel, and are oriented at right angles to the organ's surface. The trabecules alternate with sinusoidal capillaries (s), which have the same shape and orientation. Adrenal cortex, dog, HE. **Fig. 4.7.10.** (middle left) The endocrine cells of the adrenal cortex, especially so those of the zona fasciculata (f), have a vacuolated, spongy aspect, which is why they are sometimes called spongiocytes. This aspect is directly related to the storage of steroid droplets in their cytoplasm. g = zona glomerulosa, s = sinusoidal capillaries. Adrenal cortex, cat, 1-micrometer plastic section, toluidin blue. **Fig. 4.7.11.** (bottom left) The endocrine cells of the adrenal cortex, such as those of the zona fasciculata, are steroid hormone-secreting cells with a well-developed smooth endoplasmic reticulum (s). The cytosolic steroid droplets (d) contain cholesterol, a precursor of the steroid hormones that are synthesized and secreted by these cells. The smooth endoplasmic reticulum's membranes may touch these droplets, but they are not contained in a membrane. The mitochondria are rounded and display tubular cristae (t). The dense dots, lying in groups, are glycogen granules (g). Adrenal cortex, rabbit, TEM. **Fig. 4.7.12.** (bottom right) The endocrine cells of the adrenal cortex lie close to sinusoidal capillaries (fenestrations, f). They contain abundant smooth endoplasmic reticulum (s) and numerous mitochondria with tubular cristae (m). Steroid droplets are absent in this area of the cell, where the synthesized hormones diffuse towards the blood circulation. This indicates that these hormones do not accumulate in the cell, and that the steroid droplets do not contain hormone, only its precursor substance. Adrenal cortex, hamster, TEM.

of glycogen and a number of lipid droplets. These substances are readily dissolved during tissue preparation, which explains the translucent look of the principal cells. They are the parathyroid's only hormonally active cell type.

The oxyphilic cells are relatively large, rounded, and contain numerous mitochondria, which explains their eosinophilic granulation under the light microscope. Cells with a structure intermediate between principal cells and oxyphilic cells have been observed. The clear cells are loaded with glycogen, most of which they lose during tissue preparation, and have a flattened, eccentric nucleus. Clear cells may be derived from principal cells by crinophagocytosis of secretory vesicles and accumulation of glycogen. Although the function of both cell types is unknown, they may be inactive stages in the life cycle of the principal cells.

Parathormone, the secretory product of the principal cells, regulates the calcium level of the blood, and is antagonistic to calcitonin. When calcium levels drop below a critical value, parathormone is released and stimulates the osteoblasts to produce a humoral factor that, in turn, stimulates osteoclastic activity in the bone tissue. It also stimulates resorption of calcium by the epithelia of the intestine, the renal tubules, and the sweat glands. As a result of this, the blood calcium level increases and the secretion of parathormone stops. In addition to calcium, parathormone also regulates the blood's phosphate level. The principal cells are not influenced by the hypothalamus and hypophysis.

IV.7.4. Adrenal glands.

The adrenal glands lie close to the cranial pole of a kidney, embedded in the retroperitoneal adipose tissue. Both glands are slightly different in volume, shape, and location. Like other endocrine glands, the adrenals contain several cell types, but in this case these are carefully segregated: the adrenals display a peripheral **cortex** and a central **medulla** (Fig. 4.7.8.). Both have a different embryological origin. The cortex is one of the rare glandular tissues that are derived from mesoderm. The medulla is derived from neurectoderm. The close association of cortex and medulla probably signifies that the first is able to regulate the activity of the second. In fact, both cortex and medulla are drained by the same vein, implying that the medulla comes into contact with cortical hormones.

The cells of the **adrenal cortex** not only differ from those of the medulla, they also differ, to a much lesser extent, from each other. The cortex is built of concentric layers, each containing a slightly different cell type. Three cortical layers can be distinguished according to the arrangement of the cells (Fig. 4.7.9.). The outer layer is the **zona glomerulosa**, the cells of which are arranged in globular trabecules or cords. This layer accounts for some 15 percent of the cortex's volume. Next is the **zona fasciculata**, in which the cells form elongated, fascicular cords, oriented at right angles to the cortex's surface. Between the cords course parallel sinusoidal capillaries, intensifying the striated aspect of the zona fasciculata. This layer accounts for 75 percent of the cortical volume. The thickness of the zona fasciculata, and the distinctive shape and arrangement of its cell cords, make it the most conspicuous layer of the cortex. The deepest cortical layer is the **zona reticularis**, the cells of which form anastomosing cords and are more deeply pigmented than the other layers. This zone is relatively thin, accounting for only 5 percent of the cortical volume.

The cortical cells are steroid-secreting endocrine gland cells (II.2.1.5.2.). Their cytoplasm is loaded with smooth endoplasmic reticulum and steroid droplets (Fig. 4.7.11.). The steroid droplets cause the spongy look of these cells under the light microscope (Fig. 4.7.10.). This is especially conspicuous in the zona fasciculata. The high steroid content confers a yellowish hue to fresh adrenals. In addition, the cytoplasm contains lipofuchsin pigment and mitochondria with tubular cristae. These cells are in close contact with sinusoidal capillaries (Fig. 4.7.12.). In the different layers, the cortical cells show minor differences. The cells of the zona fasciculata, with their diameters of some 20 micrometers, are clearly larger than those of the other layers. The most extensive accumulations of lipofuchsin are found in the cells of the zona reticularis, explaining its darker color. Ultrastructurally, this pigment is endosomal and lysosomal material. Tubular mitochondrial cristae are most prominent in the zona fasciculata.

The adrenal cortex secretes various types of steroid hormones. The mineralocorticoids, secreted by the zona glomerulosa, regulate the concentrations of certain ions, particularly sodium. The glucocorticoids, secreted by the zona fasciculata and zona reticularis, regulate the metabolism of carbohydrates, lipids, and proteins. Some of these have an anabolic effect (they stimulate synthesis of substances), others a catabolic effect (they stimulate break down of substances). Glucocorticoids also inhibit certain cells of the immune system, inhibiting inflammatory processes. Small amounts of sex hormones are synthesized along with glucocorticoids, the chemical structure of both only differing in details. The secretion of glucocorticoids, but not of mineralocorticoids, is under hypothalamic hormonal control via the adrenocorticotrophs of the anterior pituitary gland. Thus, the cortex may be regarded, in a functional sense, as a double endocrine gland, one of which is under hypothalamic control, while the other one isn't.
The most important mineralocorticoid is aldosterone. This hormone stimulates resorption of sodium from the lumen of the renal distal contorted tubules. Sodium ions are extremely hydrophilic, so that water molecules come with them. Therefore, sodium retention results in conservation of body fluids, resulting in a relatively elevated blood pressure. When blood pressure drops

beneath a critical level, various pressure sensitive mechanoreceptors are stimulated, such as the kidney's juxtaglomerular cells (IV.8.1.3.). These secrete renin, an enzyme that acts on a plasma protein, angiotensinogen. Angiotensinogen is converted to angiotensin I, which is converted, by angiotensin converting enzyme of the pulmonary capillary endothelium, to angiotensin II. Angiotensin II contracts the vascular smooth muscle fibers, so that the blood pressure rises. In addition, it stimulates secretion of aldosterone by the zona glomerulosa, resulting in sodium and water resorption.
The most important glucocorticoid is cortisol. It stimulates breakdown of glucose, fatty acids, and proteins, increasing the level of energy production. This catabolic effect is accompanied by an anabolic one: polymerization of glucose to glycogen, in the liver parenchyma. Cortisol both ensures increased energy production and building up of energy stores. During periods of prolonged stress, such as cold exposure, malnutrition, and infection, the hypothalamus incites the anterior pituitary's adrenocorticotroph cells to produce adrenocorticotrope hormone, which stimulates production of cortisol. Cortisol inhibits the hypothalamus.

The endocrine cells of the **adrenal medulla** can be stained with chromium salts, earning them the name of chromaffin cells. Ultrastructurally, these cells have the cytological structure of amine hormone-secreting gland cells (Fig. 2.22.). Their secretory vesicles have diameters of 100 to 300 nanometers. Some cells contain secretory vesicles with very dark cores, others with lighter cores (Fig 4.7.13.). These contain adrenalin and noradrenaline, respectively. Between the cell cords lie numerous sinusoidal capillaries (Fig. 4.7.14.). In addition, nerve terminals of the cholinergic type may be encountered.

The adrenal medulla activates the body's metabolism, like the thyroid and the adrenal cortex, but this activation is short-lived and very intense. The medulla is active during periods of brief, excessive stress, such as anger and panic. In general terms, it enables the body to produce large amounts of energy and to generate excessive force during periods of sudden, intensive stress. Noradrenaline, one of the medullary hormones, is also an important neurotransmitter in postsynaptic orthosympathetic motor nerves, which have the same effects. Adrenalin is derived from noradrenaline and acts in the same way. The enzyme that induces the conversion of noradrenaline to adrenalin is activated by glucocorticoids. Each medullary cell is innervated by a motor nerve fiber from the central nervous system. In fact, the medullary cells are postsynaptic orthosympathetic nerve cells

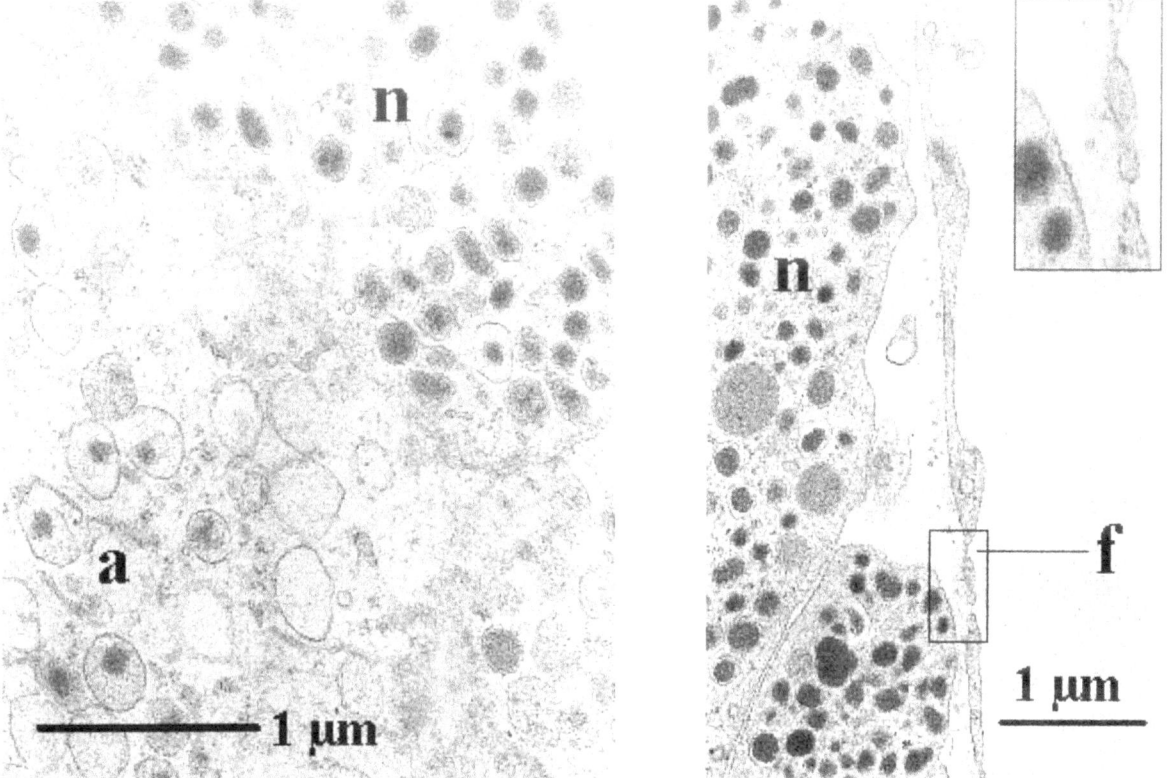

Fig. 4.7.13. (left) The adrenal medulla contains two kinds of amine hormone-secreting cells. The cells that secrete adrenaline (a) contain somewhat larger vesicles with a relatively small core. The cells that secrete noradrenaline (n) contain somewhat smaller vesicles with a relatively large core. Adrenal medulla, rabbit, TEM. Fig. 4.7.14. (right) The amine hormone-secreting cells of the adrenal medulla (noradrenaline-secreting cells, n, in this image) closely contact sinusoidal capillaries (fenestrations, f). Adrenal medulla, cat, TEM.

(IV.4.2.1.) that have never developed processes. The adrenal medulla is a modified orthosympathetic ganglion and its cells, like those of the hypothalamic nuclei, are neurosecretory cells. The innervation of the medullary cells by motor nerves implies that they are under direct nervous influence of the central nervous system, which accounts for the fact that the adrenal medulla can react very rapidly, more rapidly so than other endocrine glands.

References.

Carmichael S.W., Winkler H.: The adrenal chromaffin cell. Sci. Am. 1985, august: 30-39.

Fujita H.: Fine structure of the thyroid gland. Int. Rev. Cytol. 1975, 40: 197-280.

Hazard J.B.: The C cells (parafollicular cells) of the thyroid gland and medullary thyroid carcinoma. Am. J. Pathol.1977, 88: 214-249.

Inoue K., Couch E., Takano K., Ogawa S.: The structure and function of folliculo-stellate cells in the anterior pituitary gland. Arch. Histol. Cytol. 1999, 62: 2052-218.

Isono H., Shoumura S., Emura S.: Ultrastructure of the parathyroid gland. Histol. Histopath. 1990, 5: 95-112.

Kobayashi S., Coupland R.E.: Morphological aspects of chromaffin tissue: the differential fixation of adrenaline and noradrenaline. J. Anat. 1993, 183: 223-235.

Nussdorfer G.G.: Cytophysiology of the adrenal zona glomerulosa. Int. Rev. Cytol. 1980, 64: 307-368.

Nussdorfer G.G., Mazzocchi G., Meneghelli V.: Cytophysiology of the adrenal zona fasciculata. Int. Rev. Cytol. 1978, 55: 291-365.

Wild P., Setoguti T.: Mammalian parathyroids: morphological and functional implications. Microsc. Res. Tech. 1995, 32: 120-128.

IV.8. Excretory system.

The excretory system consists of the kidneys and their excretory ducts: the urethers, the urinary bladder, and the urethra. Essentially, the kidneys are organs that remove waste substances from the blood and regulate the volume and concentration of the body fluids. As a direct consequence of the second function, the kidneys regulate blood pressure.

The kidneys consist of a compact mass of renal tubules or **nephrons**. The nephrons drain into intrarenal ducts, the **collecting ducts**. Both nephrons and ducts are made of **epithelium**, which has, rather unusually, a mesodermal origin. The blind end of each nephron is closely associated with a capillary tuft or **glomerulus**, made of **endothelium**. The glomerulus and the nephron terminal form a renal corpuscle, which submits the blood plasma to a filtering process. The

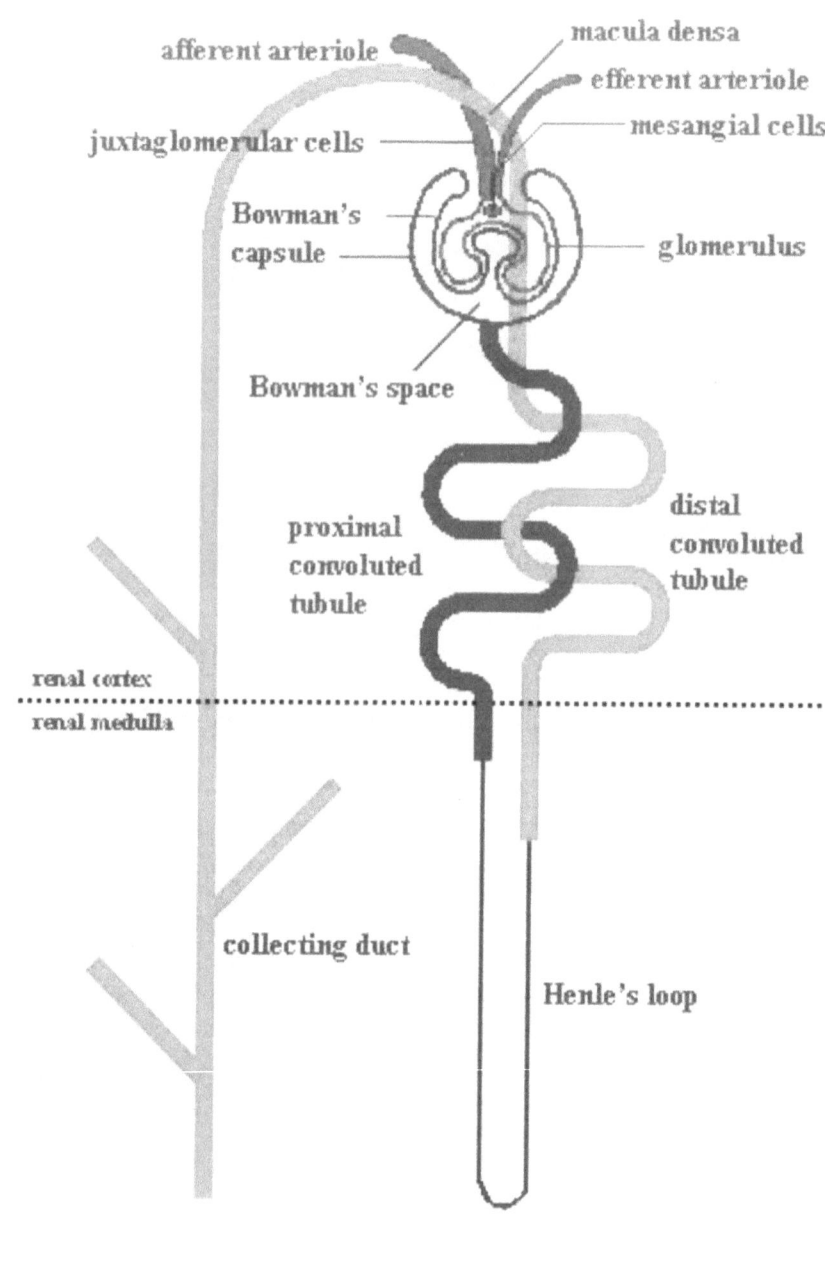

afferent arteriole

macula densa

efferent arteriole

juxtaglomerular cells

mesangial cells

Bowman's capsule

glomerulus

Bowman's space

proximal convoluted tubule

distal convoluted tubule

renal cortex

renal medulla

collecting duct

Henle's loop

Fig. 4.8.1. The kidney is a collection of nephrons. A nephron is a blind tubule, the end of which is expanded, like a vesicle. A capillary network indents this vesicle, transforming it into a double-walled cup: Bowman's capsule. The outer, or parietal, wall of Bowman's capsule has a smooth contour, while the inner, or visceral, wall, is draped over the convoluted capillaries. The capillary network and the visceral wall constitute a glomerulus. The capillaries are supplied with blood by an afferent arteriole, and drained by an efferent one. The glomerulus functions as a filter of blood plasma. The filtration fluid is collected in Bowman's space, between visceral and parietal walls, and conducted through the rest of the nephron. The proximal convoluted tubule lies in the renal cortex, the thin-walled loop of Henle in the medulla (Fig. 4.8.2.). The distal convoluted tubule returns to the cortex, and runs through the fork formed by the afferent and efferent arterioles of the nephron it belongs to. At the level of this fork, the epithelium forms the macula densa, composed of endocrine cells. In addition, the smooth muscle fibers making up the afferent arteriole's media locally differentiate into endocrine cells, the juxtaglomerular cells. A third type of endocrine tissue are the mesangial cells, located in the interstitial tissue between the capillary convolutions. These 3 types of endocrine tissue make up the juxtaglomerular apparatus. The distal convoluted tubules of several nephrons drain into a collecting duct, which opens at the surface of the renal papilla (Figure 4.8.14.).

plasma filtrate is collected in the nephron's lumen. The nephron reabsorbs specific substances from the filtrate. The end result is the fluid called urine, in which the waste products of the body's protein metabolism are concentrated. The filtration and reabsorption processes are essential to the body's osmoregulation: the regulation of the volume and concentration of the body fluids. In addition, the nephrons contain a few types of endocrine and receptor cells. These are strongly modified smooth muscle fibers, epithelial cells, and matrix producing cells. They form the **juxtaglomerular apparatus**.

Urine is drained from the kidneys by means of extrarenal ducts. It reaches the **urinary bladder** via the two **urethers** and is periodically removed via the **urethra**. The extrarenal ducts are constructed mainly of epithelium and visceral muscle tissue.

IV.8. 1. Kidneys.

The structural and functional kidney unit is the nephron. A human kidney numbers about a million of these.

A nephron (Fig. 4.8.1.) is a blindly terminating tubule, the wall of which is formed by a simple epithelium. During embryological development, the blind terminal expands and contacts a spherical capillary tuft with a diameter of some 200 micrometers. The capillary tuft deeply indents the terminal, in such a fashion that it is completely enveloped by a double-layered capsule, **Bowman's capsule.** The outer layer is the parietal epithelium, the inner layer is the visceral epithelium. Both are simple epithelia. The parietal epithelium does not greatly specialize and remains cuboidal. The visceral one becomes a highly specialized squamous epithelium. The visceral epithelium forms numerous folds, which carefully drape the capillaries of the tuft, now called a **glomerulus**. The glomerulus is supplied with blood by a relatively wide afferent arteriole and drained by a relatively narrow efferent arteriole. The difference in diameter between both explains the relatively high glomerular blood pressure, which supplies the necessary filtration pressure.

The rest of the nephron is a narrow tubule, in which selective reabsorption and secretion takes place. The initial tubular part of the nephron is the **proximal convoluted tubule**, which derives its name from its tortuous course. The proximal convoluted tubule drains into a very narrow nephron segment, **Henle's loop.** This segment runs more or less straight, forms a hairpin bend and runs back in the direction from where it came. It expands again, forming the final segment of the tubular nephron, which resumes a tortuous course, the **distal convoluted tubule**. The distal tubule courses back to the renal corpuscle from which it ultimately arises and passes through the fork formed by the afferent and efferent glomerular arterioles. Eventually, it drains into a straight collecting duct. The collecting ducts of several nephrons merge.

The kidney (Fig. 4.8.2.) is enveloped by a thin fibrous capsule and is embedded in the retroperitoneal adipose

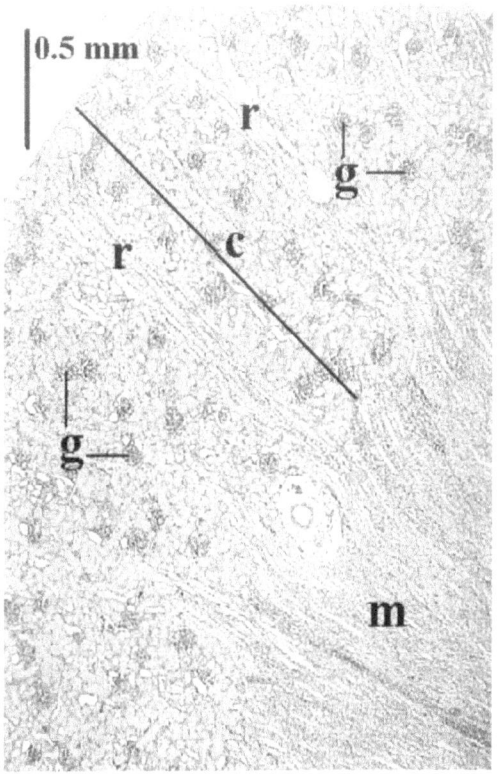

Fig. 4.8.2. The renal cortex (c) contains numerous globular glomeruli (g) and convoluted tubules. The medulla (m) is dominated by the straight segments of the nephrons, Henle's loops, as well as by collecting ducts. A few medullary rays (r) penetrate into the cortex. Kidney, goat, HE.

tissue. The organ is has a concave side, which points towards the body's midline. Here lies the hilus, where the urether arises and where the large veins and arteries connect to the kidney. The renal corpuscles and the convoluted tubules, both proximal and distal, are situated at the periphery of the kidney and form a cortex. The straight elements, Henle's loops, collecting ducts, and the specialized capillaries forming the vasa recta follow a radial course in the medulla. The medulla is made up of several, more or less separate, conical units or renal **pyramids**. Their tips point to the renal hilus, their bases are associated with part of the cortical region. A renal pyramid, with its associated cortex, is a renal lobe. In some places, the straight elements of the medulla penetrate into the cortex, forming **medullary rays**. At the hilus, each pyramid protrudes somewhat and forms a renal **papilla** (Fig. 4.8.14.). The largest collecting ducts open at the tip of each papilla. Before it connects to the kidney, the urether widens, forming a renal **pelvis**. The pelvis is subdivided into smaller renal **chalices**, each of which collects fluid from a single papilla.

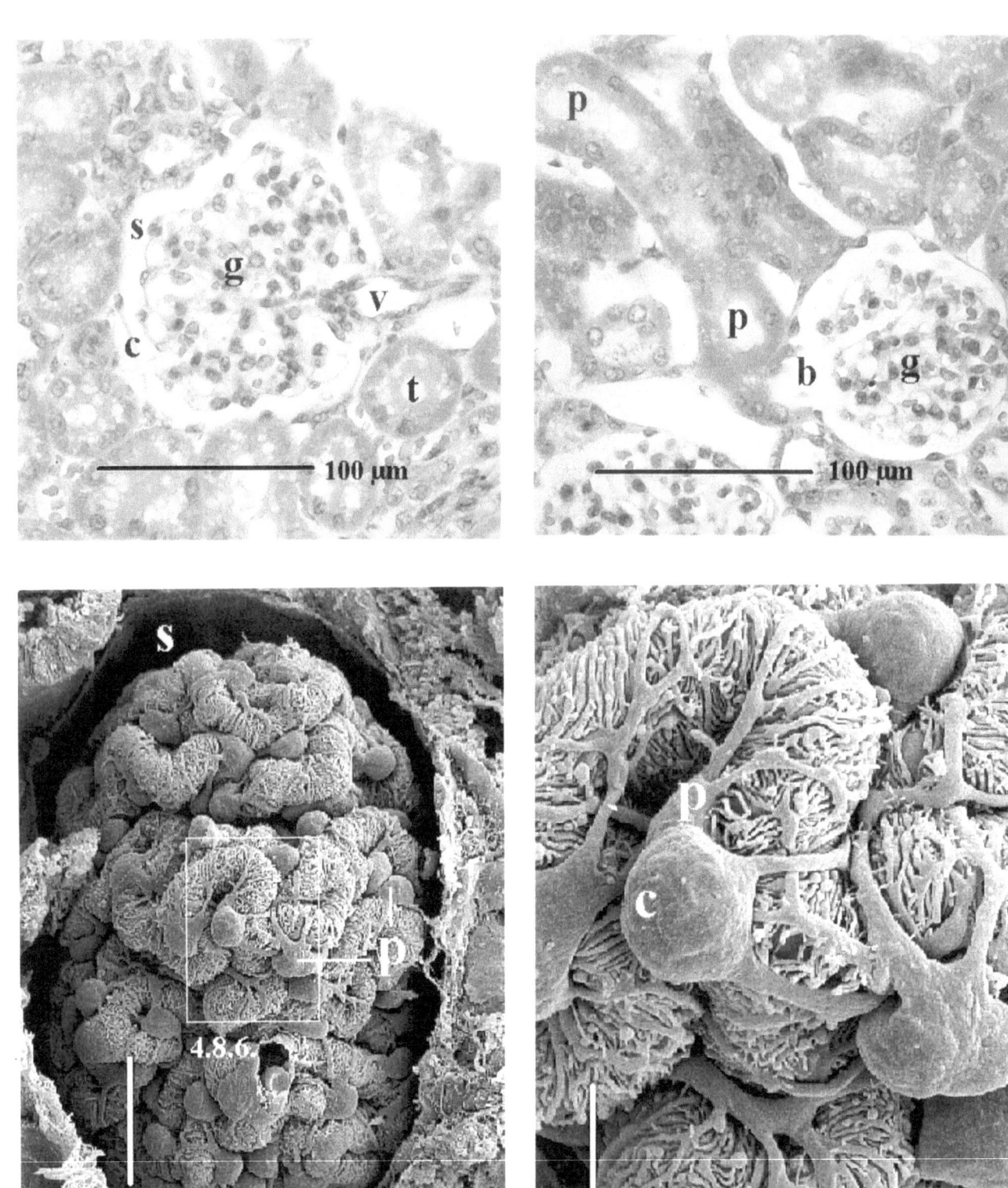

Fig. 4.8.3. (top left) At the vascular pole of the glomerulus (g), a blood vessel (v) enters the capillary network. s = Bowman's space, c = Bowman's capsule. The glomerulus is surrounded by convoluted tubules (t). Kidney, rabbit, HE. **Fig. 4.8.4.** (top right) At the urinary pole of the glomerulus (g), Bowman's space (b) is confluent with the proximal convoluted tubule (p), the wall of which is a simple prismatic epithelium. Kidney, rabbit, HE. **Fig. 4.8.5.** (bottom left) The glomerulus has been uncovered by removal of the parietal leaflet of Bowman's capsule. The glomerulus is a capillary network, draped with the visceral layer of Bowman's capsule. This visceral layer is a specialized epithelium, made of podocytes (p). s = Bowman's space. Kidney, rabbit, SEM. **Fig. 4.8.6.** (bottom right) Podocytes are epithelial cells with a cell body (c) and a number of branched processes (p), which eventually give rise to pedicelles. One podocyte's processes interdigitate with those of another. Kidney, rabbit, SEM.

IV.8.1.1. Nephrons.

IV.8.1.1.1. Renal corpuscles.

Renal corpuscles can be regarded as specialized interfaces between blood vessels and nephrons. Each renal corpuscle has both a vascular pole and a urinary pole. At the vascular pole (Fig. 4.8.3.), the glomerulus receives blood from an afferent arteriole and is drained by an efferent arteriole. At the urinary pole (Fig. 4.8.4.), the filtration fluid enters the tubular part of the nephron, beginning with the proximal convoluted tubule.

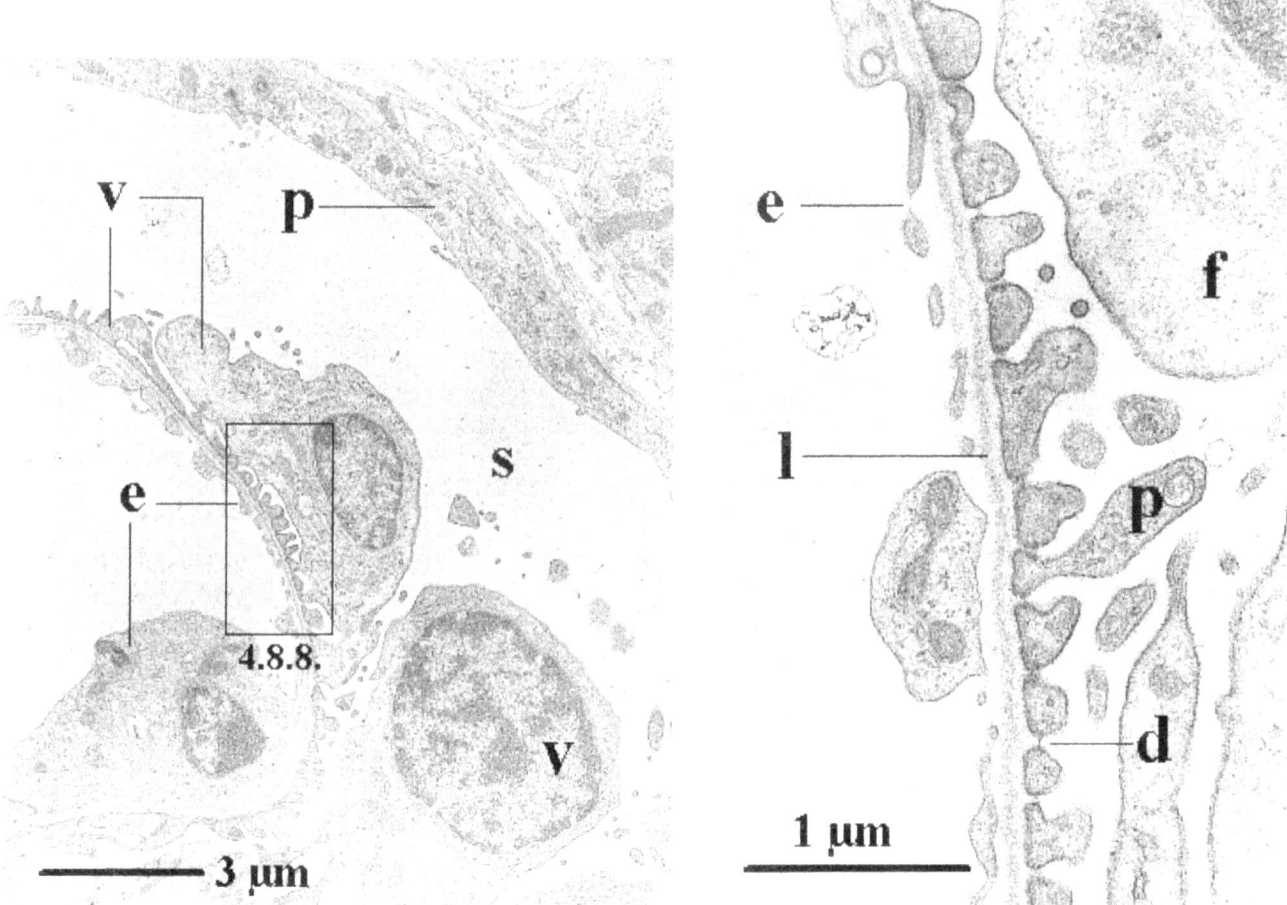

Fig. 4.8.7. (left) A section of Bowman's capsule (p = parietal wall) and the glomerulus shows the extremely narrow association between the podocytes of the visceral wall (v) and the endothelial cells (e) of the capillaries. Thus, a glomerular filter for blood plasma is formed. s = Bowman's space. Kidney, cat, TEM. **Fig. 4.8.8.** (right) The glomerular filter, on closer inspection, is made up of 3 components. One of them is a densely fenestrated endothelium (e). Next is a thick basement membrane, whose dense lamina (l) is shared by the adjoining endothelium and epithelium. The third component is epithelial: the pedicelles (p) of the podocytes, interconnected through diaphragms (d). Mark the presence of filaments (f) in the podocyte's cytoplasm. Kidney, cat, TEM.

In the renal corpuscle, the glomerular endothelium is closely associated with the visceral epithelium of Bowman's capsule, which consists of specialized lining cells, the podocytes (Figs. 4.8.5.-7.). The glomerular endothelium (Fig. 4.8.8.) is of the fenestrated type. The fenestrations contain no diaphragm, or a very thin one at most. The endothelium rests on a strongly developed basement membrane, the dense lamina of which can have a thickness of 300 nanometers or more. The basement membrane is shared with the podocytes, which lie at the other side of the dense lamina (Fig. 4.8.8.).

Podocytes are very specialized epithelial cells, which have developed tentacle-like processes. They have a cell body, containing the nucleus, which bulges into Bowman's space, the narrow space between the parietal and the visceral layers of the capsule. The cell body forms several primary processes (Fig.4.8.5., 4.8.6.) that carry short, parallel, transverse secondary processes. In a similar way, the secondary processus form tertiary processes. Each process carries basal end feet or pedicels. These rest on the basement membrane and interdigitate with pedicels of other processes. Between adjacent pedicels is a narrow space or filtration slit, which is spanned with a diaphragm (Fig. 4.8.8.). In this way, histological sections produce an image that is superficially similar to a fenestrated endothelium.

Endothelium, basement membrane, and podocytes constitute a blood plasma filter. The filter's permeability depends on the endothelial fenestrations, the mesh of the basement membrane and the podocyte's filtration slits. This filter allows passage of water, ions, and small organic molecules, but stops blood cells and high molecular weight substances such as plasma proteins. Only albumin is able to pass the filter, in small quantities, which allows the conclusion that the filter's largest meshes have about the size of an albumin molecule. Each 24-hour period, both kidneys together produce almost 200 liters of filtrate. This volume is greatly reduced before it is discharged. Most of the water and the useful substances it contains are reabsorbed during passage of the filtrate down the tubular part of the nephron. Only the nitrogenous waste products of protein metabolism, such as urea, are not reabsorbed and are discharged in the urine.

IV.8.1.1.2. Proximal convoluted tubules.

The parietal epithelium of Bowman's capsule is confluent with that of the proximal convoluted tubule (Fig. 4.8.9.), which is, with its length of about 15 millimeters, the longest segment of the nephron.

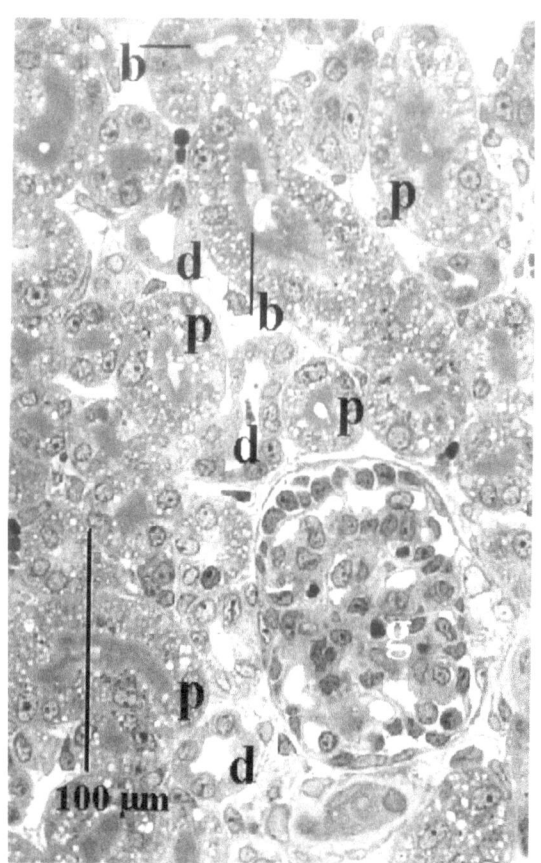

Fig. 4.8.9. In tissue sections, the proximal convoluted tubules (p) may be recognized by the apical brush border (b) of their epithelial cells, which appears, light optically, as a clear layer surrounding the tubular lumen. The distal convoluted tubules (d) have a lower epithelium, lacking a brush border. g = glomerulus. Kidney, cat, 1-micrometer plastic section, toluidin blue.

Its wall is a simple cuboidal to prismatic epithelium, composed of absorbing brush border cells (II.2.2.2.1., Fig. 4.8.10.). The brush border consists of long, slender microvilli and is coated with a glycoprotein layer, the glycocalyx. The glycocalyx is actively maintained by the cells: they secrete glycoproteins at the basis of the microvilli. The glycocalyx may contribute to the cell membrane's selective permeability. At the base of the microvilli, endocytosis takes place (Fig. 2.23.) and the apical cytoplasm contains lysosomes. The lateral cell membrane forms crests, which are highest where they contact the basement membrane and contribute to the broadening of the cell basis. They are not unlike the supporting buttresses at the base of rain forest tree trunks. The crests interdigitate with those of adjacent cells. The basal cell membrane forms deep, narrow, perpendicular folds. The lateral crests and the basal folds greatly increase the membrane surface available to exchange processes. The necessary energy for these is supplied by numerous mitochondria.

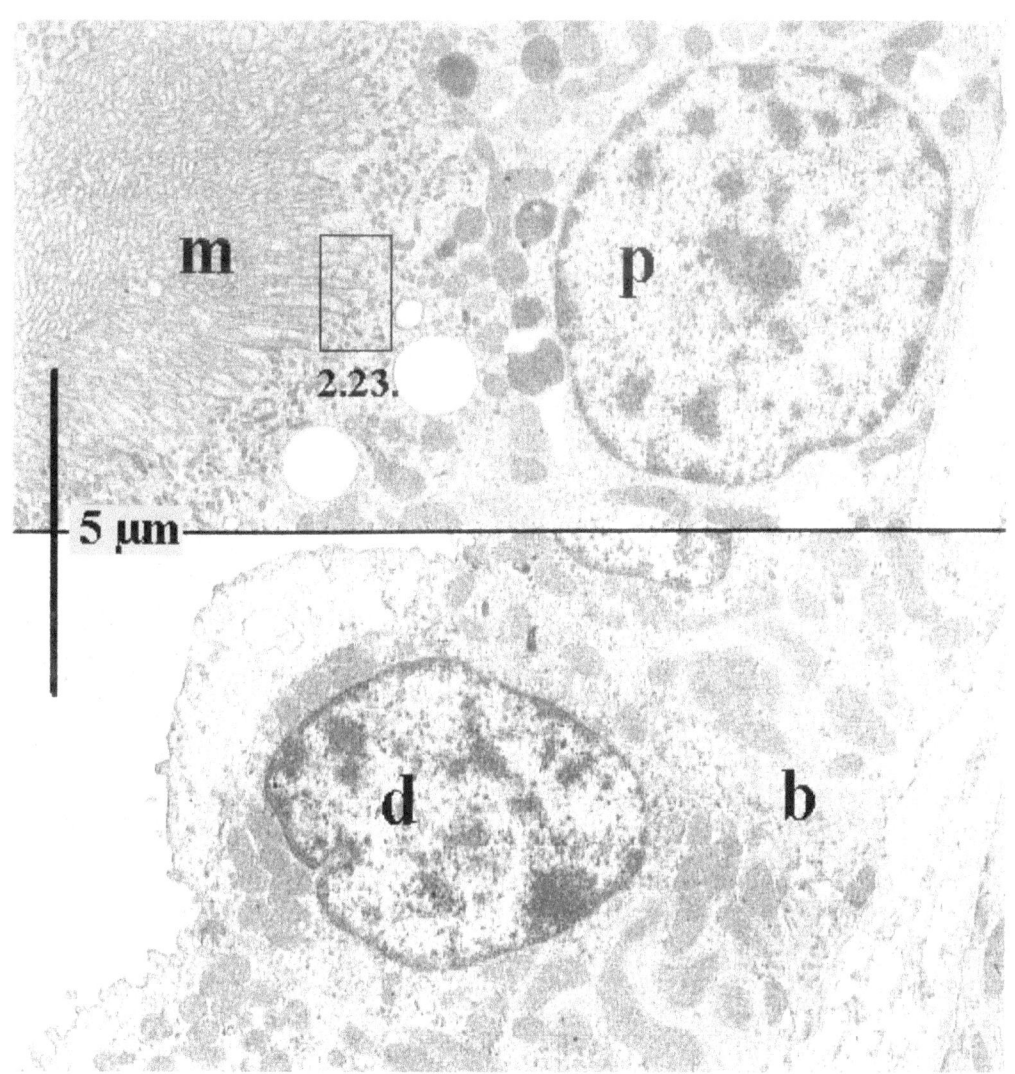

Fig. 4.8.10. A proximal convoluted tubule cell (p) is shown next to a distal convoluted tubule's (d). In the proximal tubule cell, the microvilli of the brush border (m) are very prominent. In the distal tubule, microvilli are poorly developed. Mark the position of the nuclei: those of the proximal tubule lie basally, while those of the distal tubule lie apically, making room for a large amount of basal cytoplasm (b) that houses a number of deep membranous folds, where ion transport takes place. Kidney, cat, TEM.

The epithelium is highest in the proximal third of the convoluted tubule. In the distal part, its height is halved. The apical brush border is likewise most strongly developed in the proximal segment. The distal segment is not as intensively convoluted as the proximal segment. The very last stretch is straight. At the cortico-medullary junction, it is confluent with Henle's loop.

About 75 percent of the glomerular filtrate's volume is reabsorbed in the lumen of the proximal convoluted tubules, enabling the body to recuperate large amounts of water and useful substances.
Sodium ions are reabsorbed by active uptake. The brush border and the lateral and basal cell membranes contain the necessary pumps to ferry sodium ions from the tubular lumen to the interstitial spaces. During transport of sodium ions, water molecules follow passively because of sodium's hydrophylic properties. Amino acids and monosaccharides are actively reabsorbed as well. Blood plasma proteins that happen to pass the glomerular filter are endocytosed and lysosomally degraded.

IV.8.1.1.3. Henle's loops.

Except for the final stretch of its "ascending" limb, Henle's loop is a very thin walled segment of the nephron. Its epithelium is, over most of its length, simple squamous, changing into simple cuboidal in the terminal, thick segment of the "ascending " limb. The squamous epithelial cells are moderately to extremely flattened and their nucleus causes a bulge towards the lumen, giving the thin segments of Henle's loops a deceptive likeness to capillaries, such as the vasa recta (Figs. 4.8.11.-12.). The cells carry a few microvilli. Their edges form complex interdigitations with adjacent cells.

Henle's loop is a powerful device for recuperation of water and concentration of the luminal fluid, i.e. the urine, thus limiting water loss. The cells of the final, thick part of the "ascending" limb actively reabsorb sodium ions. They have distinct characteristics of epithelial cells involved in ion transport: deep, narrow infoldings of the basal cell membrane, with numerous mitochondria in the cytoplasm between them. There is

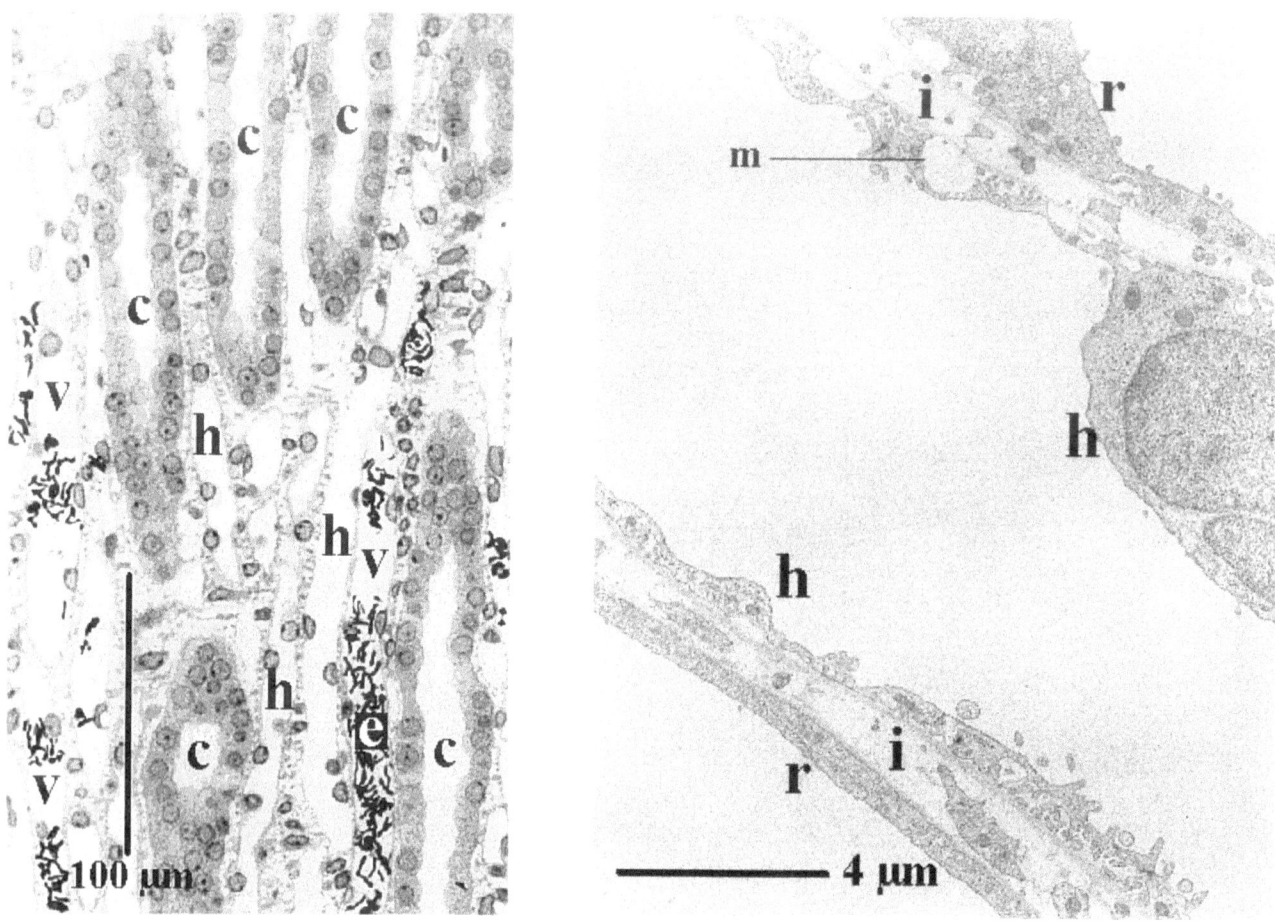

Fig. 4.8.11. (left) When the renal medulla is sectioned parallel to the plane of the straight tubules it contains, longitudinal sections through Henle's loops and collecting ducts show. Henle's loops (h) are lined with simple squamous epithelium, which closely resembles the capillary endothelium of the vasa recta (v). Characteristically, Henle's loops do not contain erythrocytes (e) and their nuclei may be somewhat less flattened than those of the capillaries. The collecting ducts (c) are lined with simple cuboidal epithelium. Kidney, hamster, 1-micrometer plastic section, toluidin blue. **Fig. 4.8.12.** (right) In the renal medulla, Henle's loops (h) run alongside capillaries, the vasa recta (v). The epithelium of the former and the endothelium of the latter are separated by a thin layer of interstitial tissue (i). The basal cell membranes of both types, especially so those of the epithelial cells (m), undulate. Kidney, hamster, TEM.

an essential difference, however, with the sodium transport that takes place in the proximal convoluted tubules: the wall of the loop's thick "ascending" limb is impermeable to water. Consequently, only sodium ions are reabsorbed and the interstitial fluid of the renal medulla becomes hypertonic in comparison to the luminal fluid of the loops. On the other hand, the thin "descending" and "ascending" segments of Henle's loops are permeable to water. Because of the medullary interstitial fluid's hypertonicity, caused by the activity of the thick segment of the "ascending" limbs, water molecules are passively drawn from the lumen of the thin segments and enter the interstitial space. Parallel to Henle's loops, and consequently having a straight course as well, are capillaries called vasa recta, which allow the reabsorbed water to enter the blood circulation. Thus, the relatively uncomplicated cellular structure of the thin segments

corresponds to the absence of an active transport function.

IV.8.1.1.4. Distal convoluted tubules.

The distal convoluted tubules have a length of about 5 millimeters, making them much shorter than the proximal ones. Consequently, they are less frequent in histological sections (Fig. 4.8.9.).

The epithelium is simple cuboidal to prismatic. The distal tubules are a little narrower than the proximal ones. The epithelium, however, is lower, so that their lumen appears wider. They only show part of the characteristics of actively absorbing cells (Fig. 4.8.10.). A distinct brush border is lacking, but the basal cell membrane shows deep, narrow, perpendicular infoldings, the lateral cell membrane

190

develops folds which interdigitate with those of adjacent cells, and the cytoplasm contains numerous mitochondria. The nucleus often occupies an apical position, making room for the basal membrane folds. The final stretch of the distal tubule contains dark, mitochondria-rich, intercalated cells.

Like the proximal tubules, but less intensively so, the distal tubules actively reabsorb sodium and, passively, water. Reabsorption of sodium by the distal convoluted tubules is selectively stimulated by the hormone aldosterone of the adrenal cortex (IV.7.4.), which explains the hormone's ability to raise blood volume and blood pressure. The distal tubules also reabsorb calcium ions. The intercalated cells secrete protons or bicarbonate ions.

IV.8.1.2. Collecting ducts.

The collecting ducts are lined by a simple epithelium, which initially is cuboidal (Fig. 4.8.11.), but progressively heightens as the ducts course to the renal papilla. The epithelium consists of principal clear cells and, especially so in the proximal segments of the ducts, intercalated dark cells (Fig. 4.8.13.). The clear cells contain few organelles, which explains their translucent aspect in the light microscope. The apical cell membrane forms a few short microvilli. Their basal cell membrane may show numerous narrow infoldings. The dark cells contain numerous mitochondria. Their apical cell membrane forms short, meandering outfoldings.

The collecting duct's epithelium is permeable to water. It is not entirely clear which aspects of their cytological structure explain this characteristic, however. Since the medullary interstitial fluid is hypertonic as a consequence of the activity of Henle's loops, large amounts of water are reabsorbed from the collecting duct's lumen and returned to the blood circulation at the level of the vasa recta. In contrast to Henle's loop, the collecting duct's permeability is variable, and can be regulated by the antidiuretic hormone of the neurohypophysis (IV.4.6.). Antidiuretic hormone increases the collecting duct's permeability, allowing for increased water reabsorption and, consequently, decreased urine volume. This is the antidiuretic effect that gives the hormone its name. Increased reabsorption of water way raise blood pressure by increasing the blood's volume, which explains antidiuretic hormone's older name, vasopressin. The dark intercalated cells secrete protons into the duct lumen.

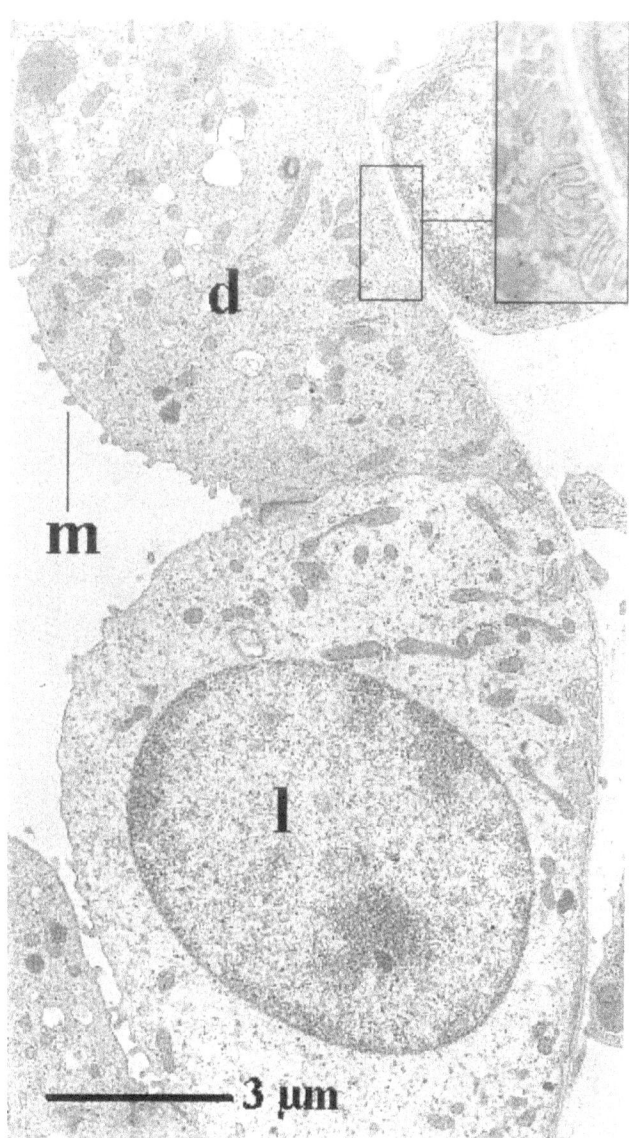

Fig. 4.8.13. The simple epithelium of the collecting ducts is composed of light (l) and dark (d) cells. The apical membrane forms a few stubby microvilli (m) or folds. The basal cell membrane is folded (rectangle). Kidney, hamster, TEM.

IV.8.1.3. Juxtaglomerular apparatus.

The juxtaglomerular apparatus is a collection of specialized cells of the afferent arteriole of the glomerulus, the distal convoluted tubule, and the mesangial interstitial tissue that fills the spaces between the glomerular capillaries and the visceral epithelium of Bowman's capsule.

Immediately prior to its entry in the glomerulus, the smooth muscle fibers in the afferent arteriole's tunica media are modified to **juxtaglomerular cells** (Fig. 4.8.15.). The muscle fiber origin of these cells is still

191

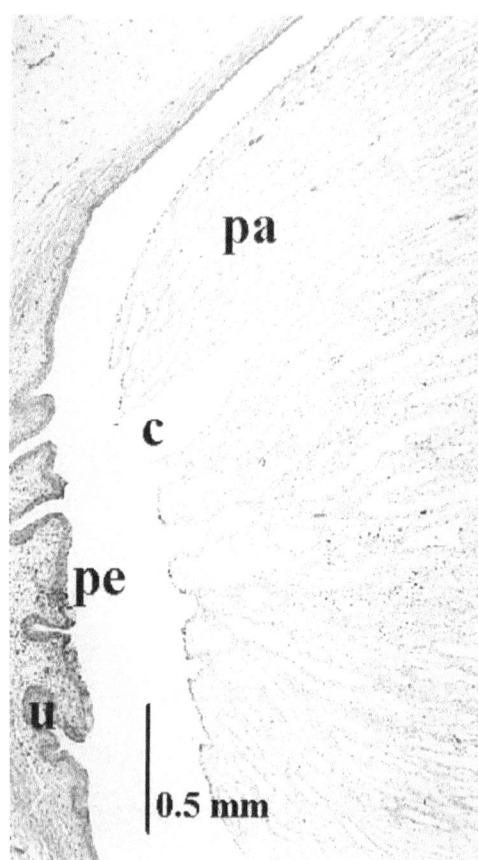

the beginning of the tubule, the tubule's epithelial cells facing the glomerulus are higher and narrower than the others. This causes a certain concentration of nuclei, so that this part of the tubule appears denser or darker than the rest of the epithelium: it forms a **macula densa** (Fig. 4.8.16.). The cytological structure of these cells is different from that of the rest of the tubular epithelium. The apical microvilli and the infoldings of the basal cell membrane are not well developed. Deep intercellular canals separate these cells, up to the level of the apical junctional complexes. These cells also contain a number of secretory vesicles.

Like the juxtaglomerular cells, these cells are thought to regulate blood pressure via the renin-angiotensin system. It is likely that they are stimulated by changes in the concentration of vascular sodium ions, rather than to changes in blood pressure.

The mesangial interstitial tissue contains a specialized cell type: mesangial cells or **Goormaghtig's cells** (Fig. 4.8.17.) They are elongated, flattened cells with numerous thin processes. They contain secretory vesicles and microfilaments. Their function is uncertain, but they are considered as having a regulatory influence on blood pressure.

Fig. 4.8.14. The collecting ducts (c) open at the renal papilla (pa), discharging into the renal pelvis (pe). The pelvis, in its turn, is drained by the urether (u). Kidney, cat, HE.

apparent from the remaining microfilaments and fusiform densities. Instead of these, the cells accumulate numerous secretory vesicles with an opaque content.

The juxtaglomerular cells are baroreceptors, sensitive to slackening of the blood vessel wall as a consequence of decreased blood pressure. When the blood pressure drops below a critical level, the juxtaglomerular cells liberate renin by exocytosis of their dense vesicles. Renin is a proteolytic enzyme, which converts the blood plasma protein angiotensinogen to angiotensin. Angiotensinogen is converted first to angiotensin I, which is in its turn converted, by angiotensin converting enzyme of the pulmonary capillary endothelium, to angiotensin II. Angiotensin II contracts the vascular smooth muscle fibers, so that the blood pressure rises. In addition, it stimulates secretion of aldosterone by the zona glomerulosa of the adrenal cortex (IV.7.4.), resulting in sodium and water resorption, which also has the effect of raising blood pressure.

The course of the distal convoluted tubule leads it through the fork formed by the afferent and efferent arterioles of its nephron's glomerulus. At this point, at

IV.8.2. Urethers, urinary bladder, and urethra.

Urine drains from the kidneys at the tips of the papillae, and is collected in the widened part of the **urether**, the pelvis. The urether conducts the urine to the urinary bladder. The lumina of pelvis and urether are lined with **transitory epithelium** (III.4.1.3.3.). With a relatively dense lamina propria, the epithelium makes up a mucosa. Underneath the mucosa, there is a double **muscularis**, made up of visceral muscle tissue. The smooth muscle fibers of the inner layer run more or less longitudinally, those of the outer layer run circularly. In the distal third of the urether, a third layer of longitudinal muscle fibers is added to the outside of the other two. The muscularis shows peristaltic contractions, which force urine towards the urinary bladder. The muscularis is enveloped with a relatively loose fibrous adventitia containing blood vessels and nerve fibers.

The wall of the **urinary bladder** (Fig. 4.8.18.) has the same composition as the urether's distal third: a mucosa with transitory epithelium, a triple musculosa and an adventitia. The muscularis contains relatively large amounts of elastic tissue and contracts periodically, during micturition. The middle, circular muscle layer forms a sphincter at the origin of the urethra. The adventitia contains a plexus of motor

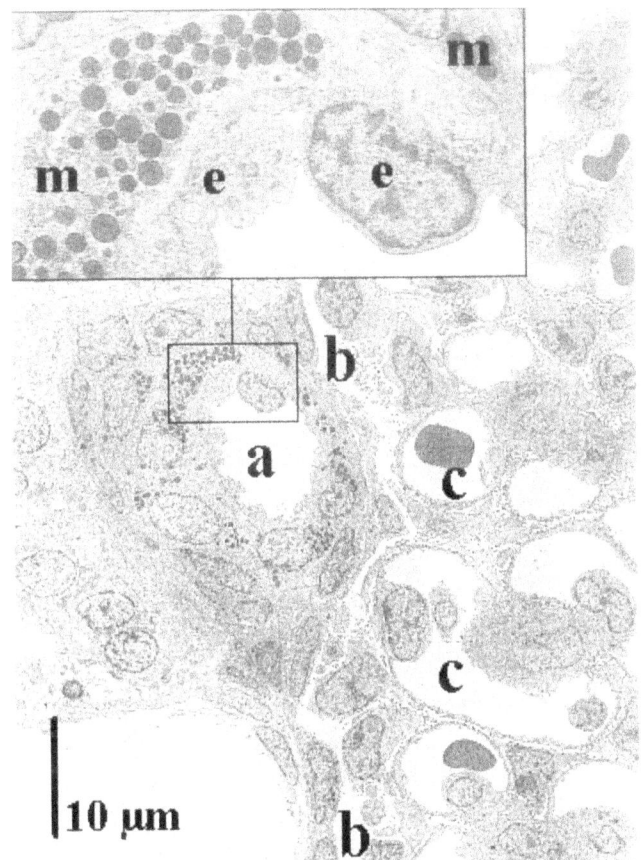

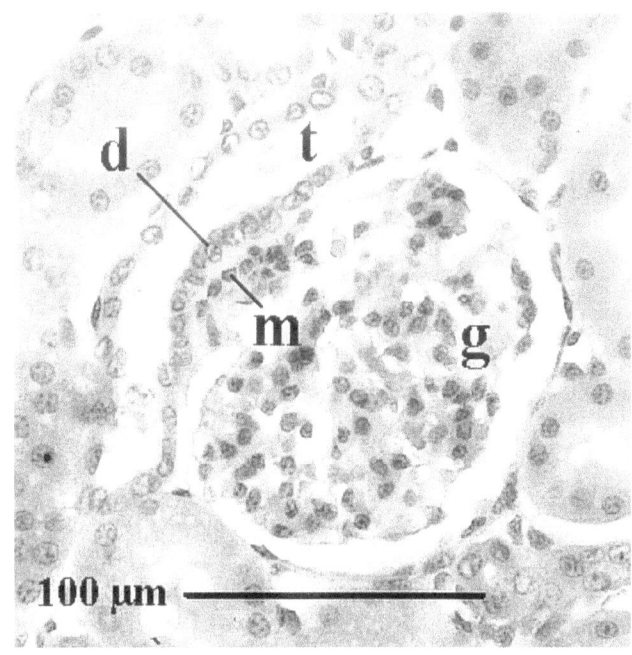

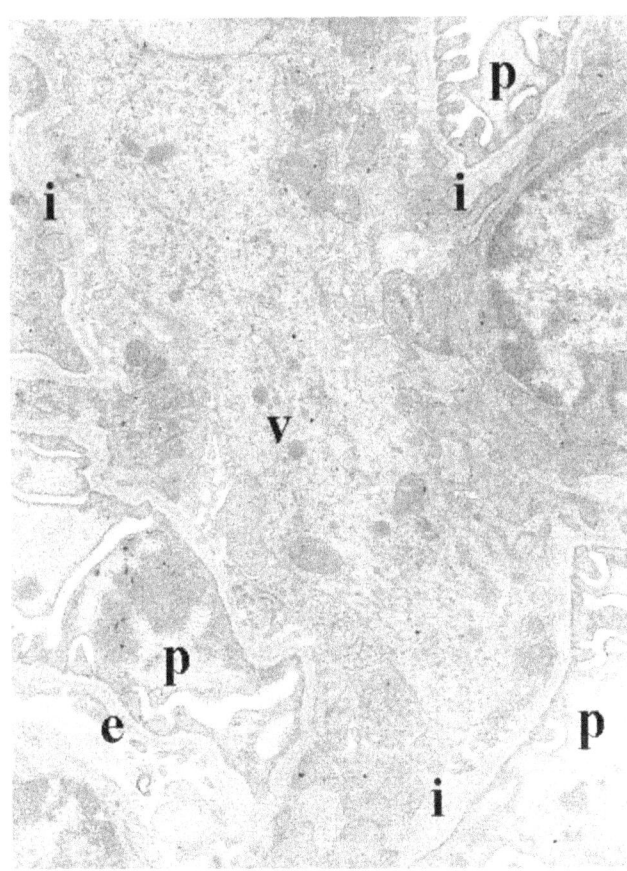

Fig. 4.8.15. (top left) At the base of a glomerulus (c = capillaries, b = Bowman's space) a section of the afferent arteriole (a) can be seen. The smooth muscle fibers making up its media (m) develop into juxtaglomerular cells. These are endocrine cells with dense secretory vesicles. e = endothelium of the afferent arteriole. Kidney, cat, TEM. Fig. 4.8.16. (above) Upon passing by the glomerulus (g) it is connected with, the epithelium of the distal convoluted tubule (t) facing the glomerulus develops into a macula densa (d) of endocrine cells. The epithelium becomes distinctly prismatic and, from a distance, its numerous slender, closely packed nuclei give it a "dense" look. A few mesangial cells (m) are also present. Kidney, cat, HE. Fig. 4.8.17. (bottom left) The interstitial tissue (i) filling the spaces between the capillary loops and the visceral wall of Bowman's capsule locally contains Goormaghtigh's mesangial cells. These are endocrine cells containing secretory vesicles (v). p = podocytes, e = endothelium. Kidney, hamster, TEM.

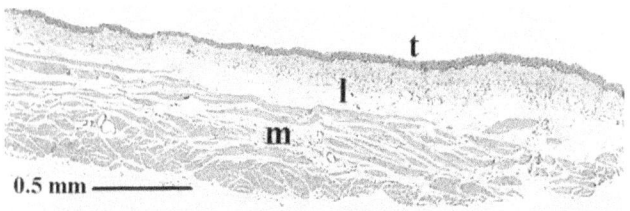

0.5 mm

Fig. 4.8.18. The uretheral (and bladder) lumen is lined with transitory epithelium (t), which, in combination with the underlying fibrous tissue lamina propria (l), forms a mucosa. Peripheral to the mucosa is a layer of visceral muscle tissue and fibrous tissue, the muscularis (m). Urether, cat, HE.

nerves, which can induce contraction of the muscularis and relaxation of the sphincter, enabling micturition.

The **urethra** conducts urine from the urinary bladder to the exterior of the body. It is longest, more than 20 centimeters, in the male, where it runs inside the penis. At its origin, where the prostate gland lies, the lumen is still lined with transitory epithelium. Distally, the epithelium changes to a compound prismatic or pseudostratified one, which forms mucus-secreting paraurethal glands. Beneath this epithelium is the erectile tissue of the penis. At its mouth, the urethra is lined with Malpighian epithelium. The female urethra is much shorter, only a few centimeters, and is largely lined with Malpighian epithelium. In addition to visceral muscle tissue, the uretheral muscularis also contains striated muscle tissue, forming a sphincter that is under voluntary control.

References.

Bulger R.E., Dobyan D.C.: Recent advances in renal morphology. Ann. Rev. Physiol. 1982, 44: 147-179.

Evan A.P., Gattone V.H., Connors B.A.: Ultrastructural features of the rabbit proximal tubules. Arch. Histol. Cytol. 1992, 55: S139-S145.

Madsen K.M., Verlander J.W., Tisher C.C.: Relationship between structure and function in distal tubule and collecting duct. J. Electron. Microsc. Tech. 1988, 9: 187-208.

Taugner R., Hackenthal E.: On the character of the secretory granules in juxtaglomerular epithelioid cells. Int. Rev. Cytol. 1988, 110: 93-131.

Verlander J.W.: Normal ultrastructure of the kidney and lower urinary tract. Toxicol. Pathol. 1998, 26: 1-17.

IV.9. Skin.

The skin is composed mainly of **epithelium** and **fibrous tissue**. The epithelium is the extremely specialized keratinized epithelium (III.4.1.3.5.). In combination with a few other cell types, it forms the **epidermis**. Locally, the epidermis forms **glandular tissue**: sweat glands, mammary glands, and sebum glands. It also forms strongly keratinized **appendages**: hairs and nails. The epidermis rests on a thick fibrous tissue layer, the **dermis**. The dermis rests on a hypodermis, which may be rich in adipose tissue, and which joins the skin to the underlying muscles or bones. The dermis and hypodermis contain a number of extensive vascular plexi, made of endothelium. A little visceral muscle tissue is associated with the hair roots. The skin is rich in nerve tissue: it contains numerous sensory nerve fibers which often participate in the formation of complex receptor organs: Ruffini's corpuscles, Meissner's corpuscles, and Vater-Pacinian corpuscles, among others.

IV.9.1. Epidermis.

The epidermis is derived from keratinized epithelium and the great majority of its cells are keratinocytes (III.4.1.3.5.). This epithelium forms a tough, impregnable coat that protects the body against mechanical damage, dessication, and infection. In addition to keratinocytes, the epidermis contains a few other cell types, which are much less numerous, but also have important protector as well as receptor functions: **melanocytes, Merkel's cells** and **Langerhans's cells**.

The structure of the epidermis is not uniform. It varies from place to place and is adapted to local requirements.
At the level of the palms of the hands and the soles of the feet (Fig. 4.9.1.), where the epidermis participates in the formation of naked, glabrous skin, it may reach a thickness of about 1 millimeter. The stratum corneum, the most resistant layer, is particularly thick and, when it experiences strong frictional forces, forms callosities. The epidermis is not smooth, but forms papillae which alternate with corresponding dermal papillae. Thus, the dermo-epidermal junction undulates, which lengthens it and allows for more intensive contact and tighter cohesion of the two. As a consequence of the epidermal undulation, its surface shows ridges and grooves. These form a characteristic pattern, which is genetically determined and forms a fingerprint, unique to each single person. This

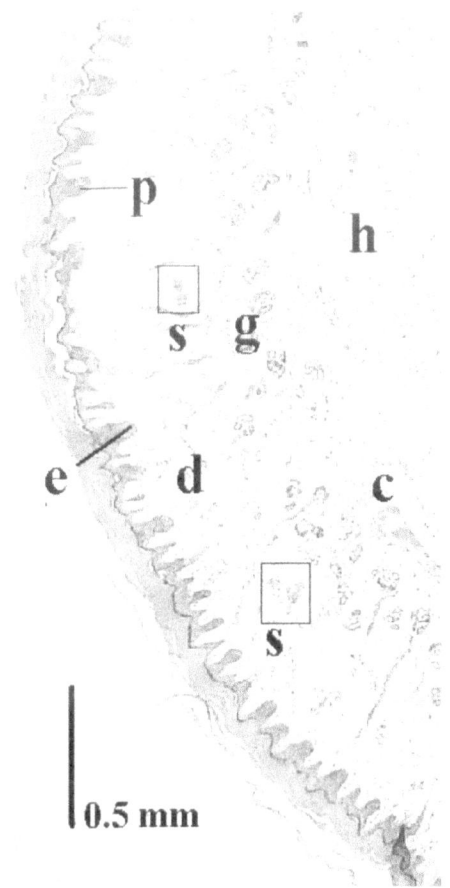

Fig. 4.9.1. The skin consists of a stratified and keratinized epithelium (Figure 3.4.13.) forming the epidermis (e), and a fibrous tissue dermis (d). The underside of the epidermis undulates: it forms epidermal papillae (p), which alternate with dermal papillae. Beneath the dermis is an adipose hypodermis (h). The boundary between dermis and hypodermis is indicated by the secretory coils of the sweat glands (g) and a plexus of relatively wide capillaries, the rete cutaneum (c). At a higher level of the dermis lies a second vascular plexus of narrower capillaries, the rete subpapillaris (s). Glabrous skin, foot sole, human baby, HE.

epidermis of the glabrous skin forms many sweat glands, but no hairs at all.
In most other places, the epidermis is much thinner. The stratum corneum is less well developed and the dermo-epidermal junction is more or less smooth, as is the epidermal surface. This thin epidermis always forms hairs. The hair's density is largest in the scalp, and may decrease to almost nothing elsewhere.

IV.9.1.1. Melanocytes.

Melanocytes are specifically adapted to the production of pigment, **melanin**, by means of which they protect the underlying tissues against energetic

195

Electromagnetic waves, i.e. ultraviolet light. Originally, these cells do not reside in the epidermis. They arise in the neurectoderm (Fig. 4.1.) and are, in an embryological sense, nerve cells. During embryological development, they migrate to the epidermis. They lodge in the stratum germinativum. In colored people, they are also found in more superficial epidermal strata.

In principle, melanocytes are homogeneously distributed over the entire surface of the body. In fair-skinned people, they are encountered in a ratio of one melanocyte to about forty keratinocytes. In some places, notably the thick epidermis of hand palms and foot soles, they are completely absent. In other places, such as the nipples and the surrounding areola, they

may be somewhat more numerous. Melanocytes also occur in the stratum germinativum of the hair follicles.

A functional melanocyte (Fig. 4.9.2.) shows, like a nerve cell, characteristics of both membrane-bearing and fiber-bearing cells. It has a cell body, which houses the nucleus, as well as a well-developed rough endoplasmic reticulum and Golgi-complex. The cell body carries numerous filamentous, branched processes, supported by microtubules and filaments, which run between adjacent keratinocytes and may penetrate as far as the stratum granulosum. The fact that melanocytes do not form junctions with keratinocytes illustrates the fact that they are cells that do not originally belong in the epidermis.

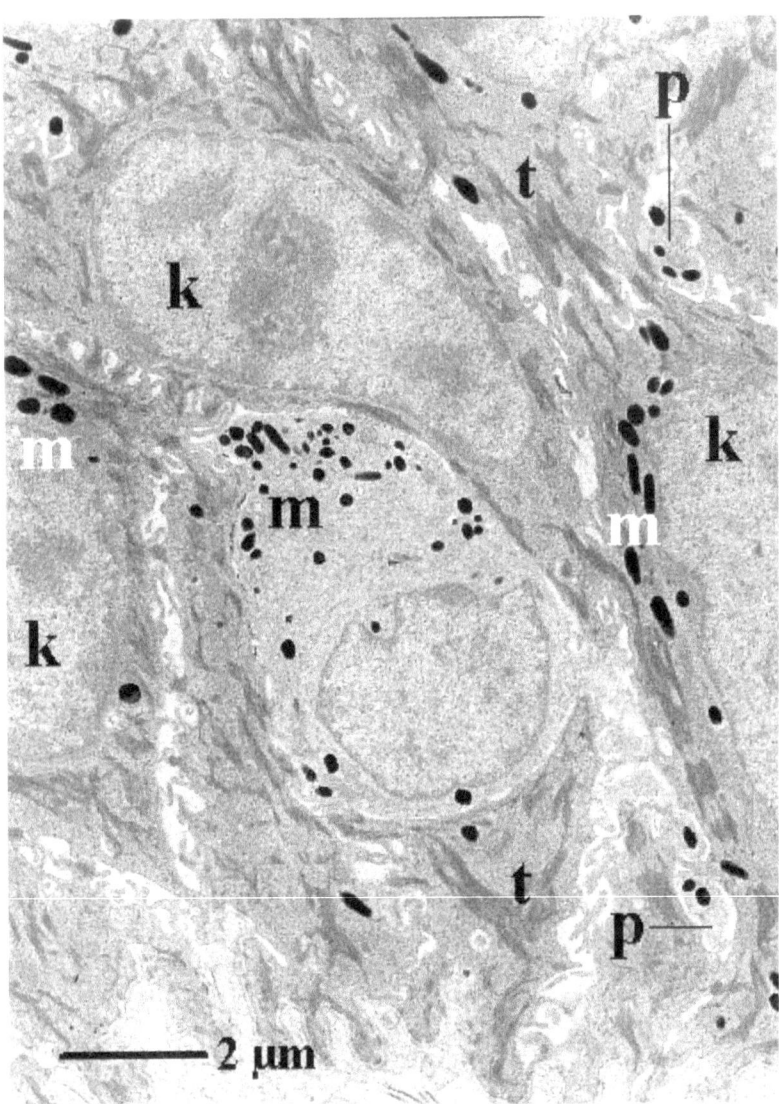

Fig. 4.9.2. Apart from keratinocytes, the epidermis contains melanocytes, predominantly so in the deeper layers of the epidermis. Their cytoplasm is rich in melanosomes (black m). They form processes (p) that penetrate between the keratinocytes (k), which engulf the melanosomes (white m), a process called cytocriny. Mark the presence of intermediary tonofilaments (t) in the keratinocytes, and their absence in the melanocytes. Foot sole, cat, TEM.

Melanocytes synthesize the enzyme protyrosinase, stored in cytoplasmic vesicles, the premelanosomes. Premelanosomes are elongated vesicles with a length of some 500 nanometers and a diameter of about 300

nanometers. They may be somewhat larger in colored skin. Premelanosomes also contain filaments, which run parallel to their long axis. Since the premelanosomes deviate from the spherical shape, these filaments in all likelihood support them. In addition, they contain protyrosinase. The amino acid tyrosine is stored in these vesicles as well. Under the influence of ultraviolet light, protyrosinase is activated to tyrosinase, which modifies and polymerizes tyrosine to melanin. This process is adaptable, and multiple different molecular variants of melanin exist. Melanin is bound to protein carriers. In the course of its synthesis, it gradually fills the premelanosomes, progressively obscuring their internal structure. A completely filled vesicle is called a **melanosome** and is homogeneously opaque. Melanosomes are actively transported into the melanocyte's processes (Fig. 4.9.2.). Their content is liberated, merocrine fashion, by exocytosis. Subsequently, the liberated melanin granules are endocytosed by keratinocytes. It is as though the melanocyte injects its melanin into a keratinocyte, a process called **cytocriny**. Thus, melanin is distributed over the entire stratum germinativum and stratum spinosum.

IV.9.1.2. Merkel's cells.

Merkel's cells (Fig. 4.9.3.) are found in small numbers in the stratum germinativum. They probably originate from undifferentiated keratinocytes in the embryonic epidermis. The presence of desmosomes joining Merkel's cells to keratinocytes is a strong indication for an intraepidermal origin. They also obtain melanin from the melanocytes. They form only short processes. Merkel's cells have the cytological structure of endocrine, amine or peptide hormone-secreting gland cells (II.2.1.3.). They contain dense cored secretory vesicles with a diameter of about 100 nanometers. Some of these cells are known to form synaptic junctions with the terminals of mitochondria-rich sensory nerve fibers. The dense cored vesicles are often asymmetrically distributed, as they tend to converge toward these junctions. Merkel's cell-nerve terminal complexes are mechanoreceptors that are sensitive to deformation of the epidermis. In this way,

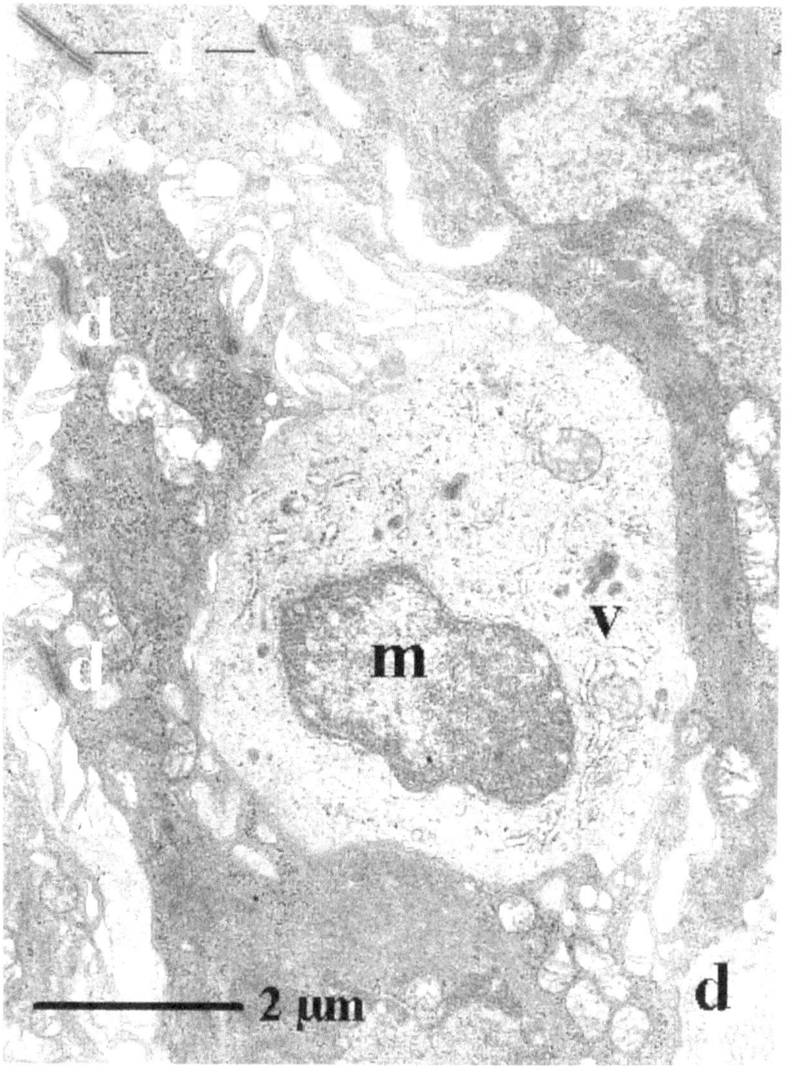

Fig. 4.9.3. Merkel's cells (m) occur in the deeper layers of the epidermis. They contain dense vesicles (v), the contents of which may be liberated by exocytosis (merocrine secretion), to diffuse into the dermis (black d), or to stimulate the terminals of sensory nerve fibers (not visible here). In the first case, Merkel's cells function as endocrine, hormone-secreting cells. In the second case, they function as receptors, sensitive to mechanical stimuli. Mark the desmosomes (white d) that join adjacent keratinocytes, and which are lacking at the level of Merkel's cell. Skin, hamster, TEM.

they contribute to the skin's sensitivity to tactile stimuli. In all probability, deformation of the epidermis is transmitted to the resident Merkel's cells, since they are joined to the keratinocytes, and this induces Merkel cell depolarization and merocrine liberation of a neurotransmitter substance, which depolarizes a sensory nerve cell terminal. The uninnervated cells may secrete hormones that regulate certain aspects of epidermal maturation and maintenance.

IV.9.1.3. Langerhans's cells.

Langerhans's cells are usually found in the intermediate epidermal strata. They represent a few percent of the total number of epidermal cells. They are dendritic cells with a flattened cell body, which forms long and slender processes. Cell body and processes lie parallel to the epidermal surface.

The cell's processes are supported by microtubules and microfilaments. Langerhans's cells do not form junctions with keratinocytes. The nucleus may have an irregular shape. An unusual type of secondary organelles in the cytoplasm are oddly shaped vesicles, the **Birbeck granules**. These vesicles have a disk shape, but in histologic sections they usually appear as rods. The interior of the rods contains regular cross striations, making them look like zip-fasteners. Frequently, this zip-fastener is open at one end, and here the vesicle expands. The whole structure now superficially resembles a tennis racket. At the moment, there is no ready explanation for this unique vesicular structure. Concerning their function, it is supposed that the Birbeck granules are very specialized endosomes, by means of which antigenic material is internalized.

Langerhans's cells help to defend the body against foreign intruders that might succeed in penetrating the epidermis. They descend from precursor cells in the bone marrow and reach the skin via the blood circulation. When they come into contact with antigenic material, they internalize it by means of receptor-mediated endocytosis. Subsequently, they migrate out of the epidermis, enter the dermal lymph capillaries and are carried to the peripheral lymph nodes. Here, the antigenic material that they have processed is presented to the T-lymphocytes of the paracortex, thus initiating an immune response.

IV.9.1.4. Glands.

During embryonic development, the epidermis forms invaginations into the underlying dermis, which develop into glands.

IV.9.1.4.1. Sweat glands.

Sweat glands come in two variants: merocrine glands and apocrine glands. Actually, these names are not entirely accurate but are kept from tradition.

Merocrine glands are simple tubular glands (III.5.1.) with a straight duct and a compactly coiled secretory part or tubulus (Fig. 3.5.4.). By convention, the position of the secretory parts of these glands determines the border between dermis and hypodermis (Fig. 4.9.1.). They are distributed over virtually the entire surface of the body, but are not associated with hair follicles. They are absent in only a few places, such as the lips and the glans penis.

The coiled, secretory tubulus has a relatively narrow lumen and is lined with a simple cuboidal to prismatic epithelium (Fig. 4.9.4.), which consists of clear cells and a few dark cells.

Confusingly, the **clear cells** are in fact not gland cells in the strict sense, because they do not synthesize the material they secrete. They are secretory brush border cells (Fig. 4.9.5.). Their lateral cell membranes are not tightly joined over most of their length, giving rise to intercellular canals. The central nucleus is surrounded on all sides by numerous mitochondria and large amounts of glycogen granules. During preparation for light microscopy, this glycogen is easily dissolved, causing the translucent look of these cells.

Clear cells actively pump sodium ions into the tubular lumen, which are passively followed by water molecules. Using this mechanism, the merocrine glands produce a watery fluid, isotonic at first, which will vaporize on the surface of the skin, thus withdrawing heat from it: sweat. In this way, the merocrine glands contribute to the body's thermoregulation. Since sweat is a watery, ion-containing fluid, they also have osmoregulatory functions.

A much rarer cell type, intercalated sporadically between the clear cells, are the **dark cells** (Fig. 4.9.5.). These cells are real gland cells, since they synthesize the material they secrete. They have the cytological structure of enzyme-secreting gland cells, with a basal cell nucleus, perinuclear rough endoplasmic reticulum, and apical secretory

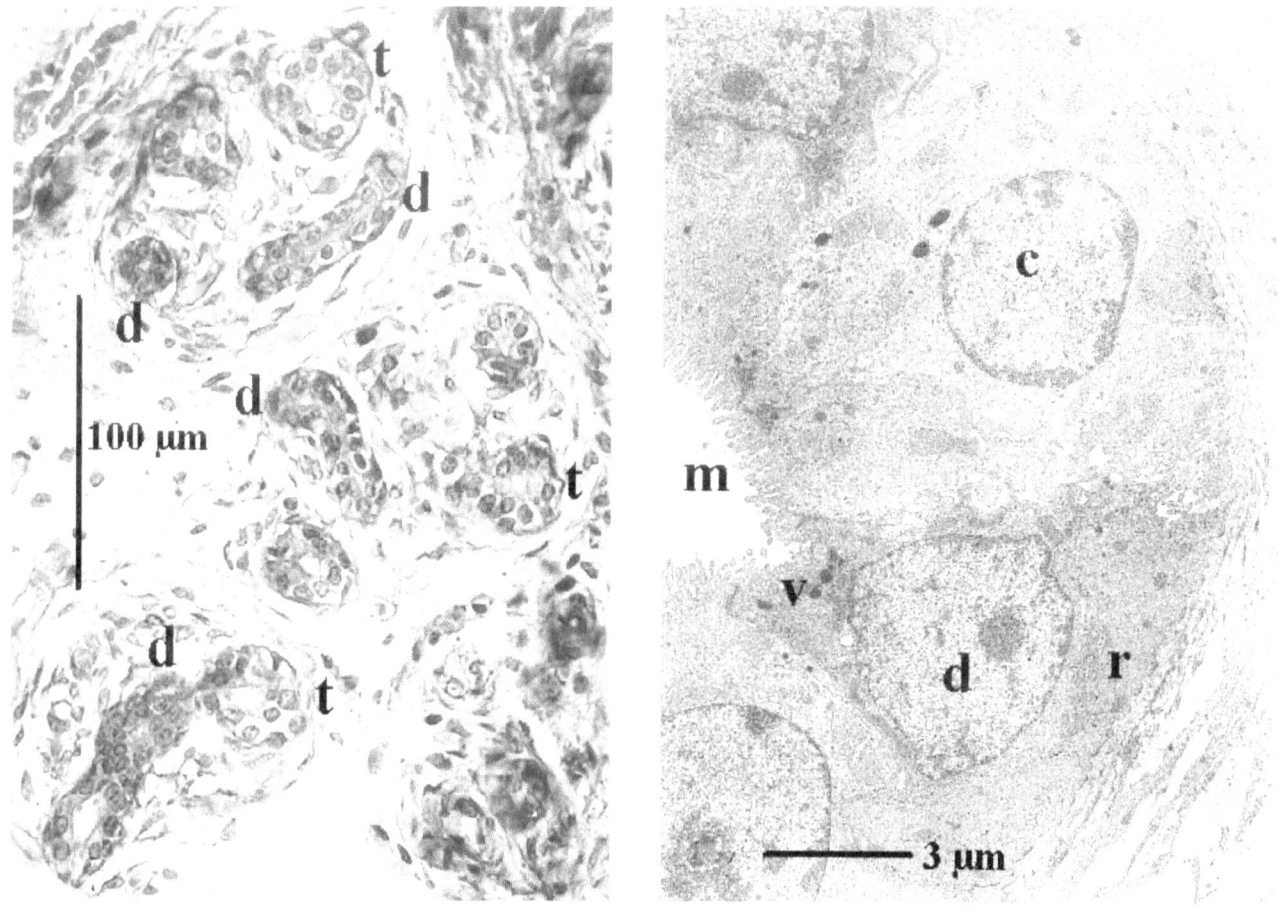

Fig. 4.9.4. (left) In sweat glands, the terminal secretory tubule and a short stretch of duct form a coil. The secretory tubule (t) has a relatively large diameter, with a tall prismatic epithelium and a wide lumen. Because of their large amount of cytoplasm, these cells look paler than those of the duct. The duct's cells (d) are relatively small and cuboidal. The duct's diameter is small, and its lumen is narrow. Foot sole, human baby, Masson stain. **Fig. 4.9.5.** (right) The clear cells (c) of sweat glands are in fact not gland cells at all in the strict sense of the word, but ion-transporting cells. They have a fairly well developed apical brush border of microvilli (m). Dark cells (d) also occur. These are real exocrine gland cells, with basal rough endoplasmic reticulum (r), and apical secretory vesicles (v). Skin, cat, TEM.

vesicles. The exact nature of the proteins they produce is not well known, but it is assumed they are similar to those produced by the apocrine glands. These cells have a merocrine mechanism of secretion.

Underneath the epithelium, flattened myoepithelial cells are found. Especially when they are numerous and form a continuous layer, they can cause the impression that the tubular epithelium is double. Contraction of the myoepithelial cells helps to expel sweat from the glandular lumen.

The duct has a smaller diameter and a narrower lumen than the secretory tubulus (Fig. 4.9.4.). It is lined with a double cuboidal epithelium of dark cells. The superficial cells carry a few microvilli and reabsorb part of the sodium ions secreted with sweat, making it hypotonic. The duct proper runs to the base of the epidermis. In the epidermis, sweat is evacuated through a pore, continuous with the ductal lumen of the sweat gland. The pore has a spiral course and opens at the epidermal surface. It is lined with keratinocytes in various degrees of development.

The **apocrine glands** are compound tubular glands (III.5.1.) and have a limited distribution. They are mainly found in the areola, the armpits and the ano-genital region. Most often, they are associated with a hair follicle.

Apart from their branched ducts, apocrine glands differ from merocrine glands mainly in the structure of the secretory tubules, which have a large diameter and a wide lumen. It is lined with a simple cuboidal epithelium, composed of cells with the cytological structure of enzyme-secreting gland cells. The structure of their vesicles is very variable. These cells shed portions of their apical cytoplasm, which is similar to the apocrine secretory mechanism of other cells. It is not clear, however, what the content of the various vesicles is, nor how this content is liberated.

Apocrine glands only develop at the onset of puberty and are strongly influenced by sex hormones. They produce body odors and are analogous to the scent glands of animals. The large lumen may serve as a temporary storage space of secretory material, which is expelled periodically when the underlying myoepithelial cells contract.

IV.9.1.4.2. Mammary glands.

Mammary glands or milk glands are essentially strongly modified apocrine sweat glands. In the female, mammary glands start to develop at the onset of puberty, under the stimulus of hypophyseal hormones and sex hormones. Not only the glandular tissue develops, the underlying dermal tissue participates as well, resulting in the formation of a pronouncedly elevated breast. In the course of the menstrual cycle, and in particular during pregnancy and lactation, the mammary glands undergo profound changes.

In fact, each breast contains about twenty independent mammary glands, embedded in adipose tissue and separated from each other by dense fibrous tissue

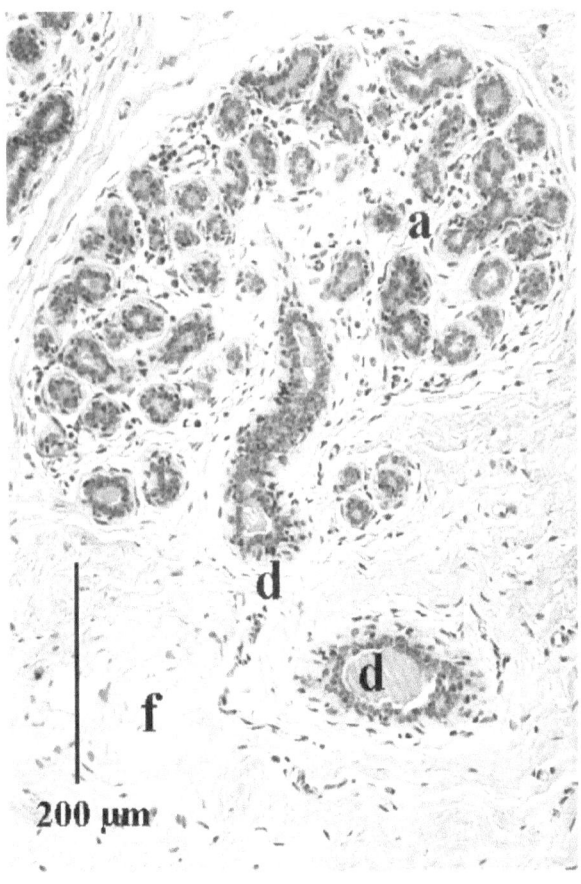 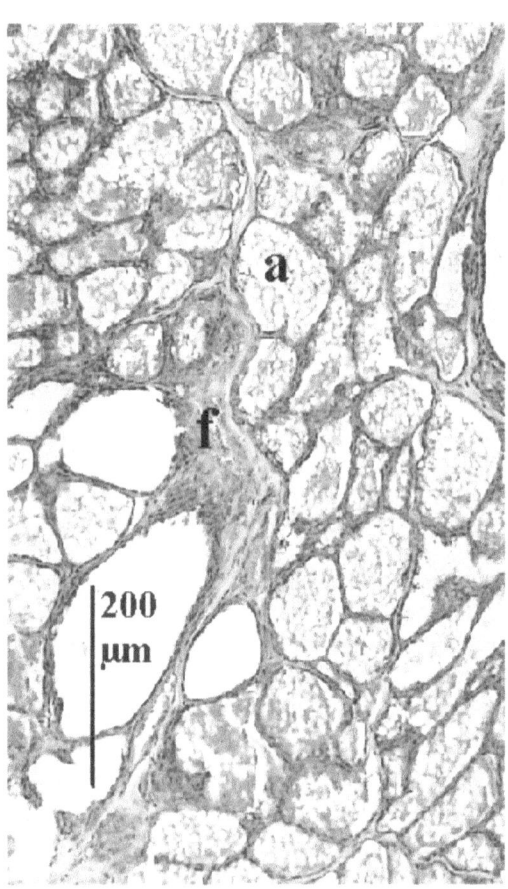

Fig. 4.9.6. (left) The mammary gland is a large, compound, acinar or tubulo-acinar gland. In an inactive mammary gland, there is little difference between the alveolar gland cells (a) and the ductal epithelial cells (d). The amount of glandular tissue is small and the glandular lobes are separated from each other by thick septa of fibrous tissue (f). Mammary gland, human, HE. **Fig. 4.9.7.** (right) In a lactating mammary gland, the amount of glandular tissue has spectacularly increased, at the expense of the fibro-adipose tissue (f). The alveoli (a) are very numerous, strongly dilated, and filled with secretory product. Mammary gland, human, HE.

septa. Each mammary gland is a compound tubulo-acinar gland (III.5.1.), invaded by fibrous tissue septa that partition it into lobes and lobules. Its main duct, or **lactiferous duct**, discharges into the exterior at the top of the nipple. Just before its mouth, the lactiferous duct widens to form a **lactiferous sinus**, the wall of which is thrown into longitudinal folds.

Below the lactiferous sinus, the lactiferous duct repeatedly branches, forming a great number of **alveolar ducts**, which eventually connect to the mammary gland's secretory units (Fig. 4.9.6.). The secretory units or **alveoli** have a globular to elongated shape and are lined with a simple cuboidal epithelium. Below this is a single layer of myoepithelial cells, forming a loose network. In a resting mammary gland, the alveolar epithelium shows few secondary organelles and its cytological structure hardly differs from that of the duct epithelium. In a lactating mammary gland (Fig. 4.9.7.), the epithelium changes into a glandular epithelium and the distinction between alveoli and ducts becomes blurred, since the terminal parts of the ducts expand and differentiate to glandular tissue.

The smallest alveolar ducts are lined with a simple cuboidal epithelium, which changes into a double one in the lactiferous sinus and duct. In the smaller ducts, the myoepithelial cells are star-shaped and form a network, parallel to the epithelium. In the larger ducts, they become fusiform and oriented with their long axis parallel to the duct axis. The terminal part of the lactiferous sinus is lined with epidermal, keratinized epithelium.

During pregnancy, the mammary glands undergo profound changes as a consequence of the actions of the sex hormones estrogen and progesterone, and the hormone prolactin of the anterior pituitary. In early pregnancy, estrogen and progesterone will induce proliferation of ducts and alveoli, at the expense of the surrounding adipose and fibrous tissue. Towards the end of pregnancy, the alveoli, under prolactin influence, will start to show signs of milk synthesis, in the form of cytoplasmic inclusions. The initial secretion of the mammary glands is colostrum, a protein-rich fluid that, contrary to real milk, is poor in lipids. Milk secretion proper only begins shortly after birth. A lactating mammary gland (Fig. 4.9.7.), has wide alveoli that tend to suppress the surrounding fibrous tissue. Although the epithelial cells are now actively synthesizing and secreting gland cells, they retain their relatively low, cuboidal shape. This is mainly a consequence of the secretory mechanism, which is partly apocrine, resulting in loss of cytoplasm. The milk that fills the alveolar and duct lumen is an eosinophilic mass containing numerous lipid droplets. The myoepithelial cells contract under the influence of the hormone oxytocin, produced by the neurohypophysis, stimulating milk evacuation. Oxytocin is released in reflectory fashion, following mechanical stimulation of the nipple during suckling.

During lactation, mammary gland cells show a mixture of characteristics of protein-secreting and lipid-secreting gland cells. Milk proteins, such as lactalbumin and casein, are synthesized in the well-developed rough endoplasmic reticulum. Via the Golgi-complex, relatively large secretory vesicles are formed with a rounded shape and variable dimensions. In each of these vesicles, a few dense protein granules form by condensation, and are liberated at the cell apex by merocrine secretion, through simple exocytosis.

The Golgi-complex adds carbohydrates, such as lactose, to the vesicular content. A third milk component, lipid, accumulates as lipid droplets. Lipids are partly synthesized by the cell itself, although its smooth endoplasmic reticulum is not well developed. Lipids are also taken up from the blood. The largest lipid droplets produce pronounced bulges at the apical cell pole. Eventually, each bulge constricts at its base, separating the lipid droplet, surrounded by a narrow rim of cytoplasm, from the rest of the cell. This method of secretion is apocrine.

IV.9.1.4.3. Sebum glands.

Sebum glands (Fig. 4.9.8.) are acinar glands, sessile (III.5.1.) or with a very short duct, which most often arise from the epidermis of a hair follicle, although solitary sebum glands are not rare. A sebum gland's peripheral cells are undifferentiated keratinocytes, which form in effect a stratum germinativum. In this case, however, they do not develop into fiber-bearing, lining cells, but in stead into lipid-secreting gland cells. This development is gradual, and as development advances, the cells end up progressively closer to the center of the acinus.

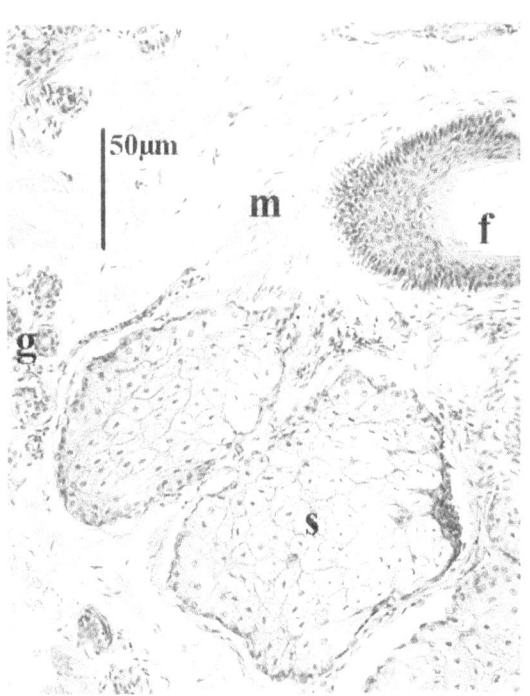

Fig. 4.9.8. Sebum glands (s) are most often associated with a hair follicle (f). They are composed of lipid-secreting exocrine gland cells. The spongy look of these cells is caused by the presence of lipid droplets. A few sweat glands (g) and an arrector muscle (m) are also seen. Hairy skin, human, HE.

The developing gland cells acquire a spherical shape and initially contain a central nucleus, surrounded by an extensive smooth endoplasmic reticulum and some rough endoplasmic reticulum. They are not clearly polarized, although they are exocrine cells. This is a direct consequence of their mechanism of secretion. As they synthesize lipids, the cytoplasm is gradually loaded with lipid droplets. The nucleus involutes and becomes pycnotic. Eventually, it is lost completely. The other organelles also degenerate and the cell ends up as little more than a bag of lipid droplets. Lipids are easily dissolved during preparation for light microscopy. Consequently, mature sebum gland cells acquire a spongy aspect. The lipid droplets tend to coalesce, and their diameter can attain large values, up to a few micrometers. Eventually, the cell membrane gives way and the lipids are released. This secretory mechanism, which involves loss of the whole cell, is called **holocrine**. Lost cells are continuously replaced from the stratum germinativum.

The largest sebum glands, and the largest number of them, a few hundred per square centimeter, are found in the scalp and the skin of the face. These glands are influenced by sex hormones, especially during puberty. At late ages, they involute somewhat.

The secretory product, a complex mixture of lipids, is discharged in the hair follicle and ends up on the skin surface. The functional significance of sebum is not well understood. It mainly contains apolar lipids, which in principle do not mix well with the epidermal lipids, which carry strongly polar heads.

IV.9.1.5. Hairs.

Hair development starts in the same way as gland formation: as tubular invaginations of the epidermis in the underlying dermis, the **hair follicles** (Figs. 4.9.9.-10.). The apex of the hair follicle is swollen, forming a **hair bulb**. It is indented at its top by a dermal papilla, rich in blood vessels. In the hair bulb, the keratinocytes of the stratum germinativum proliferate and enter their developmental pathway. As in the epidermal keratinocytes, differentiation and keratinization finally results in complete loss of primary organelles and cell death. Depending on their position, they enter different pathways of keratinization. Each pathway produces a concentric layer of keratinized cells around the long axis of the hair follicle, resulting in the formation of a thread-like, keratinized growth, a **hair shaft** (Fig. 4.9.10.). The hair shaft lengthens by continuous cell proliferation and differentiation in the bulb.

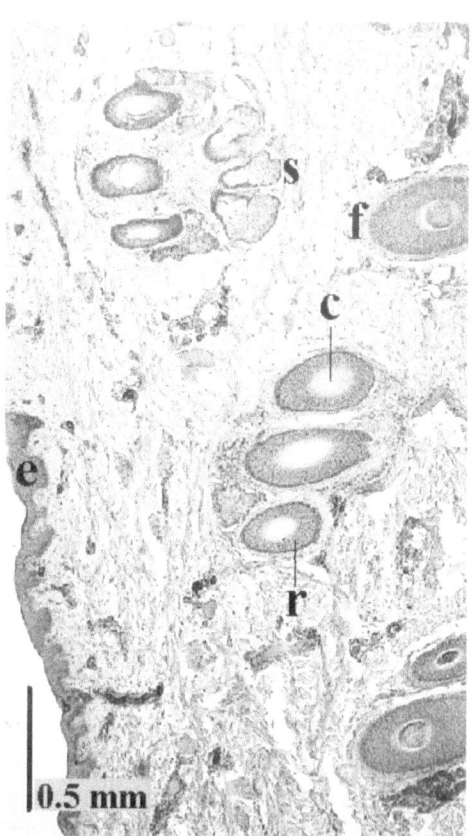

Fig. 4.9.9. Hairy skin is characterized by the presence of hair follicles (f). These are inpocketings of the epidermis (e), which lack a stratum corneum. They are composed of an epithelium, the internal root sheath (r), which corresponds to the deeper layers of the epidermis. In the center of a follicle, a hair shaft develops. In a few follicles, the hair shaft's cortex (c) is seen. The follicular epithelium locally forms sebum glands (s). Hairy skin, human, HE.

The keratinocytes at the bottom of the hair bulb show four different patterns of differentiation and keratinization, resulting in four concentric layers of keratinized cells (Fig. 4.9.11.). Since the differentiation process takes time, this pattern is not clearly visible until continuous addition of cells from below has shifted the differentiating cells to a certain distance from the hair bulb.

In the center of the hair shaft, the keratinocytes have differentiated to form the **medulla**. The medullary keratinocytes do not form filaments, but granules, which are analogous to the keratohyalin granules of the epidermal keratinocytes. Eventually, these coalesce, and the whole cell is filled with an amorphous mass. The medulla is surrounded by a **cortex**, produced by keratinocytes that have followed another pathway of differentiation (Fig. 4.9.12.). The cortex is made up of several layers of squamous cells, filled with filaments and dense granules. It is the thickest layer of the hair shaft and its most important structural component. In its turn, the cortex is surrounded by a few layers of

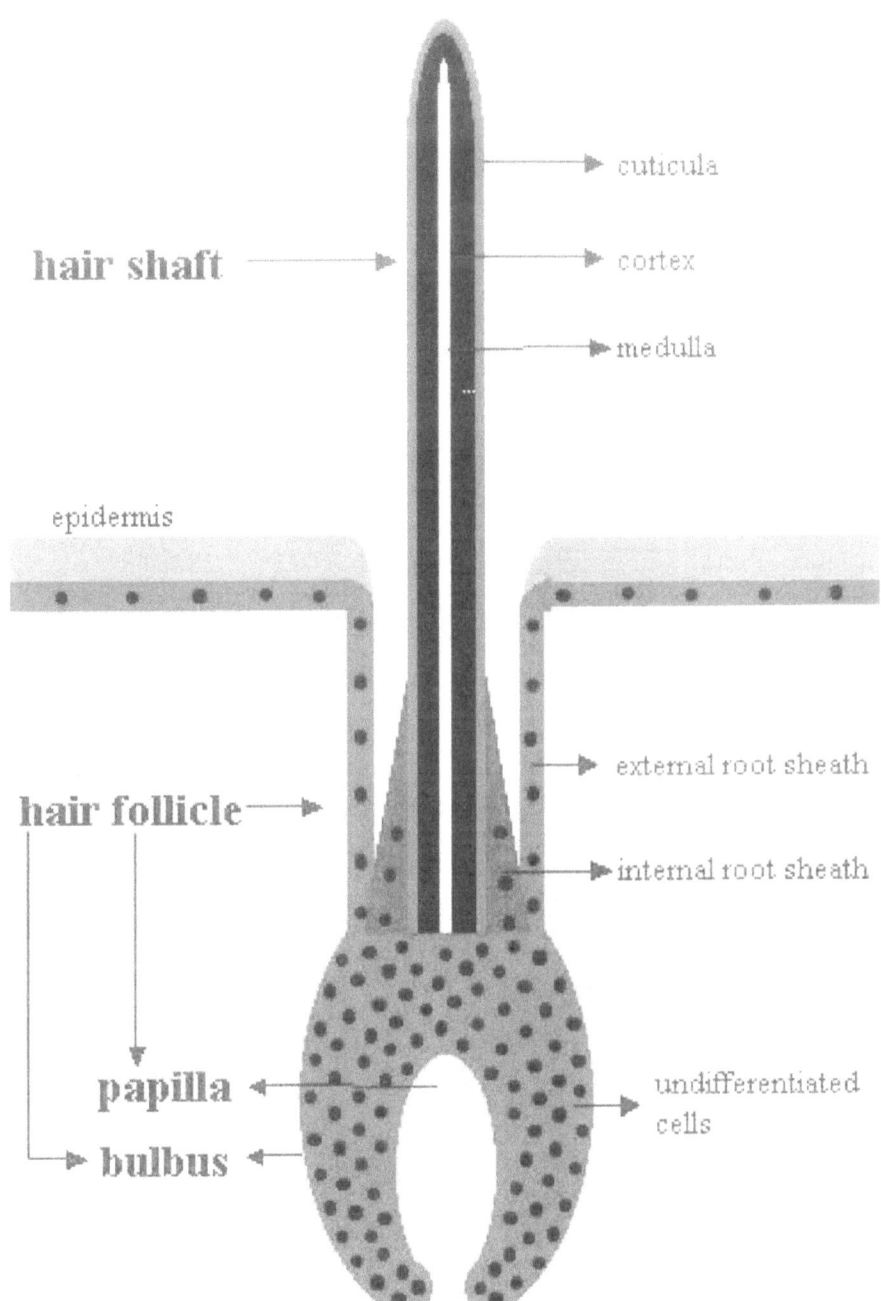

hair shaft

cuticula

cortex

medulla

epidermis

hair follicle

external root sheath

internal root sheath

papilla

bulbus

undifferentiated cells

Fig. 4.9.10. A hair shaft grows out of a hair follicle. The bottom of this follicle is expanded, forming a hair bulb, which is indented at its apex by a dermal papilla. By cell multiplication in the bulb, a hair shaft arises and grows. The hair shaft is made up of several concentric layers, each having its own characteristic pattern of differentiation and keratinization. Beginning at its center, the hair shaft is made up of a medulla, a cortex and a cuticula. The stretch that is within the follicle is additionally enveloped in an internal root sheath. The external root sheath is continuous with the epidermis.

squamous cells, which form the **cuticula**. The cuticular keratinocytes contain, like the medullary ones, mostly dense granules. At a relatively short distance from the hair bulb, the medullary keratinocytes will shift to the cortical pathway. In this way, the stretch of hair shaft containing a medulla is very short. For most of its length, the hair shaft is made up of cortex (central position!) and cuticula only. Finally, the cuticula is surrounded by an **internal root sheath** (Fig. 4.9.13.). The keratinocytes that have formed it contain tonofilaments, as well as trichohyalin granules, which are analogous to the keratohyalin granules of the epidermis. Like the medulla, the internal root sheath occupies only a short stretch of hair shaft. It is limited to the subepidermal part of the hair stem, the root. The **external root sheath** is the wall of the hair follicle. It corresponds to the stratum germinativum and the stratum spinosum of the epidermis, and is continuous with these at the mouth of the hair follicle. Since the internal root sheath is lost, the external root sheath does not adhere to the hair shaft.

The basal membrane anchoring the external root sheath to the dermis may be so thick that it is visible in the

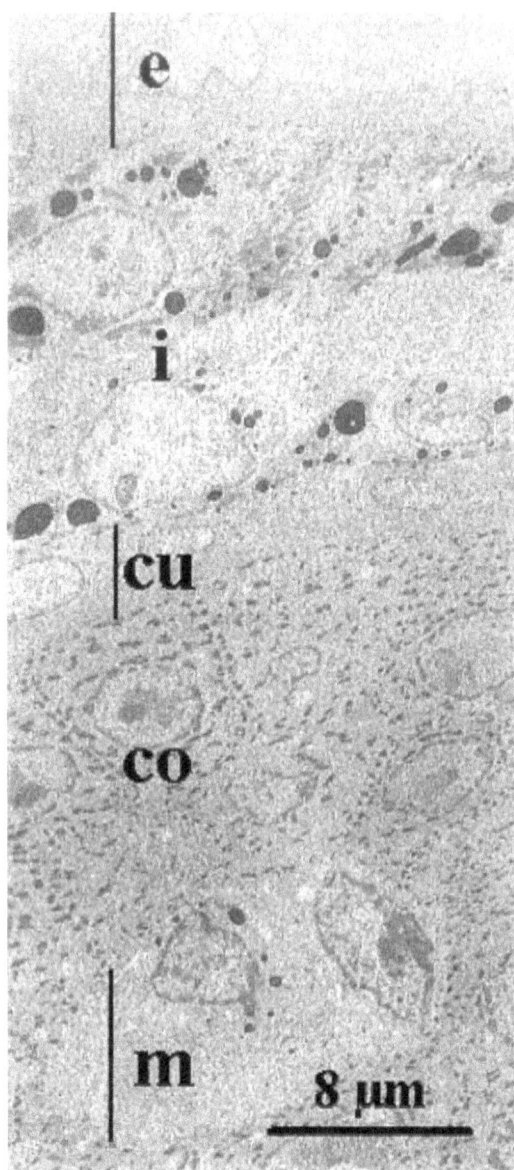

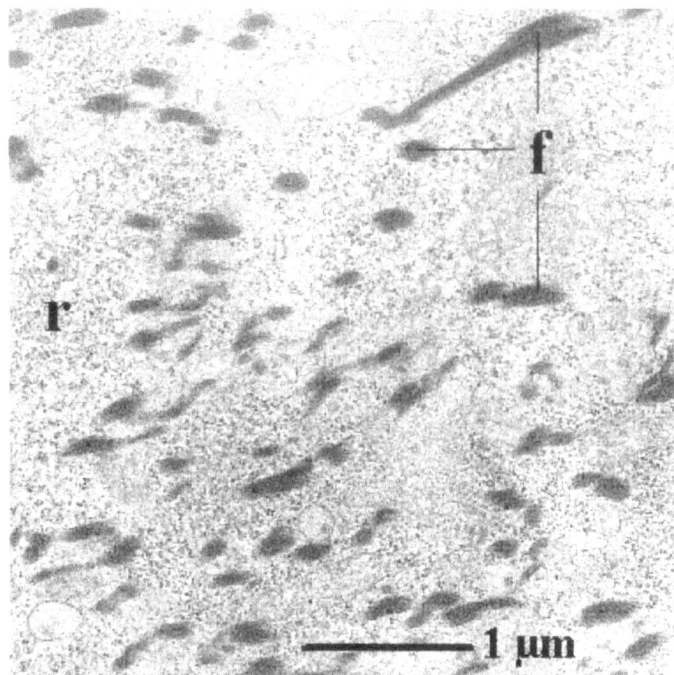

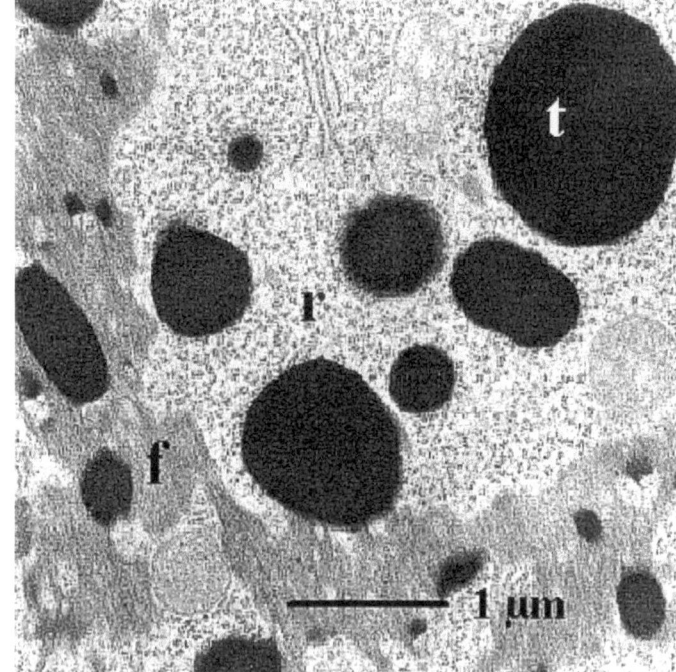

Fig. 4.9.11. (above) A hair follicle, transversely sectioned near the bulb, consecutively shows the thin medulla (m), the thick cortex (co), and the cuticula (ca) of the hair shaft. The hair shaft is enveloped in an internal root sheath (i) and an external root sheath (e). The first 4 layers are composed of keratinocytes in different stages of keratinization, while the last layer is the hair follicle's germinative stratum. Skin, rabbit, TEM. **Fig. 4.9.12.** (top right) The keratinocytes making up the hair shaft's cortex contain numerous filament bundles (f), the presence of which indicates that a specific keratinization process is going on. The cytoplasm is loaded with ribosomes (r). Hair shaft, rabbit, TEM. **Fig. 4.9.13.** (right) The keratinocytes of the internal root sheath contain filament bundles (f) and trichohyalin granules (t), indicative of a specific keratinization process. The cytoplasm is loaded with ribosomes (r). Hair shaft, rabbit, TEM.

light microscope as a so-called glassy membrane.

The hair cortex contains variable amounts of different types of melanin, creating black and brown hair colors. This melanin is synthesized by melanocytes, which are lodged between the proliferating cells of the hair bulb. Blonde hairs contain little or no melanin. Gray hairs are caused by minuscule air bubbles in the cortex.

Hair follicles usually reach deeper into the dermis than sweat glands do. Close to the epidermis, the hair follicle frequently forms a lateral bulge that develops into a sebum gland. In some body parts, apocrine sweat glands empty into the follicles.

The dermis surrounding the follicle is rich in sensory nerve fibers, which are stimulated by movements of the hair shaft, and thus function as mechanoreceptors. These are the so-called peritrichal receptors.

Many hair follicles are associated with a bundle of smooth muscle fibers, which are attached to the follicle's terminal at one end, and anchored in the subepidermal dermis at the other end. Frequently, hair follicles are inclined and can be pulled upright by contraction of these muscle fibers. Therefore, they are called **arrector muscles** (Fig. 4.9.8.). Arrector muscles are innervated and contract during exposure to cold or as a consequence of strong emotions. The resulting upright position of the hair shaft causes goose flesh.

The dimensions of the hair follicles and the hairs they produce, as well as their relative numbers, differ in various regions of the skin. Hair follicles are completely absent in the glabrous skin of hand palms and feet soles. Over most of the rest of the body surface, the skin contains few and short (length of 2 to 3 millimeters) hair follicles. On the other hand, hair follicles are very numerous and moderately long (length of 4 to 5 millimeters) in the scalp. In a few places, such as the armpits, the genital zone, the eye lashes, the eye brows and the beard, hair follicles are moderately numerous but very thick and long (length exceeding 5 millimeters). The dimensions of the hairs are proportional to those of the follicles that produce them.

When they are sufficiently numerous, hairs are able to trap a layer of air close to the skin, which thermically isolates the body, immobile air being an inefficient conductor of heat. In the human being, this physiological function of hair is taken over by the adipose tissue of the hypodermis.

IV.9.1.6. Nails.

At the dorsal side of the tips of fingers and toes, the epidermis forms a horizontal, flattened, rearward invagination, which produces a strongly keratinized sheet, a nail. The nail keratin is harder even than that of the hairs and differs, in the details of its physical and chemical structure, from both hair keratin and epidermal keratin. The deepest part of the invagination, the nail matrix, consists of proliferating keratinocytes. Part of it is visible at the base of the semitransparent nail as a whitish area, in the shape of a half moon, the lunula. Proliferation and progressive keratinization produce the nail plate, or nail proper. As the nail lengthens, it gradually moves over the underlying tissue, the nail bed, which is covered with a thin epidermis.

IV.9.2. Dermis and hypodermis, including mechanoreceptors.

The dermis is a layer of fibro-elastic fibrous tissue. It is thickest underneath the thick epidermis of hand palms and feet soles, where it forms papillae. The superficial part of the dermis, the region of the papillae, is the pars papillaris. It is a relatively loose fibrous tissue, with diffusely distributed fibrils. It rests on a much thicker pars reticularis, which consists of denser fibrous tissue, in which the fibrils tend to form bundles. The underlying hypodermis consists of loose fibrous tissue, which locally forms large accumulations of white adipose tissue. The level occupied by the secretory coils of the merocrine sweat glands conventionally defines the transition of dermis to hypodermis. The hypodermis joins the skin to the underlying tissues. The presence of a hypodermis means that human skin adheres rather tightly to the body and that, in contrast to most other mammals, it is a little more difficult to skin a human being.

At the transition of pars papillaris and pars reticularis lays a network of capillaries, the rete subpapillaris (Fig. 4.9.1.). Deeper, at the transition of dermis and hypodermis, i.e. at the same level as the secretory coils of the merocrine sweat glands, is another capillary bed, the rete cutaneum. In this network, the capillaries clearly have a larger diameter than those forming the upper bed (Fig. 4.9.1.). Both networks supply the dermis with blood. The epidermis is avascular and, consequently, has to rely on diffusion from the dermis. An even deeper capillary network, situated in the hypodermis, is the rete hypodermale.

The capillary beds of the skin are interconnected through thin blood vessels, which may form arteriovenous anastomoses. When opened, these allow part of the blood to pass directly from arteries to veins, bypassing the superficial capillary networks. During exposure to cold or warmth, this mechanism helps to limit or to promote, respectively, the loss of body heat through the skin and contributes to the skin's thermoregulatory function. In exposed parts of the body, such as the finger tips and the external ear, an arteriovenous anastomosis may develop into a glomus. A glomus is a highly coiled, spherical part of the anastomosis. Before it enters the coil, the tunica media of the arterial segment of the anastomosis thickens and its smooth muscle fibers shorten and expand, assuming the aspect of epithelial cells. These epitheloid cells may control the arterial diameter, and the amount of blood that can enter the glomus.

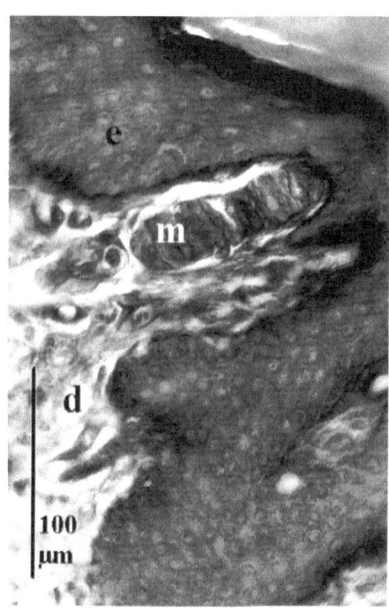

Fig. 4.9.14. In the dermal papillae of the tips of fingers and toes lie Meissner corpuscles (m). They are mechanoreceptors, the most prominent component of which is a stack of epitheloid cells, which can be regarded as modified glia cells. e = epidermis, d = dermis. Foot sole, human baby, Masson stain.

The exposed position of the skin makes it ideally suited to capture stimuli from the outside world. In fact, the skin is densely supplied with sensory nerve fibers and it is an important sense organ. Apart from free nerve terminals, which may penetrate the epidermis, and the peritrichal receptors associated with hairs, the dermis and hypodermis contain a number of highly specialized receptor organs. The most frequently encountered of these are Meissner's corpuscles, Ruffini's corpuscles, and Vater-Pacinian corpuscles. The last two are also found in other organs than the skin. Much rarer and more controversial are Krause's spherical end bulbs and Golgi-Mazzoni

corpuscles. These corpuscles are mechanoreceptors, with the sheathing of the nerve fiber terminal by a capsule consisting of modified Schwann cells, perineural cells, and fibrous tissue, as a characteristic property. These capsules may be deformed mechanically, and this deformation is transmitted to the sensory nerve terminals inside, which depolarize and initiate action potentials. The nature and the mechanical properties of the capsule largely determine exactly which kind of stimulus the nerve terminals are sensitive to.

IV.9.2..1. Ruffini's corpuscles.

Ruffini's corpuscles are encountered in both the dermis and the hypodermis. They are fusiform corpuscles, up to a few millimeters in length, and enveloped by a dense fibrous connective tissue capsule. Inside this capsule is an intensively branched sensory nerve fiber, the terminals of which are filled with mitochondria and enveloped in one or more layers of modified Schwann cells as well as collagen fibrils. Between the Schwann cell coat and the capsule is a broad space or amorphous layer, which contains a few collagen fibrils. The nerve terminals form characteristic finger-like processes, or filipodia, up to a micrometer long, which penetrate between the Schwann cells and reach the amorphous layer. It is probably these processes that, upon deformation of the fibrous tissue coat, initiate the formation of action potentials

IV.9.2.2. Meissner's corpuscles.

Meissner's corpuscles (Fig. 4.9.14.) have a very localized distribution, predominating in the most sensitive areas of the skin, such as the tips of fingers and toes, the nipples, the eyelids, the lips and the genitals. They lie immediately underneath the epidermis, preferentially so at the apex of the dermal papillae. The corpuscles are composed of a number of modified, more or less flattened Schwann cells, which form a stack, lying at right angles to the local skin surface. The cells in the middle of the stack are wider than those on top or at the bottom, resulting in an ellipsoid overall shape. The cell nuclei lie at the periphery of the stack. The Schwann cells form numerous horizontal lamellae, which interdigitate with the lamellae of adjacent cells. One or a few sensory nerve fibers penetrate the capsule at its base, losing their myelin sheath in the process, and insinuate themselves between the Schwann cells or their lamellae. They form branches, the tips of which expand into wide, flattened terminals, filled with mitochondria. The nerve terminals also form filipodia.

206

The Schwann cell stack is enveloped by a thin fibrous tissue capsule, containing perineural cells (IV.4.1.). Collagen fibrils link this capsule to the basement membrane of the overlying epidermis.

IV.9.2.3. Vater-Pacinian corpuscles.

Vater-Pacinian corpuscles are widely distributed over the body, but are limited to the hypodermis (Fig. 4.9.15.). They are very conspicuous because of their size: their dimensions may reach values of about a millimeter.

In histological sections, the most striking part of a Vater-Pacinian corpuscle is its capsule, which accounts for more than 99 percent of the corpuscle's volume. It has a concentrically layered structure, like a sliced onion. The capsule is ellipsoid and, on closer inspection, consists of an inner capsule and an outer capsule (Fig. 4.9.16.). The whole structure is enveloped with a fibrous tissue layer. The outer capsule is continuous with the perineurium of a peripheral nerve. It numbers several tens of concentric lamellae, made up of perineural cells (Fig. 4.9.17.), many of which are joined with tight junctions. These lamellae are widely spaced and fluid circulates in the interlamellar spaces, probably secreted by the perineural cells. Capillaries run between these lamellae. At one of its poles, the outer capsule is penetrated by a single sensory nerve fiber, which soon loses its myelin sheath and follows a straight course along the corpuscle's long axis until it reaches the vicinity of the opposite pole. Here, it expands and forms a terminal, filled with mitochondria (Fig. 4.9.18.). This terminal, and the final preterminal stretch of nerve fiber, are enveloped by successive layers of modified, flattened Schwann cells, closely packed, and joined with gap junctions, forming the inner capsule. In fact, the inner capsule consists of two symmetrical halves, each of both made up of concentric hemilamellae. They flank both faces of the enclosed nerve terminal, which is somewhat flattened. Between the two halves of the inner capsule is a cleft, in which the nerve terminal extends short processes or filipodia. These are especially numerous at the tip of the terminal.

References.

Bell J., Bolanowski S., Holmes M.H.: The structure and function of pacinian corpuscles: a review. Prog. Neurobiol. 1994, 42: 79-128.

Borradori L., Sonnenberg A.: Structure and function of hemidesmosomes: more than simple adhesion complexes. J. Invest. Dermatol. 1999, 112: 411-418.

Chu T., Jaffe R.: The normal Langerhans cell and the LCH cell. Br. J. Cancer 1994, 70: S4-S10.

Hirobe T;: Structure and function of melanocytes: microscopic morphology and cell biology of mouse melanocytes in the epidermis and hair follicle. Histol. Histopathol. 1995, 10: 223-237.

Hogan A.D., Burks A.W.: Epidermal Langerhans' cells and their function in the skin immune system. Ann. Allergy Asthma Immunol. 1995, 75: 5-10.

Iggo A., Andres K.H.: Morphology of cutaneous receptors. Ann. Rev. Neurosci. 1982, 5: 1-31.

Munger B.L., Ide C.: The structure and function of cutaneous sensory receptors. Arch. Histol. Cytol. 1988, 51: 1-34.

Ogawa H.: The Merkel cell as a possible mechanoreceptor cell. Prog. Neurobiol. 1996, 49: 317-334.

Kurosumi K., Shibasaki S., Ito T.: Cytology of the secretion in mammalian sweat glands. Int. Rev. Cytol. 1984, 87: 253-329.

Tachibana T.: The Merkel cell: recent findings and unresolved problems. Arch. Histol. Cytol. 1995, 58: 379-396.

Teunissen M.B.M.: Dynamic nature and function of epidermal Langerhans cells in vivo and in vitro: a review, with emphasis on human Langerhans cells. Histochem. J. 1992, 24: 697-716.

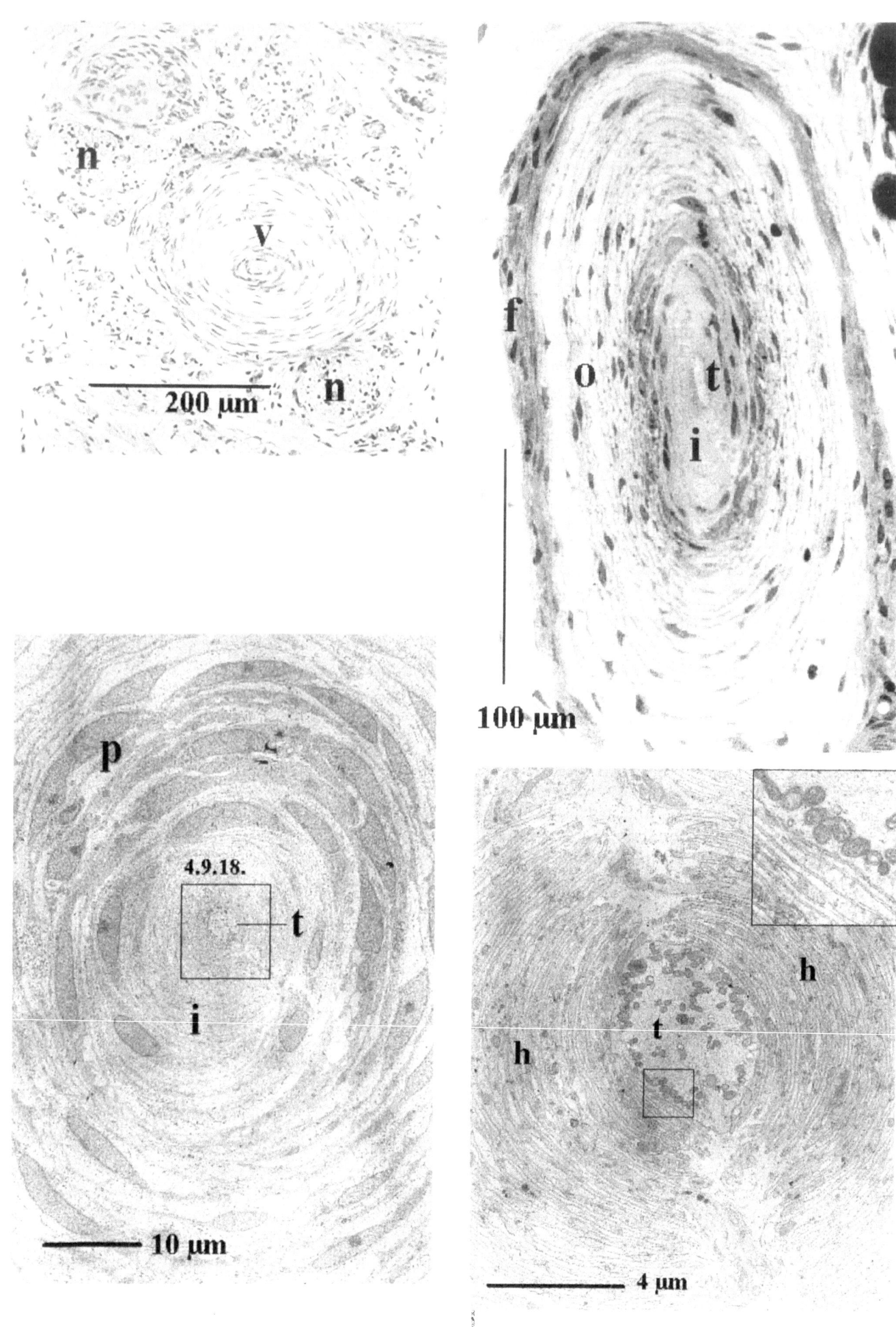

Fig. 4.9.15. (top left) In the hypodermis, Vater-Pacinian corpuscles (v) are frequently encountered. They are mechanoreceptors, having a prominent capsule of multiple, concentric lamellae. n = nerve fiber bundles. Foot sole, human baby, HE. Fig. 4.9.16. (bottom left) The capsule of Vater-Pacinian corpuscles has a complex, concentric, structure. In the center is the terminal (t) of a sensory nerve fiber. This terminal is ensheathed by, consecutively, an inner capsule (i), an outer capsule (o), and a fibrous tissue layer (f). Skin, cat, 1-micrometer plastic section, toluidin blue. Fig. 4.9.17. (top right) The outer capsule of a Vater-Pacinian corpuscle is made of perineural cells (p), derived from a peripheral nerve perineurium. In the center is the sensory nerve terminal (t), enveloped by the inner capsule (i). Skin, cat, TEM. Fig. 4.9.18. (bottom right) The sensory nerve terminal (t) of a Vater-Pacinian corpuscle is loaded with mitochondria. It is slightly ellipsoid, indicating that it (and the entire corpuscle) is not spherical, but somewhat flattened. The inner capsule is made of squamous Schwann cells, which form concentric hemilamellae (h) at both sides of the terminal. Skin, cat, TEM.

IV.10. Male reproductive system.

The male reproductive system consists of the testes, a number of ducts, the accessory glands, and the penis. In the seminiferous tubules of the testes, the male gametes, or spermatozoa, develop. The testicular interstitium synthesizes testosterone, the male sex hormone. The ducts conduct and temporarily store the spermatozoa. The accessory glands contribute to the synthesis of fluids in which the spermatozoa are suspended. The penis is the copulatory organ.

The dominant tissues that participate in the formation of the male reproductive tract are epithelium, glandular tissue, and visceral muscle tissue. **Epithelium** forms the seminiferous tubules and lines the ducts. In the accessory glands, it develops into **exocrine glandular tissue**. The testicular interstitium contains **endocrine glandular tissue**. Both epithelium and glandular tissues have, rather unusually, a mesodermal origin (Fig. 4.1.). Visceral muscle tissue contributes to the formation of the walls of the larger ducts and is found profusely in the accessory glands.

IV.10.1. Testes.

The testes are enveloped in a thick capsule of dense fibrous connective tissue, the tunica albuginea. The tunica's surface and the inside of the scrotum are coated with a serosa, the tunica vaginalis. The deeper layers of the tunica albuginea are vascularized, and constitute a tunica vasculosa. The tunica covering the posterior part of the upper testicular pole is locally thickened, forming the mediastinum. Starting from the mediastinum, the tunica vasculosa forms thin, incomplete, radiating septa, which partition each testis into some 250 incompletely defined, conical lobules. Each lobule contains one to a few convoluted **seminiferous tubules** (Fig. 4.10.1.), which drain into a duct at the level of the mediastinum. Usually, the seminiferous tubules have the shape of a loop, both ends converging towards the mediastinum. They are often branched and adjacent tubules or branches may merge. Seminiferous tubules have a diameter of about 200 micrometers, and a length of about 80 centimeters. The intertubular spaces are filled with a very loose interstitial tissue, collectively forming the interstitium. It contains accumulations of endocrine cells, **Leydig's cells** (Fig. 4.10.1.).

At the level of the mediastinum, the seminiferous tubules drain into the first segment of the intratesticular ducts.

IV.10.1.1. Seminiferous tubules.

Seminiferous tubules resemble tubular glands, the walls of which consist of stratified epithelium (Fig. 4.10.2.). This stratified epithelium, or seminiferous epithelium, is made up of **spermatogenic cells** and **Sertoli's cells.**

Spermatogenic cells are the precursors of the spermatozoa, in different stages of development. The least differentiated cells, the spermatogonia, form the most basal cell layer of the epithelium. They proliferate by mitosis and some of their daughter cells will start their differentiation to spermatozoa. The more superficial layers of this epithelium correspond to successive stages of spermatogenesis: primary spermatocytes, secondary spermatocytes, spermatids, and spermatozoa.

Sertoli's cells are not gametes, but ordinary somatic cells, the functions of which promote the development of spermatozoa.

The seminiferous epithelium rests on a basement membrane, followed by one to several layers of myoid cells (Fig. 4.10.3.) that form a peritubular sheath. They are the local variant of myoepithelial cells. Their contractile, peristaltic activity helps to propel the tubular contents. In this way, the spermatozoa, which are not yet actively motile at this stage, can be transferred to the ducts.

IV.10.1.1.1. Meiosis.

Spermatogenesis, the formation of spermatozoa, is a complex process. At the heart of it is a unique kind of nuclear division: **meiosis**.

In order to understand what meiosis is primarily about, it is important to realize that chromosomes normally come in homologous pairs. The number of chromosomes found in the nucleus of a non-reproductive body cell is always even, because it is a double, or **diploid**, number. For example, human cell nuclei contain 46, or two times 23, chromosomes. They make up 23 homologous pairs. In each pair, one partner has a paternal origin, having been contributed by a spermatozoon, while the other has a maternal origin, having been contributed by an ovum. They came together during fertilization, when a spermatozoon and an ovum merged. The primary objective of meiosis is easy to understand: it is the separation of both partners of each pair, in order to produce gametes with a halved, **haploid**, number of chromosomes. This is an anticipation to fertilization, when diploid chromosome numbers will be restored.

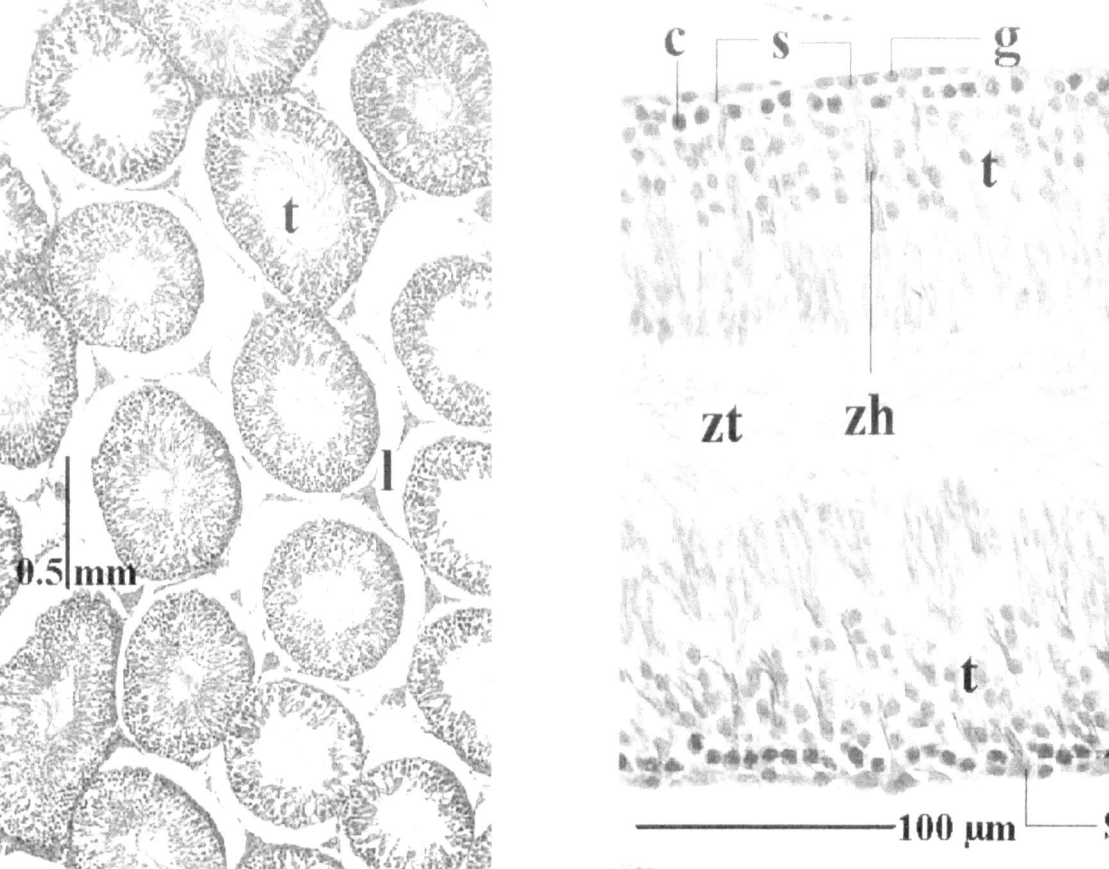

Fig. 4.10.1. (left) The testis contains a large number of seminiferous tubules (t), in which spermatozoa are formed. The interstitium contains groups of endocrine cells, Leydig cells (l), which produce the male sex hormone, testosterone. Testis, rat, HE. **Fig. 4.10.2.** (right) A seminiferous tubule wall is an epithelium, made of spermatogenic cells in different stages of development, and Sertoli cells. The most primitive spermatogenic cells are the relatively small, cuboid spermatogonia (g) on the epithelium's deepest levels. Towards the tubular lumen lie the large primary spermatocytes (c), which enter the first division of meiosis. Secondary spermatocytes immediately continue into the second meiotic division, and are consequently very rare. Spermatids (t) are the end result of the second meiotic division and enter the successive stages of spermiogenesis: the morphological and functional development into spermatozoa. The tails of the spermatozoa (zt) lie in the tubular lumen, their heads (zh) are associated with Sertoli cell cytoplasm. Sertoli cells (s) are very tall cells, which cover the entire thickness of the epithelium. Their nucleus lies in a conical cell body at the periphery of the seminiferous tubule. Testis, rat, HE.

Meiosis is such a complicated affair because, prior to separation of the partners of a chromosomal pair, one chromatid of each partner (as in mitosis, the chromosomes are themselves double) exchanges genes with a chromatid of the other partner. Both partners carry, at the same locations, homologous genes, which code for the same characteristic (eye color, to give a simplistic example), but are not necessarily identical, because each has been contributed by another parent (e.g. one may code for blue eyes, the other for brown eyes). When segments of chromosome carrying genes are exchanged, the genes will end up in combination with different genes than before. This mechanism increases the amount of genetic variation among the gametes to be produced, and ultimately among the offspring. This is essentially what sexual reproduction is about. A double consequence of this mechanism being operational is that it actually takes two subsequent nuclear divisions to complete meiosis and that the prophase of the first division is unusually prolonged and complex.

It is during the prophase of this first meiotic division, **prophase I**, that exchange of genes between homologous chromosome partners takes place. For this reason, prophase I takes much more time and is much more complex than the prophase of an ordinary mitotic division. In addition, the nuclear envelope remains intact, so that prophase I is entirely an intranuclear affair. For convenience, prophase I has been subdivided in subphases.

During the first subphase, the **leptotene**, the chromosomes condense out of the chromatin and appear as slender threads. In the next subphase, the **zygotene**, each chromosome lines up with its homologous partner and is joined with it. The coupled

211

partners shorten and thicken, initiating the third subphase, the **pachytene**. It is during the pachytene, the longest subphase, that homologous chromosome segments are exchanged between two chromatids of a chromosome pair, one of each partner. The number of exchanged segments, as well as the length and the location of each, are in principle random. This means that they are different for each nucleus that divides meiotically. Consequently, the exchange pattern will nowhere exactly be repeated and in different nuclei chromatids result with ever changing combinations of paternal and maternal genes. During **diplotene**, the last subphase of prophase I, the tight joining of the chromosome partners is ended, but for the time being they stay together. The nuclear envelope is broken down and a microtubular spindle forms.

During **metaphase I**, the chromosome pairs are positioned in the cell's equatorial plane. During **anaphase I**, the homologous partners are separated, and moved to opposite poles. The halving of the chromosome number, which is the primary objective of meiosis, thus takes place during this phase. A telophase proper does not take place because the chromosomes remain intact, in anticipation of the second meiotic division. Cell division does take place, however, producing two daughter cells with a halved chromosome number, each of which will enter the second division.

As a direct consequence of the exchange of genes between one chromatid of each of the partners of a chromosome pair during prophase I, the two chromatids of a particular chromosome may no longer be identical. If they are not separated, problems may arise after fertilization. When the fertilized ovum starts to multiply mitotically, the chromatids of a particular chromosome will end up in separate cells. The end result would be an organism, the constituent cells of which differ in their genetic content. This may fatally interfere with a proper functioning of the organism. This complication is avoided by the introduction of a second meiotic division, which separates each chromosome's chromatids.

The second meiotic division has no prophase proper, because the chromosomes are already formed. Metaphase II, anaphase II and telophase II are identical to those of a mitotic division: each chromosome's chromatids end up in one of both daughter cells.

The end result of meiosis is that one diploid cell has produced four haploid cells, each with a different genetic pattern. The number of possible genetic patterns among the gametes of a single organism, and the zygotes which result from their union, is truly astronomic. This is the reason why brothers and sisters, although born form the same parents, are different from each other. The genetic differences between population members which are not so closely related are even greater. This genetic variation, supplied and maintained by meiosis and sexual reproduction, is the raw material of natural selection, and the motor of evolution.

IV.10.1.1.2. Spermatogenic cells.

The most primitive spermatogenic cells are the **spermatogonia** (Fig. 4.10.3.). They form the basal layer, often only one cell thick, of the seminiferous epithelium. They are small cuboidal cells, with a diameter of about 12 micrometers. The small amount of cytoplasm contains little secondary organelles and most of it is occupied by a round nucleus. Some spermatogonia have a homogeneously heterochromatic nucleus and multiply infrequently. They have to be considered as a population of reserve cells. Others have a euchromatic nucleus and multiply mitotically. In part of their offspring, the nucleus tends to revert to a heterochromatic condition. These spermatogonia are destined to grow into primary spermatocytes. Cell division in spermatogonia is often incomplete, resulting in cytoplasmic bridges between the cells. These bridges may be maintained until the differentiation stage of the spermatids. The existence of these bridges partly explains why spermatogenesis is synchronous in large groups of cells.

Primary spermatocytes (Fig. 4.10.4.) appear by growth of spermatogonia. They are polyhedral cells with a final diameter that is twice that of spermatogonia. The nucleus has grown proportionally and has an extremely variable aspect. This is a direct consequence of the fact that it is the primary spermatocytes that undergo the prophase of the first meiotic division. Prophase I being a complicated, prolonged affair, primary spermatocytes exist for prolonged periods of time and have ample opportunity to accumulate. They are the most conspicuous cells of the seminiferous epithelium, both because they are the largest and because they form several layers. Starting from the zygotene stage, the nucleus shows synaptonemal complexes, each of which corresponds with a section of a coupled homologous chromosome pair. A synaptonemal complex consists of two parallel, dense bands, probably made of chromatin, separated from each other by a translucent space in which a third, more slender parallel band is seen, which is interpreted as a connecting structure. Frequently, synaptonemal complexes appear to be connected to the inner face of the nuclear envelope.

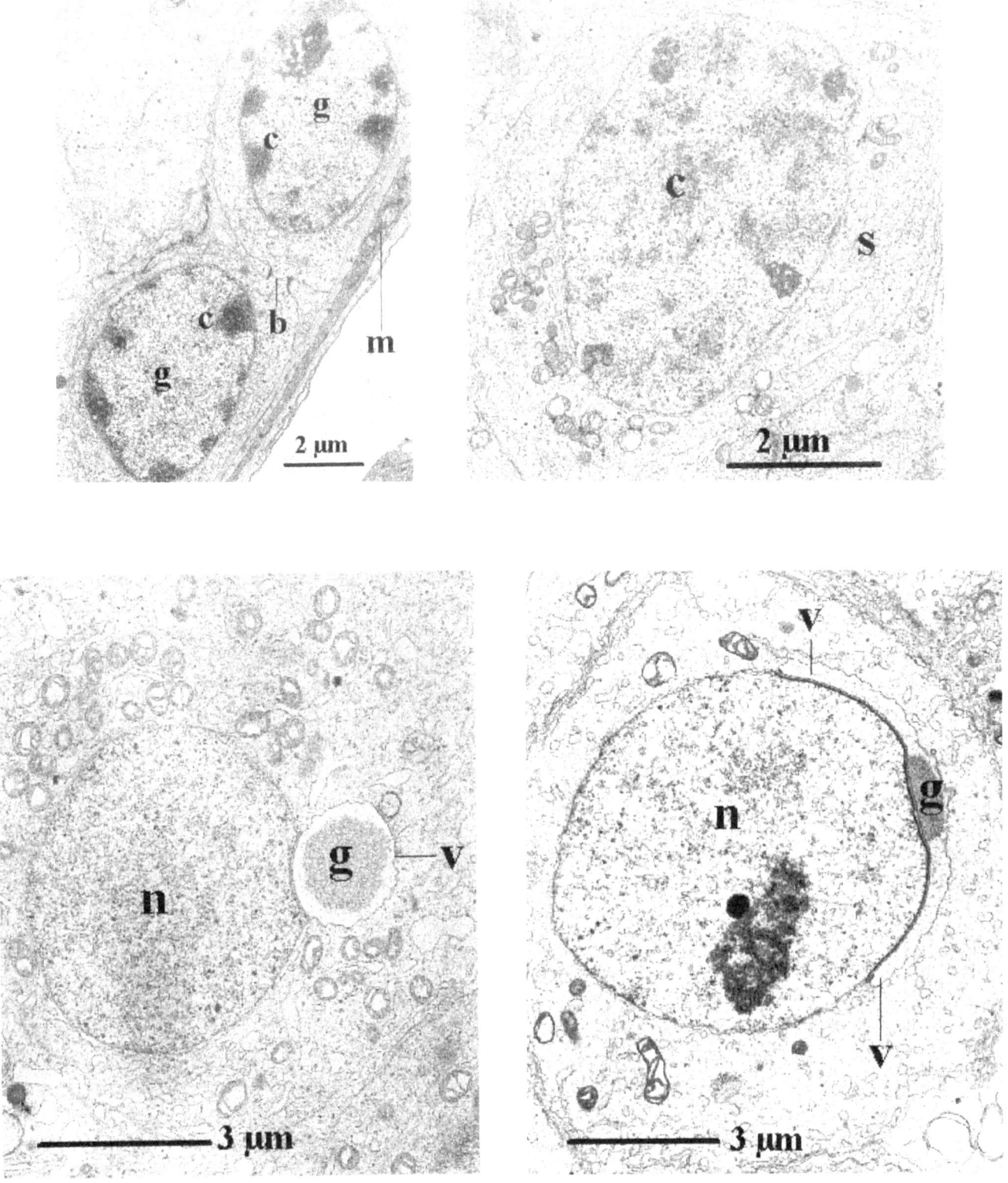

Fig. 4.10.3. (top left) Spermatogonia (g) have little cytoplasm, poor in organelles, a characteristic of undifferentiated cells. Frequently, their mitotic divisions are incomplete, resulting in temporary cytoplasmic bridges, interconnecting them (b). The irregular clumps of chromatin (c) in the nucleus indicate that these particular cells are destined to further differentiation. Beneath the spermatogenic epithelium, a myoid cell is seen (m). Testis, hamster, TEM. **Fig. 4.10.4.** (top right) Primary spermatocytes (s) have abundant cytoplasm. The nucleus contains numerous moderately dense lumps of chromatin (c). Their presence indicates the formation of synaptonemal complexes, in which the partners of homologous chromosome pairs are joined during the prophase of the first meiotic division. Testis, hamster, TEM. **Fig. 4.10.5.** (bottom left) At one of the poles of a spermatid's nucleus (n), an acrosomal vesicle (v) containing a dense acrosomal granule (g), is forming. Testis, hamster, TEM. **Fig. 4.10.6.** (bottom right) In the next stage of development, the acrosomal vesicle (v) flattens, its membrane covering part of the spermatid nucleus (n). The acrosomal granule (g) stays in place. Testis, hamster, TEM.

The first meiotic division produces two secondary spermatocytes from each primary spermatocyte. The **secondary spermatocyte** has a relatively small diameter, about 9 micrometers, as a consequence of the preceding cell division. It almost immediately enters the second meiotic division, which is relatively rapidly completed, so that secondary spermatocytes have no opportunity to accumulate and are infrequently observed. The second meiotic division results in 2 spermatids per secondary spermatocyte, 4 per primary spermatocyte.

When only genetic criteria are taken into account, the **spermatid** is a fully developed gamete, both meiotic divisions having been completed. Functionally, however, the spermatid is still very immature, in the sense that it is not yet able to fertilize an ovum. To be able to do this, the spermatid must be transformed into a motile cell, which is equipped to penetrate into an ovum: a spermatozoon.

The differentiation of a spermatid to a spermatozoon begins with the appearance of secondary organelles: a Golgi-complex and microtubules. The Golgi-complex produces an acrosomal vesicle, which progressively enlarges and in the interior of which an acrosomal granule appears (Fig. 4.10.5.). The acrosomal vesicle migrates towards the nucleus and spreads itself over the nuclear envelope, changing into a flattened vesicle with the acrosomal granule in its center (Fig. 4.10.6.). Together, they form the acrosome. A considerable part of the nuclear surface is covered, in this way, with what amounts to a double membrane. The position of the acrosomal granule determines the anterior nuclear pole. At the posterior pole, a centrosome appears. Its distal centriole, which is oriented at right angles to the nucleus, induces assembly of microtubules, which are arranged in the standard manner of a cilium. Acrosomal granule and distal centriole determine the head-tail axis of the later spermatozoon.

In the course of subsequent differentiation stages, the spermatids orient themselves with their acrosomal granule pointing to the base of the seminiferous epithelium. The cells are stretched along an axis that points towards the tubular lumen and that is determined by the ever-lengthening microtubules. At first, the result is a very elongated cell with an eccentric nucleus. Gradually, the cell membrane will follow ever closer the contours of the cell nucleus and the microtubular bundle, transforming the spermatid into a cell with a head and a flagella, respectively. Meanwhile, a substantial portion of the cytoplasm is shed. The nucleus becomes elongated and undergoes progressive condensation of the chromatin, until it is uniformly heterochromatic. Peripheral to the microtubules of the growing flagella, 9 longitudinal outer dense fibers develop. Distal to the centrosome, where the microtubules originate, the mitochondria fuse, forming a spiral at the periphery of the outer dense fibers. Where the mitochondrial spiral ends, a fibrous sheath is formed at the periphery of the outer dense fibers. This development, form spermatogonia to spermatozoa, has taken about 64 days.

A fully developed **spermatozoon** is a complex, whip-like cell with a length of about 60 micrometers, which shows a head and a flagellum. In its turn, the flagellum can be further subdivided in a neck, a middle piece, a tailpiece, and an end piece (Fig. 4.10.7.).

The **head** (Fig. 4.10.8.) has an ellipsoid contour and is flattened. It is approximately 5 micrometers long, 3 micrometers wide, and 1 micrometer thick. The nucleus is a homogeneously compact chromatin mass, occupying the available space almost completely. The anterior two thirds of the nucleus are covered with the membranous portion of the **acrosome**, while the acrosomal granule occupies the anterior nuclear pole. The posterior nuclear pole is slightly concave, forming the **implantation fossa** of the flagella.

The **neck** is a very short piece (Fig. 4.10.7.). It contains the **capitellum**, a conical, fibrous structure, the basis of which contacts the **basal plate** at the bottom of the implantation fossa. The capitellum looks like some kind of articulation surface between the basal plate and the outer dense fibers of the flagellum. It encloses the centrosome's proximal centriole. The distal centriole has largely degenerated.

The **middle piece** (Fig. 4.10.9.) is about 6 micrometers long and has a diameter of about 1 micrometer. From the center towards the periphery, it contains the characteristically arranged **microtubules**, the nine **outer dense fibers**, and spirally arranged **mitochondria**. In sections, the outer dense fibers have a teardrop shape, oriented with their points towards the flagellum's center.

The **tailpiece** (Fig. 4.10.9.) is about 45 micrometers long and slightly more slender than the middle piece. The microtubules in the center are surrounded by seven, not nine, outer dense fibers, which are surrounded, in their turn, by a **fibrous sheath**. The fibrous sheath is made up of circumferential fibrous rings. On both sides of the flagellum, the fibrous sheath is thickened, forming a **longitudinal column**. It will be remembered that the nucleus is flattened, defining a dorsoventral plane. One longitudinal column lays dorsally, the other ventrally. They partition the tailpiece in two longitudinal, lateral compartments, one of which contains three outer dense fibers, the other four. It is assumed that the longitudinal columns represent the missing two outer dense fibers.

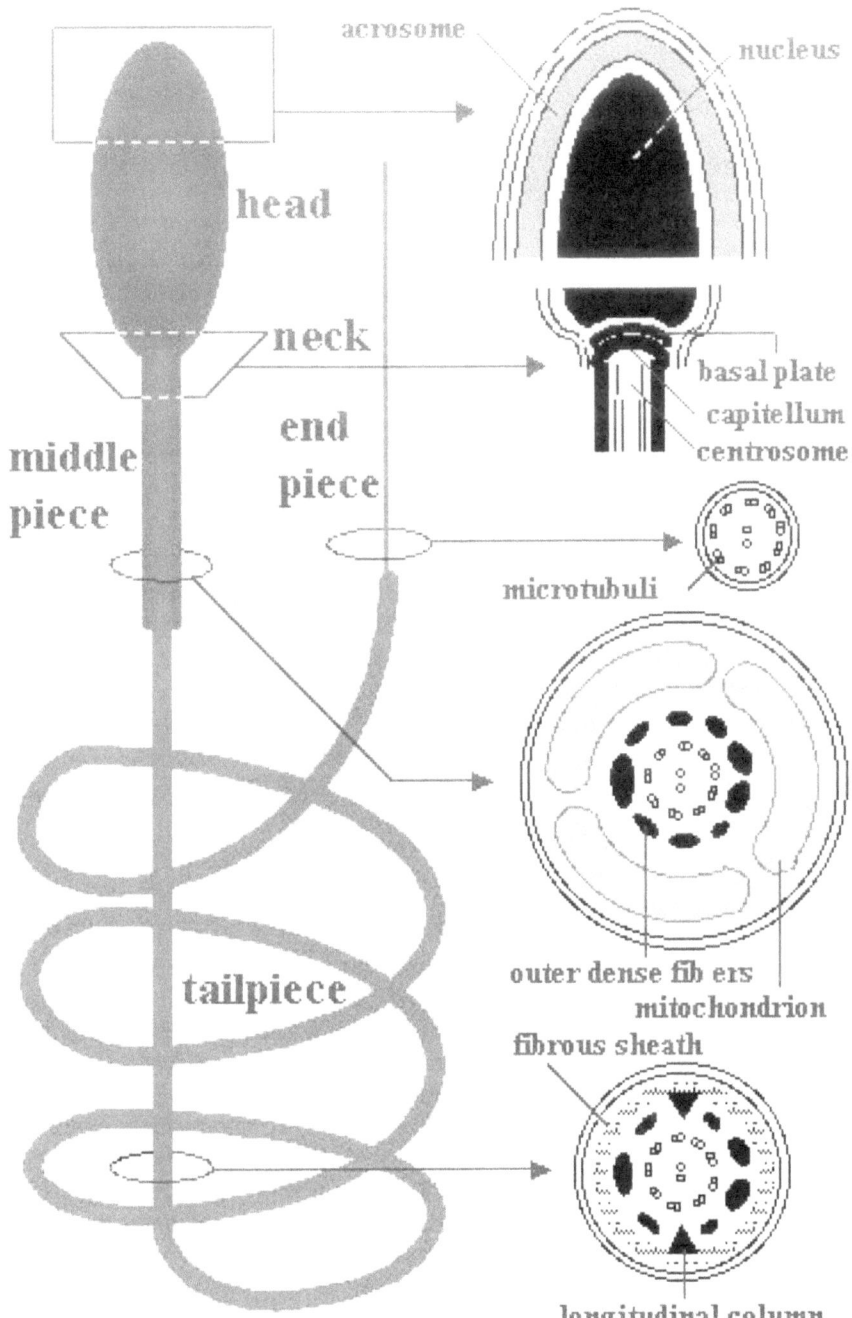

acrosome

nucleus

head

neck

basal plate
capitellum
centrosome

middle
piece

end
piece

microtubuli

tailpiece

outer dense fibers
mitochondrion
fibrous sheath

longitudinal column

Fig. 4.10.7. A spermatozoon has a head and a tail. The tail includes a neck, a middle piece, a tailpiece, and an end piece. The head is little more than a dense, extremely heterochromatic nucleus, its apex covered with the acrosome. At its base, the nucleus is concave. In the neck lie a centrosome, which gives rise to the microtubules of the tail, and a capitellum, which functions as the basis of the other fibrillar components of the tail. The middle piece contains a central ring of microtubules in the characteristic arrangement of a cilium (Figure 2.37.), surrounded by a ring of outer dense fibers (mark their variable sizes and asymmetric arrangement) and a spiral mitochondrion. In the tailpiece, the mitochondrion is no longer present. In its place is found a fibrous sheath, composed of 2 longitudinal columns with a triangular cross section. The end piece has the same structure as a cilium.

The **end piece** (Fig. 4.10.9.) is only about 5 micrometers long, very slender, and contains nothing but the microtubular bundle. Thus, its structure is identical to that of a cilium.

The spermatozoon is one of the most specialized cell types of the body. It is little more than a dense, streamlined lump of genetic material, the head, propelled by an outboard motor, the flagellum. Once deposited in the female genital tract, the spermatozoa have to travel upstream in order to have a slight chance to meet an ovum, which is moved in the opposite direction. This voyage may take a few days. The flagellum beats back and forth in the same dorsoventral plane, which is determined by the flattening of the head and the position of the longitudinal columns. The asymmetric structure of the tail piece, a consequence of the uneven number of outer dense fibers, may explain why the flagellum beats more powerfully in one direction than in the other. As in a cilium, the active movements of the flagellum originate in the microtubules, while energy is supplied by the mitochondrial spiral. The dense outer fibers and the fibrous sheath are probably reinforcing elements. Only few spermatozoa succeed in reaching an ovum. Their ordeal is not yet over. In order to fertilize the ovum, they have to break a number of barriers. The ovum is

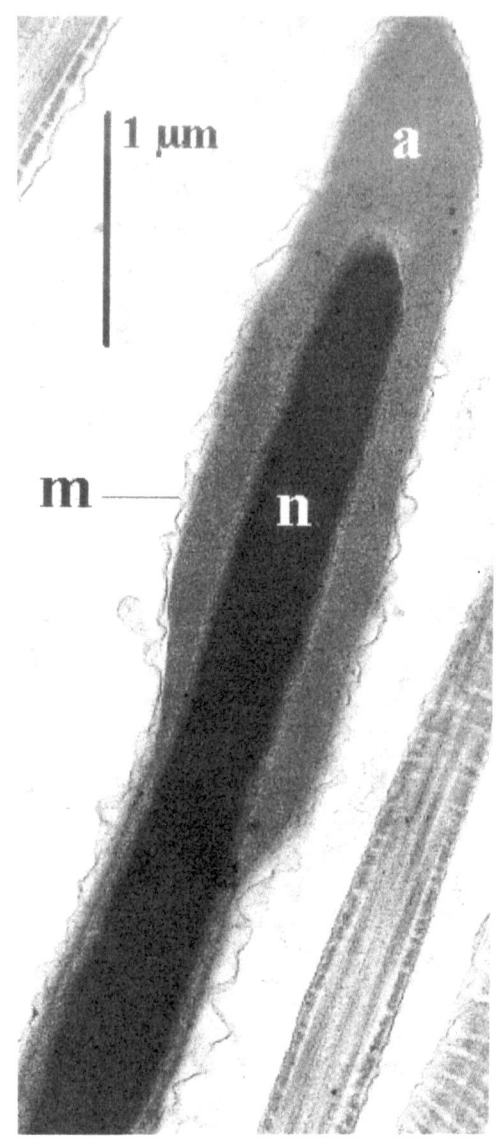

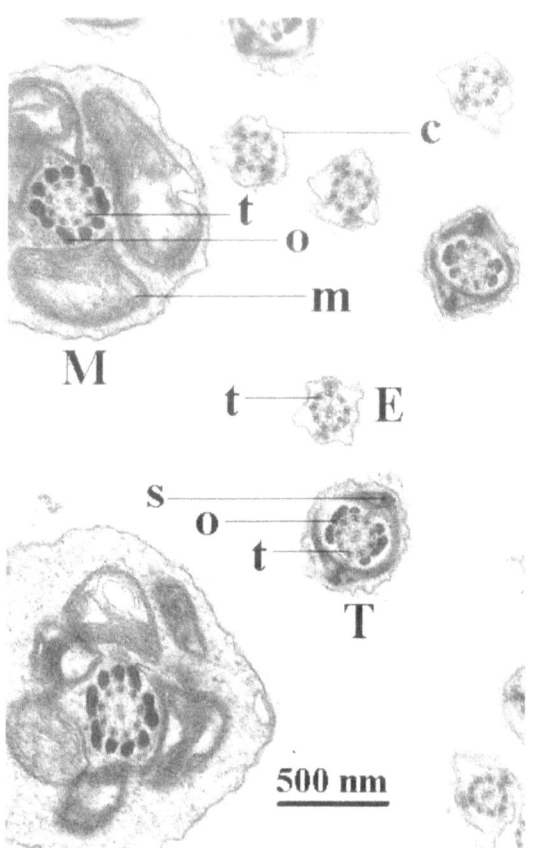

Fig. 4.10.8. (left) The flattened head of a spermatozoon, with its extremely heterochromatic nucleus (n), its apex covered by an acrosome (a). m = cell membrane. Spermatozoon, hamster, TEM. **Fig. 4.10.9.** (above) The middle piece (m), tail piece (t), and end piece (e) of spermatozoa, in cross section (compare with Figure 4.10.7.). Starting in the center, the middle piece contains a ring of microtubules (t), a ring of outer dense fibers (o), and a spiral mitochondrion (m). The tailpiece contains, starting in the center, a ring of microtubules (t), a ring of outer dense fibers (o), and a fibrous sheath with the longitudinal columns (s). The end piece only contains a microtubular ring (t). c = cell membrane. Spermatozoa, hamster, TEM.

enveloped by an acellular zona pellucida and a cellular corona radiata. It is only now that the acrosome comes into play. It contains hydrolytic enzymes, which are liberated by exocytosis, and by means of which the cells of the corona radiata can be detached and the zona pellucida degraded. Finally, the cell membrane of the spermatozoon's head fuses with the ovum's cell membrane. The nucleus, as well as the flagellar cytoplasm, penetrates into the ovum's cytoplasm.

IV.10.1.1.3. Sertoli's cells.

Sertoli's cells are relatively high, pyramidal cells, which rest on the basement membrane of the seminiferous epithelium. Their apex extends towards the lumen of the seminiferous tubule (Fig. 4.10.2.). They have a large, ellipsoid, euchromatic nucleus. In the light microscope, their cytoplasm is not conspicuous. The spermatids and the heads of the developing spermatozoa are closely associated with the apices of the Sertoli's cells.

The contours of the Sertoli cells are extremely wavy: the cell membrane closely follows the contours of the adjacent spermatogenetic cells. Sertoli's cells touch at their lateral cell membranes and at the ends of long processes. They are joined by means of gap, tight, and adhering junctions. Tight junctions are more numerous at the basal cell pole, the other types predominate at the apical cell pole. These junctions create the blood testis barrier: substances from the blood do not freely penetrate into the seminiferous tubule lumen and vice versa. The barrier is situated between the spermatogonia and pre-meiotic spermatocytes, and the other spermatogenic cell types. An obvious function of the barrier is to seal off the central compartment of the

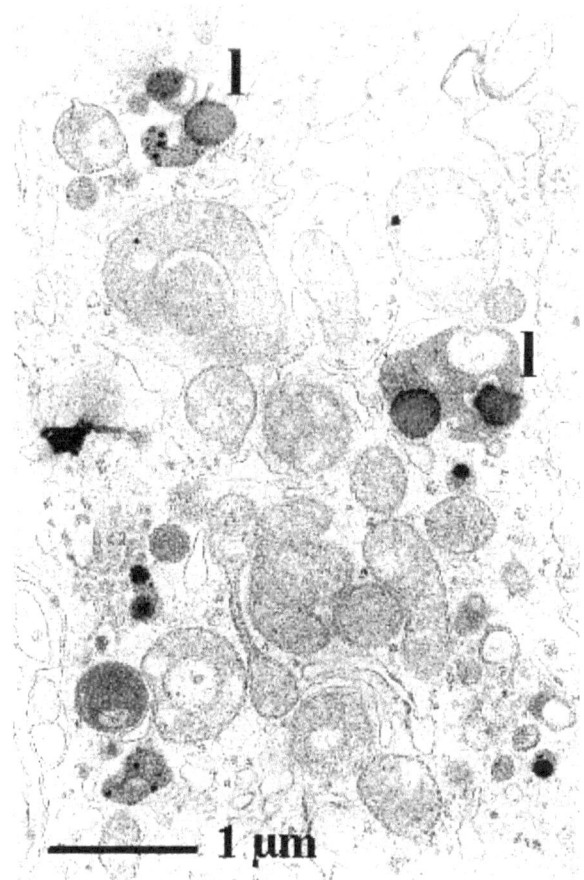

rich in smooth endoplasmic reticulum, particularly so at the periphery. This may indicate that Sertoli cells secrete hormones that regulate spermatogenesis. They probably regulate the transfer of food substances to the spermatogenetic cells, since the seminiferous epithelium is avascular. They also phagocytose and degrade the cytoplasm shed by the spermatids.

IV.10.1.2. Interstitium.

In the testicular interstitium, as well as in the mediastinal fibrous tissue, groups of **Leydig's cells** are frequently encountered (Figs. 4.10.1., 4.10.11., 2.28.). These cells have the typical cytological structure of endocrine, steroid hormone-secreting gland cells (II.2.1.5.2.). Human Leydig cells may contain a proteinaceous, crystalloid inclusion, Reinke's crystal.

Leydig's cells synthesize and secrete **testosterone**, the male sex hormone. Testosterone stimulates spermatogenesis and induces development of the secondary male sexual characteristics. They are hormonally stimulated by the gonadotroph cells of the anterior pituitary and inhibit the hypothalamus by means of testosterone.

Fig. 4.10.10. Sertoli cells function, among others, as macrophages: their cytoplasm contains phagosomes and secondary lysosomes (l). Testis, hamster, TEM.

seminiferous tubules, which contain haploid cells (spermatids and spermatozoa) and to separate it from the peripheral compartment, where those cells reside which are still diploid. Haploid cells may not contain the same combinations of genes as the ordinary diploid cells of the body. There is a chance that their presence will alarm the immune system. Some forms of male infertility may have such an autoimmune reaction as their ultimate cause, the consequence of a defective blood testis barrier. The junctions are flexible, however. Occasionally they come apart, enabling an underlying spermatogenetic cell to shift towards the lumen, and then close again. This system works like a sluice, allowing passage of cells and at the same time ensuring the integrity of the barrier.

The Sertoli cell cytoplasm is rich in filaments, smooth endoplasmic reticulum and lipid droplets, and phagosomes or secondary lysosomes (Fig. 4.10.10.). Thus, Sertoli's cells show a mixture of characteristics of membrane-bearing and fiber-bearing cells. The intracellular filaments reinforce them, allowing them to function as supportive cells to the seminiferous epithelium. The apical cytoplasm, which is deeply indented with the heads of developing spermatozoa, is

IV.10.1.3. Intratesticular ducts.

The seminiferous tubules are drained by short **straight tubules** or tubuli recti (Fig. 4.10.11.), one for each testicular lobule. The straight tubules branch and merge, forming a complex network, the **rete testis** (Fig. 4.10.12.), in the mediastinum. Both tubules and rete are lined with a simple cuboidal epithelium, the cells of which carry a few microvilli and a single cilium. The cytoplasm contains few secondary organelles. In the underlying fibrous tissue, the lamina propria, myoid cells are found. It is assumed that the epithelial cilia, as well as the myoid cells, contribute to the propulsion of the intraluminal liquid, in which spermatozoa are suspended.

IV.10.2. Extratesticular ducts.

The rete testis is drained by about ten **efferent ductules** (Fig. 4.10.13.), which form the cranial part of the epididymis.

Their epithelium is simple, and consists of groups of prismatic cells, alternated with groups of cuboidal cells. Consequently, the epithelium's outer perimeter is smooth, the inner one undulates. Both cell types

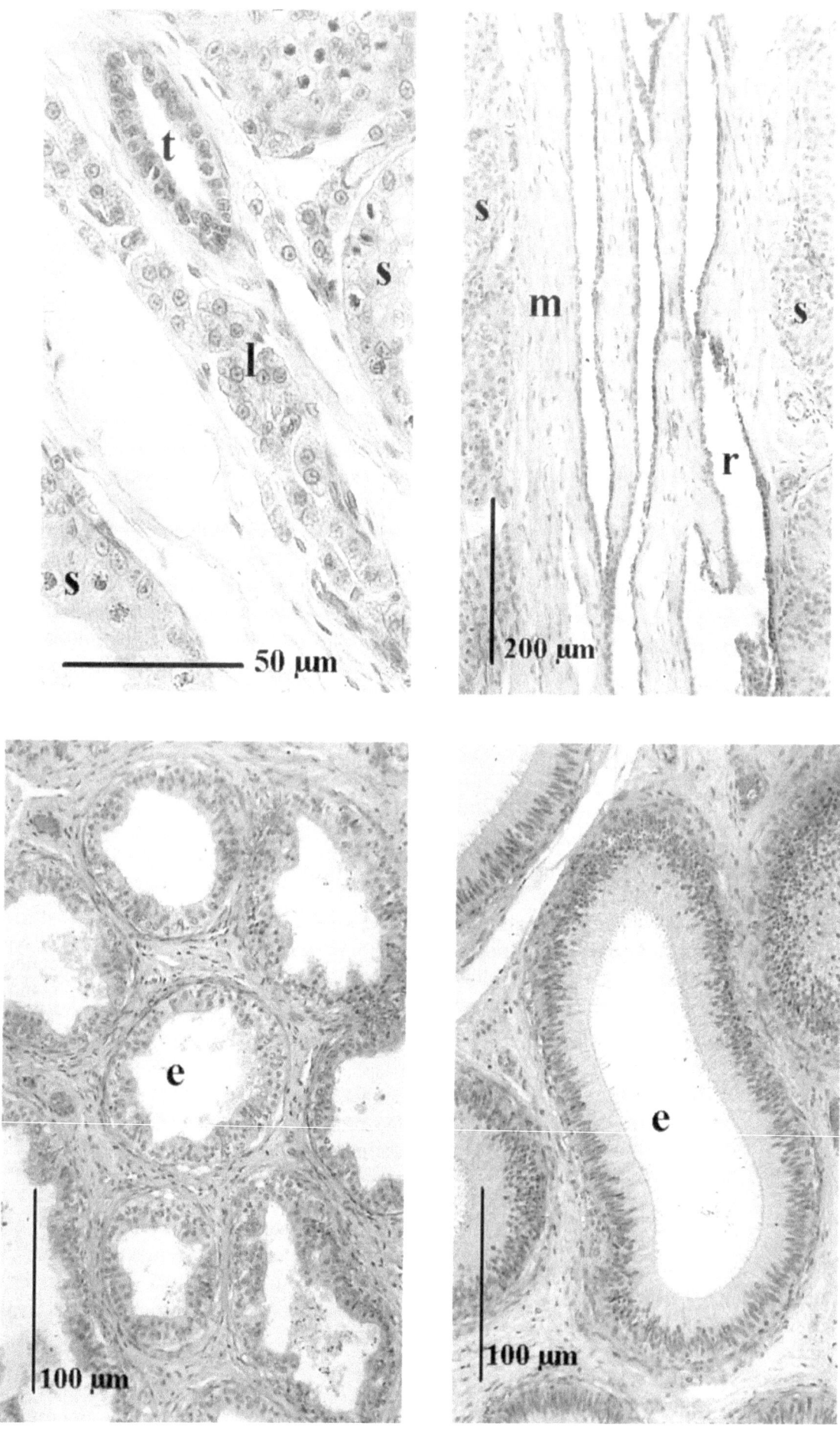

Fig. 4.10.11. (top left) Spermatozoa are conducted through the straight tubules (t), which enter the testicular mediastinum. The wall of these ducts is a simple cuboidal epithelium. Numerous Leydig cells (l) are observed, with the vacuolated cytoplasm that is typical for steroid-secreting endocrine cells. s = seminiferous tubules. Testis, cat, HE. **Fig. 4.10.12.** (top right) The straight tubules merge into a network of ducts in the testicular mediastinum, the rete testis (r). The mediastinum (m) is dense fibrous tissue. s = walls of seminiferous tubules. Testis, cat, HE. **Fig. 4.10.13.** (bottom left) From the rete testis, the spermatozoa are conducted into the efferent ductules (e), which form the head of the epididymis. Their epithelium is characteristically undulating, since it consists of groups of tall cells that alternate with groups of low cells. Epididymis, human, HE. **Fig. 4.10.14.** (bottom right) The efferent ductules merge into a single epididymal duct (e). This duct has a characteristic epithelium: it is pseudostratified, with very tall prismatic cells of equal height, equipped with stereocilia. See Figure 3.4.8. for a detailed view of the epithelium. Epididymis, human, HE.

contain apical inclusions. The majority of the prismatic cells are ciliated, while most of the cuboidal cells carry a brush border. The brush border cells contain the largest numbers of inclusions. These assume different shapes: relatively large membranous spaces and smaller vesicles with a variably opaque content. The first are most likely endosomes, the second lysosomes. In addition, the rough endoplasmic reticulum and the Golgi-complex are fairly well developed. Thus, the brush border cells show characteristics of macrophages.

The efferent ductules are the first testicular duct segment where the lamina propria contains smooth muscle fibers.

The efferent ductules conduct spermatozoa to the epididymis. This transport depends on various mechanisms. The ciliated cells propel the luminal fluid with their ciliary movements. The non-ciliated cells absorb fluid and particles, inducing a fluid stream that originates in the seminiferous tubules, carrying spermatozoa with it. The ciliated cells may possess secondary absorptive properties and contribute to this mechanism. The smooth muscle cells generate peristaltic waves, which propel the luminal fluid.

The efferent ductules drain into a single, very long (meters), intensively convoluted duct, which forms the rest of the epididymis, the **epididymal duct** (Fig. 4.10.14.).

The epididymal duct is lined with a pseudostratified epithelium (Fig. 3.4.8.). Its functional, prismatic cells carry very long (tens of micrometers), light optically visible microvilli, called **stereocilia**. The epithelium's height and the length of the stereocilia are maximal at the beginning of the epididymal duct and decrease progressively further on. The cytoplasm contains variably dense apical vesicles, which are probably lysosomes, a strongly developed Golgi-complex, as well as smooth and rough endoplasmic reticulum. The basal cells predominantly contain primary organelles. Smooth muscle fibers occur in large numbers, and form a distinct musculosa underneath the lamina propria. It is relatively thin at the beginning of the epididymal duct, but thickens progressively.

The initial segment of the epididymal duct is absorptive, contributing to the transport of spermatozoa. The more terminal segments form a reservoir for temporary storage of spermatozoa during the final stages of their maturation. It is during this stay that they acquire active motility. In all probability, the epithelium secretes substances that promote their maturation. The musculosa shows peristaltic contractions.

The **ductus deferens** (Fig. 4.10.15.) has the same epithelium, be it somewhat lower and less distinctly pseudostratified, as the epididymal duct. The lamina propria is rich in elastic fibers. The musculosa is very thick (more than a millimeter) and consist of multiple layers: a circular layer sandwiched between an inner and an outer longitudinal layer. The ductus deferens, like the epididymal duct, is a reservoir of spermatozoa. In contrast to the epididymal duct, the musculosa is densely innervated by adrenergic motor nerve fibers (Fig. 4.10.16.), and contracts with great force upon neural stimulation. This results in ejaculation, the forceful expulsion of luminal fluid, carrying spermatozoa, through the urethra. The final segment of the ductus deferens is called the ejaculatory duct.

IV.10.3. Accessory glands.

The most important accessory glands are the **seminal vesicles** and the **prostate gland.**, which empty into the ductus deferens. The accessory glands produce viscous fluids, in which the spermatozoa are suspended. This suspension is sperm or semen. The fluids contribute to the protection of the spermatozoa once they have been deposited in the female genital tract, and have other functions that aid them in their task.

IV.10.3.1. Seminal vesicles.

Both seminal vesicles have to be regarded as an outpocketing of the ductus deferens, partitioned into lobes by means of fibrous tissue septa. Although spermatozoa may be seen in its lumen, the seminal vesicle, in contrast to the epididymal duct and the ductus deferens, does not store them. The epithelium

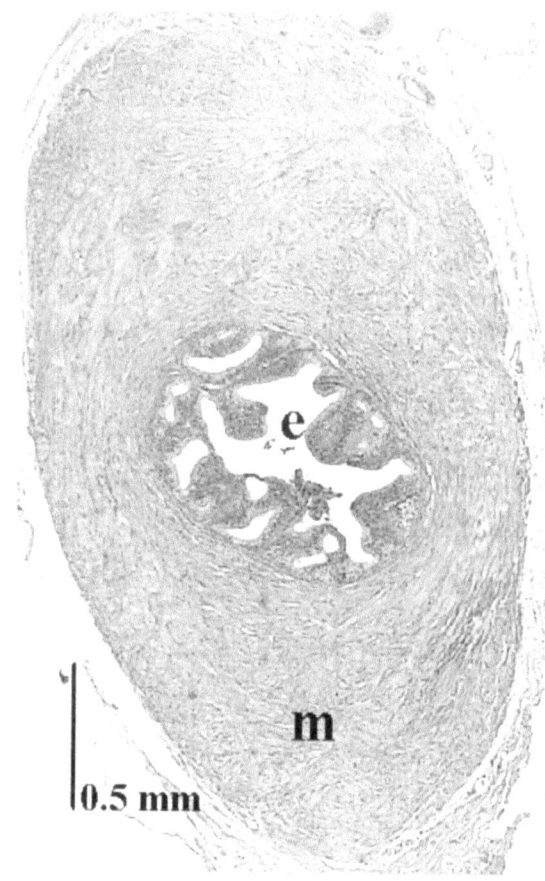 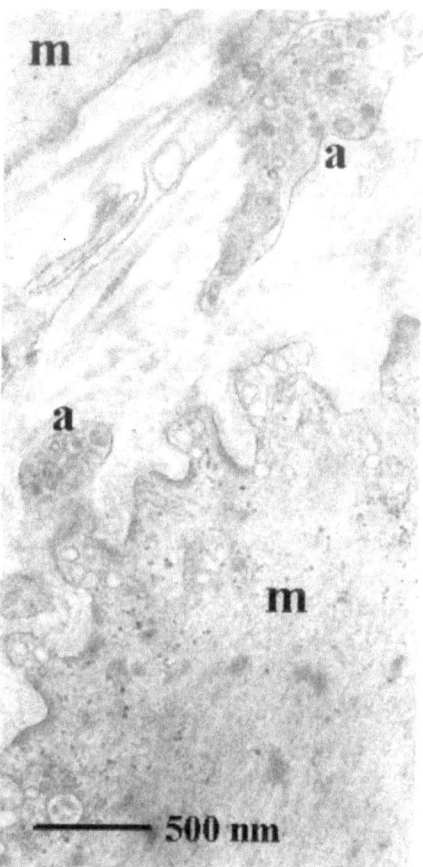

Fig. 4.10.15. (left) The ductus deferens has, in principle, the same epithelium (e) as the epididymal duct, be it that it is less tall. There is a prominent muscularis (m) of visceral muscle tissue. Ductus deferens, dog, HE. **Fig. 4.10.16.** (right) Between the smooth muscle fibers (m) of the muscularis of the ductus deferens run adrenergic nerve fibers (a) of the autonomic nervous system, characterized by dense synaptic vesicles. Ductus deferens, hamster, TEM.

is pseudostratified (III.4.1.3.2.) and its functional, prismatic cells have the cytological structure of protein-secreting cells. In addition, these cells have distinctive phagocytic properties. They produce a basic, viscous secretion with a very complex composition. The basic properties of this fluid may help to temporarily neutralize the acid environment of the vagina, promoting the survival of spermatozoa. The fluid also contains carbohydrates, such as fructose, and prostaglandins. Fructose is an energy source for the spermatozoa. Prostaglandins induce contraction of the smooth musculature of the female genital tract, which may stimulate internalization of spermatozoa. There is a well-developed musculosa with an inner circular and an outer longitudinal layer of smooth muscle fibers. The motor innervation of the musculosa is dense, and it contracts forcefully during ejaculation.

IV.10.3.2. Prostate gland.

The prostate gland is a relatively complex organ, which is in fact made up of three different glands, concentrically arranged around the urethra. It is enveloped in a fibro-elastic capsule, which forms a number of incomplete septa, partitioning the organ in some fifty lobes. The septal fibrous tissue and the interstitial tissue enveloping the glandular tissue are rich in smooth muscle fibers (Fig. 4.10.17.). This mixture of glandular tissue with visceral muscle tissue, resulting in a musculo-glandular organ, is very characteristic and fairly unique to the prostate gland. During ejaculation, this visceral muscle tissue contracts.

The majority of the prostatic glands are of the compound tubulo-acinar type (III.5.1.). The principal glands occupy the peripheral two thirds of the prostate gland. They drain into the urethra through some 20 long ducts. The submucosal or inner periurethal glands occupy the inner third of the prostate. They have short ducts. The very small mucosal or inner periurethal glands are in fact sessile glands, which drain directly into the urethra.

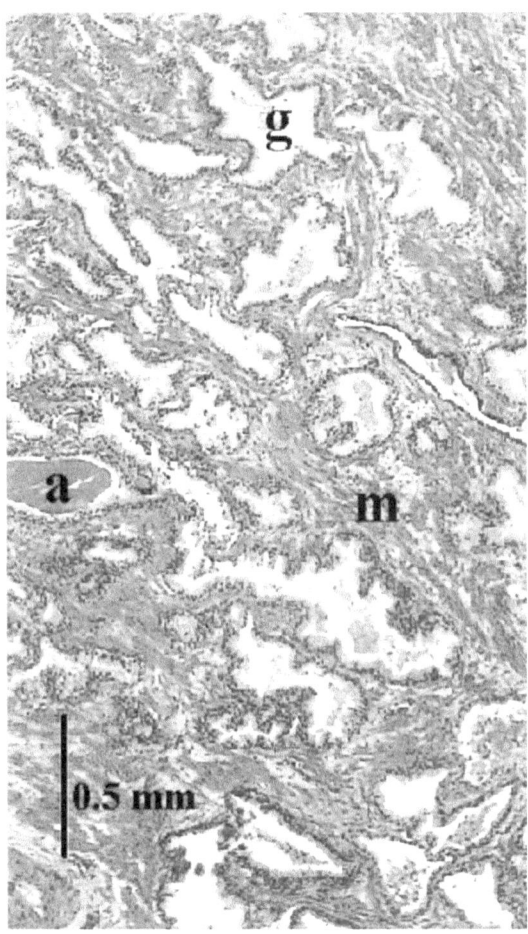

Fig. 4.10.17. The prostate's glandular tissue (g) consists of irregular secretory units, interwoven with visceral muscle tissue (m). In a few places, the glandular lumen contains corpora amylacea (a). Prostate gland, human, HE.

The glandular epithelium is wavy, consisting of cells of variable height. The cells have the cytological structure of enzyme-secreting gland cells (II.2.1.1.1.). Their secretion is a thin, milky fluid, rich in glycoproteins, which constitutes about half of the ejaculate's volume. It also contains citrate, which the spermatozoa can utilize as an energy source, various proteolytic enzymes, and fibrinolysin, which counteracts clumping and clotting of the ejaculate. With increasing age, condensed masses appear in this secretion, which show layering and may calcify: corpora amylacea or prostatic liths (Fig. 4.10.17.). Occasionally, the epithelium contains endocrine cells of the polarized type, with basal secretory granules. The ductal epithelium is not clearly different from that of the secretory units. Close to their mouths, the ducts are lined with transitory epithelium.

IV.10.4. Penis.

The penis consists of three elongated masses of erectile tissue, the cavernous bodies. The unpaired urethral cavernous body lies ventrally and envelops the urethra. The top of the penis, the glans, is a continuation of the urethral cavernous body. The paired and partly fused penile cavernous bodies lie dorsolaterally. The cavernous bodies are enveloped in a dense fibro-elastic capsule. The skin of the penis forms an anterior, circular fold, the prepuce, which covers the glans. Its inside face, as well as the glans, are lined with Malpighian epithelium. The rest of the penis is lined with skin.

The erectile tissue of the cavernous bodies consists of an extensive network of venous sinuses. During sexual stimulation, the arteries supplying these sinuses with blood dilate under neural inhibitory influence. The sinuses then fill with blood and the erectile tissue is inflated. This mechanism is reinforced by compression or constriction of the veins that drain the sinuses. The result is that the penis swells, draws itself up, and becomes rigid, a phenomenon called erection. The erection confers enough rigidity to the penis to enable it to penetrate into the vagina during copulation. The erected penis is the only body part that is supported, not by a bony or cartilaginous skeleton, but by a hydrostatic skeleton. The glans penis, which also shows erection, has a dense sensory innervation.

References.

Griswold M.D.: Interactions between germ cells and Sertoli cells in the testis. Biol. Reprod. 1995, 52: 211-216.

Guraya S.S.: The comparative cell biology of accessory somatic (or Sertoli) cells in the animal testis. Int. Rev. Cytol. 1995, 160: 163-220.

Manandhar G., Simerly C., Schatten G.: Highly degenerated distal centrioles in rhesus and human spermatozoa. Hum. Reprod. 2000, 15: 256-263.

Mata L.R.: Dynamics of the seminal vesicle epithelium. Int. Rev. Cytol. 1995, 160: 267-302.

Noordzij M.A., van Steenbrugge G.J., van der Kwast T.H., Schröder F.H.: Neuroendocrine cells in the normal, hyperplastic and neoplastic prostate. Urol. Res. 1995, 22: 333-341.

Pelletier R.M., Byers S.W.: The blood-testis barrier and Sertoli cell junctions: structural considerations. Microsc. Res. Tech. 1992, 20: 3-33.

Piomboni P.: Microanatomy of the epididymis and vas deferens. J. Submicrosc. Cytol. Pathol. 1997, 29: 583-593.

Prince F.P., Fraser H.M., Mann D.R.: A Reinke-like inclusion within Leydig cells of the marmoset monkey (*Callithrix jacchus*). J. Anat. 1999, 195: 311-313.

Zamboni L.: Sperm structure and its relevance to infertility. Arch. Pathol. Lab. Med. 1992, 116: 325-344.

IV.11. Female reproductive system.

The primary female reproductive organs, which produce female gametes or ova and which secrete the female sex hormones, are the **ovaries**. The female gametes, or ova, are conducted through **oviducts**, in the course of which they may be fertilized. Left and right oviducts distally merge to a muscular organ, the **uterus**, in which a fertilized ovum, already developed into a blastocyst, may be implanted to continue its development. The narrow lower part of the uterus, the **cervix**, opens into the **vagina**. At the mouth of the vagina lie the external genitalia, which constitute the **vulva**. The female reproductive system consists mostly of **epithelium**, mainly of mesodermal origin, which may form exocrine as well as endocrine **glandular tissue**, and **muscle tissue**.

The female reproductive system shows a cyclic activity, with a period of some 28 days. The cycles are marked by menstrual bleeding. Conventionally, a cycle starts on the first day of a menstrual bleeding. Menstrual bleeding is a consequence of the degradation of the uterine mucosa, the endometrium. This happens every time when there is no beginning of pregnancy. During the first half of a menstrual cycle, the endometrium, which was degraded at its beginning, is gradually restored. It grows thicker under the influence of a female sex hormone, **estrogen**, produced in the ovaries: the endometrium shows a proliferative, or growth phase. In the ovaries, estrogen is produced by the ovarian **follicles**, a tissue closely associated with developing ova: parallel to the endometrial growth phase, there is a follicular phase in the ovaries. The follicles develop under the influence of the gonadotroph cells of the anterior pituitary, which produce follicle-stimulating hormone. When the menstrual cycle is about half way, follicular development is complete, and the ovum is set free, a phenomenon called **ovulation**. It is collected in an oviduct's mouth and conducted towards the uterus. It may be fertilized during this passage. Under the influence of the gonadotrophs of the anterior pituitary, which produce luteinizing hormone, the remaining follicle develops into a **corpus luteum**, an endocrine tissue which secretes another female sex hormone, **progesterone**, in addition to estrogen. Under the influence of progesterone, the endometrium starts to secrete various substances and prepares itself for the eventual implantation of a blastocyst. Postovulatory, the endometrium thus shows a secretory phase, parallel to the ovarian luteal phase. The corpus luteum is under the control of the gonadotrophs, which secrete luteinizing hormone. If the ovum has been fertilized and if the blastocyst succeeds in implanting itself, a pregnancy begins. The blastocyst produces hormones that will further stimulate the corpus luteum and induces the endometrium enveloping the blastocyst to develop into a decidua. The decidua will be contacted by the placenta, which will take over the hormonal production of the corpus luteum. The endometrium remains intact and a menstrual bleeding will not occur. The menstrual cycle has been interrupted. If fertilization does not occur, or if implantation of the blastocyst fails, there will be no hormonal stimuli to keep the corpus luteum going. This means that the endometrium cannot be maintained. It is degraded, which causes a menstrual bleeding, starting the next cycle.

VI.11.1. Ovaries.

The ovaries are ellipsoid organs, enveloped with a dense fibrous tunica albuginea, lined with mesothelium (Fig. 4.11.1.). Internally, an ovary consists of a well-developed cortex, incompletely delineated from a much less prominent medulla. The cortex consists of a very cellular interstitial tissue, cytogenic stroma (Fig. 4.11.11.). Embedded in this stroma, numerous **follicles** (Fig. 4.11.1.) are found, each of which contains an ovum. The medulla contains blood vessels, lymph vessels, nerve fibers and a number of interstitial cells. These have the typical cytological structure of endocrine, steroid-secreting gland cells and produce female sex hormones. They already mature in the fetal ovaries and play their most important part before the onset of puberty, when their hormonal activity contributes to the development of the body and the ovaries. During the time of sexual maturity, they are much less numerous. Their continual activity contrasts them with the cortical endocrine cell types, the activities of which are cyclic, and in phase with the menstrual cycle.

IV.11.1.1. Meiosis, oogenesis, and fertilization.

As it is in spermatogenesis, meiosis is an essential part of oogenesis, the production of ova. There are, however, a few differences. The most primitive ovum precursors are the **oogonia**. In the fetal ovaries, they multiply mitotically, but only until the sixth month of fetal development. Then, they enter the first meiotic division, and at this stage they can be regarded as **primary oocytes**. The entire stock of oogonia enters the first meiotic division, so that none of them remain. This is the first difference with spermatogenesis, where the testes continue to maintain a stock of spermatogonia. The first meiotic division progresses as far as the diplotene, then it is halted. At birth, the

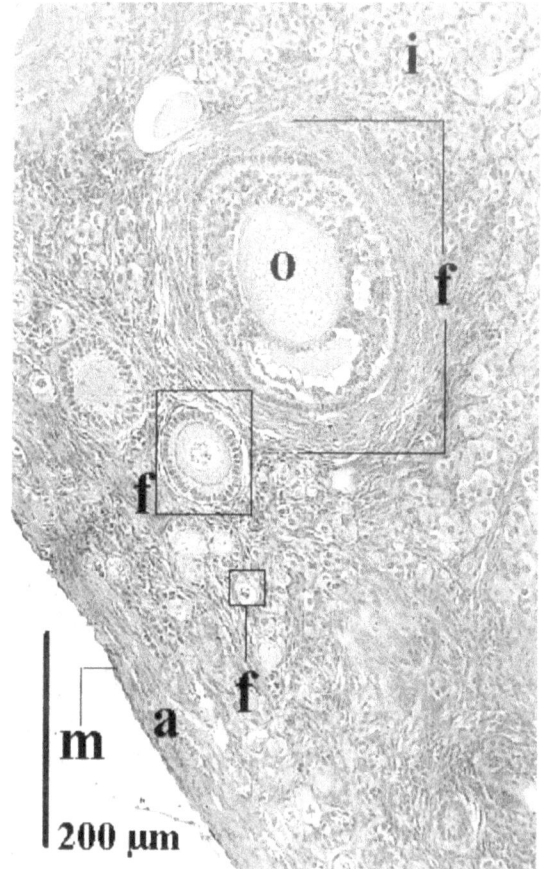 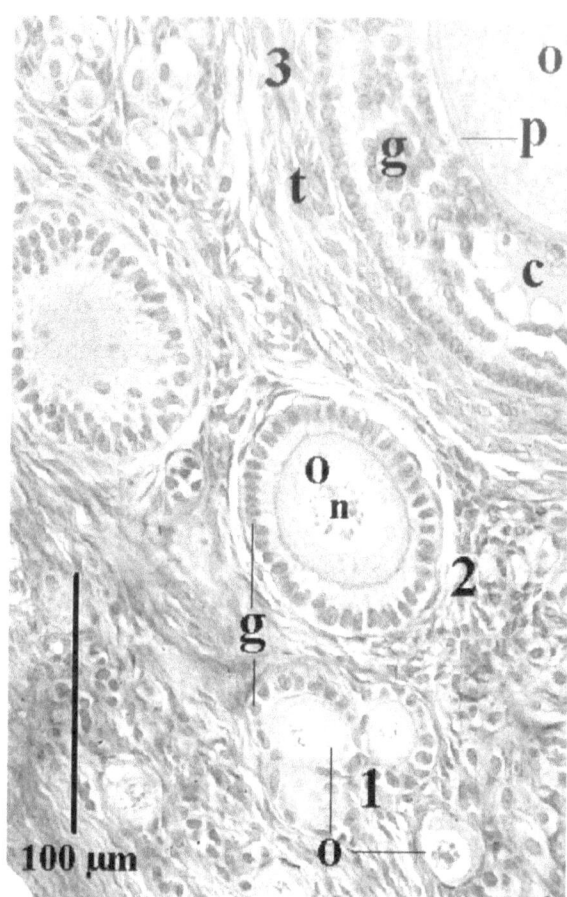

Fig. 4.11.1. (left) The ovarian cortex contains follicles (f) in various stages of development. Each follicle contains a ripening ovum (o). Apart from follicles, large numbers of interstitial cells (i) are seen, which produce the female sex hormone estrogen. The dense fibrous tunica albuginea (a) is lined with mesothelium (m). Ovary, rabbit, HE. **Fig. 4.11.2.** (right) The most primitive ovarian follicles are the primordial follicles (1). The comparatively minute ovum (o) is encased in a single layer of flattened granulosa cells. Somewhat more developed primordial follicles have cuboidal granulosa cells (g). In growing follicles (2) the ovum's volume has increased considerably, while the enveloping granulosa cells have become prismatic. The ovum contains a prominent nucleolus (n). In the next stage, the ovum has grown larger still, and has developed a prominent "membrane", the zona pellucida (p). Between the granulosa cells, now present in multiple layers, spaces appear, filled with follicular fluid, the Call-Exner bodies (c). This stage is called the cavitary follicle (3). The cavitary follicle is enveloped in a fibrous tissue theca (t). Ovary, rabbit, HE.

ovaries contain hundreds of thousands of these primary oocytes, part of which are lost during childhood. From the onset of puberty onwards, and during each menstrual cycle, a small part of the primary oocytes will continue their development. Usually, only a single one of them will complete its development and be set free at ovulation. This means that, during the entire fertile part of a women's life, a few hundred, at most, ripe ova will be formed, in contrast to the astronomical numbers of spermatozoa produced in the male. Just before ovulation, the first meiotic division is completed, and the single ovum that is set free can be regarded as a **secondary oocyte**. This division is asymmetrical: the oocyte does not divide in two equal halves, but in stead ejects a minuscule **polar body**. The polar body is a miniature daughter cell, which contains one partner of each homologous chromosome pair, but only very little cytoplasm. This mechanism reconciles the necessity of reducing chromosome number with the requirement that most of the ovum's cytoplasm, the later embryo, must be retained. The second meiotic division follows immediately after the first, but it is likewise halted, in the metaphase stage. It is a secondary oocyte that is collected in the oviduct, where it may be fertilized. Strictly speaking, it is an unripe gamete that will be fertilized. Only when fertilization effectively takes place is the second meiotic division completed. A second polar body is ejected, and an **ootid** results. Thus, the result of two meiotic divisions is a single gamete, not four as in the male. The other cells are the three (the first one usually enters the second meiotic division) abortive polar bodies. A final contrast with spermatogenesis is that after this stage, there is no further development:

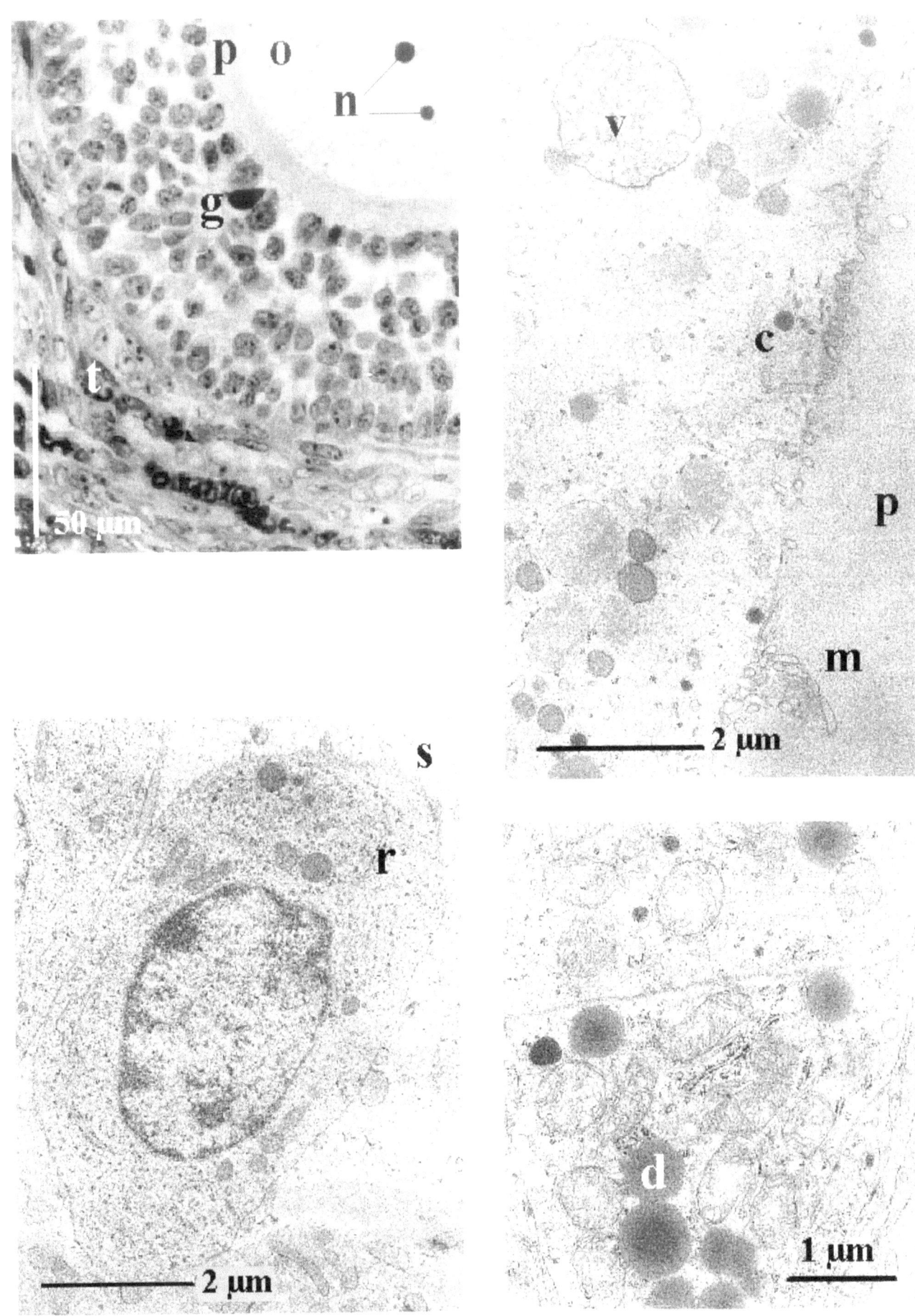

225

Fig. 4.11.3. (top left) A growing follicle, just prior to developing into a cavitary follicle, contains multiple layers of granulosa cells (g), as yet closely joined. The ovum (o) is enveloped in a thick zona pellucida (p). Its cytoplasm is granular. The nucleus has become relatively small as a result of the growth of the cytoplasm, but it is euchromatic and contains 2 dense nucleoli (n). The fibrous tissue sheathing the follicle develops into a vascularized (erythrocytes!) theca (t). Ovary, cat, 1-micrometer plastic section, toluidin blue. Fig. 4.11.4. (top right) The zona pellucida (p) is not a cell membrane at all, but a featureless, extracellular layer separating the ovum (o) from the granulosa cells. The developing ovum forms microvilli (m). It engulfs various materials, resulting in cytoplasmic growth. The presence of multivesicular bodies (v) indicates that certain organelles, which are no longer needed, are being degraded. It already contains a few cortical granules (c), which will undergo exocytosis in the event of fertilization. Ovum, rabbit, TEM. Fig. 4.11.5. (bottom left) Granulosa cells have a rather euchromatic nucleus and ample cytoplasm, rich in ribosomes (r). These are characteristics of metabolically active cells. In between the cells, spaces (s) appear, indicating the accumulation of follicular fluid. Ovarian follicle, rabbit, TEM. Fig. 4.11.6. (bottom right) In this picture, the endocrine cells of the internal theca contain little smooth endoplasmic reticulum (they do contain rough endoplasmic reticulum), but steroid droplets (d) are present. Ovarian follicle, rabbit, TEM.

the ootid is the functional female gamete, the **ovum**. Fertilization occurs during the stage when the ovum is halted in its second meiotic division. When the sperm nucleus enters the cytoplasm, there is a massive exocytotic reaction of the cortical granules (IV.11.1.2.). Their contents interact with the zona pellucida, and a physical block is formed to the penetration of other spermatozoa. The sperm nucleus now lies in the ovum's cytoplasm. It decondenses and a new nuclear envelope appears, giving rise to a male pronucleus. The second meiotic division is completed, and a female pronucleus appears. Both nuclei are closely apposed, and their chromatin recondenses, forming chromosomes, while the nuclear envelopes are broken down. A mitotic spindle is formed, which arranges male-derived and female-derived chromosomes in homologous pairs. The centriole that is at the basis of the spindle has been contributed by the spermatozoon. The ensuing anaphase can be regarded as being part of the first mitotic division of the zygote.

IV.11.1.2. Follicles.

An ovarian follicle consists of an ovum, enveloped by one or more layers of granulosa cells. The granulosa cells form an epithelium, and rest on a basement membrane.

The ovarian cortex contains a large amount of **primordial follicles** (Fig. 4.11.2.). These are the most primitive follicles, containing a primary oocyte, stopped in its tracks in prophase I of meiosis. The primary oocyte is relatively small, having a diameter of about 40 micrometers. The surrounding granulosa cells form a simple squamous epithelium. The oocyte contains predominantly primary organelles: ribosomes and mitochondria. The nucleus lies centrally, is euchromatic, contains a well-developed nucleolus and its envelope has numerous pores, which are characteristics of a metabolically active cell.

During the preovulatory, follicular phase of each menstrual cycle, a number of these primordial follicles, under the influence of follicle stimulating hormone of the anterior pituitary, start a maturation process. Only a single one will normally complete it, the others will drop out at an earlier or a later stage. The granulosa cells grow, becoming cuboidal and later prismatic. They also multiply, and envelop the oocyte with a stratified epithelium. This stage is the **growing follicle** (Figs. 4.11.2.-3.). Since granulosa cell proliferation is more intense on one side of the oocyte than on the other, the oocyte shifts to an eccentric position. The oocyte grows and between it and the granulosa cells appears a translucent "membrane", which eventually reaches a thickness of a few micrometers, the **zona pellucida**. Ultrastructurally, the zona pellucida has a homogeneous, finely granular look (Fig. 4.11.4.).The granulosa cells develop the cytological structure of protein-synthesizing cells (Fig. 4.11.5.). They secrete, among others, glycoproteins, which contribute to building up of the zona pellucida. They are joined with junctions, at first only desmosomes, followed later in development by growing numbers of gap junctions. Those granulosa cells bordering the zona pellucida form apical microvilli, which extend into zona pellucida and may interdigitate with microvilli of the oocyte. Both may be joined with desmosomes. The granulosa cells may even form long, slender processes, which penetrate into the oocyte cytoplasm. The granulosa cells form what amounts to an epithelium, the purpose of which is to seal the developing ovum hermetically from the rest of the body. The oocyte, being on its way to become a haploid cell, differs from the ordinary diploid body cells, and must be shielded from the immune system. In the oocyte of a growing follicle, the smooth and rough endoplasmic reticula and the Golgi-complex start to develop. The Golgi-complex contributes to the formation of the zona pellucida. It also forms the **cortical granules**, which are required at fertilization. These are characterized by their dense content. The oocyte develops microvilli (Fig. 4.11.4.). At the basis

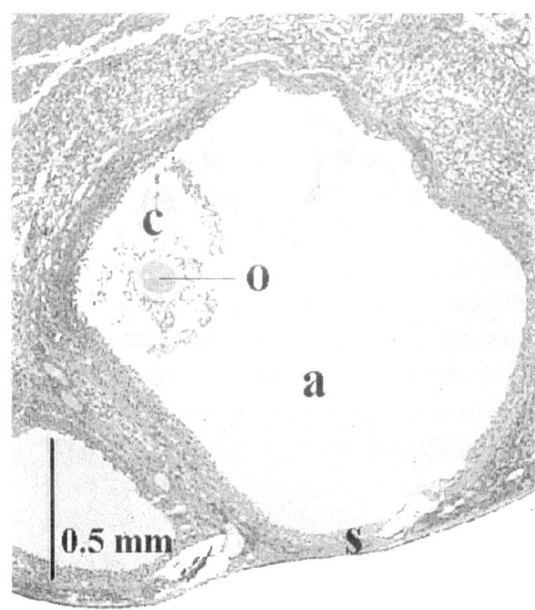

Fig. 4.11.7. In a Graafian follicle, the spaces between the granulosa cells have merged into a single follicular cavity or antrum (a), filled with follicular fluid. The ovum (o) is now relatively minute because of the enormous growth of the follicle. In addition, it now occupies an eccentric position. The bulging granulosa cell mass that holds it is the cumulus oophorus (c). The follicular wall has thinned, especially so at the stigma (s), where it bulges into the abdominal space. This, in combination with the incipient degradation of the cumulus, indicates that ovulation is imminent. Ovary, rabbit, HE.

of the microvilli, pinocytotic vesicles arise. This indicates that the oocyte is actively taking up substances and that the microvilli are the sites of active exchange processes between oocyte and granulosa cells. During development, glycogen granules, protein granules, and lipid droplets accumulate. Various structures appear which can be interpreted as endocytotic vesicles, autophagosomes, and multivesicular bodies (II.2.1.4., Fig. 4.11.4.). The presence of the last two indicates that the oocyte is recycling part of its "old" cytoplasm to build new substances and organelles. As the oocyte develops, unique organelles appear, which are made up of stacks of nuclear envelope membrane, including pores: the **annulate lamellae**. After fertilization, these will be incorporated into the nuclear envelopes of the male and female pronuclei. In the younger oocyte, the organelles tend to cluster around the nucleus, forming the "yolk" nucleus or Balbiani body. As development proceeds, the organelles disperse towards the periphery. This is especially evident in the cortical granules. The number of Golgi-complexes and the amount of rough endoplasmic reticulum decline in maturing oocytes.

In a later stage, the granulosa cells start to secrete a proteinaceous fluid, which accumulates in small cavities: **Call-Exner bodies**. This stage is called a **cavitary follicle** (Fig. 4.11.2.). Gradually, the cytogenic stroma surrounding the follicle develops into a capsule or theca. The fusiform interstitial tissue cells bordering the follicle acquire a cuboidal to polyhedral shape. They develop the cytological structure of endocrine, steroid-secreting gland cells (Fig. 4.11.6.). This endocrine tissue is the **internal theca**. It secretes estrogen, in increasing quantities as the menstrual cycle progresses. The peripheral theca cells develop into matrix-secreting cells and deposit large amounts of collagen fibrils. Thus, an **external theca** is formed. The theca is separated from the granulosa cells by a thick basement membrane, visible in the light microscope, **Slavjanski's glassy membrane**. Contrary to the area of the granulosa cells, the theca is vascularized (Fig. 4.11.3.).

Eventually, all the cavities between the granulosa cells merge into a single central cavity or antrum (Fig. 4.11.7.), bordered by only a few layers of granulosa

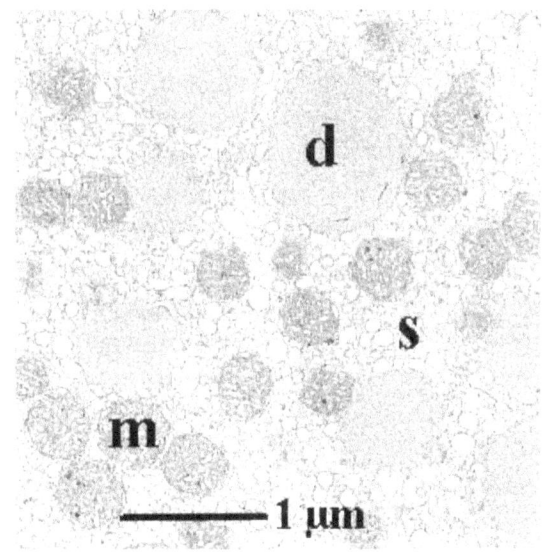

Fig. 4.11.8. Interstitial cells contain smooth endoplasmic reticulum (s), steroid droplets (d), and mitochondria with tubular cristae (m), each of which are characteristic of steroid hormone-secreting endocrine cells. Ovary, rabbit, TEM.

cells. The follicle now has dimensions in the order of a centimeter. The (still primary) oocyte has grown to impressive dimensions, up to 150 micrometers in diameter. It is enveloped in a thick zona pellucida and lies, eccentrically, at the tip of a "peninsula" that bulges into the antrum: the **cumulus oophorus**. It may be separated from the antrum by only a few layers of granulosa cells, often a single one which forms a simple prismatic epithelium, the **corona radiata**. Both the internal and external theca have developed accordingly. This stage, the mature follicle, is the **Graafian follicle**.

Most often, only one Graafian follicle is formed. The others sooner or later interrupt their development and in stead develop into endocrine tissue: **atretic follicles**. In this case, the oocyte and the granulosa cells undergo apoptosis, while the internal theca cells grow in size and number. Their structure of steroid hormone-secreting cells is developed to further extremes and they are called **interstitial cells** (Figs. 4.11.1., 4.11.8.). Follicular atresia not only takes place during the menstrual cycles, but in smaller measure in the prepubertal period and during menopauze. At the end of a cycle, atretic follicles degenerate and their places are taken over by matrix-secreting cells of the stroma. These form fibrous scar tissue, a **corpus fibrosum**.

A Graafian follicle is so large that it forms a clear bulge at the surface of the ovary (Fig. 4.11.7.). When the time of ovulation is near, the granulosa cells produce proteolytic enzymes that locally degrade the follicular wall, the theca and the tunica albuginea. An opening or **stigma** results, through which the oocyte, still enveloped in its zona pellucida and corona radiata, leaves the ovary: ovulation.

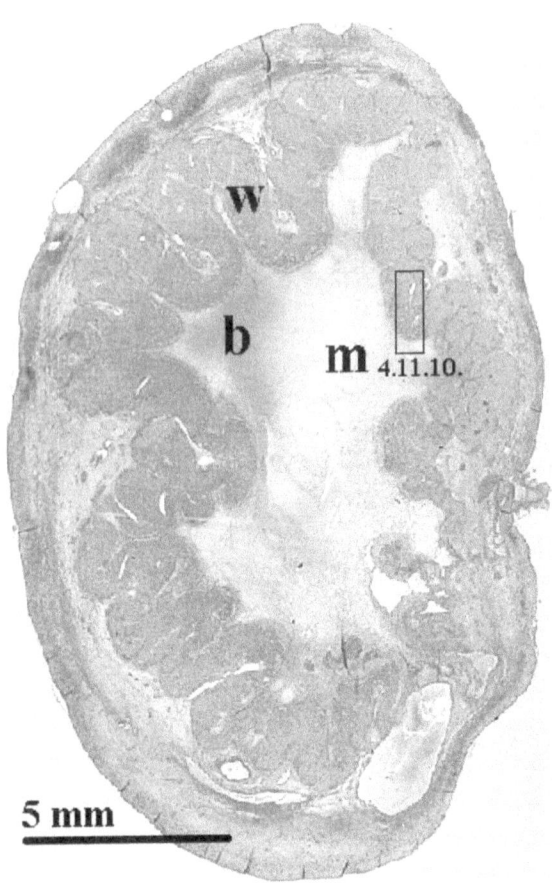

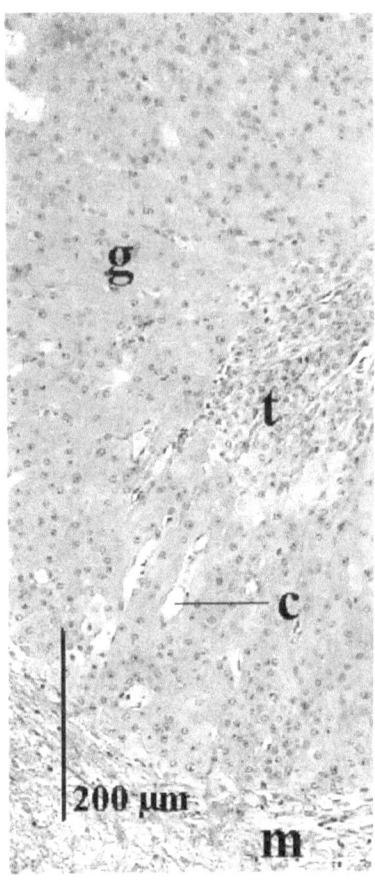

Fig. 4.11.9. (left) After ovulation, what is left of the Graafian follicle develops into an endocrine gland: the corpus luteum. In contrast to the Graafian follicle, its wall (w) is deeply folded, since the follicle has been emptied of follicular fluid. The lumen still contains some blood (b), as a consequence of the wall's rupture during ovulation. Most of the lumen is already occupied by young mesenchymal tissue (m). Both characteristics indicate that the developmental stage reached by this corpus luteum is between a younger corpus rubrum and a fully mature corpus luteum. Ovary, human, HE. **Fig. 4.11.10.** (right) The lumen of the corpus luteum is filled with mesenchymal tissue (m). Its wall is made of a thick, deeper layer of granulosa lutein cells (g) and a thin, peripheral layer of theca lutein cells (t). Granulosa lutein cells are derived from granulosa cells, which have developed into steroid hormone-secreting endocrine cells. This development has been accompanied by vascularization of the original follicular wall: capillaries (c) are now present. The theca lutein cells are derived from theca interna cells, which have not been greatly modified. They are only about half as large as granulosa lutein cells, so that their nuclei are much more densely packed than those of granulosa lutein cells. Corpus luteum, human, HE.

IV.11.1.3. Corpus luteum.

After ovulation, the Graafian follicle, minus the ovum, remains in the ovary and develops into an endocrine tissue, the **corpus luteum** (Fig. 4.11.9.). Initially, the granulosa cells increase in number. Upon rupture of the follicular wall at ovulation, the antrum has emptied and the follicular wall has collapsed. Another consequence of the follicular wall's rupture is bleeding, and the greatly diminished antrum may contain some blood. Therefore, this stage of corpus luteum development may be called corpus rubrum. Soon, this blood is removed by macrophages, and replaced with mesenchymal tissue. The basement membrane, Slavjanski's glassy membrane, is degraded and capillaries penetrate into the hitherto avascular area occupied by the granulosa cells. The granulosa cells gradually change into endocrine, steroid hormone-secreting gland cells (II.2.1.5.2.), characterized by a well-developed smooth endoplasmic reticulum and accumulated lipid droplets. They also accumulate carotene, an orange pigment, with a chemical structure that has a few aspects in common with that of steroids. The granulosa cells are now called **granulosa lutein cells**, or simply lutein cells. The cells of the internal theca, which have increased in number and carried their differentiation to steroid-hormone secreting cells to further extremes, are now called **theca lutein cells**, or paralutein cells. A mature corpus luteum has dimensions in the order of a centimeter or more, and is colored intensively orange-yellow by the presence of carotene. Its deeply infolded wall consists largely of granulosa lutein cells. Peripheral to these, there is a thinner layer of theca lutein cells. The theca lutein cells tend to concentrate in the crypts formed by the infolding of the wall. Granulosa lutein cells are about twice as large as theca lutein cells. Consequently, their nuclei appear more spaced than those of the theca lutein cells (Fig. 4.11.10.). When the oocyte liberated at ovulation is not fertilized or fails to implant, the corpus luteum will degenerate towards the end of the menstrual cycle. The granulosa and theca lutein cells are lost, and the antral mesenchyme is progressively replaced with dense woven fibrous tissue. In the end, a fibrous scar, the **corpus albicans** (Fig. 4.11.11.), is all that remains. When the oocyte is fertilized, develops into a blastocyst and successfully implants in the endometrium, the corpus luteum survives for a longer time. The blastocyst produces a hormone with luteotrope effects, maintaining the corpus luteum until the third month of pregnancy, after which its functions are taken over by the placenta. With dimensions in the order of 2 to 3 centimeters, such a corpus luteum of pregnancy is much bigger than an ordinary menstrual

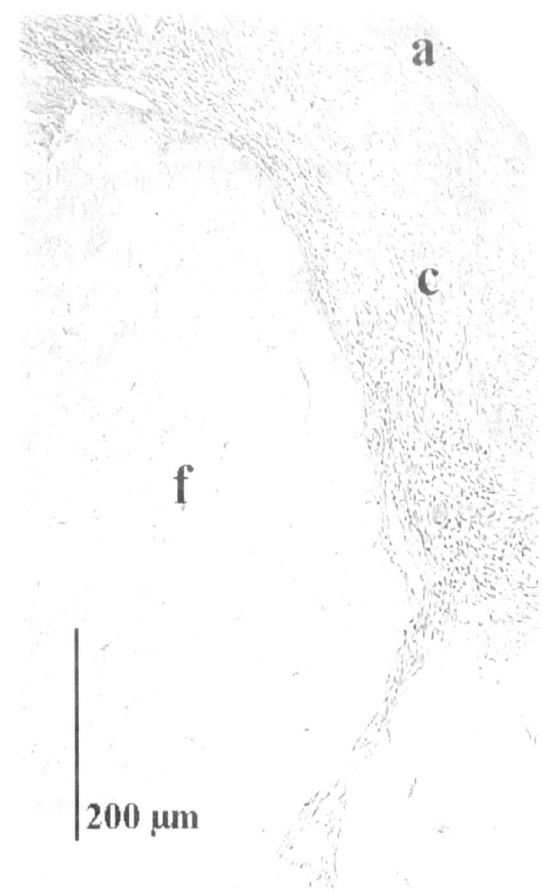

Fig. 4.11.11. The corpus albicans is the final stage in the degeneration of a corpus luteum. The cellular wall of the corpus luteum has disappeared, and the original mesenchymal tissue has been replaced with dense fibrous woven tissue (f). c = cytogenic stroma of the ovarian cortex, a = tunica albuginea. Ovary, human, HE.

corpus luteum. The corresponding corpus albicans is also much bigger and survives for much longer periods of time.

IV.11.2. Oviduct.

The oviduct is a tube with a funnel-like mouth, situated next to an ovary. The rim of this expanded mouth, the **infundibulum**, carries frill-like fimbriae. Behind the infundibulum comes a lengthy, thin-walled segment, the **ampulla**, followed by a short, narrowed, thick-walled segment, the **isthmus**, which contacts the wall of the uterus. The wall of the oviduct consists of a mucosa, a musculosa, and a serosa. The **mucosa** is thrown into a complex, branched pattern of luminal folds, especially so at the level of the ampulla. In cross section, this gives a labyrinthine aspect to the lumen (Fig. 4.11.12.). The epithelium is simple prismatic to pseudostratified and rests on a vascularized, loose fibrous tissue (Fig. 4.11.13.). It is under hormonal

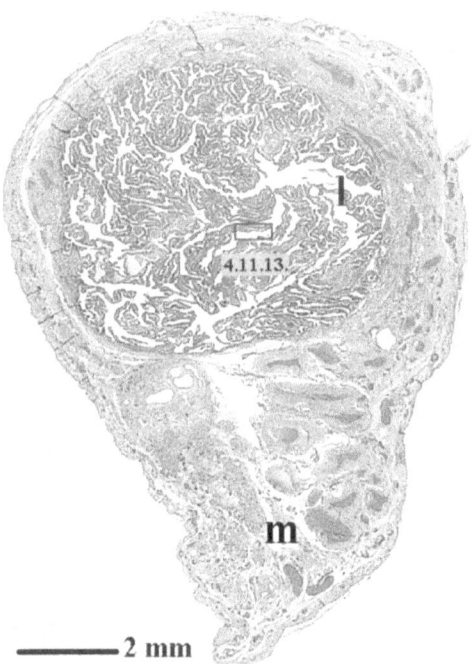

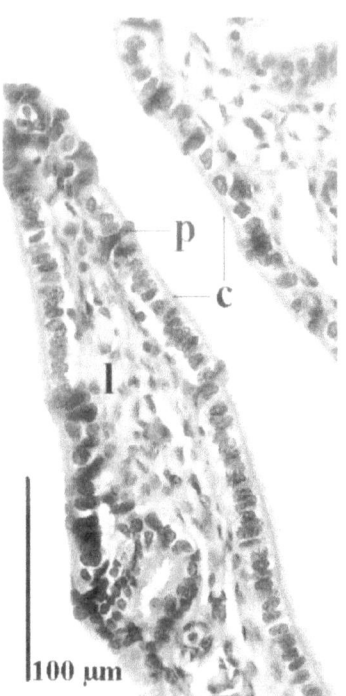

Fig. 4.11.12. (left) The longest stretch of the oviduct, with the thinnest wall, is the ampulla. The mucosa is thrown into long, branched folds, so that the lumen (l) looks like a labyrinth. Part of the mesovarium (m) is also seen. This is a fibrous tissue ribbon, carrying numerous blood vessels and lined with mesothelium, which suspends the oviduct to the abdominal wall. Oviduct, human, HE. **Fig. 4.11.13.** (right) The epithelium of the ampullar mucosa is simple prismatic, and contains ciliated cells (c: cilia), as well as slender peg cells (p). l = lamina propria. Oviduct, human HE.

influence and is slightly higher around the time of ovulation. It contains three types of prismatic cells: ciliated cells, gland cells and narrow, elongated peg cells. The **ciliated cells** (II.2.2.1.) are most numerous in the infundibulum and decrease in frequency in the direction of the isthmus. Their exact function is unclear. Some beat with their cilia in the direction of the uterus, and may generate fluid streams that carry the ovum with them. Others beat in the opposite direction, and may facilitate the displacement of spermatozoa. It is also possible that the spermatozoa move upstream, against the beat direction of the cilia. The **gland cells** increase in number towards the isthmus. Their apical pole is filled with vesicles. They secrete carbohydrates and proteins, which probably help to maintain ova and spermatozoa during their passage through the oviduct. They are especially prominent in the postovulatory period, when an ovum or blastocyst may pass. The **peg cells** may be inactive or undifferentiated cells.

The **musculosa** is made up of visceral muscle tissue and is thickest at the level of the isthmus. Elsewhere, it is incoherent or almost missing. In addition, the isthmus musculosa is double, consisting of an inner circular layer and an outer longitudinal layer. The peristaltic movements of the musculosa may contribute

to the conduction of the ovum or blastocyst towards the uterus.

IV.11.3. Uterus.

The uterus is a part of the female reproductive system that has no equivalent in the male: it is the part in which a very young embryo, or blastocysts, implants itself to continue its development until a mature baby can be born. The uterus consists of a distended, very muscular part, the corpus, and a narrow mouth, the cervix, which opens into the vagina.

Most of the uterine wall (Fig. 4.11.14.) of the corpus consists of visceral muscle tissue, which forms bundles, running in various directions, interwoven with loose fibrous tissue. It forms a thick musculosa or **myometrium**. At the outside, the myometrium is coated with a thin serosa, or **perimetrium**, consisting of a thin layer of loose fibrous tissue, lined with mesothelium. At the inside of the myometrium, bordering the uterine lumen, is a mucosa, the **endometrium**, consisting of a very cellular fibrous tissue, lined with epithelium. The epithelium regularly forms exocrine glands. Locally, the endometrium penetrates somewhat into the myometrium. During

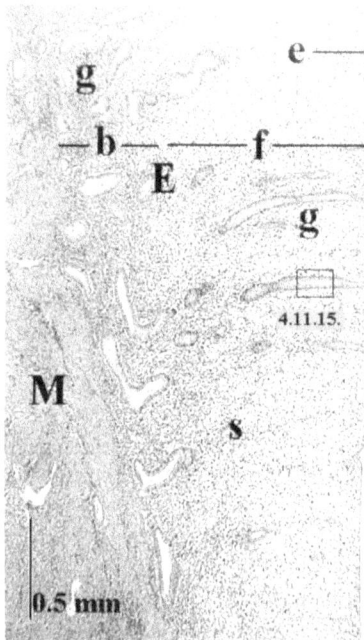

Fig. 4.11.14. The uterine wall consists of 3 concentric layers: the endometrium (a mucosa) on the inside, followed by the myometrium (a muscularis) and the perimetrium (a serosa). The endometrium (E) is a simple epithelium (e) which rests on a lamina propria of very loose fibrous tissue, the cytogenic stroma (s). Locally, the epithelium gives rise to sessile tubular glands (g). Initially, these follow a straight course but, in the deeper layers of the endometrium, they start to coil. In these deeper layers, the cytogenic stroma is exceptionally rich in cells. From a distance, their nuclei give the deeper endometrium a dark aspect. This deeper layer is basal layer (b), which essentially survives successive menstrual cycles and, at the onset of a new menstrual cycle, allows the endometrium to regenerate, forming a superficial, clearer, functional layer (f). The basal layer rests on the myometrium (M). Uterus, Preovulatory endometrium, human, HE.

each menstrual cycle, the endometrium undergoes profound changes in anticipation of the implantation of a blastocyst.

IV.11.3.1. Preovulatory endometrium.

At the end of a menstrual bleeding, and as a result of it, the endometrium has largely been sloughed off. Only in those places where the endometrium penetrates into the myometrium, a few more or less intact pieces are left. Starting form these leftovers, the endometrium gradually recovers and eventually forms a renewed, continuous coating of the myometrium. It consists of a very cellular loose fibrous tissue or **cytogenic stroma**, lined with a simple cuboidal to prismatic **epithelium**. In many places, this epithelium grows into sessile (III.5.1.), tubular **endometrial glands** (Fig. 4.11.15.).

Initially, the glandular epithelium is not fundamentally different from the superficial, lining epithelium.

Under the influence of estrogen, secreted by the interstitial cells and the developing follicles (Graafian and atretic) of the ovarium, the stromal as well as the epithelial cells start to proliferate, resulting in growth of the endometrium. Another factor contributing to endometrial expansion is edema, a consequence of the permeability of the endometrial capillaries. Since epithelial growth is apparently more rapid than stromal growth, the glands temporarily develop a convoluted course. In addition, the epithelium tends to develop pseudostratification. About the time of ovulation, two layers can be distinguished in the endometrium (Fig. 4.11.14.). A **basal layer** rests on the myometrium. This layer is more or less permanent: the deepest parts of it survive the successive menstrual bleedings and form "nests" out of which the endometrium regenerates. It has a dark aspect because of the dense concentration of stromal cell nuclei, and contains the distal parts of the glands, which have a convoluted course. On top of this layer, and out of it, a second layer has grown during the preovulatory, proliferative phase. This layer has a paler aspect because of the less pronounced concentration of stromal cells, and the glands have resumed their straight course. The glandular epithelium is again simple. In two respects, this layer is not permanent. In the first place, it will undergo profound changes during the postovulatory secretory phase. In the second place, if no pregnancy is initiated, it will be broken down during the next menstrual bleeding. It is called the **functional layer**. About the time of ovulation, the endometrium reaches a total thickness of 2 to 3 millimeters.

The superficial epithelial cells of the endometrium carry microvilli and occasionally a few cilia, especially at the mouths of the glands.
The glandular cells gradually become tall prismatic and develop the cytological structure of protein-secreting exocrine gland cells. They also carry apical microvilli. The nucleus acquires the euchromatic aspect of a metabolically active cell. Lysosomes are present throughout the cytoplasm. Towards the time of ovulation, the rough endoplasmic reticulum and the Golgi-complex have reached their maximum level of development. The cytoplasm also abounds with free ribosomes.

IV.11.3.2. Postovulatory endometrium.

After ovulation, the endometrium's functional layer undergoes further changes, under the influence of estrogen and progesterone of the corpus luteum. During the first half of the postovulatory or secretory phase, the endometrial glands produce secretions. During the second half, the most profound changes are in the stroma. The stromal edema increases and the endometrium reaches its maximum thickness of 5 to 6 millimeters.

Shortly after ovulation, the gland cell nucleus develops a unique structure that facilitates the transport of ribosomal RNA to the cytoplasm. Locally, the nuclear envelope folds inward and contacts the nucleolus. Then, the inner membrane of the nuclear envelope forms a lengthy tube, which penetrates the nucleolus and forms numerous coils inside. This is the **nucleolar canal system** (Fig. 4.11.17.). The membranous tubule pronouncedly increases the available membrane surface over which transport of RNA to the cytoplasm may take place. Giant mitochondria appear, with a diameter of several micrometers. The most conspicuous secretory product of the endometrial glands is glycogen, impressive amounts of which accumulate in the subnuclear region. Strangely, the smooth endoplasmic reticulum is not strongly developed. Glycogen is easily dissolved during preparation of histological slides for light microscopy. Consequently, the endometrial gland cells develop an infranuclear lucid zone, situated at he periphery of the glands (Fig. 4.11.16.). Later, glycogen shifts to the cell apex and is secreted in the glandular and endometrial lumen. Secretion is apocrine: substantial parts of the cell apex, filled with glycogen, protrude in the glandular lumen and are pinched off (Fig. 4.11.18.). Disruption of the membrane liberates glycogen. Glycogen may serve as a food source to the developing embryo, which may implant itself around this time. Around the 21st day of the menstrual cycle, secretion is at its maximum, decreasing dramatically afterwards. At this time, the gland cells have lost their apical cytoplasm, resulting in widening of the glandular lumen, which contains rests of cells and secretions.

During the second half of the postovulatory phase, roughly from the 23rd day onwards, the cytogenic stroma is transformed into a predecidua. The stromal cells lose their spindle shape and change into polyhedral cells. Their nucleus becomes euchromatic and the cytoplasm develops additional intermediary filaments, consisting of cytokeratin. They begin to store glycogen. These epitheloid cells are called predecidua cells. They transform the superficial functional layer to a **compact zone**. The deeper functional layer remains more or less unchanged and is now called the **spongious zone**. In the compact zone, the glands acquire an unusual saw tooth course. This decidual transformation is another anticipation of the implantation of a blastocyst, which might take place around this time. Metrial cells appear, also called endometrial granulocytes. These cells contain opaque granula and superficially resemble eosinophilic granulocytes, except for their unlobed nucleus. The function of these immune cells is taken to be the suppression of other immune cells. This contributes to the protection of the embryo, which differs genetically from the maternal organism, against immunological defense reactions.

In the event that a pregnancy begins, i.e. when a blastocysts succeeds in implantation, the differentiation of the predecidua cells surrounding the blastocyst is carried on to greater extremes. They develop into decidua cells, which will be contacted later by the developing placenta.

When no pregnancy is started, the corpus luteum degenerates, which in turn seals the fate of the endometrium's functional layer. Through a combination of factors, this part of the endometrium dies and fragments. The shreds of tissue, sloughing off and mixed with blood, are discharged through the vagina and constitute the menstrual bleeding. Today, **menstruation** is essentially seen as an inflammatory process. When progesterone levels fall, the endometrium is invaded with macrophages and immune cells, such as mast cells, eosinophils, and neutrophils. The chemical mediators released by these cells have multiple effects: constriction of endometrial blood vessels, degradation of cell junctions, autophagocytosis and apoptosis of endometrial cells, and secretion of lytic enzymes by endometrial cells.

IV.11.3.3. Cervix.

The uterine cervix protrudes into the vagina and encloses an endocervical canal, which connects the uterine lumen with the vaginal lumen.
The mucosa bordering the canal shows complex folds. It is lined with a simple prismatic epithelium of mucous cells, the **endocervical epithelium**. Towards the uterus, this epithelium gradually changes into that of the endometrium. Towards the vagina, this epithelium is brusquely replaced by a Malpighian epithelium, the exocervical epithelium, which lines the bulging mouth of the cervix and continues into the vagina. The junction between these two epithelia is called the squamo-columnar junction. Its exact location differs with age. In the newborn, the junction often has an exocervical position. During the years of sexual maturity, it coincides with the mouth of the

232

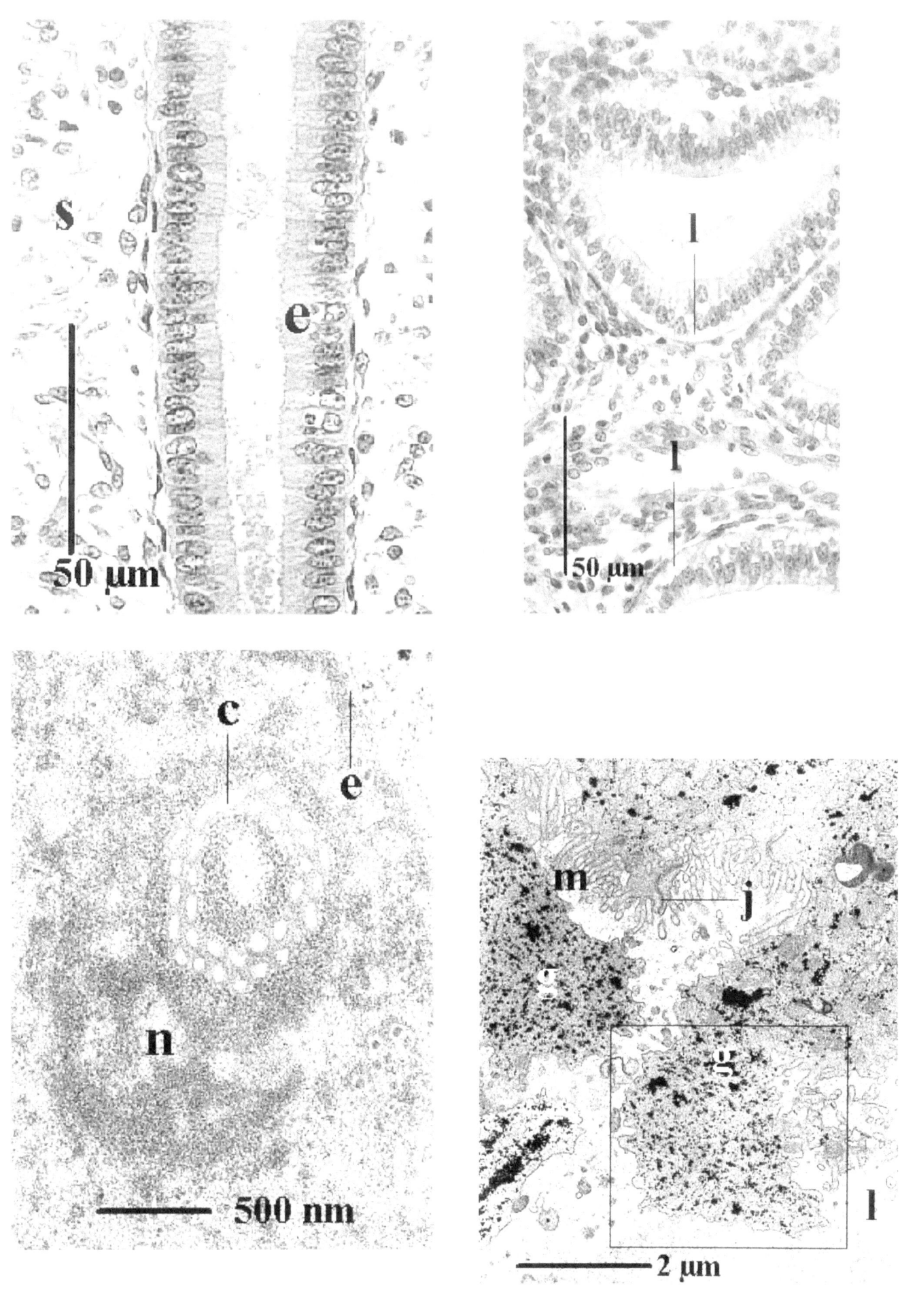

Fig. 4.11.15. (top left) An endometrial gland is lined with a simple prismatic epithelium (e), which rests on an extremely cellular cytogenic stroma (s). Preovulatory endometrium, human, HE. **Fig. 4.11.16.** (top right) During the early postovulatory stage, the endometrial glands accumulate glycogen in the basal part of their cells. This glycogen is dissolved during tissue preparation for light microscopy, giving rise to a characteristic, peripheral lucid zone (l). The nuclei have shifted towards the middle of the cells (compare with Figure 4.11.15., where the nuclei lie basally.). Postovulatory endometrium, human, HE. **Fig. 4.11.17.** (bottom left) The inner membrane of the nuclear envelope (e) of an endometrial gland cell gives rise to a tubular, convoluted inpocketing, which penetrates into the nucleolus (n): the nucleolar canal system (c). This increases the available surface for exchange of substances between nucleus and cytoplasm. Endometrium, human, TEM. **Fig. 4.11.18.** (bottom right) During the postmenstrual secretory phase, the basally accumulated glycogen (g) migrates to the apical cell pole (mark the junctional complexes, j, and the microvilli, m), and is secreted into the lumen (l) of the endometrial glands. This happens through apocrine secretion: areas of cytoplasm, lined with membrane and loaded with glycogen, are pinched off (rectangles). Postovulatory endometrium, human, TEM.

cervix. After the menopauze, it often recedes into the endocervical canal.

In sections, the complex shape of the folds of the endocervical mucosa may give the impression of sessile, branched tubular glands. The epithelium produces a mucous secretion, the composition of which depends on the stage of the menstrual cycle. Preovulatory, under estrogen influence, this secretion is thin and fluid, allowing passage of spermatozoa on their way to the oviducts. Postovulatory, under added progesterone influence, the secretions become viscous, plugging the cervix mouth. Occasionally, the secretion dilates the spaces enclosed within the mucosal folds, creating so-called Naboth's follicles.

The endocervical mucosa contains a very cellular stroma, rich in elastic fibers. Beneath the stroma, or lamina propria, is a musculosa, much thinner and less coherent than the myometrium. The surrounding fibrous tissue merges with the tissues of the body wall.

IV.11.4. Vagina.

The vagina is a fibro-muscular canal, lined with a Malpighian epithelium that rests on a dense lamina propria, rich in elastic fibers. Beneath this mucosa is a musculosa, the smooth muscle fibers of which course in various directions. A fibrous tissue adventitia connects the vaginal wall with the surrounding tissues. The vagina does not contain glands, but is lubricated by the cervical secretions. The epithelium produces glycogen, which is fermented to lactate by specialized, local bacteria. This acid environment protects the vagina against infection.

During the menstrual cycle, the vaginal epithelium undergoes changes. About four layers of cells can be distinguished. The basal layer is a simple, prismatic layer in which cell proliferation takes place. On top of this lie, in succession, a parabasal layer, an intermediary layer, and a superficial layer, which represent successive differentiation stages of basal cells. The superficial layer shows extremely flattened cells with pycnotic nuclei and numerous cytokeratin

filaments. The most superficial of these cells slough off. Preovulatory, under estrogen influence, the basal cells proliferate and differentiate into superficial cells. Postovulatory, under added progesterone influence, the differentiation process is interrupted when the stage of the intermediary cell is reached.

IV.11.5. Vulva.

The vulva lies at the mouth of the vagina. The urethra opens here as well. At both sides of the vulva, the skin forms a pair of folds, the inner and outer labiae, or lips. The inner lips are lined with a thin, hairless epidermis. They also contain sebaceous glands and are richly vascularized. The outer lips have a much thicker epidermis, the outer face of which forms hair follicles. At the frontal junction of the lips is the clitoris, an erectile corpuscle with a rich sensory innervation, which contains two cavernous bodies and a glans. The vestibular glands of Bartholin are tubulo-acinar glands with prismatic cells that produce a mucous, lubricating fluid.

References.

Abe H.: The mammalian oviductal epithelium: regional variations in cytological and functional aspects of the oviductal secretory cells. Histol. Histopathol. 1996, 11: 743-768.

Cornillie F.J., Lauweryns J.M., Brosens I.A.: Normal human endometrium. An ultrastructural survey. Gynecol. Obstet. Invest. 1985, 20: 113-129.

Gosden R., Krapez J., Briggs D.: Growth and development of the mammalian oocyte. Bioessays 1997, 19: 875-882.

Ferenczy A.: Ultrastructure of the normal menstrual cycle: a review. Microsc. Res. Tech. 1993, 25: 91-105.

Gulyas B.J.: Cortical granules of mammalian eggs. Int. Rev. Cytol. 1979, 63: 357-392.

McGaughey R.W., Racowsky C., Rider V., Baldwin K., DeMarais A.A., Webster S.D.: Ultrastructural correlates of meiotic maturation in mammalian oocytes. J. Electron Microsc. Tech. 1990, 16: 257-280.

Motta P.M., Nottola S.A., Familiari G., Macchiarelli G., Vizza E., Correr S.: Ultrastructure of human reproduction from folliculogenesis to early embryo development. A review. Ital. J. Anat. Embryol. 1995, 100: 9-72.

Salamonsen L.A., Lathbury L.J.: Endometrial leukocytes and menstruation. Hum. Reprod. Update 2000, 6: 16-27.

Sathanantnan A.H.: Ultrastructure of the human egg. Hum. Cell 1997, 10: 21-38.

Verma V.: Ultrastructural changes in human endometrium at different phases of the menstrual cycle and their functional significance. Gynecol. Obstet. Invest. 1983, 15: 193-212.

IV.12. Eyes.

The eyes, the organs of sight, are complex organs, at the core of which are extremely specialized, light sensitive photoreceptor cells. Essentially, photoreceptor cells are nerve cells. Consequently, the most important tissue of the eyes is **nervous tissue**. Other tissues, such as **fibrous tissue** and **epithelium**, also have important functions. The structure and function of the eye are closely mimicked by those of a camera. Because of its location inside an orbit and the presence of an internal pigment coat, the eye is a dark chamber. The light sensitive film, the retina, is nervous tissue and is sensitive to electromagnetic radiation from a narrow band of wavelengths, making up the visible spectrum. Perhaps a closer analogy still would be an electronic camera, which stores its images digitally, instead of on film. The retina does not store pictures either, this happens in the brain. In addition to light sensitive elements, the eyes contain a diaphragm,

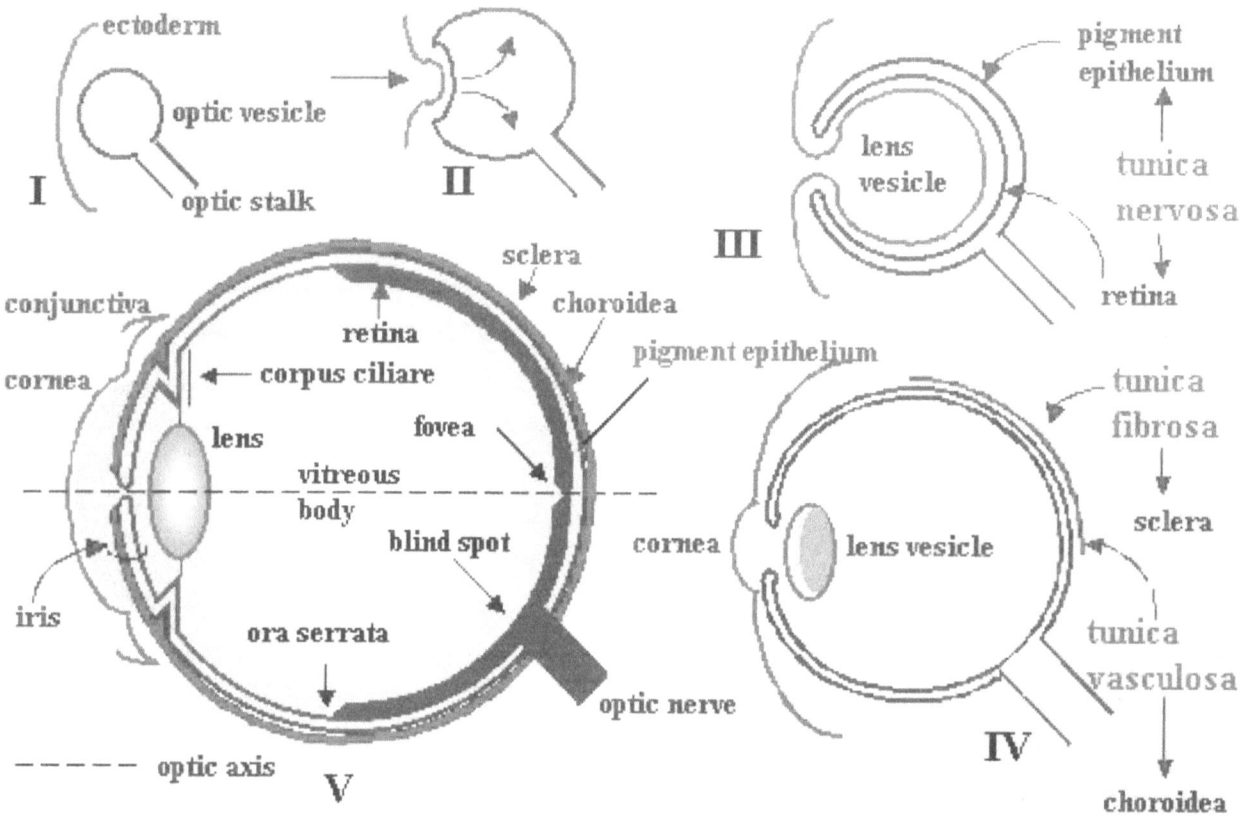

Fig. 4.12.1. The eye originates as an outpocketing of the embryonic brain, the optic vesicle (I). Where it touches the ectoderm, this forms a corresponding inpocketing, which indents the optic vesicle, transforming it into an optic cup (II). The rim of the cup constricts, so that the ectodermal inpocketing is gradually separated from the overlying ectoderm. As a result of its transformation from a vesicle into a cup, the wall of the optic cup, the tunica nervosa, is a double epithelium. The central epithelium will partly develop into the light-sensitive retina, the peripheral epithelium into a pigment epithelium (III). The ectodermal inpocketing, after having been separated from the overlying ectoderm, transforms into a lens vesicle, completely enclosed by the optic cup. Its posterior wall will form the lens fibers. The overlying ectoderm will develop into the cornea. The tunica nervosa is enveloped, consecutively, by a vascular coat or tunica vasculosa, which will give rise to the later choroidea, and a fibrous coat or tunica fibrosa, later to become the sclera (IV). Section V shows a horizontal section through the mature right eye, seen from above. The light sensitive part of the retina is at the back of the eyeball and is substantially thickened. The blind spot is the starting point of the optic nerve, which is itself derived from the base of the optic cup, the optic stalk (I). The fovea is a depression at the end of the eye's optic axis. Here, the light sensitivity of the retina, as well as its visual acuity, are at their maximum. The light sensitive part of the retina abruptly ends at the ora serrata, although the tunica nervosa continues into the anterior parts of the eyeball, the ciliary body and the iris. The lens is suspended to the ciliary body by means of Zinn's fibers. The space behind the lens is filled with a viscous matrix, the vitreous body. Between the lens and the iris is the posterior eye chamber, between the iris and the cornea the anterior eye chamber. The corneal epithelium continues into the conjunctiva.

the iris, as well as an accommodation system to focus incoming bundles of light. This system consists of the cornea, and the lens, attached to the ciliary body. The cornea is largely made up of fibrous tissue. The corpus ciliare, as well as the iris, are made up largely of epithelium. The lens is also an epithelium, but so extremely modified that its epithelial nature is hardly evident.

During embryonic development (Fig. 4.12.1.), the eye arises as a tubular outpocketing of the primitive brain, the wall of which is a simple layer of neurectodermal cells. The tip of this outfolding dilates, giving rise to an **optic vesicle**. Subsequently, the distal part of the optic vesicle is pushed in, forming a double-walled **optic cup**. The optic cup touches the overlying ectoderm, which infolds locally. The mouth of the optic cup narrows and eventually the ectodermal infolding is pinched off, closes, and forms a **lens vesicle**, consisting of a simple epithelium, inside the optic cup. The progressive narrowing of its mouth transforms the optic cup into a spherical structure, but now its wall consists of two epithelia whose apical faces virtually touch, the **tunica nervosa**. The tunica nervosa is analogous to the brain's cortex. The enclosed space fills with a specialized, avascular interstitial tissue, the **vitreous body**. The ground substance of this interstitial tissue is a transparent material containing numerous fine collagen fibrils. Peripheral to the tunica nervosa, the mesoderm develops into a fibrous tissue sheath. The deeper layers of this sheath are penetrated by numerous blood vessels, for which reason it is called the **tunica vasculosa**. The peripheral layers develop into a dense fibrous connective tissue, the **tunica fibrosa**. The narrow stalk connecting the optic vesicle to the brain becomes the **optic nerve**. Strictly speaking, the optic nerve is no nerve at all, but part of the brain's white matter.

The **tunica fibrosa** coats the largest part of the eyeball as a tough fibrous layer, called the **sclera** (Fig. 4.12.2.). The sclera protects the weaker parts of the eye and offers insertion points to the eye muscles, made up of skeletal muscle tissue, which enable the eye ball to move inside its orbit.
In front, the tunica fibrosa is thin and transparent and assumes a much stronger curvature. This part is the **cornea**. Its surface is lined with an epithelium of ectodermal origin (Fig. 4.12.1.).

The **tunica vasculosa** is a vascular fibrous tissue layer which provides for the metabolic needs of the overlying and underlying layers, which contain much less blood vessels. In addition, this layer is pigmented.

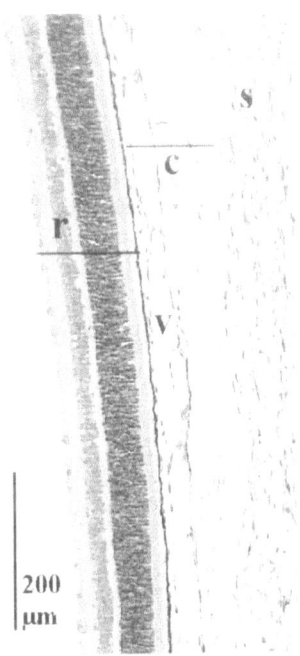

Fig. 4.12.2. The eyeball is composed of 3 concentric layers. Starting from the outside, they are the sclera (s), the choroidea (c), and the retina (r). The sclera is dense fibrous tissue. The choroidea is especially rich in blood vessels (v) in its deeper layer, where it touches the retina. This layer is the choriocapillaris. The retina is nervous tissue. It has a complex, layered structure. Eye, rabbit, HE.

The most extensive and most specialized part of the tunica vasculosa is the **choroidea** (Fig. 4.12.2.). The most superficial blood vessels, grazing the sclera, are relatively wide. In the deeper parts of the choroidea lies an extensive network of capillaries, the **choriocapillaris**. The endothelial cells that face the tunica nervosa carry numerous fenestrations with a diaphragm. These are directly related to the choroidea's nutritive function. The fibrous tissue stroma contains numerous **melanocytes**.
In front, the choroidea thickens and develops into a **ciliary body**, which tapers into the **iris** (Fig. 4.12.1.). The iris is situated behind the cornea and its pigment is visible as eye color. The space between cornea and iris is the anterior eye chamber. The iris has a central opening with a variable diameter, the **pupil**. The lens is suspended to the ciliary body. The space between iris, ciliary body and suspensory ligaments of the lens is the posterior eye chamber.

As a consequence of its embryological development, the **tunica nervosa** consist of two epithelia, a central one and a peripheral one. Their apical faces are turned to one another and come into close contact. The peripheral epithelium's basal face is turned to the outside of the eyeball, the central epithelium's to the center of the eyeball. At the front of the eyeball, both epithelia extend to the pupil's rim, where they are continuous.

The peripheral epithelium is thin and simple (Fig 4.12.1.). It is the **pigment epithelium**, the basement membrane of which rests on the choroidea.

At the back of the eyeball, the central epithelium is thick and stratified. Here, it is photosensitive and forms the **retina** (Fig. 4.12.2.). The fully developed retina does not retain much of its original epithelial structure: it is in fact nervous tissue. The retina's basement membrane rests on the vitreous body. In the anterior part of the eyeball, the central epithelium remains thin and simple and is not photoreceptive (Fig. 4.12.22.). It coats the ciliary body and the posterior face of the iris. At the level of the iris, it is pigmented.

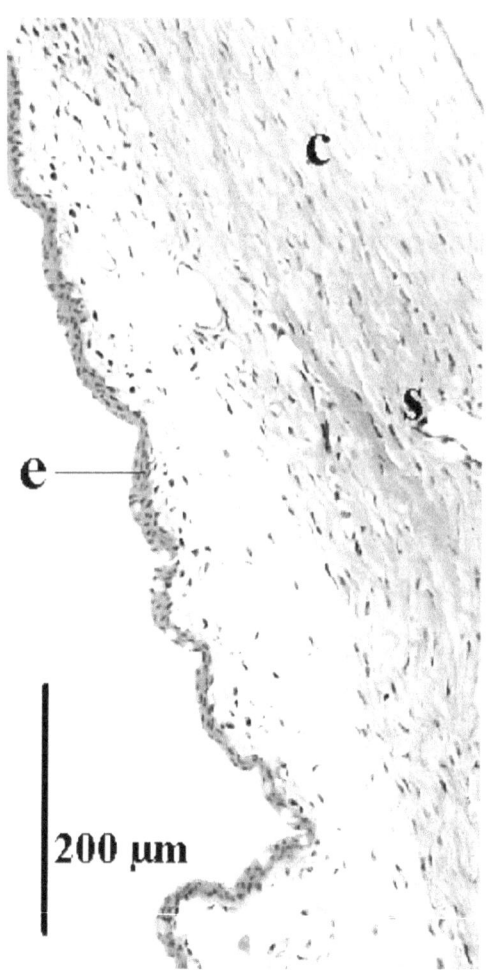

Fig. 4.12.3. The conjunctiva is fibrous tissue (c). Its epithelium (e) is a continuation of the cornea's. At the junction of both is Schlemm's canal (s). Eye, cat, HE.

Various accessory structures surround the eyeball or are associated with it and contribute to its protection.

The **conjunctiva** (Fig. 4.12.3.) is a mucosa that coats the inside of the eyelids and the exposed part of the sclera (the white of the eye). Its epithelium should be typically Malpighian, but this is not so: the superficial

stratum consists of prismatic cells, some of which are goblet cells. The secretions produced by this epithelium contribute to the protection of the exposed part of the eyeball.

At the rim of the eyelids are hair follicles that form the eyelashes. These are associated with sebaceous glands, Zeis's glands, and modified apocrine sweat glands, Moll's glands. The fibro-elastic tissue of the local conjunctiva contains modified sebaceous glands with ducts, Meibom's glands.

The tear gland or **lacrimal gland** is in fact a collection of several glands, each of which drains into the orbit through its own duct. Each gland is a compound tubulo-acinar gland, the secretory units of which consist of serous cells. Tears are isotonic with blood plasma and contain an enzyme, lysozyme, with antimicrobial properties. Through a nasolacrimal duct, tears drain to the nasal cavity.

IV.12.1. Cornea.

The cornea (Fig. 4.12.4.) is mostly **stroma**: a layer of dense fibrous, highly ordered connective tissue. The collagen fibrils of the stroma form several hundred lamellae, each a few tens of micrometers thick, which lie parallel to the surface. In each lamella, the fibrils are arranged in parallel, but in successive lamellae, their orientation changes (Fig. 4.12.5.). The fibrils have fairly constant diameters, between 20 and 30 nanometers. They are embedded in a matrix that regularly spaces them at about 60 nanometers. The cornea's transparency is a consequence of the diminutive dimensions, smaller than the wavelength of visible light, of the fibrillar diameters and the interfibrillar spaces. The regular spacing of the fibrils is maintained by the matrix, the hydratation of which is carefully regulated by the cornea's endothelium.

The stroma's superficial layer, **Bowman's membrane**, has a different structure. Its collagen fibrils are shorter and irregularly arranged. It is about 10 micrometers thick, and appears, in the light microscope, as an amorphous layer underneath the corneal epithelium.

At the surface of the eye, the stroma is lined with **Malpighian epithelium**, about five cell layers thick, which is continuous with the epithelium of the conjunctiva at the edge of the cornea. This epithelium is analogous to the epidermis, but shows no keratinization. The superficial cells carry short microvilli. The cells are joined by means of desmosomes and gap junctions. Hemidesmosomes attach the basal epithelial layer to the dense lamina of the basement membrane (Fig. 4.12.5.).

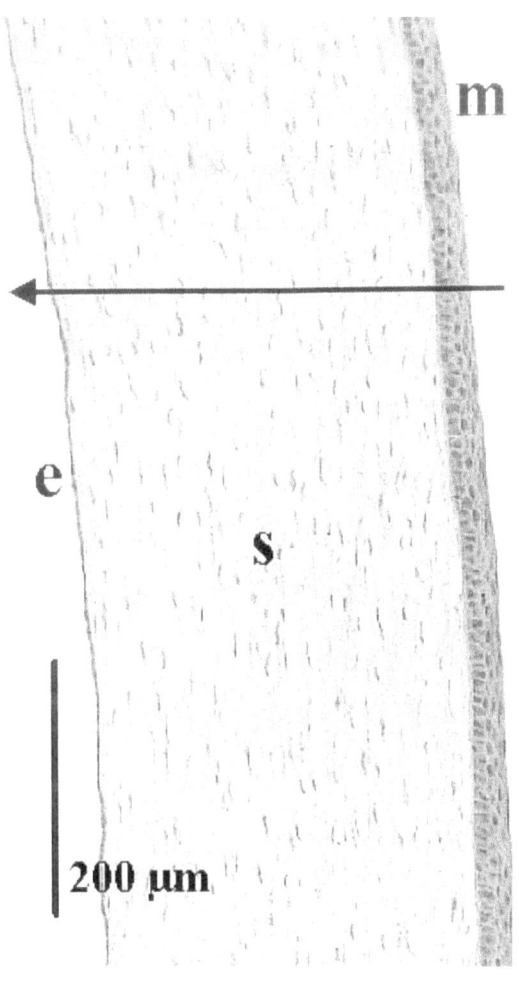

m

e

s

200 µm

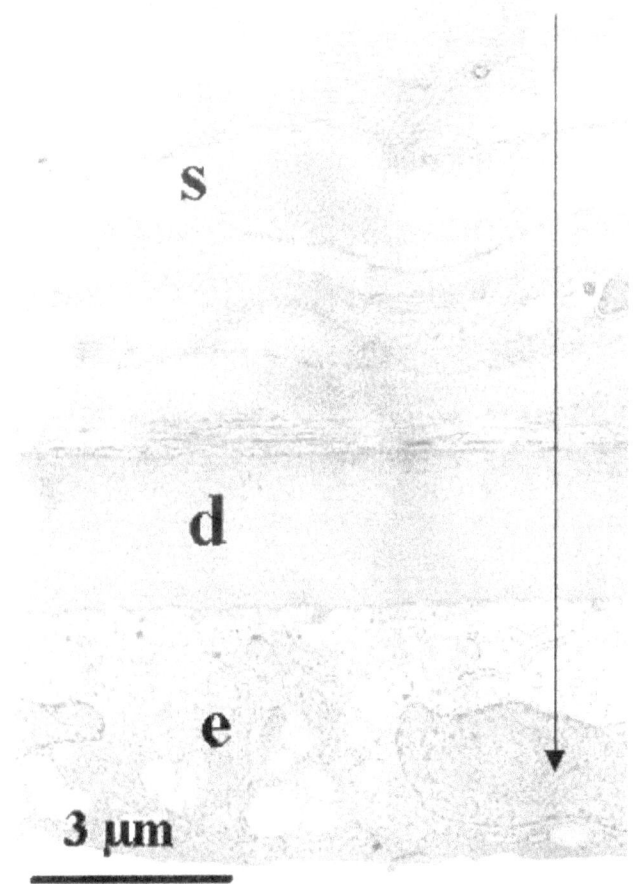

s

d

e

3 µm

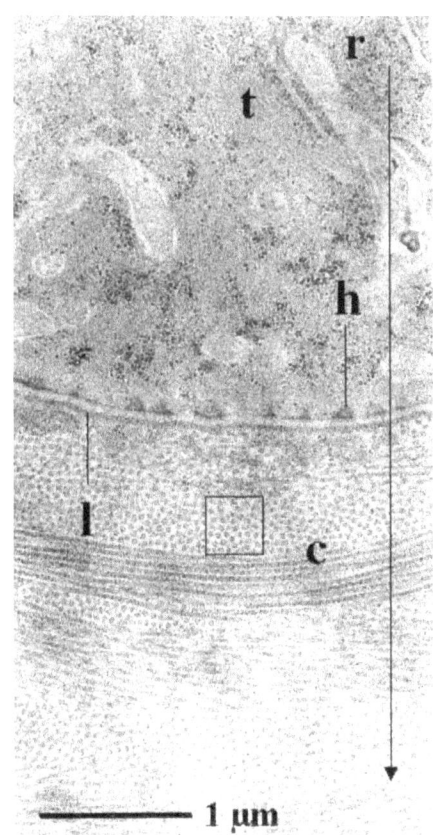

r

t

h

l

c

1 µm

Fig. 4.12.4. (top left) The cornea is largely made of dense fibrous tissue, the stroma (s), derived from the sclera. At the anterior surface, the stroma is lined with Malpighian epithelium (m), while its posterior surface is lined with endothelium (e). The arrow indicates the direction of incoming light rays. Cornea, rabbit, HE. **Fig. 4.12.5.** (left) The epithelial cells lining the cornea are rich in (intermediate) tonofilaments (t) and ribosomes (r). Hemidesmosomes (h) join them to the dense lamina (l) of the basement membrane, Bowman's membrane. Bowman's membrane may be so thick that it becomes visible light optically. The corneal stroma consists of successive layers of collagen fibrils (c). In each layer, the fibrils have a different orientation. Where the fibrils are sectioned transversely, their regular spacing (square) is apparent. This is one of the factors accounting for the cornea's transparency. Arrow: direction of a ray of incident light. Cornea, rabbit, TEM. **Fig. 4.12.6.** (above) The posterior surface of the collagen stroma (s) is lined with a thick basement membrane, Descemet's membrane (d), and an endothelium (e). Exceptionally, this endothelium is made of tall cells: the nuclei, to the left and right, do not bulge. Arrow: direction of a ray of incident light. Cornea, rabbit, TEM.

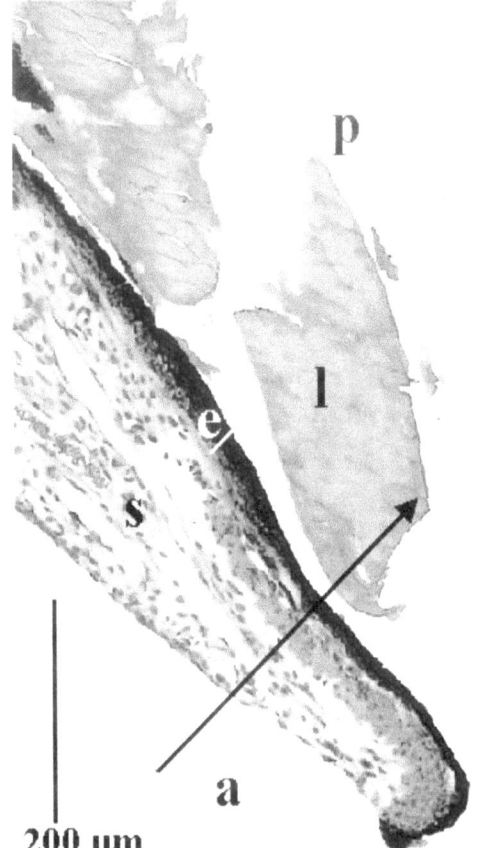

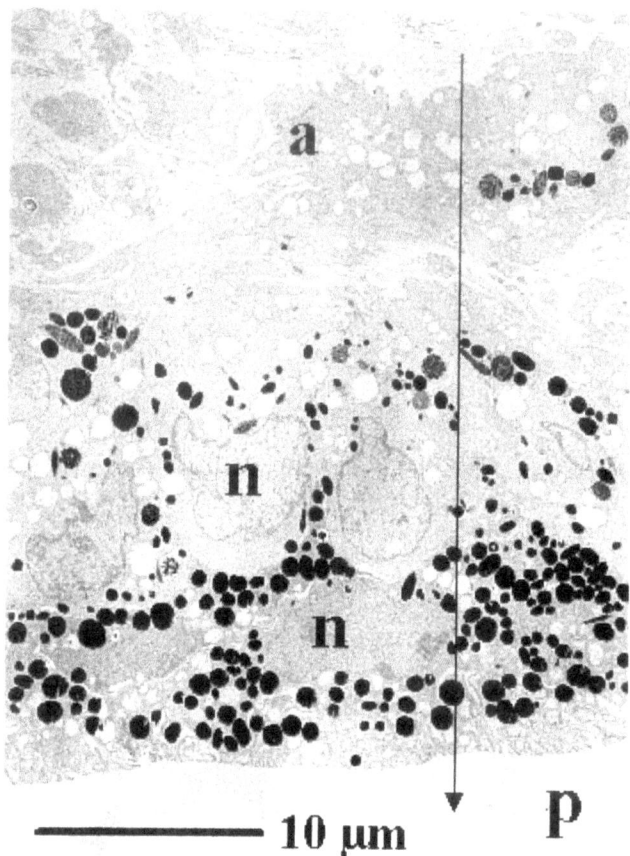

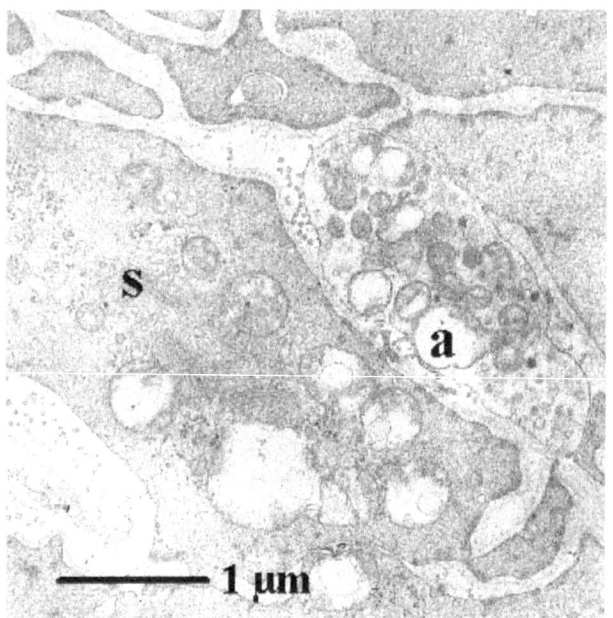

Fig. 4.12.7. (top left) The iris is made of a vascular stroma (s), derived from the tunica vasculosa, the posterior surface of which is covered with a double pigment epithelium (e). The iris is a septum, separating the anterior eye chamber (a) from the posterior eye chamber (p). An arrow at the level of the pupil indicates the direction of an incident light beam. Some parts of the lens (l), damaged during dissection, are seen. Iris, rabbit, HE.

Fig. 4.12.8. (above) Both layers (mark the double layer of nuclei, n) of the double pigment epithelium of the iris are loaded with dense pigment granules. The anterior epithelium forms processes (a), which extend into the stroma and are contractile. For this reason, the cells of the anterior epithelium are called myoepithelial cells. They form a dilator muscle, which is able to enlarge the pupil's diameter. The posterior epithelium, lined with a basement membrane (it was on the outside of the original optic cup), contacts the posterior eye chamber (p). The exposed cell membrane forms numerous folds, which is typical of cells that transport ions and fluid. Arrow: direction of a ray of incident light. Iris, rabbit, TEM.

Fig. 4.12.9. The stroma of the iris contains smooth muscle fibers (s), innervated by adrenergic (mark the dense vesicles) autonomic motor nerve fibers (a). They form a constrictor muscle, which is able to decrease the pupil's diameter. Iris, rabbit, TEM.

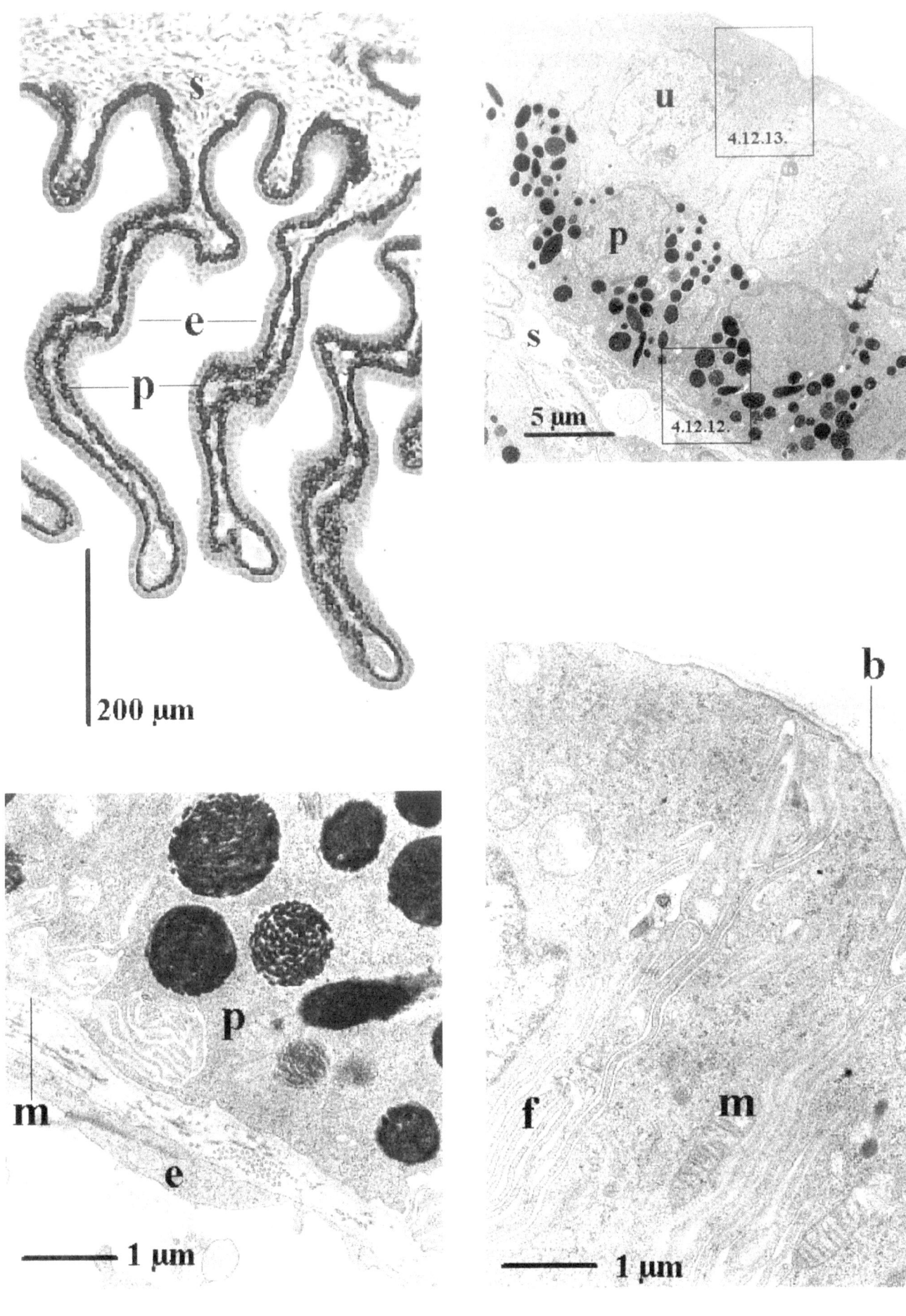

Fig. 4.12.10. (top left) In the ciliary body, the stroma (s) forms numerous folds, lined with a double epithelium. The basal epithelium, which rests on the stroma, is pigmented (p), whereas the superficial epithelium (e) is unpigmented. Eye, rabbit, HE. **Fig. 4.12.11.** (top right) The ciliary body's pigmented epithelium (p), which rests on a vascular stroma (s), was part of the outer wall of the embryonic optic cup. It is loaded with pigment granules. The unpigmented epithelium (u) is derived from the optic cup's inner wall. Consequently, its basal pole points away from the stroma. Ciliary body, rabbit, TEM. **Fig. 4.12.12.** (bottom left) Magnification of Figure 4.12.11.. The basal pole of the pigmented epithelium (p) can be identified as such because it rests on a basement membrane (m). Beneath this is a stroma, rich in blood capillaries, lined with endothelium (e). Ciliary body, rabbit, TEM. **Fig. 4.12.13.** (bottom right) Magnification of Figure 4.12.11.. The cell membrane at the unpigmented epithelium's basal pole, lined with basement membrane (b), forms numerous deep folds (f). Numerous mitochondria (m) are also seen. These are typical characteristics of cells that transport ions and fluid. Ciliary body, rabbit, TEM.

At the interior face of the cornea, bordering the anterior eye chamber, the stroma is lined with a single layer of squamous cells, which is an **endothelium**. It rests on a basement membrane, which may be so thick that it can be observed with the light microscope: **Descemet's membrane** (Fig. 4.12.6.). The endothelial cells contain numerous mitochondria and large amounts of rough endoplasmic reticulum, but are poor in filaments. Adjacent cells form interdigitations and tight junctions. Descemet's membrane usually has a homogeneously filamentous structure, even in the electron microscope. Nevertheless, it has distinct elastic properties. The corneal endothelium is metabolically very active and continuously pumps fluid out of the stroma, thereby maintaining its degree of hydratation between narrow limits. This is vital to the regular spacing of the stromal collagen fibrils and thus to corneal transparency.

The cornea has the largest refractory power of all parts of the eye and contributes greatly to the focusing of incoming light bundles on the retina.

IV.12.2. Iris.

The iris (Fig. 4.12.7.) consists of a vascular **stroma**, derived from the tunica vasculosa, which is coated, at its posterior face, with a double, pigmented **epithelium** that is part of the tunica nervosa. During embryological development, the anterior face of the stroma, which borders the anterior eye chamber, is lined with endothelium, which is lost later on. Consequently, the stroma comes in direct contact with the fluid circulating in the anterior eye chamber.

The stroma contains smooth muscle fibers and cellular structures resembling myoepithelial cells (III.5.1., Fig. 4.12.8.). The smooth muscle fibers are arranged concentrically around the pupil. The myoepithelial "cells" are in fact the basal processes of the peripheral epithelial cells, which have the same structure as ordinary myoepithelial cells. These processes are

arranged radially with respect to the pupil. Between the smooth muscle fibers and myoepithelial processes, numerous nerve fibers course. In addition, the stroma may contain melanocytes, the pigment of which, **stromal pigment**, contributes to the coloring of the eye. Increasing amounts of pigment result in green, brown, and black eye colors.

The double, cuboidal epithelium (actually, they are two simple epithelia) is also pigmented, both layers of it (Fig. 4.12.9.) This **epithelial pigment** causes, in the absence of stromal pigment, blue or gray eye colors.

The pigmentation of the iris contributes to the regulation of light intensity inside the eyeball, enabling it to function as a dark chamber. The concentric smooth muscle fibers form a constrictor muscle or sphincter, which decreases the pupil's diameter when stimulated by motor nerve fibers. The radial myoepithelial processes form a dilator muscle, which can, under motor nerve influence, increase the pupil's diameter. In this way, the pupil's diameter can be accurately adapted to the intensity of the incoming light, enabling the iris to function as a diaphragm.

IV.12.3. Ciliary body.

Like the iris, the ciliary body is composed of a fibrous, vascular stroma, derived from the tunica vasculosa, which is coated, on the inside of the eye ball, with a double epithelium, derived from the tunica nervosa. The surface of the ciliary body shows folds (Figs. 4.12.10.), the stroma of which is rich in fenestrated capillaries. In contrast to the iris and the choroidea, this stroma does not contain melanocytes. The eye lens is suspended from the ciliary body, by means of a number of collagen fibrils, which collectively form **Zinn's ligament**. The stroma contains circular and radial smooth muscle fibers, innervated by motor nerve fibers.

Of both epithelia, only the peripheral one, bordering

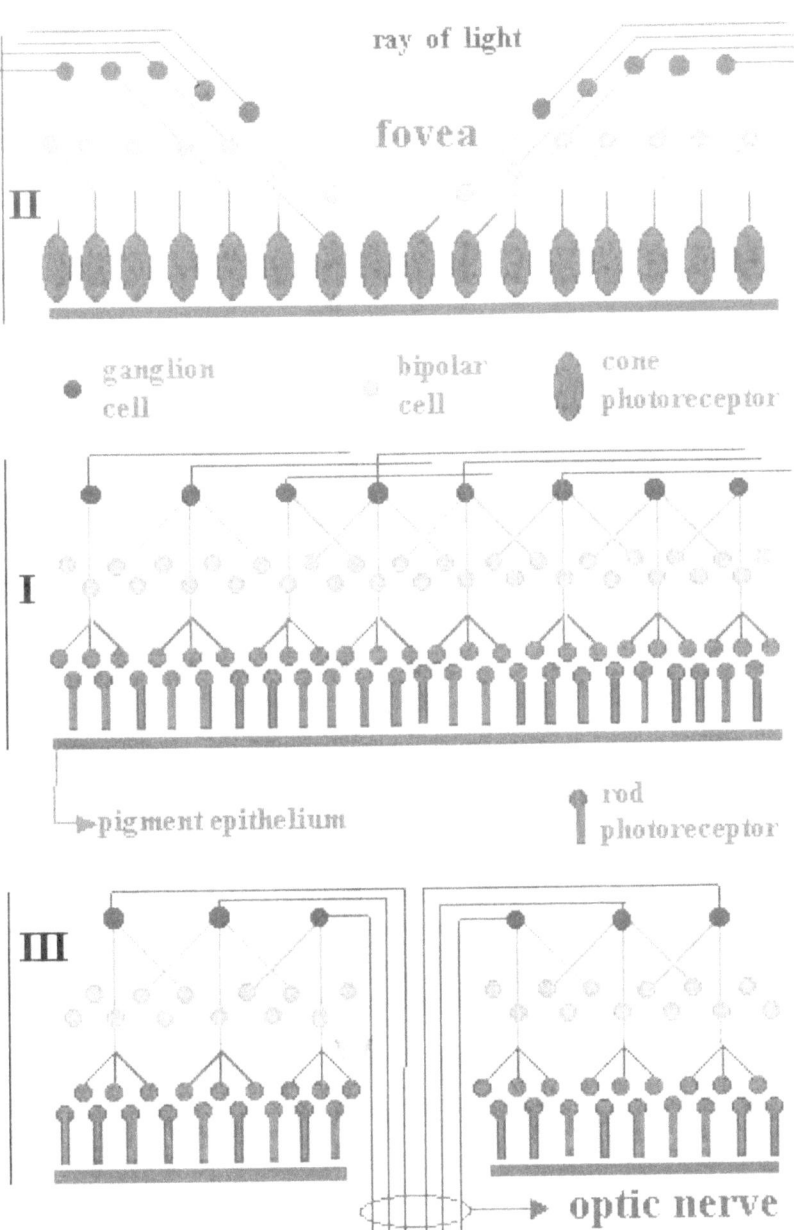

ray of light

fovea

II

ganglion cell   bipolar cell   cone photoreceptor

I

pigment epithelium   rod photoreceptor

III

optic nerve

Fig. 4.12.14. I: Interneurons, most of them bipolar cells, connect the retinal photoreceptor cells with ganglion cells. II. At the end of the eye's optic axis lies the fovea. Here, most photoreceptors are cones. The other nerve cells making up the retina retreat from the optic axis, forming a depression. There is little convergence: each photoreceptor is connected to a single ganglion cell (compare with I.). III. The axons of the ganglion cells course to the brain via the optic nerve. Where they penetrate the retina, a blind spot is formed.

the stroma, is pigmented (Figs. 4.12.11.-13.).

The basal cell poles of the central epithelium, which face the eyeball's interior, show deep, narrow, more or less parallel infoldings of the cell membrane. In the cytoplasm between the folds, numerous mitochondria are found (Fig. 4.12.13.). A structure like this is typical for cells that actively displace fluids and ions. In the lamina densa of this epithelium's basement membrane, the fibrils of Zinn's ligament are anchored.

The ciliary body is contractile, enabling it to control the tensile forces that, through Zinn's ligament, are transmitted to the equator of the lens. These tensile forces, in turn, determine the curvature of the lens and, consequently, its refractive power. Thus, the lens contributes to the formation of focused images on the retina. The circular smooth muscle fibers, when they contract, diminish the tension in Zinn's ligament, allowing the lens to increase its curvature. Contraction of the radial fibers increases tension in Zinn's ligament, which decreases the curvature of the lens.

A second function of the ciliary body is the production of eye chamber fluid. Ultimately, this fluid is derived from blood plasma. It reaches the ciliary body stroma through the local fenestrated capillaries. From here, it is actively secreted into the eye chambers by the central epithelium. The hydrostatic pressure that is created in this way supports the cornea and the iris and contributes to the nutrition of the cornea, which is avascular. The eye chamber fluid is conducted from the posterior eye chamber to the anterior one via the pupil. Ultimately it is drained from the anterior eye chamber into the venous blood through Schlemm's canal (Fig. 4.12.3.). This canal follows a circular course at the junction of the cornea with the sclera. It is lined with endothelium. It does not open into the anterior eye chamber. Fluid percolates through the sclera, which locally has wide meshes.

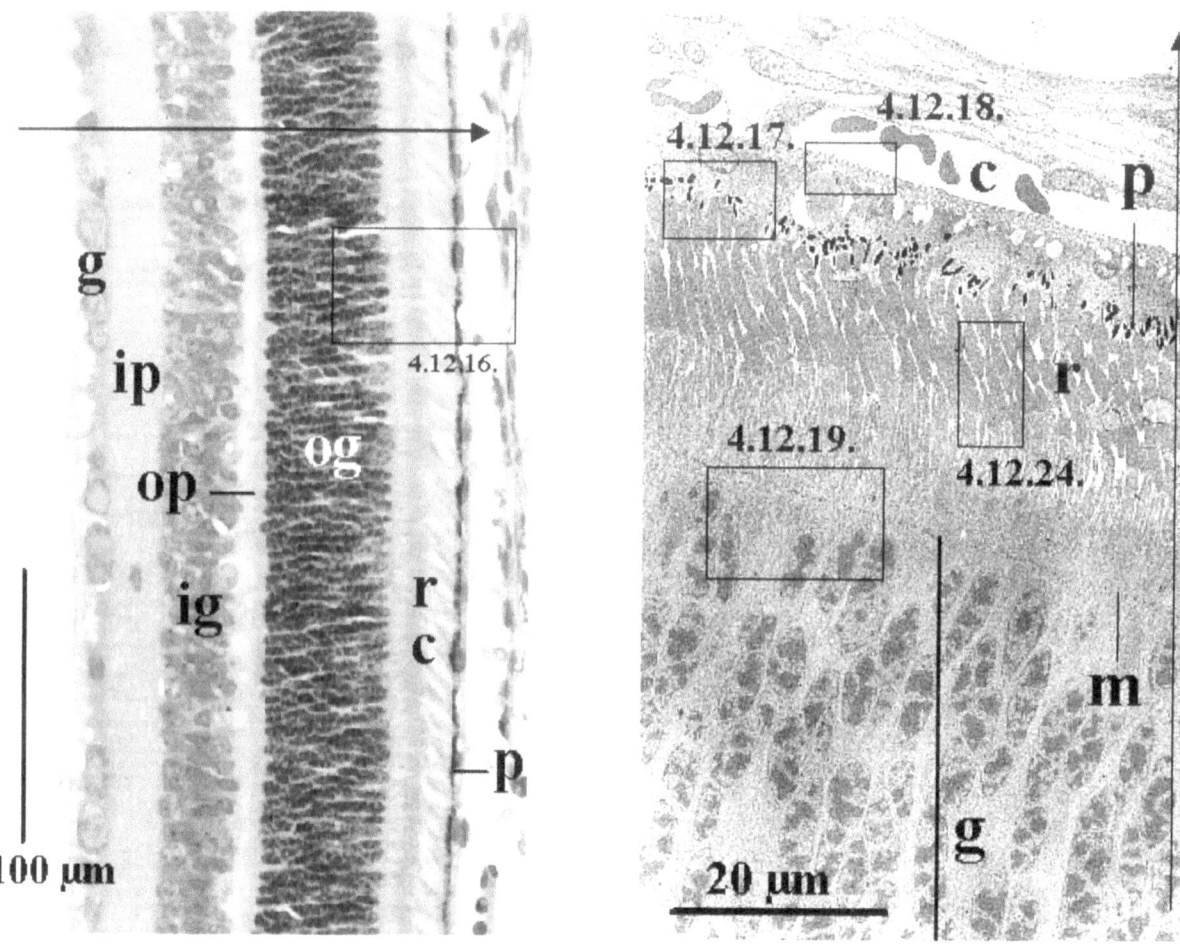

Fig. 4.12.15. (left) The retina contains a thin pigment epithelium (p), derived from the optic cup's inner wall. The other layers are derived from the optic cup's outer wall. The retinal photoreceptors, the rods and cones (r, c), touch the pigment epithelium. Their nuclei lie in the outer granular layer (og). Next is the outer plexiform layer (op), wherein the photoreceptors form synaptic junctions with interneurons, the nuclei of which accumulate in the inner granular layer (ig). In the inner plexiform layer (ip), these interneurons, in their turn, form synaptic junctions with ganglion cells (g). The arrow indicates the direction followed by an incoming light beam. Eye, rabbit, HE. **Fig. 4.12.16.** (right) The photoreceptors, in this region mostly rod cells, their cell bodies accumulating in the outer granular layer (g), form a rod-like process (r), which contacts the pigment epithelium (p). The pigment epithelium rests on the vascular choriocapillaris (c). At the junction of rod and cell body, the photoreceptor cells are joined to very slender supporting cells by means of desmosomes. These junctions form the external limiting membrane (m), which may be visible light optically. Arrow: direction of a ray of incident light. Eye, rabbit, TEM.

IV.12.4. Retina.

Posterior to the ciliary body, the retina arises as an abrupt thickening of the central epithelium of the tunica nervosa. Like nervous tissue elsewhere, it consists of nerve cells and glia cells. The most important type of glia cells are **Müller's cells**, extremely slender cells which extend through the entire retinal thickness and fill the spaces between the nerve cells. The retinal nerve cells are a varied group: the rod and cone cells, the interneurons, and the ganglion cells (Fig. 4.12.14., I). The **rod** and **cone cells** are photoreceptive nerve cells, which are able to transform electromagnetic energy in action potentials. The axons of the **ganglion cells** collectively form the optic nerve. The **interneurons** form synaptic connections between

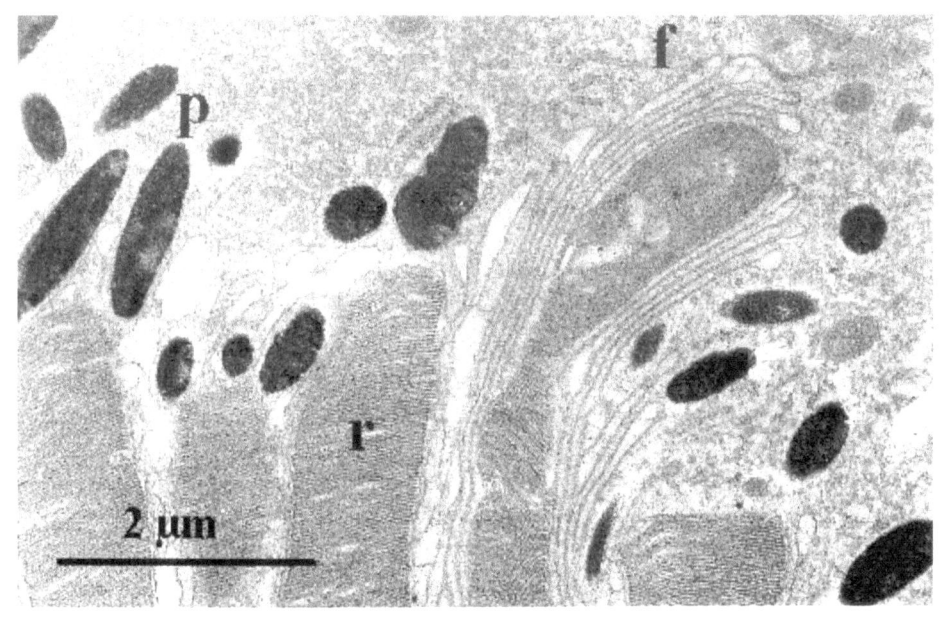

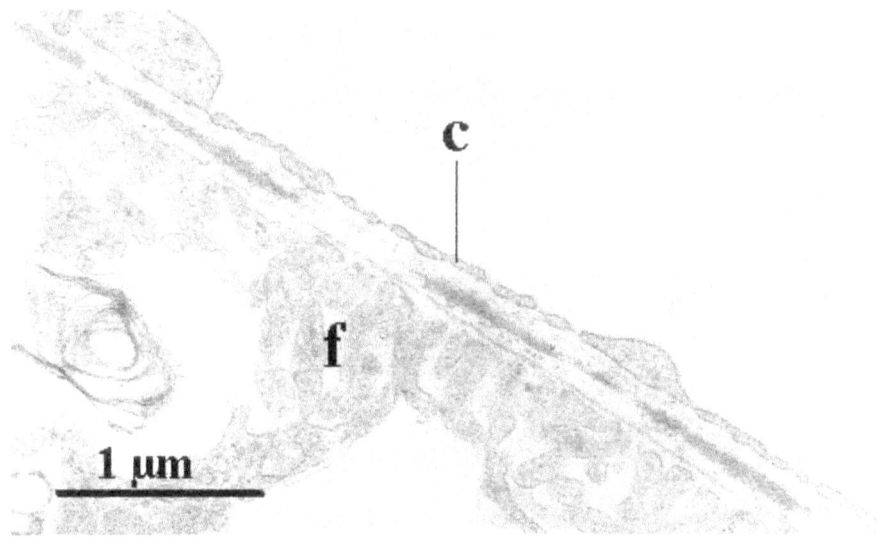

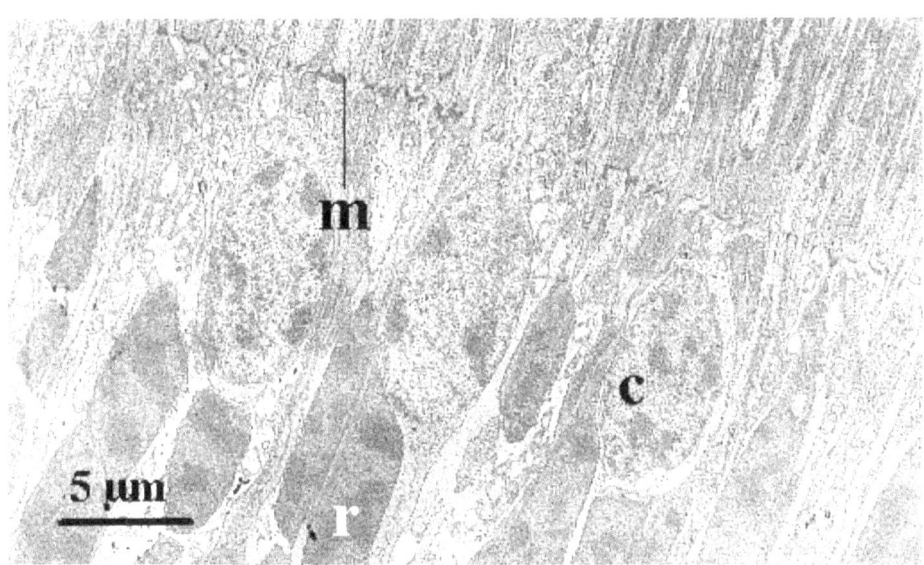

Top to bottom: **Fig. 4.12.17.** The apical pole of the pigmented epithelial cells, as it would show upon magnification of Figure 4.12.16., contains pigment granules (p), while its cell membrane is deeply folded (f). These folds envelop the rod ends (r). Retina, rabbit, TEM. **Fig. 4.12.18.** The pigmented epithelium's basal pole, as it would show upon magnification of Figure 4.12.16., shows membrane folds (f), and rests against the fenestrated capillaries (c) of the choriocapillaris. Retina, rabbit, TEM. **Fig. 4.12.19.** The outer granular layer, after magnification of Figure 4.12.16., contains the relatively slender, heterochromatic nuclei of the rod photoreceptor cells (r). Just below the external limiting membrane (m) are a few wider, euchromatic, nuclei of cone receptor cells (c). Retina, cat, TEM.

the photoreceptor cells and the ganglion cells. They also subject the visual information to preliminary processing before it is transmitted to the brain by the ganglion cells. Three types of interneurons are distinguished: **bipolar cells**, **amacrine cells**, and **horizontal cells**.

The photoreceptive rod and cone cells paradoxically lie in the deeper layers of the retina. They differentiate at the apical pole of the central epithelium and face the pigment epithelium, the peripheral epithelium of the optic cup that, in turn, borders the choroidea (Fig. 4.12.15.). Their nuclei make up the **outer granular layer**. Since cone cells are somewhat shorter than rod cells, their nuclei occupy the deeper (peripheral) parts of the outer granular layer (Fig. 4.12.19.). In the light microscope, the peripheral face of this layer is bordered by a dense line, the **external limiting membrane**. Ultrastructurally, this line corresponds to the level of the cellular junctions between Müller's cells and the photoreceptor cells (Figs. 4.12.16., 4.12.19.). The nuclei of Müller's cells and those of the interneurons occupy the **inner granular layer**. Between both layers is the **outer plexiform layer**, made up of processes of photoreceptor cells, Müller's cells and interneurons. The **ganglion cells** form a nuclear layer at the surface of the retina. Between them and the inner granular layer, the **inner plexiform layer** is found, made up of the processes of ganglion cells and interneurons. On top of the ganglion cell layer, bordering the vitreous body, is a nucleus-free region formed by the unmyelinated stretches of the ganglion cell axons, which converge towards the optic nerve, where they are myelinated. Finally, this layer is lined with the basement membrane of the retina, which is visible in the light microscope as the **internal limiting membrane**.

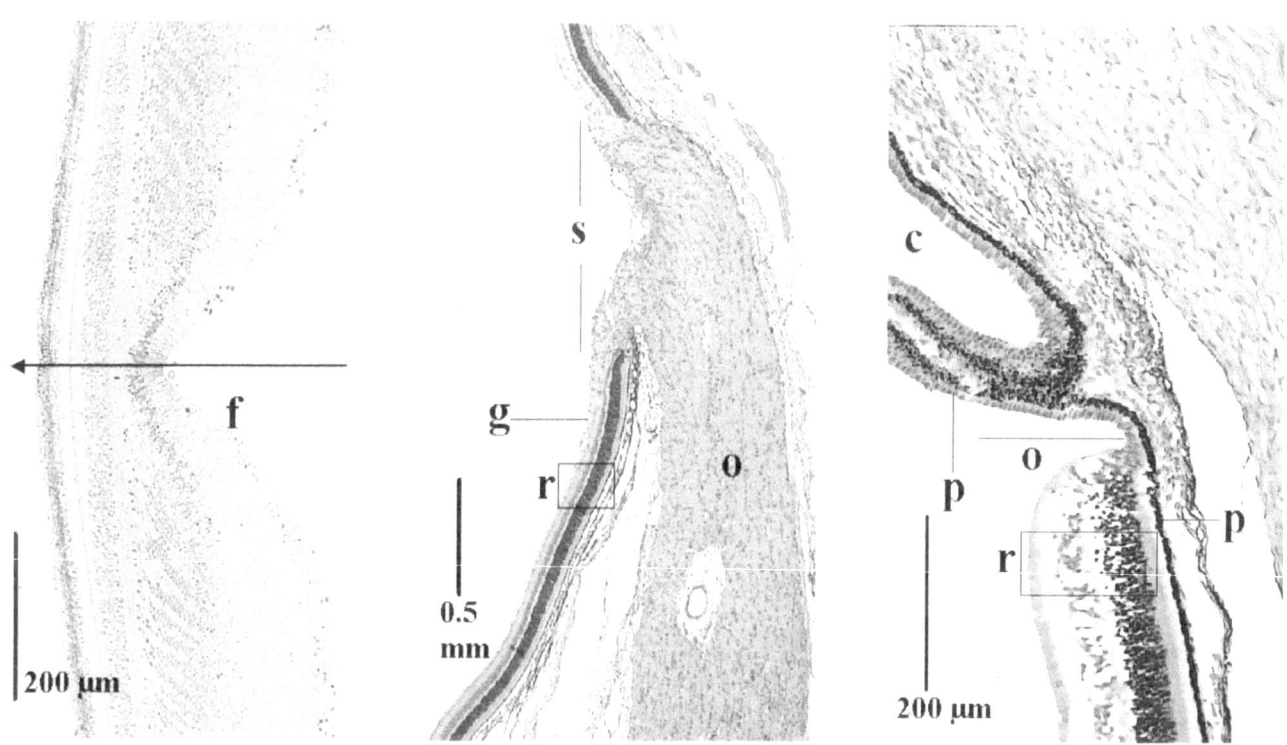

Fig. 4.12.20. At the fovea (f), the inner layers of the retina retreat from the optic axis, creating a depression. The arrow follows the eye's optic axis, and indicates the direction followed by an incoming beam of light. Retina, hamster, 1-micron plastic section, toluidin blue. Fig. 4.12.21. At the origin of the optic nerve (o), processes of the retinal ganglion cells (g) penetrate the retina (r), interrupting it and creating a blind spot (s). Eye, cat, HE. Fig. 4.12.22. The photoreceptive area of the retina ends abruptly at the ora serrata (o). The pigment epithelium (p) continues into the inner, pigmented, epithelium of the ciliary body (c). The photoreceptive epithelium (r) abruptly changes into the outer, unpigmented epithelium of the ciliary body. Eye, rabbit, HE.

Peripheral to the outer granular layer, the photoreceptive parts of the rod and cone cells, the rods and the cones, contact the peripheral **pigment epithelium** (Fig. 4.12.16.). The pigment cells are rich in mitochondria and contain large numbers of fusiform melanin granules and residual bodies with lipofuchsin pigment. Their apical pole, pointing towards the center of the eyeball, is thrown into folds, which descend over the rods and cones (Fig. 4.12.17.). Their basal pole, resting on the choriocapillaris, shows numerous clefts (Fig. 4.12.18.). The pigment epithelium absorbs light and phagocytoses cellular debris, produced by the rod and cone cells.

As already mentioned, the retina contains two kinds of **photoreceptors**: rod cells and cone cells (Fig. 4.12.19.). The human retina numbers about a hundred million of the first kind and about six million of the second kind. Rod cells allow detection of light intensity. They are synaptically connected to relatively few interneuron processes. Cone cells are selectively sensitive to the wavelength of light and come in three varieties: blue-sensitive, green-sensitive, and red-sensitive. They allow color vision. They synaptically connect to numerous interneuron processes.

Cone cells are most concentrated in an area that is called the **macula lutea** (Figs. 4.12.14.II., 4.12.20.). This is a circular area of the retina, which is transected by the optic axis formed by the cornea and the lens. The elements occupying the outer granular layer and the more central layers recede from this area, exposing the cones. Thus, a conical depression is formed, the **fovea**. The corresponding area of the choroidea is free of blood vessels, and the yellow-brown color of the melanin, present in the pigment epithelium, shines through, creating a "yellow spot". In this area, the ratio of cone cells to ganglion cells is about 1 to 1. This means that each cone cell eventually corresponds to a single nerve fiber in the optic nerve. All these properties explain why the fovea is the retinal area with greatest visual acuity. As the distance to the fovea increases, the cone cells are progressively replaced with rod cells and the number of photoreceptors per ganglion cell increases. Peripheral to the fovea, the ability to see colors and the acuity of vision decrease.

Another distinctive retinal landmark is the **blind spot** (Figs. 4.12.14.III., 4.12.21.), which lies a few millimeters medial to the fovea. Here are found no photoreceptors at all. This is a consequence of the peculiar, not to say paradoxical, structure of the retina, which illustrates that every living thing is formed by blind evolutionary forces, not conceived by an intelligent maker. The most efficient structure of the retina would be with the photoreceptor cells on the surface, directly exposed to incident light. As already mentioned however, the photoreceptor cells lie in the deep, peripheral layers of the retina, and send their axons to the surface, towards the ganglion cells. In order to form the optic nerve, the ganglion cell axons have to penetrate the retina, and the peripheral layers of the eyeball as well. This is what creates the blind spot. The corresponding area of the sclera forms the lamina cribrosa.

The retina ends abruptly in the vicinity of the ciliary body, at a zone called the **ora serrata** (Fig. 4.12.22.). Here, it abruptly decreases in thickness and continues into the epithelium of the ciliary body.

The most numerous **interneurons** are the bipolar cells. They are fairly typical bipolar nerve cells. Their perikarya lie in the middle of the inner granular layer. At both sides of the perikaryon, an axon originates, which branches intensively. In the outer plexiform layer it forms synaptic junctions with one or several photoreceptor cells, in the inner plexiform layer with one or more ganglion cells.

The horizontal cells are multipolar nerve cells, but not typical ones: several of their processes have the structure of axons. Some of these conduct action potentials towards the perikaryon, others away from it. Their perikarya occupy the periphery of the outer granular layer, bordering the outer plexiform layer. The horizontal cells interconnect photoreceptor cells.

The amacrine cells are atypical multipolar nerve cells that, like the horizontal cells, possess several axons. Their perikarya are situated somewhat more centrally than those of the horizontal cells, in the direction of the inner plexiform layer. The amacrine cells interconnect ganglion cells and the central axons of bipolar cells. Occasionally, they also contact photoreceptor cells.

IV.12.5. Photoreceptor cells.

Essentially, the photoreceptive rod and cone cells are strongly modified bipolar nerve cells (II.2.3.). Their most specialized part, which is responsible for their light sensitivity, is their peripheral process, which extends towards the pigment epithelium. The shape of this peripheral process, resembling a rod or a cone, gives the receptor cells their names.

The peripheral process of the **rod cells** (Figs. 4.12.23.-24.) is shaped as an elongated cylinder, or rod, which occupies about half of the total cell length. Halfway, the rod shows a lateral constriction, giving rise to a

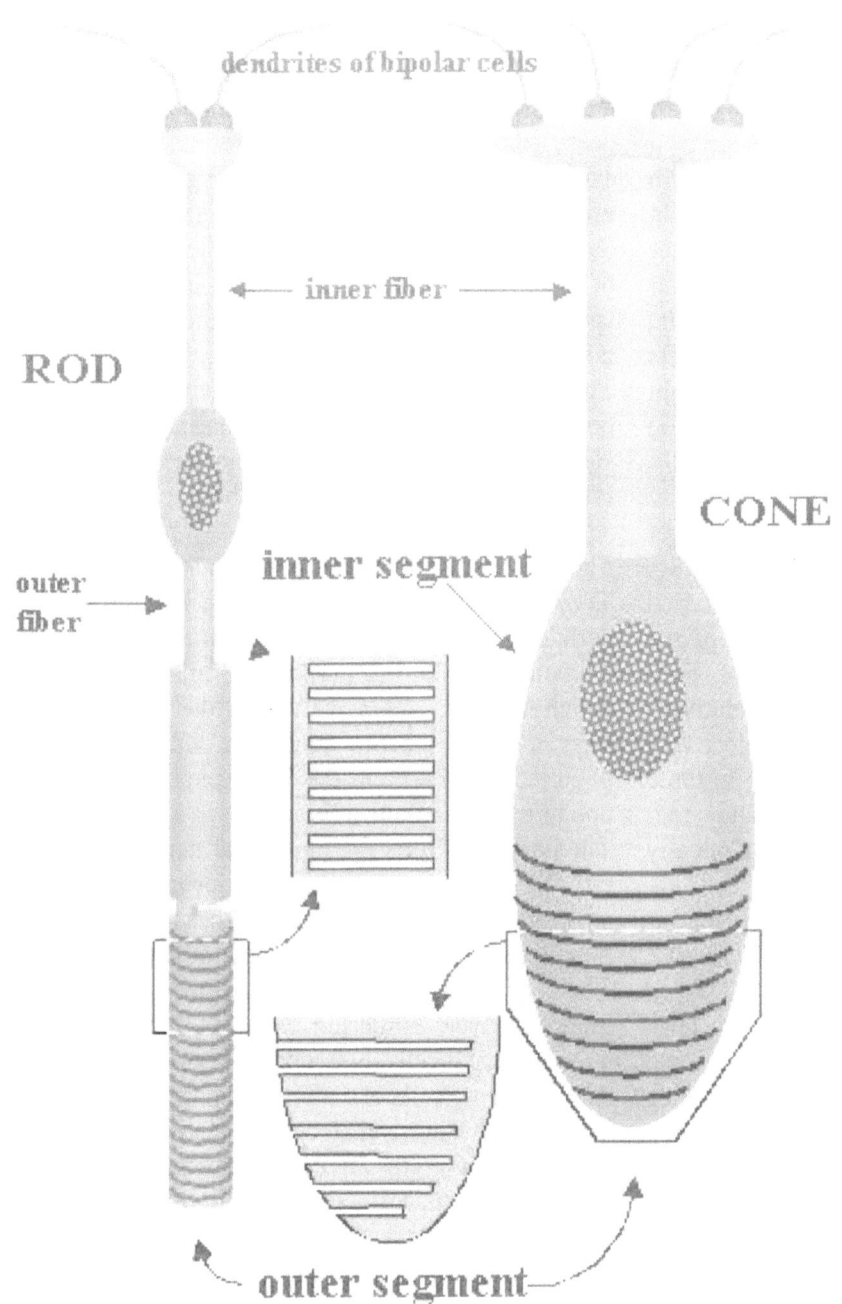

dendrites of bipolar cells

inner fiber

ROD

inner segment

outer fiber

CONE

outer segment

Fig. 4.12.23. The "rod" of a rod photoreceptor, as well as the "cone" of a cone photoreceptor, consist of both an outer segment and an inner segment. The outer segments contain a stack of discoid vesicles, the membrane of which carries photoreceptive pigments. The disks of the rod cells are completely separated from the cell membrane, those of the cone cells are confluent with it. The cone cell's inner segment contains the nucleus. The nucleus of the rod cells lies in the cell body, separated from the inner segment by means of an outer fiber. At the other pole, the cell body narrows into an inner fiber. The inner fiber terminal, which has the structure of an axon, expands into an end knob, which forms synaptic junctions with the dendrites of bipolar cells.

short, narrow stalk that divides the rod into a peripheral **outer segment** (length about 7 micrometers, diameter about 1 micrometer) contacting the pigment epithelium, and a central **inner segment**.

The outer segment is very distinctive: it is occupied by a stack of flattened, parallel membranous cisterns or disks. These disks are continuously formed at the basis of the rod, apparently by fusion of vesicles that originate in the inner segment. At the tip of the rod, these disks are continuously lost. A stack of 20-30 disks begins to curl, the rod constricts under the stack, and the whole complex detaches and is phagocytosed

by the pigment cells. The visual pigment of the rods is rhodopsin. It is an integral membrane protein, incorporated in the membrane of the disks.

The intersegmental stalk contains a cylinder of nine microtubular doublets, indicating that it is a modified cilium. The ciliary basal body is implanted in the inner segment.

The inner segment contains a well-developed Golgi-complex and numerous mitochondria. The inner segment narrows, forming a short axon, which leads into a perikaryon that contains the nucleus. At the opposite side of the perikaryon, a second axon arises and courses towards the inner granular layer.

The peripheral process of the **cone cells** (Fig. 4.12.23.) is short and conical, with a broad base and a narrow top. Like the rod, the cone is divided into an outer and an inner segment, separated from each other by a constriction. This constriction is circumferential and very shallow. The lateral cell membrane of the **outer segment** develops narrow, deep folds, perpendicular to the cone axis. These membranes resemble the stacked cisterns of the rods, but they never separate from the cell membrane. They are also lost and replaced, but at a slower rhythm than rod membrane disks. They contain visual pigments, analogous to rhodopsin. The inner segment continues into the perikaryon, without narrowing. On the opposite side of the cone, a short axon arises, directed to the inner granular layer.

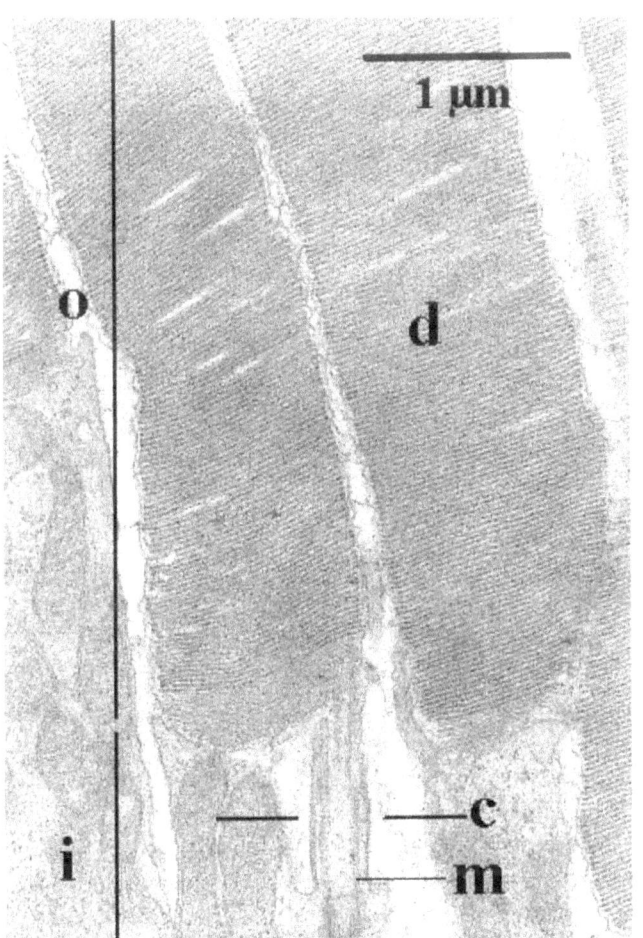 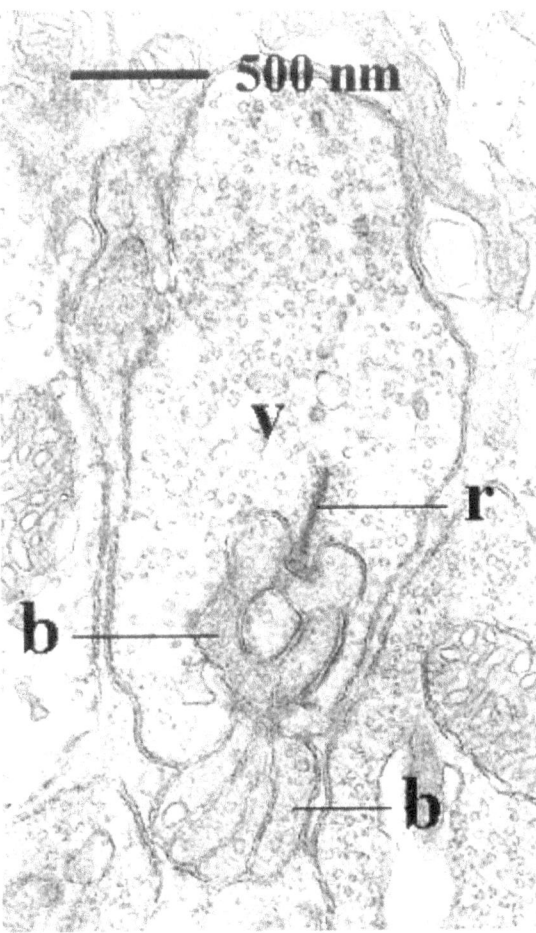

Fig. 4.12.24. (left) After magnification of Figure 4.12.16., outer (o) and inner (i) segments of a rod photoreceptor cell are seen to be separated from one another by a constriction (c), wherein lies a microtubular structure (m), as in a cilium. The outer segment contains the membranous disks (d) with photoreceptive pigments. Compare with Figure 4.12.23. Retina, rabbit, TEM. **Fig. 4.12.25.** (right) The end knob of a rod cell inner fiber or axon, in the outer plexiform layer, is indented by several dendritic end knobs of bipolar cells (b). The axonal end knob contains numerous synaptic vesicles (v), which converge towards a synaptic rod (r), oriented at right angles to the presynaptic membrane. Retina, hamster, TEM.

The peripheral axon of the photoreceptor cells dilates to a terminal, which is loaded with translucent synaptic vesicles and which is rather irregularly shaped because it is indented by one to several clusters of terminals, belonging to interneurons.

The rod cell terminal (Fig. 4.12.25.) is associated with a single cluster of interneuron terminals. The cone cell terminal is relatively wide and is associated with several clusters of interneuron terminals. In the presynaptic terminal, the one belonging to the photoreceptor cell, a **synaptic rod** is observed. A synaptic rod is a rather unusual part of a synaptic junction, which is encountered only in sensory nerve cells. In sections, it is a linear element, about 250 nanometers long and 50 nanometers wide, which lies at right angles to the presynaptic membrane, and is anchored to it by filaments. It has a trilaminar structure: a narrow, clear layer is sandwiched between two dense layers. A synaptic rod is in fact a cross section of a flattened, circular vesicle. Synaptic vesicles are linked to both faces of the rod. They are regularly spaced and at a constant distance from the rod. The function of the synaptic rod is not yet entirely clear. However, it appears to be typical to continuously, or tonically, active synaptic junctions. It apparently serves as a conveyor belt, drawing synaptic vesicles to the presynaptic membrane, where they undergo exocytosis, thus ensuring a regular, uninterrupted flow of neurotransmitter.

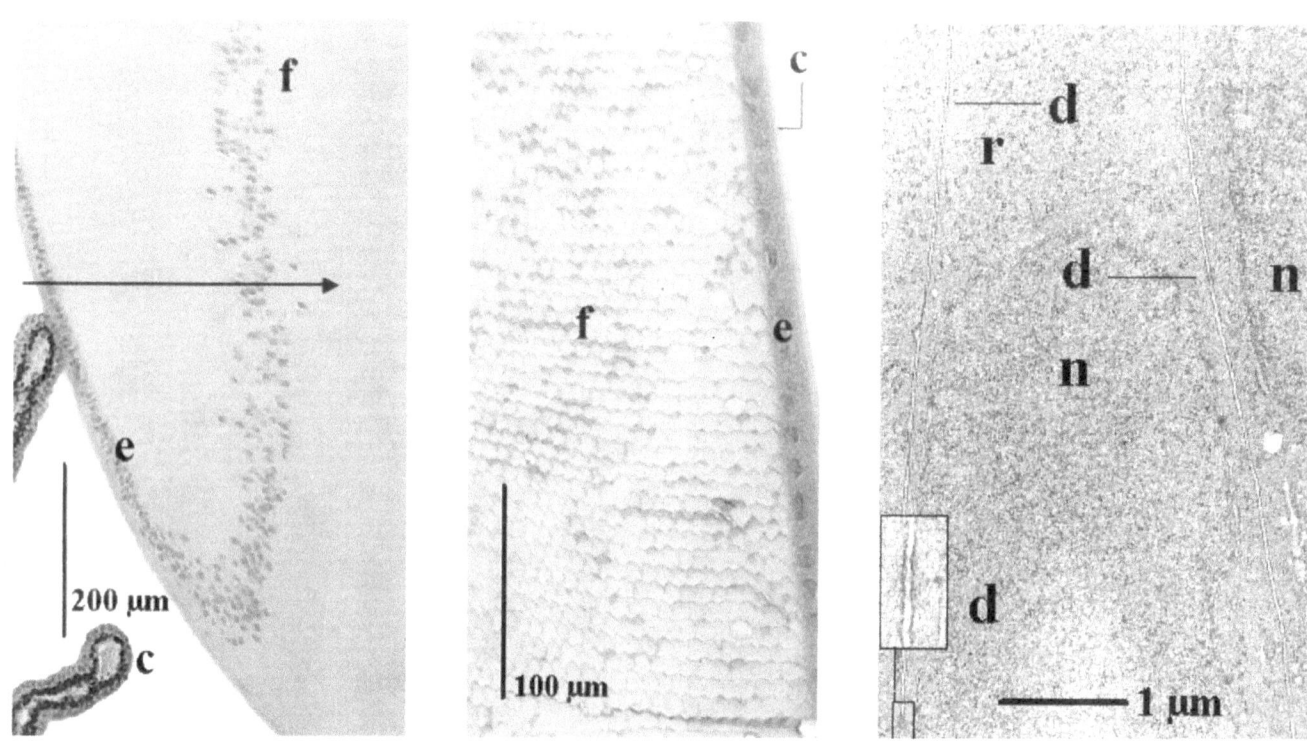

Left to right: **Fig. 4.12.26.** The anterior epithelium (e) of the lens, derived from the lens vesicle, conserves its original aspect. The posterior epithelial cells greatly lengthen, parallel to the eye's optic axis, and differentiate into lens fibers (f). c = ciliary body. The arrow shows the direction followed by an incoming light beam. Lens, rabbit, HE. **Fig. 4.12.27.** In a favorably oriented section, transverse sections of lens fibers (f) are seen. These have hexagonal shapes and are tightly packed. The anterior lens epithelium (e) is coated with a thick basement membrane, the lens capsule (c). Lens, rabbit, HE. **Fig. 4.12.28.** The lens fibers betray their epithelial origin through the presence of junctions, especially desmosomes (d). Their nucleus (n) slowly disintegrates and the cytoplasm is rich in ribosomes (r), which will synthesize a dense, crystalline, protein matrix. Eye lens, hamster, TEM.

IV.12.6. Lens.

Essentially, the lens is a highly specialized epithelium, derived from the ectodermal lens vesicle (Fig. 4.12.1.). Initially, the lens vesicle is spherical and its wall is a simple epithelium, resting on a peripheral basement membrane. The posterior cells of the lens vesicle start to lengthen, parallel to the eye's optic axis. The vesicular lumen is obliterated as a consequence of this. At the equator of the vesicle, the plane of which is perpendicular to the optic axis, cell proliferation takes place. As they are formed, these cells shift in the direction of the optic axis and start to lengthen. As the cells progress towards the optic axis, they grow into extremely elongated, slender cells, which are called **lens fibers** (Fig. 4.12.26.). Gradually, their nucleus and organelles are lost, and they accumulate an amorphous cytoplasmic matrix.

The fully developed lens consists of a few thousand of such lens fibers, which bridge almost the whole interval between both lens poles. The central fibers, close to the optic axis, are slightly curved, the more equatorial ones progressively more so. The fibers are tightly packed and have a hexagonal cross section (Fig.

4.12.27.). They form short lateral processes, which form ball and socket, as well as flap and groove, junctions with adjacent fibers. The cell membranes of adjacent fibers may fuse. The cytoplasm is loaded with an amorphous, crystalline substance (Fig. 4.12.28.), consisting of crystallin proteins.

The cells making up the anterior half of the lens vesicle have not lengthened and remain as a simple cuboidal epithelium, lining the anterior face of the lens (Fig. 4.12.26.).

In the dense lamina of the surrounding basement membrane, the **lens capsule**, the collagen fibrils of Zinn's ligament are anchored.

The crystalline substance of the lens confers refractive properties to it. After refraction by the cornea, the lens ensures finer adjustment of the focus of incident light. The degree to which the lens refracts light is variable. As already mentioned, it is the contractile state of the ciliary body that determines the curvature of the lens and its refractive power. Increasing curvature of the lens, upon contraction of the ciliary body, adjusts for near sight. Decreasing curvature, upon relaxation of the ciliary body, adjusts for far sight.

References.

Beuerman R.W., Pedroza L.: Ultrastructure of the human cornea. Microsc. Res. Tech. 1996, 33: 320-335.

Freddo T.F.: Ultrastructure of the iris. Microsc. Res. Tech. 1996, 33: 369-389.

Freegard T.J.: The physical basis of transparency of the normal cornea. Eye 1997, 11: 465-471.

Imesch P.D., Wallow I.H.L., Albert D.M.: The color of the human eye: a review of morphologic correlates and of some conditions that affect iridial pigmentation. Surv. Ophthalmol. 1997, 41 (Suppl. 2): S117-S123.

Kuszak J.R., Peterson K.L., Brown H.G.: Electron microscopic observations of the crystalline lens. Microsc. Res. Tech. 1996, 33: 441-479.

Masland R.H.: The functional architecture of the retina. Sci. Am. 1986, december: 90-99.

Nguyen-Legros J., Hicks D.: Renewal of photoreceptor outer segments and their phagocytosis by the retinal pigment epithelium. Int. Rev. Cytol. 2000, 196: 245-313.

Schnapf J.L., Baylor D.A.: How photoreceptor cells respond to light. Sci. Am. 1987, april: 32-39.

Wagner H.J.: Presynaptic bodies ("ribbons"): from ultrastructural observations to molecular perspectives. Cell Tissue Res. 1997, 287: 435-446.

IV.13. Organs of hearing and balance.

The organs of hearing and balance belong to the most delicate and complex organs of the body. They are double organs, the organs of hearing and those of balance being separate, but closely associated, entities. The organ of hearing, the **ear**, is an exteroreceptor, sensitive to stimuli that come from the exterior world. Anatomically, the ear can be divided into an external ear, middle ear, and inner ear (Fig. 4.13.1.). The actual receptor organ, which converts stimuli into neural action potentials, is the **inner ear**. The inner ear is a mechanoreceptor, sensitive to air vibrations in a limited band of frequencies, e. g. sound. The external and middle ear are not sensitive to sound, they only collect vibrations and transmit them to the inner ear.

The organ of balance is also a mechanoreceptor, but in contrast to the ear it is a proprioreceptor, sensitive to stimuli from within the body. It is stimulated by inertial fluid movements, which are caused by movements and changes in the position of the body. Anatomically, it is closely associated with the inner ear.

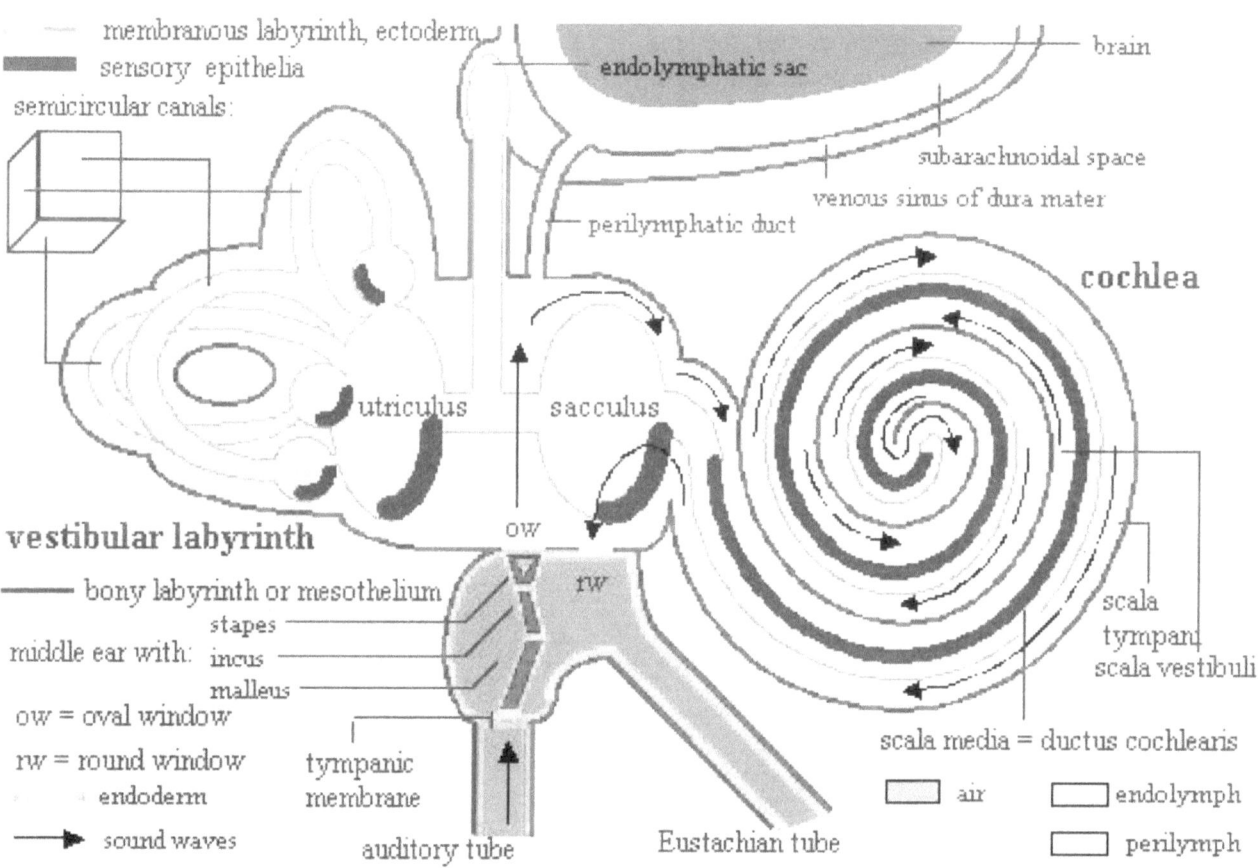

Fig. 4.13.1. To the organs of hearing and balance belong the external ear, which consists of a pinna and an auditory canal, the middle ear, and the internal ear. The middle ear contains the ossicles, which transmit vibrations of the tympanic membrane to the oval window of the inner ear. Through the Eustachian tube, the middle ear is continuous with the pharynx. It also contains the round window. Both the inner ear and the organs of balance are formed by the membranous labyrinth: a number of interconnected spaces with complex shapes, lined by an epithelium. In a few places, this epithelium is developed into a sensory epithelium. The membranous labyrinth lies in a corresponding space in the skull bones: the bony labyrinth. The sensory epithelia of the utriculus and the sacculus, the maculae ampullares, represent the organ of static balance. The utriculus gives rise to 3 semicircular canals, at right angles to one another so that there is one for each dimension of space. At one end, these canals widen to form an ampulla. In each ampulla lies a specialized sensory epithelium, a crista ampullaris. Together, they represent the organ of dynamic balance. The inner ear, the actual organ of hearing, arises from the sacculus as a blind duct, spirally coiled: the cochlear duct or scala media. The scala media is flanked by 2 spaces of the bony labyrinth (they are filled with perilymph): the scala vestibuli and the scala tympani. Both are confluent at the tip of the cochlear duct. The scala tympani ends at the round window. The junction of utriculus and sacculus gives rise to an endolymphatic duct, which ends as an endolymphatic sac in the venous sinuses of the dura mater.

The external ear originates as a local inpocketing of the ectoderm, the lumen of which remains in continuity with the exterior and which will develop into the auditory canal. The inner ear arises from another ectodermal inpocketing, but this one ends up separated from the overlying ectoderm, and forms an **auditory vesicle**. Local constrictions, elongations, expansions and fusions convert this vesicles into a hollow structure with a very complex shape. Part of the inner ear will develop into the organ of hearing, the other part into the organ of balance. Sandwiched between external ear and inner ear is an inpocketing of endoderm of the primitive pharynx, which develops into the middle ear. Its lumen remains in continuity with the pharynx and develops into the Eustachian tube.

The inner ear, i.e. the organs of hearing and balance, is essentially a specialized **epithelium**. **Nerve tissue** also participates, since the epithelium has a dense sensory innervation. In several places, specialized **fibrous tissue** structures are encountered (spiral limbus, spiral ligament, tectorial membrane). The external and middle ear are epithelia, resting on supportive tissue, and occasionally forming glands. The middle ear also contains bones, the ossicles.

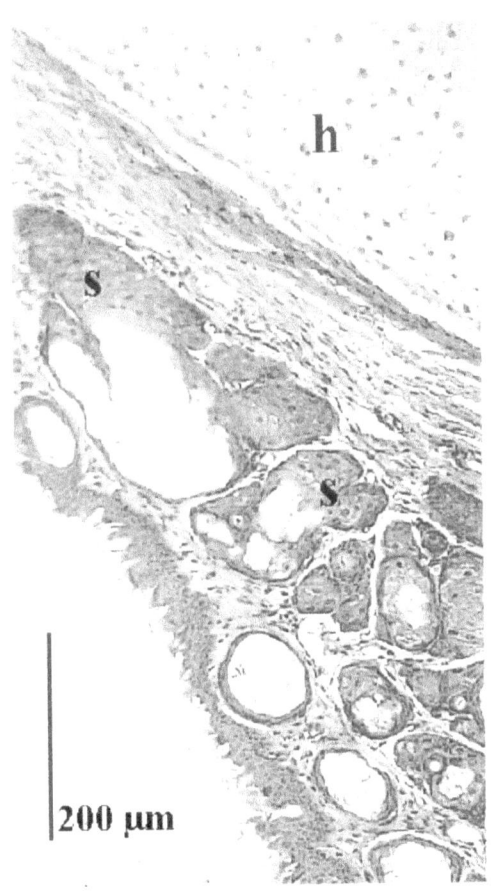
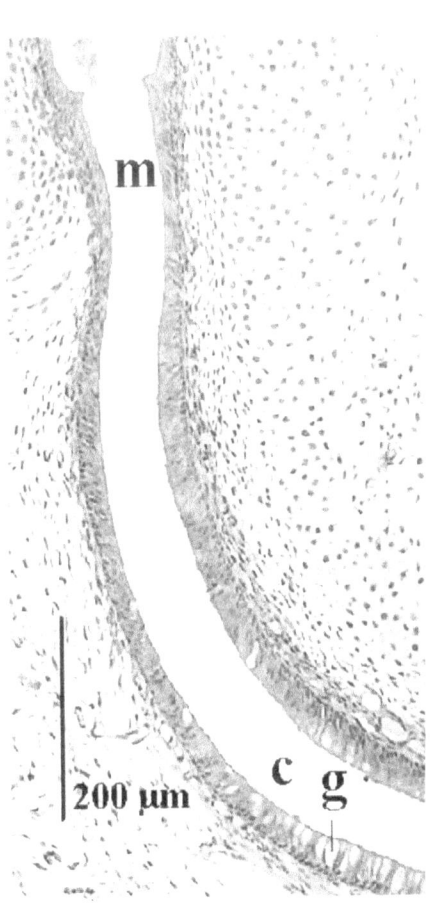

Fig. 4.13.2. (left) The auditory canal is lined with a thin epidermis, which forms sebum glands (s). h = hyaline cartilage. Ear, rabbit, HE. **Fig. 4.13.3.** (right) Towards the middle ear, the Eustachian tube is lined with ciliated epithelium (c) containing goblet cells (g). Towards the pharynx, this epithelium is gradually replaced with a Malpighian epithelium (m). Ear, rabbit, HE.

IV.13.1. External ear.

The external ear collects sound waves and guides them to deeper parts of the ear. It consists of a shell-like pinna and an auditory canal. The pinna and the outer third of the auditory canal are made of elastic cartilage, covered with skin. The inner third of the auditory canal runs in the skull wall. The epidermis of the auditory canal develops sebum glands or **ceruminous glands** (Fig. 4.13.2.).

IV.13.2. Middle ear.

The middle ear transmits vibrations to the inner ear (Fig. 4.13.1.). Essentially, it is an air-filled space in the skull wall, separated from the auditory canal by the tympanic membrane, and from the inner ear by the oval window and the round window. It is continuous with the pharynx through the **Eustachian tube** (Fig. 4.13.3.), ensuring that the air pressure inside the middle ear is the same as the external air pressure. The Eustachian tube is initially lined with pseudostratified ciliated epithelium, as is the respiratory mucosa. Towards the pharynx, this changes into a Malpighian epithelium.

The **tympanic membrane** is a thin fibrous membrane, made up of an outer cuticle, a middle fibrosa, and an inner mucosa. The **cuticle** is a thin epidermis, continuous with that of the auditory canal. The **fibrosa** is double, the outer layer consisting of radial fibrils, the inner one contains peripheral, circumferential fibrils. The **mucosa** is a continuation of the respiratory mucosa, derived from endoderm, which coats the Eustachian tube and the middle ear. It is lined with a simple squamous epithelium.

Between the tympanic membrane and the oval window is a chain of three **ossicles** (Fig. 4.13.1.). The first one, the **malleus** or hammer, has a handle, which is fastened to the center of the tympanic membrane. Its head articulates with the second ossicle, the **incus** or anvil, which articulates, in its turn, with the third ossicle, the **stapes** or stirrup. The stapes fits into the **oval window**, in which it can move up and down like a piston in a cylinder. The ossicles are enchondral bones and are made of compact bone tissue. They are coated with a thin mucosa, derived form the respiratory mucosa coating the middle ear. Sound waves, which cause vibration of the tympanic membrane, are transmitted through the ossicles and the oval window to the inner ear.

The **round window** is another opening between the middle ear and the inner ear (Fig. 4.13.1.). It is closed with a membrane that has the same structure as the tympanic membrane, since it too is derived from both endoderm and ectoderm.

IV.13.3. Inner ear.

Essentially, the inner ear is a membranous sac with a complex shape, lined with epithelium that is derived from the ectoderm of the auditory vesicle, the **membranous labyrinth** (Fig. 4.13.1.). The surrounding bone of the skull is shaped correspondingly and is called the bony labyrinth. Occasionally, the membranous labyrinth is tightly joined to the bony labyrinth. Usually, there is a

perimembranous space between the two. The membranous labyrinth, as well as the perimembranous space, contain fluid, the **endolymph** and the **perilymph**, respectively. The membranous labyrinth is a closed space. It is lined with a simple squamous epithelium, which is locally developed into innervated **sensory epithelia**. The perimembranous space is in fact a continuation of the brain's subarachnoidal space, and the perilymph is cerebrospinal fluid. Like the subarachnoidal space, the perimembranous space is bridged by fibrous tissue strands, and lined with mesothelium.

The membranous and bony labyrinths can be divided, anatomically, in two parts: the **vestibular labyrinth** and the **cochlea**. The first houses the organ of balance, the second the organ of hearing.

IV.13.3.1. Vestibular labyrinth.

The vestibular labyrinth has two parts: the vestibule and the semicircular canals (Fig. 4.13.1.).
The **vestibule** is a comparatively wide space, situated behind the oval window. Its bony component houses two membranous components, the **utricle** and the **saccule**. Both contain an area of thickened, sensory epithelium, a **macula**. The saccule extends anteriory, forming the membranous component of the cochlea. The utricle forms three tubes, which follow a circular course before opening again into the utricle. These are called the **semicircular canals**, each of which determines a plane that is at right angles to the others. Two of these planes lie vertically, the third horizontally. Each canal is widened at one of its mouths, forming an ampulla. Here, the mucosa and its thickened sensory epithelium form a crest, the **ampullar crista**, perpendicular to the tube's axis. At the base of the crest, the epithelium's basal cell membrane forms deep, narrow, parallel folds, with mitochondria in between. These cells are equipped for ion and fluid transport. They probably produce endolymph or regulate its ionic composition.
The narrow tubular connection between saccule and utricle produces a branch, the **endolymphatic sac**, which extends into the venous sinuses of the dura mater. Its epithelium has phagocytic properties and contributes to the resorption of endolymph.

IV.13.3.2. Cochlea.

The bony compartment of the **cochlea** is a spiral tubule, the convolutions of which, 2.5 in number, form a cone resembling a snail shell (Figs. 4.13.1., 4.13.4.).

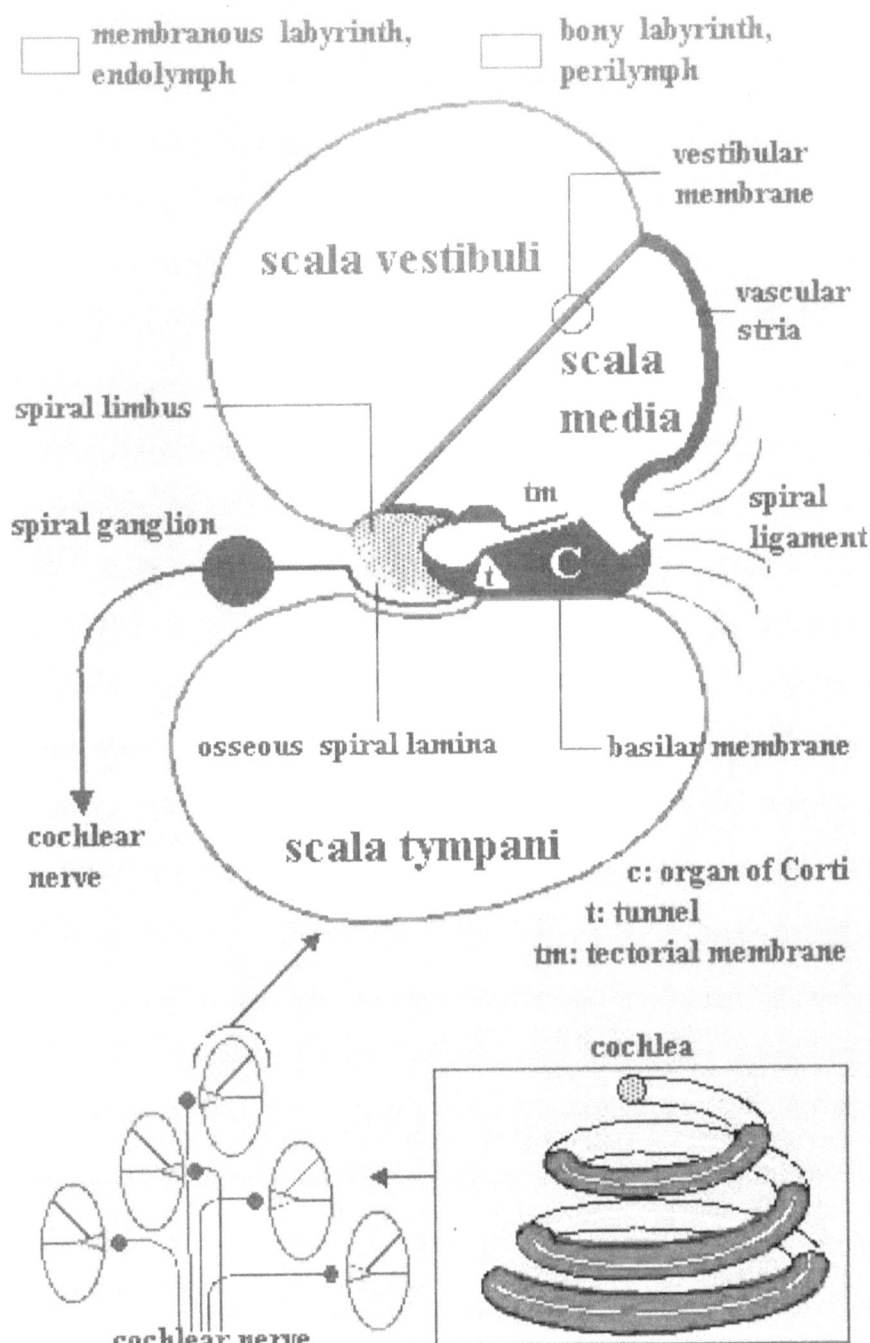

membranous labyrinth, endolymph

bony labyrinth, perilymph

scala vestibuli

vestibular membrane

scala media

vascular stria

spiral limbus

spiral ganglion

tm

spiral ligament

t

C

cochlear nerve

osseous spiral lamina

basilar membrane

scala tympani

c: organ of Corti
t: tunnel
tm: tectorial membrane

cochlea

cochlear nerve

Fig. 4.13.4. The cochlea is shaped like a snail shell, and has 2.5 coils (bottom right). In an axial section, its 3 tubular components are visible, as well as its bony axis, and parts of the spiral ganglion, which gives rise to the acoustic nerve (bottom left). In the upper part of the drawing, a single cross section of a coil is schematically represented. The scala media is the cochlear duct, a component of the membranous labyrinth. Most of its epithelium is unspecialized, such as the area participating in the formation of the vestibular membrane. At the outside of the cochlear coil, the epithelium forms the vascular stria. The local fibrous tissue is also specialized, forming the spiral ligament. The sensory area of this epithelium is Corti's organ. The tympanic membrane is an acellular matrix, originating at the spiral limbus, which is made of fibrous tissue. The peripheral axons of the bipolar nerve cells, making up the spiral ganglion, course in the bony spiral lamina. Corti's organ rests on the basilar membrane of the scala tympani, which is a specialized periost. The scala vestibuli, as well as the scala tympani, are coated with periost, which is lined with mesothelium. The vestibular periost participates in the formation of the vestibular membrane.

The cone lies on its side, its top pointing forward. The bony cochlea houses a tubular component of the membranous labyrinth, the **cochlear duct**, a continuation of the vestibular sacculus. In certain places along its perimeter, the cochlear duct touches the bony wall of the cochlea, in such a fashion that three spiral spaces are created (Fig. 4.13.4.). The middle space, the **scala media**, is the cochlear duct itself, and contains endolymph. Its cross section is triangular. "Above" it, in the direction of the cochlea's top, is the **scala vestibuli**. The scala vestibuli is continuous with the bony vestibulum and contains perilymph. In cross section, it is semicircular, bordering the "inclined" face of the scala media. At the bottom of the cochlear tube, bordering the "horizontal" face of the scala media, is another space, which is semicircular in cross section, the **scala tympani**. Like the scala vestibuli, it opens into the bony vestibulum and is filled with perilymph. Scala vestibuli and scala tympani are in continuity at the top of the cochlea.

The scala media and the scala tympani are separated from each other by the **basilar membrane** (Figs.

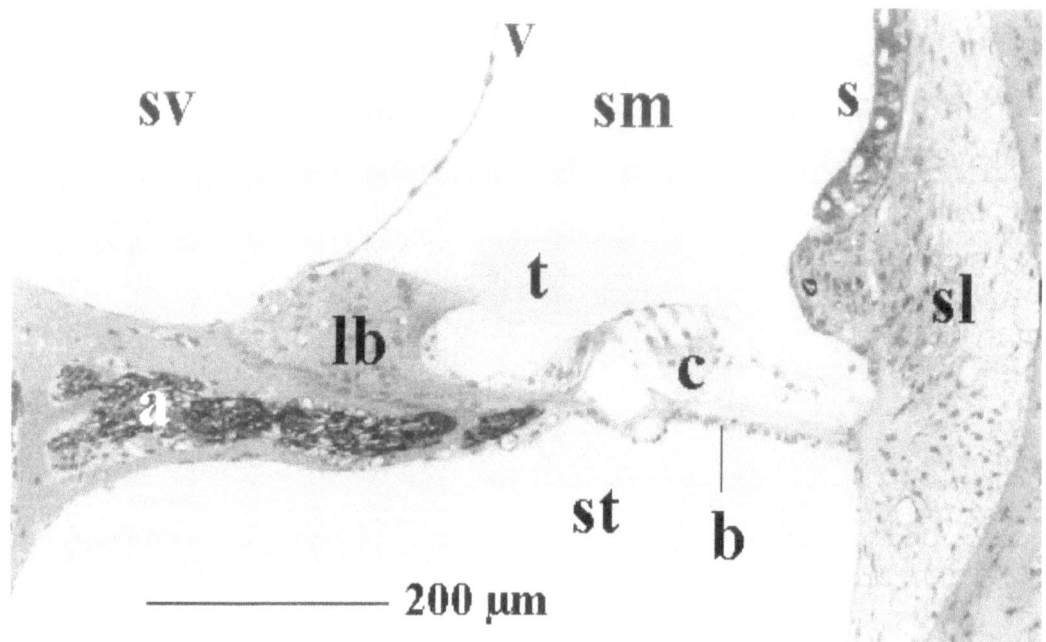

Fig. 4.13.5. The scala media (sm), contains Corti's organ (c), which rests on the basilar membrane (b), which separates scala media and scale tympani (st). Corti's organ is made of specialized epithelial cells. Corti's organ supports the acellular tectorial membrane (t). The fibrous spiral limbus (lb), the spiral ligament (sl), the vascular stria (s), and the vestibular membrane (v), which separates scala media and scala vestibuli (sv), are seen as well. In the bony spiral lamina course myelinated nerve fibers of the acoustic nerve (a). Compare with Figure 4.13.4., upper part. Cochlea, cat, 1-micrometer plastic section, toluidin blue.

4.13.4.-5.). This "membrane" is relatively thick and made of dense fibrous connective tissue. At the side of the scala tympani, it is lined with mesothelium, at the side of the scala media with epithelium. This is a very specialized epithelium, with a dense sensory innervation, which forms the organ of hearing, **Corti's organ**. The basilar membrane is attached to the outside of the cochlear convolutions by the spiral ligament, at the inside by the spiral lamina.

The spiral ligament is a thickened periost. It has a broad base that rests against the wall of the bony cochlea. The epithelium that lines it (scala media side) is specialized, forming the **vascular stria**. This epithelium is stratified and the underlying fibrous tissue is very vascular. A virtually unique characteristic of this epithelium is that it is penetrated by blood capillaries (Fig. 4.13.6.). The superficial cells of the vascular stria are prismatic. Their apex, containing the nucleus, bulges into the lumen of the scala media. Their basal cell membrane forms deep, narrow, parallel folds with numerous mitochondria in between (Fig. 4.13.7.), the characteristics of cells transporting ions and fluids. These cells probably have the same function as similar ones that are found in the cristae ampullares: production of endolymph.

The spiral lamina is a bony crest, formed by the modiolus, the axis of the bony cochlea. Near the top of the lamina, close to the attachment of the basilar

membrane, and facing the scala media, the periosteum is thickened, forming the spiral limbus. The epithelium lining the limbus give rise to a fibrous **tectorial membrane**, the top of which rests on Corti's organ. Numerous sensory nerve fibers course in the spiral lamina. They lead from Corti's organ to a spiral ganglion in the base of the lamina. This ganglion contains bipolar nerve cells.

The scala media and the scala vestibuli are separated from each other by the vestibular membrane or Reissner's membrane (Fig. 4.13.5.). This is a very thin fibrous membrane, lined with epithelium on the side of the scala media and with mesothelium on the side of the scala vestibuli.

IV.13.3.3. Sensory epithelia.

The sensory epithelia, which are at the heart of the organs of hearing and balance, are very specialized, stratified epithelia. They are found in the vestibular (utricle and saccule) maculae, the ampullar cristae, and in Corti's organ. They contain highly specialized, mechanoreceptive **hair cells** (Fig. 4.13.8.) with a sensory innervation, and supporting cells.

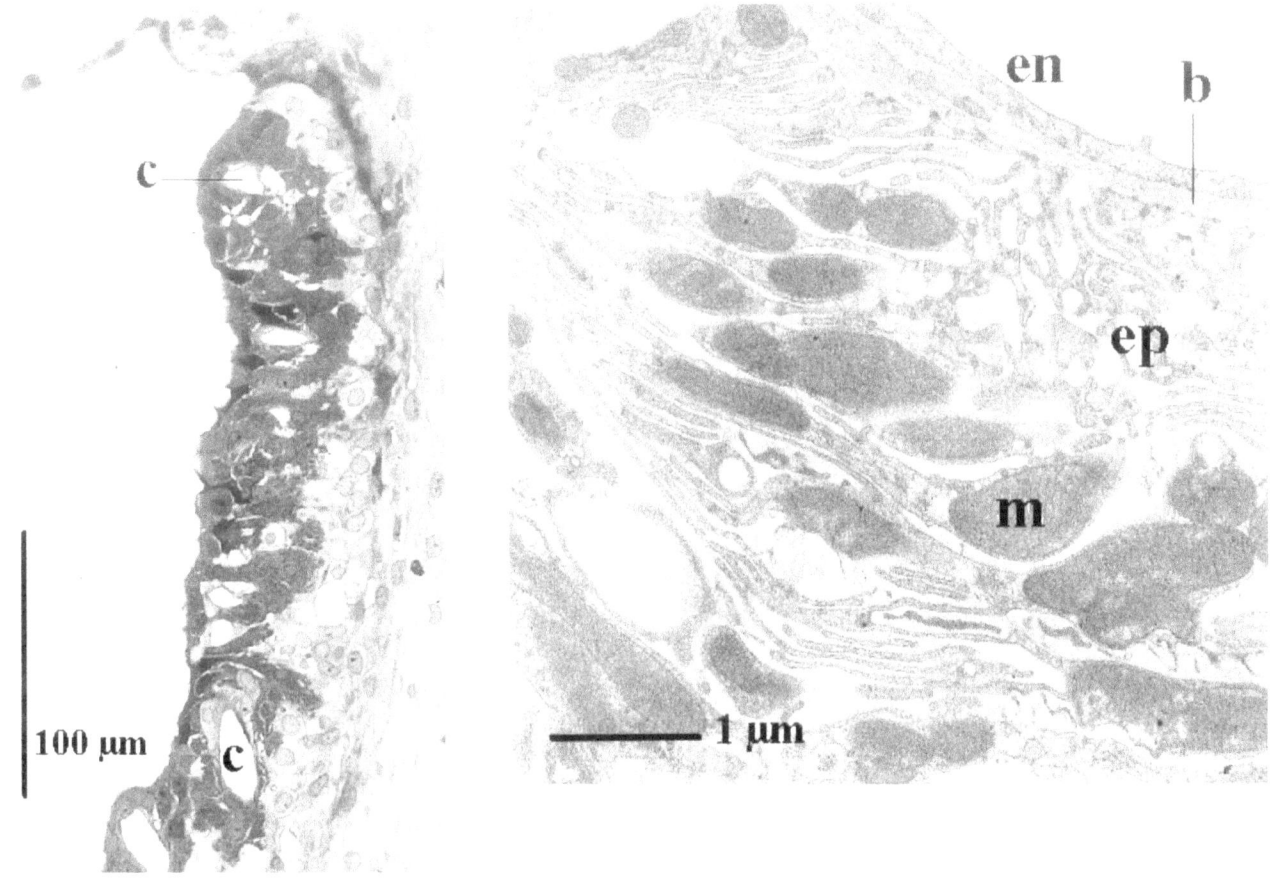

Fig. 4.13.6. (left) A unique characteristic of the vascular stria epithelium is the presence of capillaries (c). The combination of 2 tissues, epithelium and endothelium, means that the stria is actually an organ. Cochlea, hamster, 1-micrometer plastic section, toluidin blue. **Fig. 4.13.7.** (right) An endothelial cell (en) and an epithelial cell (ep) of the vascular stria, separated by their communal basement membrane (b). The epithelial cell membrane is deeply folded. The folds alternate with mitochondria (m). Both characteristics are typical of cells that specialize in the transport of ions and fluid. These cells produce endolymph. Cochlea, hamster, TEM.

IV.13.3.3.1. Vestibular maculae.

The macular **hair cells** touch the vestibular lumen, but not the basement membrane. They rest between and on top of supporting cells (Fig. 4.13.9.). Their nuclei, which are bigger and more euchromatic than those of the supporting cells, occupy a fairly high level. Hair cells are fiber-bearing cells, which carry stiff microvilli, usually called stereocilia, as well as cilia (Fig. 4.13.8.). Each hair cell carries numerous **stereocilia** and a single **cilium**, placed eccentrically (Figs. 4.13.8., 4.13.10.). The stereocilia have a constricted basis. In it runs a dense axial filament that will merge with a terminal web in the apical hair cell cytoplasm. The terminal web or **cortical plate** has the shape of a hemisphere, with its flat side parallel to the apical cell membrane. At the lateral cell membranes, the cortical plate is joined through a junctional complex to the terminal web of the adjoining supporting cells. As the stereocilia are placed closer and closer to the eccentric cilium, they grow

progressively longer. The tip of each stereocilium is linked to the body of the next, higher, stereocilium by a slender filament, or tip link. The tips of the cilium and those of the longest stereocilia are embedded in a gelatinous layer that covers the macula and is probably secreted by the supporting cells. In this layer lie a number of **otoliths**, crystals of calcium carbonate (Fig. 4.13.8.).

In fact, the macula has two kinds of hair cells (Fig. 4.13.8.). **Type 1** is bulbous, has pale cytoplasm and a basal nucleus, which occupies the middle level of the epithelium. These cells rest in the cup shaped terminal of a sensory nerve fiber (Fig. 4.13.11.), which is why they are called goblet cells. Synaptic rods are associated with the cell membrane facing the nerve terminal. Between hair cell basis and its apex is a constricted neck part, supported by microtubules. The apical appendages are well developed. **Type 2** is more slender, has a darker aspect, and the nucleus, lying in the middle of the cell, occupies a relatively high position in the macular epithelium. There is no neck

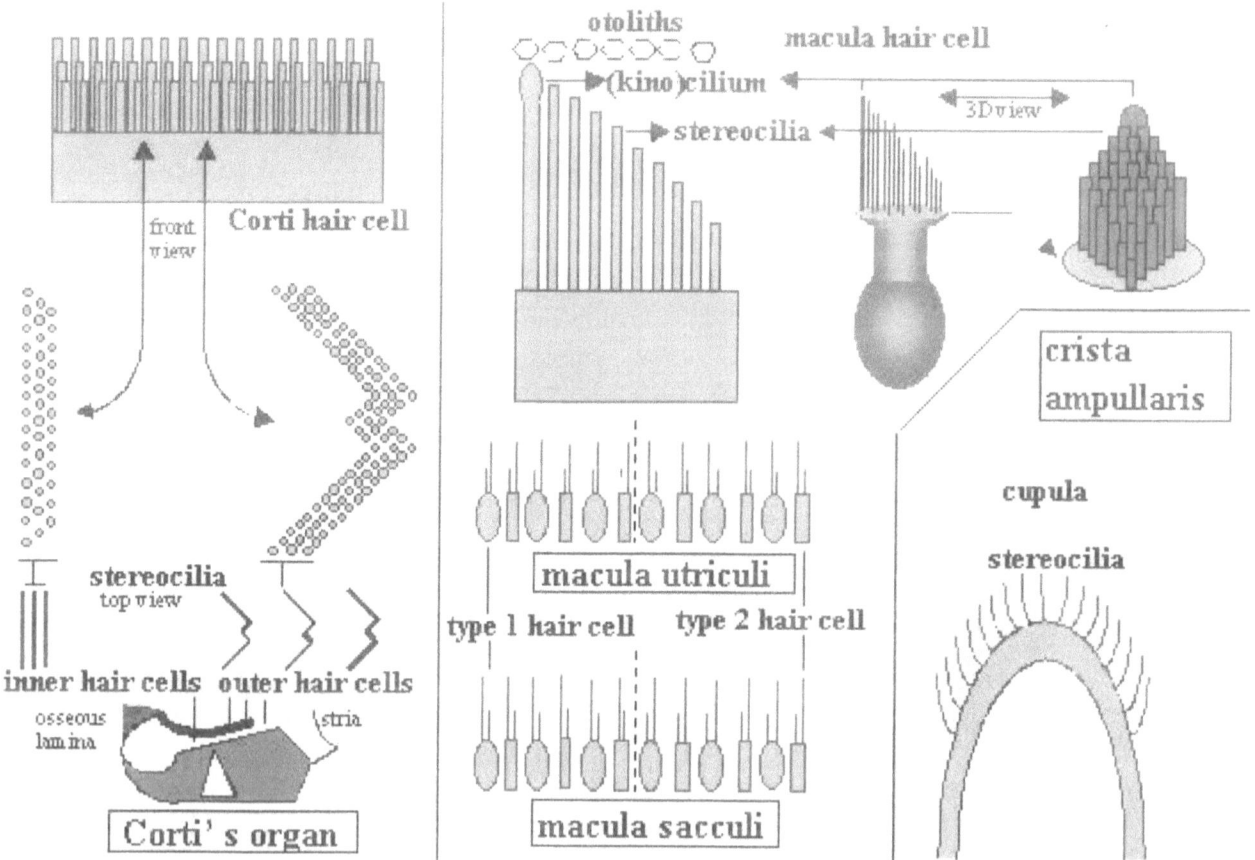

Fig. 4.13.8. The hair cells of vestibular and cochlear sensory epithelia. The inner and outer hair cells of Corti's organ carry 3 rows of stereocilia, parallel to the long axis of the cochlear duct, and supporting the tectorial membrane. While the stereocilia of the inner hair cells form straight lines, those of the outer hair cells are arranged so as to form a W, the basis of which is directed toward the outside of the cochlear coil (middle left: view from above). In frontal view (upper left), the front row of stereocilia (i.e. the row which is closest to the long cochlear axis) has the shortest stereocilia, while the back rows contain progressively longer stereocilia. The macular hair cells carry several rows of stereocilia, which progressively lengthen as they approach the single eccentric cilium, which contacts the otolithic membrane (middle right and top right). Both maculae are ellipsoid, and thus have a long axis. In the saccular macula, the hair cells on both sides of the axis orient their cilium away from it. In the utricular macula, they orient their cilium toward it. The hair cells of the cristae ampullares have very long stereocilia, which lie embedded in a mucous cupula.

and the apical appendages are a little shorter. Remarkably, the mitochondria line up at the inner face of the cell membrane. This cell is contacted, at its base, by several small nervous terminals. Apart from sensory nerve terminals, filled with mitochondria, motor nerve terminals, filled with vesicles, are observed (Fig. 4.13.12.). Facing the sensory nerve terminals, the cytoplasm of type 2 hair cells contains synaptic rods.

The **supporting cells** are slender, prismatic cells with an expanded basis that contains the nucleus. This nucleus lies at a lower level than those of the hair cells. They rest on the basement membrane and contact the vestibular lumen. These cells are clearly fiber-bearing cells. Their slightly expanded apex contains a terminal web and carries a few short microvilli, as well as a

single, underdeveloped, cilium. Internally, the cell is reinforced with a thick bundle of microtubules, which runs at one side of the nucleus and terminates in the apical web.

The maculae contribute to static balance by gathering information about the position of the head. If the head is moved from a position of balance, the otoliths will shift and deform the hair cell appendages, whereupon the hair cells will depolarize and induce action potentials in the sensory nerve fibers. The motor nerve endings associated with type 2 cells are inhibitory. Of both kinds of appendages, the stereocilia are easiest to deform. If they bend towards the cilium, the tip links are stretched and the hair cell is excited. Otherwise, the tip links slacken and the hair cell is inhibited. Both maculae, the saccular one and the utricular one, are

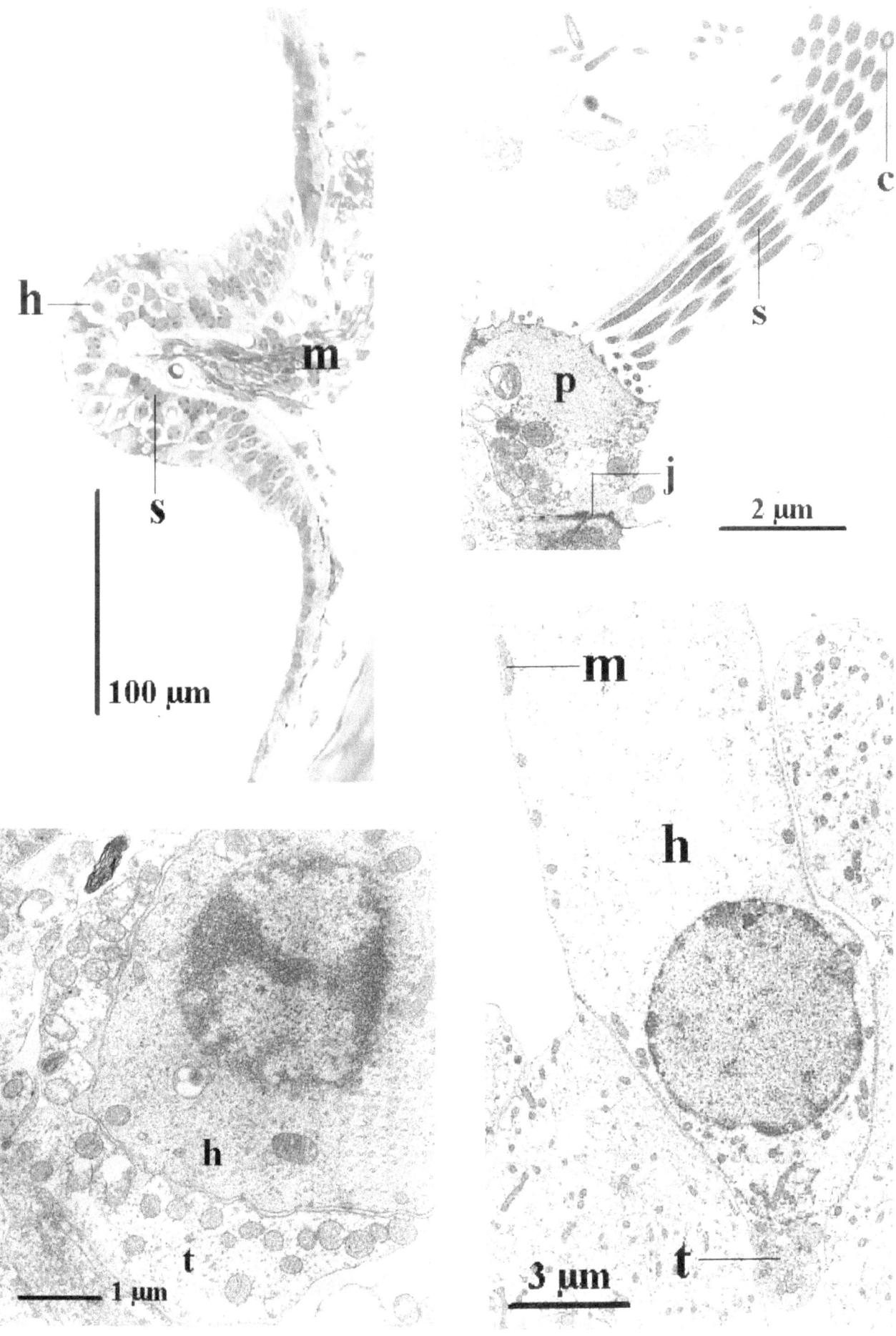

Fig. 4.13.9. (top left) The sensory epithelium of the macula (utriculi as well as sacculi) consists of specialized receptor cells, the hair cells, which alternate with supporting cells. The hair cells (h) are the voluminous, superficial cells with clear cytoplasm. The supporting cells (s) are much smaller, and their nucleus lies at the epithelial basis. Beneath the epithelium run myelinated nerve fibers (m). Vestibulum, hamster, 1-micron plastic sections, toluidin blue. **Fig. 4.13.10.** (top right) The apex of a macular hair cell, contacting 2 supporting cells. Both cell types are joined with apical junctional complexes (j). The hair cell's terminal web, called the cortical plate (p), gives rise to a bundle of stereocilia (s) with a tapering base and a widened tip. At one side of the stereociliary bundle is a single cilium (c, mark the substructure). Vestibulum, hamster, TEM. **Fig. 4.13.11.** (bottom left) The basis of a flask-shaped type 1 macular hair cell (h) rests in a cup-shaped sensory nerve terminal (t). Vestibulum, hamster, TEM. **Fig. 4.13.12.** (bottom right) A slender type 2 macular hair cell (h) is contacted by small, rounded nerve terminals (t). Mark the peripheral position of the mitochondria (m). Vestibulum, hamster, TEM.

elongated and perpendicular to each other. This way, they get stimulated when the head shifts into different positions. In the utricular macula, the hair cells on both sides of the longitudinal axis face each other with their cilium. In the saccular macula, the orientation of the hair cells is opposite.

this movement. If the head moves, the endolymph in one or more semicircular canals will be displaced because of its inertia. This movement deforms the cupula and the stereocilia. Depending on the direction in which the stereocilia are bent, towards the cilium or away from it, the hair cells are excited or inhibited.

IV.13.3.3.2. Ampullar cristae.

The sensory epithelium of the ampullar cristae (Fig. 4.13.8.) strongly resembles that of the maculae. The gelatinous glycoprotein mass covering the sensory epithelium forms a high dome or **cupula**. It does not contain otoliths. The apical appendages of the hair cells, in particular the stereocilia, are very long and are embedded in the cupula. The cristae contribute to dynamic balance by gathering information about the direction in which the head is moved and the speed of

IV.13.3.3.3. Corti's organ.

Corti's organ (Fig. 4.13.13.) is a little bit different from the vestibular and ampullar sensory epithelia because of the somewhat deviating structure of its hair cells and the presence of several types of supporting cells
At the side facing the spiral lamina, there is a space between the bases of the epithelial cells making up Corti's organ (Fig. 4.13.13.). This space forms a tunnel with a spiral course, like everything else in the cochlea. Additional intercellular spaces may occur

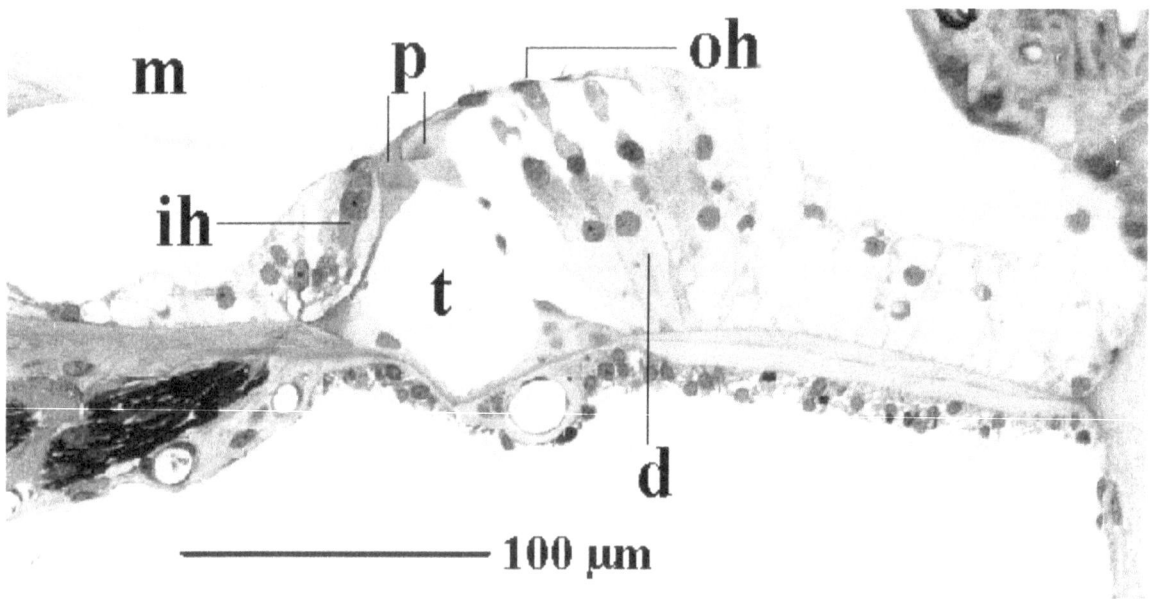

Fig. 4.13.13. Corti's organ shows a triangular extracellular space, the tunnel (t). Wide extracellular spaces also show up elsewhere. Both sides of the tunnel are bordered by pillar cells (p). The outer hair cells (oh), as well as the supporting phalangeal cells of Deiters (d), are relatively tall. The inner hair cells (ih) and phalangeal cells are less numerous and shorter. The tectorial membrane (m) rests on the apex of Corti's organ. Compare with Figure 4.13.5. Cochlea, cat, 1-micrometer plastic section, toluidin blue.

elsewhere. In cross section, the triangular tunnel is bordered, on both sides, by an inclined, prismatic supporting cell, a **pillar cell**. The pillar cell base is widened and contains the nucleus. The slender apex, or pillar, of the cell, is supported by a thick bundle of tonofilaments (Fig. 4.13.14.). The top of the pillar is slightly expanded, forming a capital. The pillar cell capitals are joined to each other and to other supporting cells by means of junctional complexes.

At greater distances from the tunnel, and on both sides of it, is a row of prismatic supporting cells of another type, the **phalangeal cells** or **cells of Deiters**. The outer phalangeal cells, facing the spiral ligament, are highest. In cross-sections, about five of them are seen. The inner ones, facing the spiral lamina, are lower and only two of them are seen in cross sections. The phalangeal cells are supported by a bundle of microtubules, which is attached to the apical junctional complex (Fig. 4.13.14.). The nucleus lies in the middle or the apex of the cell. The apical cell membrane carries microvilli.

Between the apices of the phalangeal cells, much smaller and slender **hair cells** can be made out (Figs. 4.13.13.-14.). Contrary to the supporting cells, they do not rest on the basement membrane. Between the outer phalangeal cells, about three can be seen in cross sections, a single one between the inner phalangeal cells.

The inner hair cells tend to have a globular appearance, the outer ones are more slender. They carry strongly developed microvilli or stereocilia (Fig. 4.13.15.) with lengths of a few hundred nanometers, no cilia. The inner hair cell stereocilia form three parallel rows, which lie parallel to the cochlear spiral. They are progressively longer in the direction of the spiral lamina, so that their tips appear like a series of steps. The three rows of the outer hair cell stereocilia are arranged in a W-shaped pattern (Fig. 4.13.8.), with the base of the W pointing towards the spiral ligament. The length of the stereocilia increases in the same direction.

The stereocilia are club-like, with an expanded tip. The longest touch the overlying tectorial membrane. Tip links extend from the tip of a stereocilium to the body of the next, higher one. In the stereocilary basis runs a dense axis, which merges with the hemispherical terminal web or basal plate. The cortical plate is joined to the cytoskeleton of the adjoining supporting cells through junctional complexes. Beneath the cell membrane, the smooth endoplasmic reticulum forms subsurface cisterns along the cell's perimeter. The hair cells contain numerous mitochondria in their basal and peripheral cytoplasm.

The hair cell bases are contacted by sensory nerve terminals (Fig. 4.13.16.), formed by the peripheral axons of the spiral ganglion's bipolar nerve cells. On their way to the outer hair cells, the axons cross the tunnel. The terminals are small and, rather unusually, filled with synaptic vesicles. In the hair cell cytoplasm, synaptic rods, surrounded by translucent synaptic vesicles, face these terminals.

Sound waves cause vibration of the tympanic membrane. Via the ossicles and the oval window, these vibrations are transmitted to the vestibular perilymph. From there, they are transmitted to the scala vestibuli and the vestibular membrane. Finally, they reach the endolymph of the scala media and the tectorial membrane. Through the scala tympani, vibrations reach the round window, where they decay.

The tectorial membrane, when it vibrates, deforms the hair cell stereocilia. When the stereocilia are bent towards the longest members of the group, the hair cell is activated, which ultimately leads to the induction of action potentials in the sensory nerves. When they are bent in the opposite direction, the hair cell is inhibited. The hair cells may also be inhibited by the motor functions of the sensory terminals, which contain synaptic vesicles.

The basilar membrane also contributes to the reception of sound. It is thinnest at the cochlear basis and progressively thickens towards its top. This means that vibrations of a particular frequency (pitch), will only affect a limited stretch of basilar membrane, and only stimulate the local hair cells. The highest tones are received at the cochlear basis, the lowest at the top. The range of the human ear is about eleven octaves.

References.

Hackney C.M., Furness D.N.: Mechanotransduction in vertebrate hair cells: structure and function of the stereociliary bundle. Am. J. Physiol. 1995, 268: C1-C13.

Kachar B., Parakkal M., Kurc M., Zhao Y., Gillespie P.: High-resolution structure of hair-cell tip links. Proc. Natl. Acad. Sci. USA 2000, 97: 13336-13341.

Lim D.J.: Functional structure of the organ of Corti: a review. Hear. Res. 1986, 22: 117-146.

Lysakowski A., Goldberg J.M.: A regional ultrastructural analysis of the cellular and synaptic architecture in the chinchilla cristae ampullares. J. Comp. Neurol. 1997, 389: 419-443.

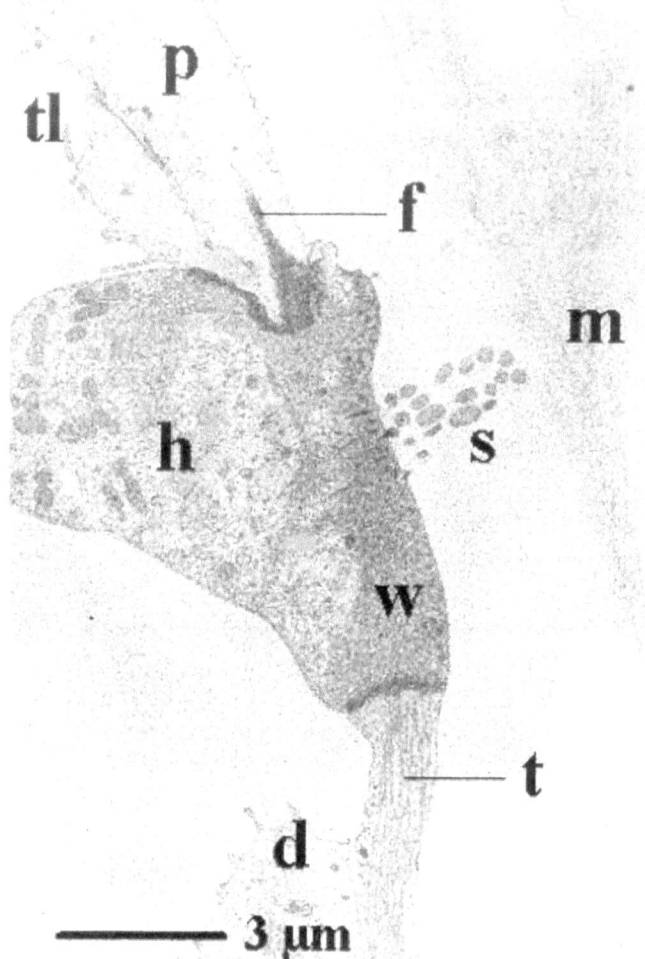

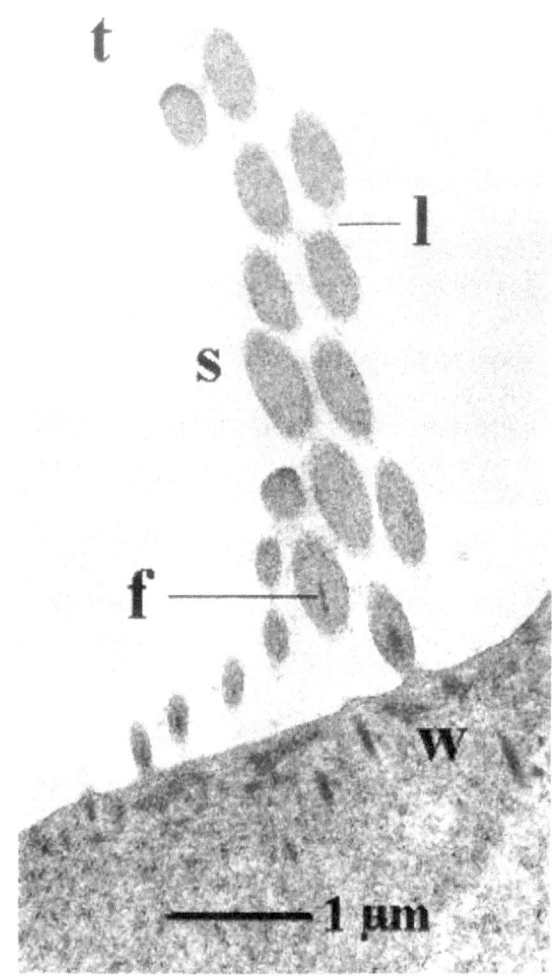

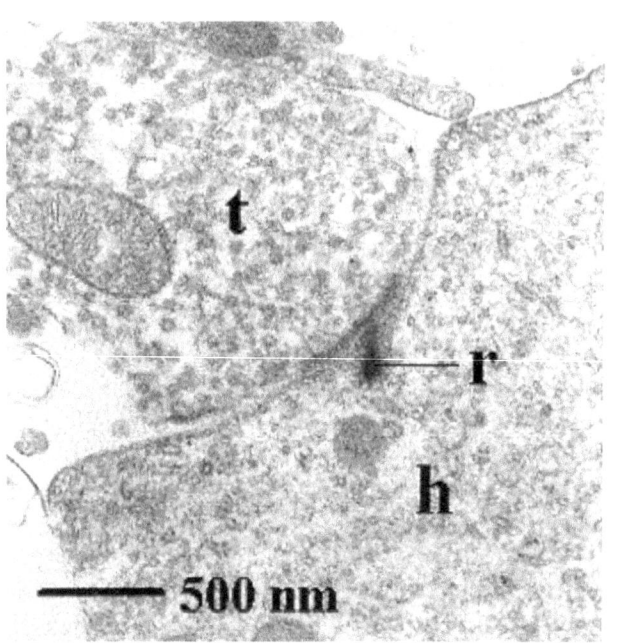

Fig. 4.13.14. (top left) The apex of a Corti hair cell (h) and 2 types of supporting cells. One of these contains a microtubular bundle (m), which identifies it as a phalangeal cell of Deiters (d). The others show a tonofilament bundle (f), and are pillar cells (p). Hair cell and supporting cells engage in junctional complexes. The hair cell carries a bundle of stereocilia (s), implanted in a terminal web or cortical plate (w). They touch the tectorial membrane (t). The intercellular spaces are extensive (artefactual?). One of them is the tunnel (tl), enclosed by the pillar cells. Corti's organ, cat, TEM. Fig. 4.13.15. (above) The stereocilia (s) of a Corti hair cell are supported by a dense microfilament axis (f), which continues into the terminal web (w). They are club-shaped: their tips are distinctly wider than their bases. Mark the links (l) between adjacent stereocilia. t = tectorial membrane. Corti's organ, cat, TEM. Fig. 4.13.16. (left) The basis of a Corti hair cell (h) is contacted by the terminal (t) of a sensory nerve fiber. In the hair cell cytoplasm is a synaptic rod (r), with synaptic vesicles clustered around it. The terminal contains numerous synaptic vesicles as well. Corti's organ, cat, TEM.

IV.14. Respiratory system.

The primary respiratory organs are the **lungs**, which take up oxygen and give off carbon dioxide. This process, called gas exchange, takes place between the inhaled air and the pulmonary blood, at the level of the **alveolar parenchyma**. Air is pumped in and out of the lungs through a system of ducts, the **airways**, the largest of which, the **trachea** and **stem bronchi**, lie outside the lungs. The trachea opens into the outside world through the **larynx** and subsequently through the oral and nasal cavities. The larynx contains the vocal cords, by means of which sounds can be produced. The **nasal cavity** houses the olfactory epithelium, in which the sense of smell resides, and the vomeronasal organ.

During embryonic development, the lungs originate as a ventral tubular outpocketing of the primitive gut epithelium. This outpocketing will produce terminal branches, as a compound gland does, which represent the later airways. The branching pattern is dichotomous and asymmetric, signifying that each branch produces, at its distal end, two narrower branches of unequal diameter, both of them lying at a different angle relative to the stem branch. The narrower of the two forms the sharpest angle. As the branches develop, they get enveloped by mesenchyme. The embryonic lung completely consists of a branched system of ducts, the primitive airways, and closely resembles a compound gland. The blind ends of the ducts eventually dilate and are compartimented by fibrous tissue septa. Thus, the alveoli are formed.

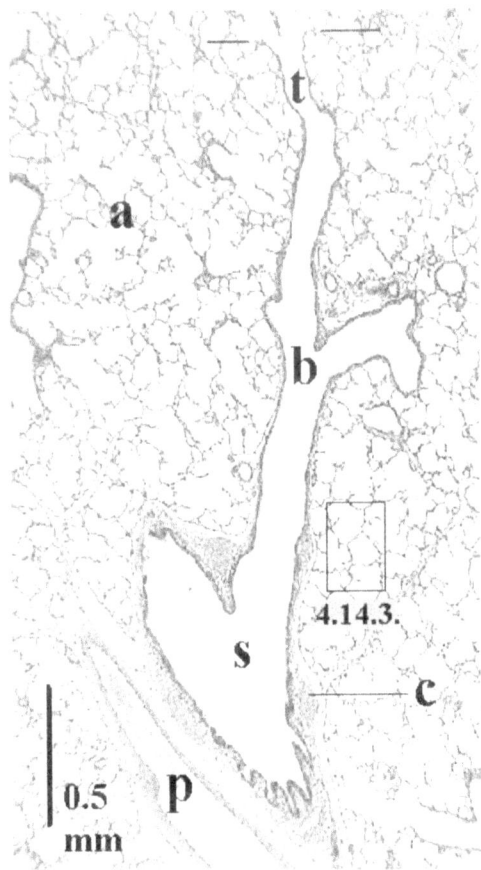
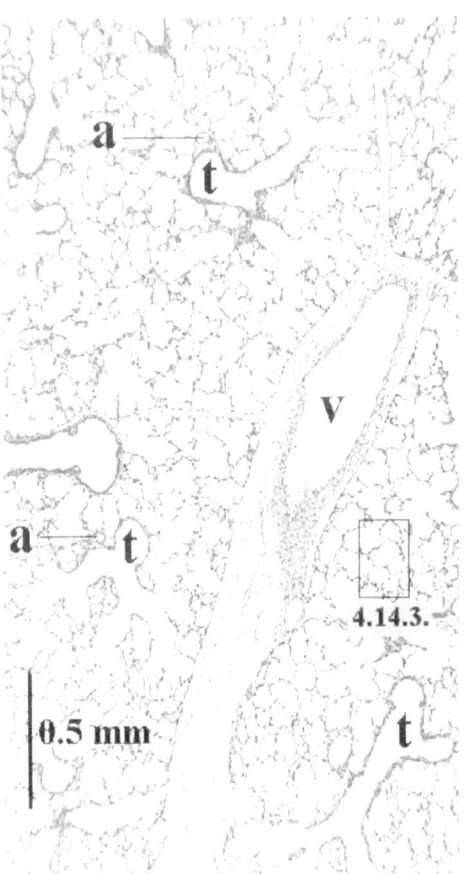

Fig. 4.14.1. (left) The lungs are mostly alveolar parenchyma (a), composed of alveoli. Gas exchange, i.e. the exchange of oxygen and carbon dioxide between the inhaled air and the pulmonary blood, occurs in the extremely thin interalveolar septa. Blood reaches the alveolar parenchyma via the pulmonary circulation (p). Air reaches it via a branched system of airways. The widest airways are the bronchi. In this picture, a segmental bronchus (s) is seen. Bronchi have a thick, complex wall, reinforced with cartilage (c). The bronchi form branches, which are narrower and have a thinner, less complex, wall: bronchioles (b). Bronchioles repeatedly branch, forming terminal bronchioles (t). These open abruptly (indicated by the horizontal lines) into the alveolar parenchyma. Lung, pig, HE. **Fig. 4.14.2.** (right) In addition to airways, this image more clearly shows the pulmonary circulation. Contrary to pulmonary arteries (a), which accompany airways (terminal bronchioles, t), pulmonary veins (v) return on their own, via the fibrous tissue septa which separate primary lung lobuli. Lung, pig, HE.

The lungs have to be regarded as extremely compartimented pouches or diverticula, derived form endoderm (Fig. 4.1.), and enveloped by mesodermal tissues. The dominant tissue of the respiratory system is **epithelium**, which lines the alveolar space and the airway lumen. The mesoderm forms the alveolar pulmonary capillaries, made of **endothelium**, as well as the other pulmonary blood vessels. The epithelium of the nasal cavity is ectodermal. The epithelium is locally transformed into **glandular tissue**. The infiltrated mesoderm also forms **fibrous** and **supportive tissue** (cartilage) and **muscle tissue**. In the airways, these tissues form concentric layers. The airways contain neural plexi and local accumulations of lymphoid tissue. As the lungs and the extrapulmonary airways lie free in the thoracic cavity, they are lined with mesothelium.

IV.14.1. Lungs.

Mature lungs largely consist of a spongy tissue mass, the **alveolar parenchyma** (Figs. 4.14.1.-3.), composed of a few hundred million alveoli, each having a diameter of a few hundred micrometers. The structure of the alveolar parenchyma reflects its function. It is the lung's gas exchange system. In a physiological sense, breathing is gas exchange between air and blood. Oxygen is taken up in the blood from the air, carbon dioxide goes the other way. Gas exchange is entirely a matter of diffusion, a passive process, driven only by the concentration gradient of the substance to be moved. Moreover, it is only effective over very short distances. As we shall see, the microscopic structure of the alveolar parenchyma is determined by the necessity to bring air and blood into very close proximity, and over enormous surfaces, so that diffusion will suffice to make gas exchange sufficiently intense to maintain the organism.

Air is conducted to and from the alveolar parenchyma by means of an extensive, intensely branched system of **airways** (Fig. 4.14.1.). This way, the alveolar parenchyma is continuously supplied with oxygen–rich air, while stale, carbon dioxide-rich air is removed. This helps to maintain the concentration gradients that are the driving forces of diffusion. Conduction of air to and from the alveolar parenchyma, or ventilation, is an active, be it largely involuntary, process. It is not the lungs that do the work, however, but the thorax, which functions as a bellows. When the respiratory muscles, the intercostals and the diaphragm, contract, the thorax expands. The intercostals elevate the ribs, while the diaphragm, which tends to bulge into the thoracic space, is pulled taut. Consequently, the intrathoracic pressure decreases and air is passively drawn in. Exhalation is largely passive, and follows upon relaxation of the respiratory muscles.

Each stem bronchus ventilates an entire lung. After entering the lung, at a spot called the hilus, the stem bronchus splits up in a number of **lobar bronchi**, each of which ventilates a lung **lobe**. The right lung has three lobes and three lobar bronchi, the left lung has only two of each. Each lobular bronchus gives rise to a number of **segmental bronchi**, which ventilate a smaller part of the lobe, a **segment**. The segments are separated from each other by fibrous tissue septa. The smaller divisions are not. The most terminal segmental bronchi have diameters of close to 1 millimeter. They split up in **bronchioles**, each of which ventilates a smaller part of the segments, a **primary lobulus**. The **terminal bronchioles** are branches of the bronchioles and, as their name implies, they are the final segments of what is called the bronchial tree. Their diameter is 0.2 millimeters at most. They ventilate a still smaller lung region, a **secondary lobulus**. Thus, it can be seen that the lungs have a fractal structure, with each pyramidal subpart split up into similarly shaped, but ever smaller subparts, their apices pointing towards the hilus, and their bases towards the periphery. From stem bronchus to terminal bronchiole, about twenty generations of airways succeed one another. This bronchial tree is the pulmonary gas conduction system. The terminal stretch of the terminal bronchioles may already carry a few alveoli. This stretch is the **respiratory bronchiole**. Most respiratory bronchioles arise after birth, by "budding" of alveoli along the terminal bronchioles. A substantial part of the terminal bronchioles, present at birth, may disappear before adulthood is reached by this process of alveolarization. Distal to the last respiratory bronchioles lie only thin walled alveoli.

Deoxygenated blood is conducted to the alveolar parenchyma through the pulmonary circulation. A branch of the pulmonary artery, which begins at the right ventricle, enters a lung at the hilus and splits up into ever-narrower branches, which follow the airways. When they reach the alveolar parenchyma, the pulmonary arterioles form a network of capillaries in the alveolar walls. Oxygenated blood is collected in the pulmonary venules and returned to the left heart through the pulmonary veins. Pulmonary venules do not accompany the airways (Fig. 4.14.2.), but course at the periphery of the primary lobuli. The largest veins run towards the hilus, in the company of the airways.

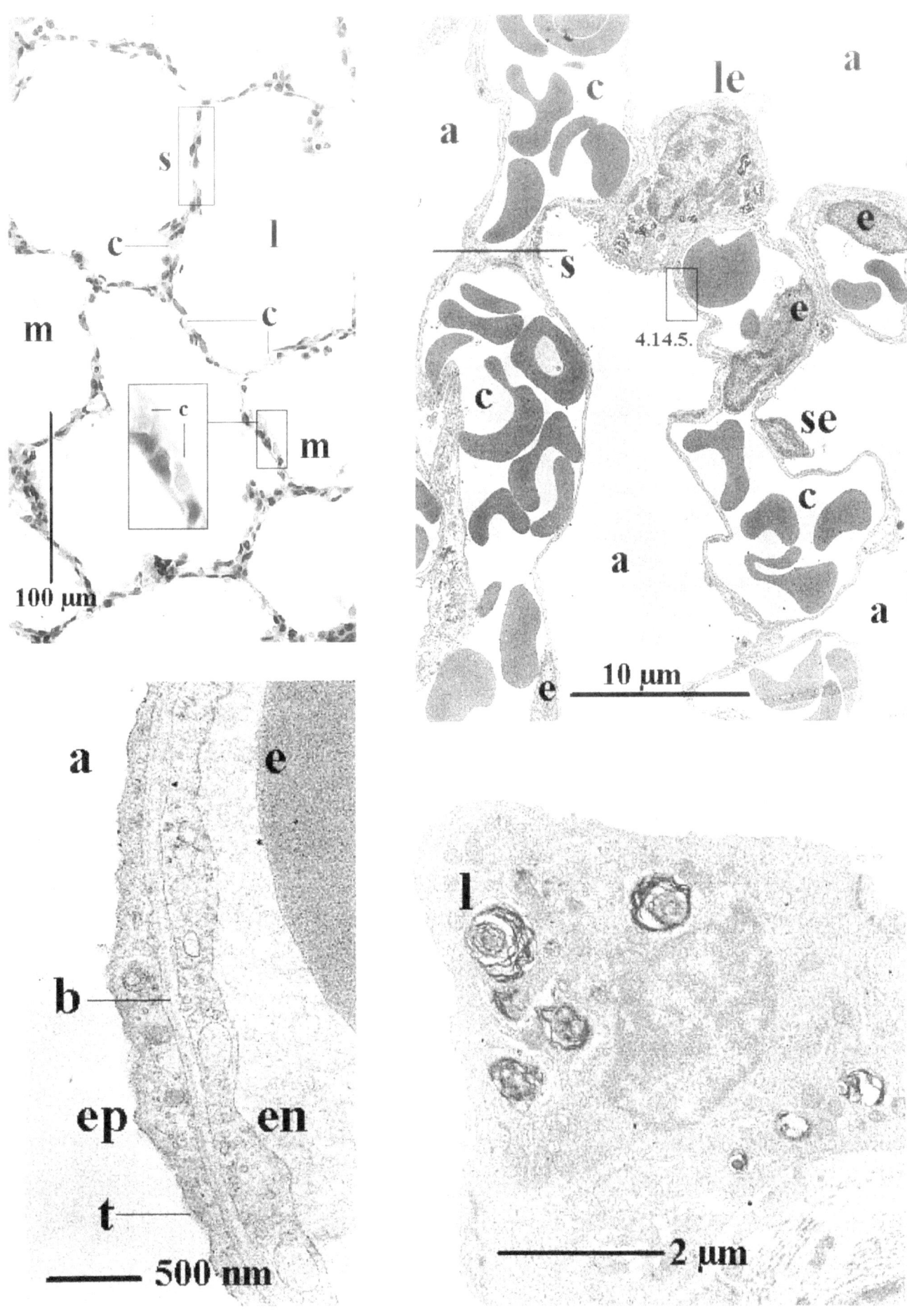

Fig. 4.14.3. (top left) In the interalveolar septa (s) run pulmonary capillaries (c). The blood (erythrocytes) that circulates through them absorbs oxygen from the air filling the alveolar lumen (l), and releases carbon dioxide into it. Two alveolar macrophages (m) are seen. Lung, pig, HE. **Fig. 4.14.4.** (top right) The interalveolar septa (s) separate the alveolar spaces (a). They are lined, on both sides, with a simple squamous epithelium of small alveolar epithelial cells (se). Occasionally, a cuboidal large alveolar epithelial cell (le) is encountered. In the fibrous tissue septum between both epithelia, capillaries (c) are seen, easily recognizable by their content of erythrocytes. They are lined with endothelium (e). The fibrous tissue layer may be locally absent, resulting in fusion of the basement membranes of both epithelia. Lung, rat, TEM. **Fig. 4.14.5.** (bottom left) Enlargement of Figure 4.14.4.. In the alveolar septa, alveolar epithelium (ep) and capillary endothelium (en), resting on their basement membranes (b), almost touch. Both layers, and the thin layer of fibrous tissue sandwiched between them, form the blood-air barrier (e = erythrocyte, a = air). Exchange of oxygen and carbon dioxide occurs by diffusion through this barrier. Mark the tensio-active film (t) that coats the epithelium. Lung, rabbit, TEM. **Fig. 4.14.6.** (bottom right) A large alveolar epithelial cell contains lamellar inclusions (l), storing the precursor substances of the tensio-active film that coats the alveolar wall. Lung, rabbit, TEM.

IV.14.1.1. Alveolar parenchyma.

Alveoli lie distal to the terminal and respiratory bronchioles. Initially, they line up to form longitudinal spaces, or **alveolar ducts**, in which they open, and which are a continuation of the terminal and respiratory bronchioles that ventilate them. More distally, they are arranged to form a dilated, blind space, the **alveolar sac**. Individual alveoli are separated from each other by very thin fibrous tissue septa, in which pulmonary capillaries run and which are lined, at both sides, with alveolar epithelium (Fig. 4.14.3.). In some places, the capillary septa are so thin that air and blood come to within less than 0.1 micrometers from each other. This thickness is of the same order as the maximal resolving power of the light microscope. Consequently, the structure of the alveolar septa is difficult to make out with light microscopy. Electron microscopic observations, on the other hand, clearly demonstrate that the alveolar lumen is lined with a continuous simple squamous epithelium. The pulmonary capillaries consist of a continuous endothelium (Fig. 4.14.4.).

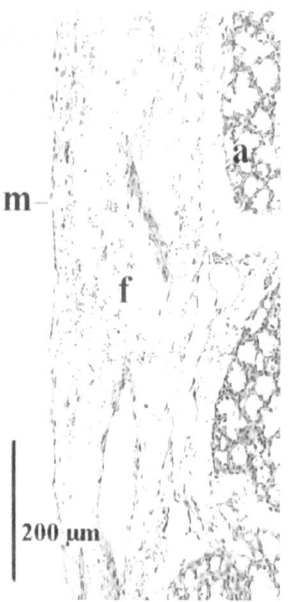

Fig. 4.14.7. The pulmonary pleura is a serosa: a mesothelium (m), lining a layer of loose fibrous tissue (f). a = alveolar parenchyma. Lung, sheep, HE.

The alveolar epithelium largely consists of cells that are extremely flattened. For this reason, and because they contain numerous micropinocytotic vesicles, they show a deceptive resemblance to endothelial cells. These are the **small** or **type I alveolar epithelial cells** (Figs. 4.14.4.-5.). Their extreme flattening is directly related to the need to allow inhaled air to come in extemely close proximity to the pulmonary blood. These cells show few secondary organelles and are relatively inert. They are joined to one another and to other alveolar epithelial cell types by means of tight junctions.

The alveolar capillary endothelium is unfenestrated. Contrary to the epithelial cells, the endothelial cells are involved in the metabolism of quite a number of substances, which is not reflected, however, in their cytological structure. The lungs function as filters, which rid the blood of certain substances and degrade

them. That this function resides in the lung is very logical: it is the only organ that receives the total amount of blood the body has to its disposal.

Sporadically, globular to cuboidal cells are encountered in the alveolar epithelium: the **large** or **type II alveolar epithelial cells** (Figs. 4.14.4., 4.14.6.). These cells carry a number of short apical microvilli. They show characteristics of protein- and lipid-secreting exocrine gland cells. Their cytoplasm contains a number of large apical vesicles with a concentrically layered content, the **lamellar bodies**. This material consists, among others, of phospholipids, as the cell membrane does. The diameters of these bodies can exceed 1 micrometer, and they resemble secondary lysosomes or residual bodies. Nevertheless, they have to be regarded as secretory vesicles, since their content is liberated in the alveolar space. The

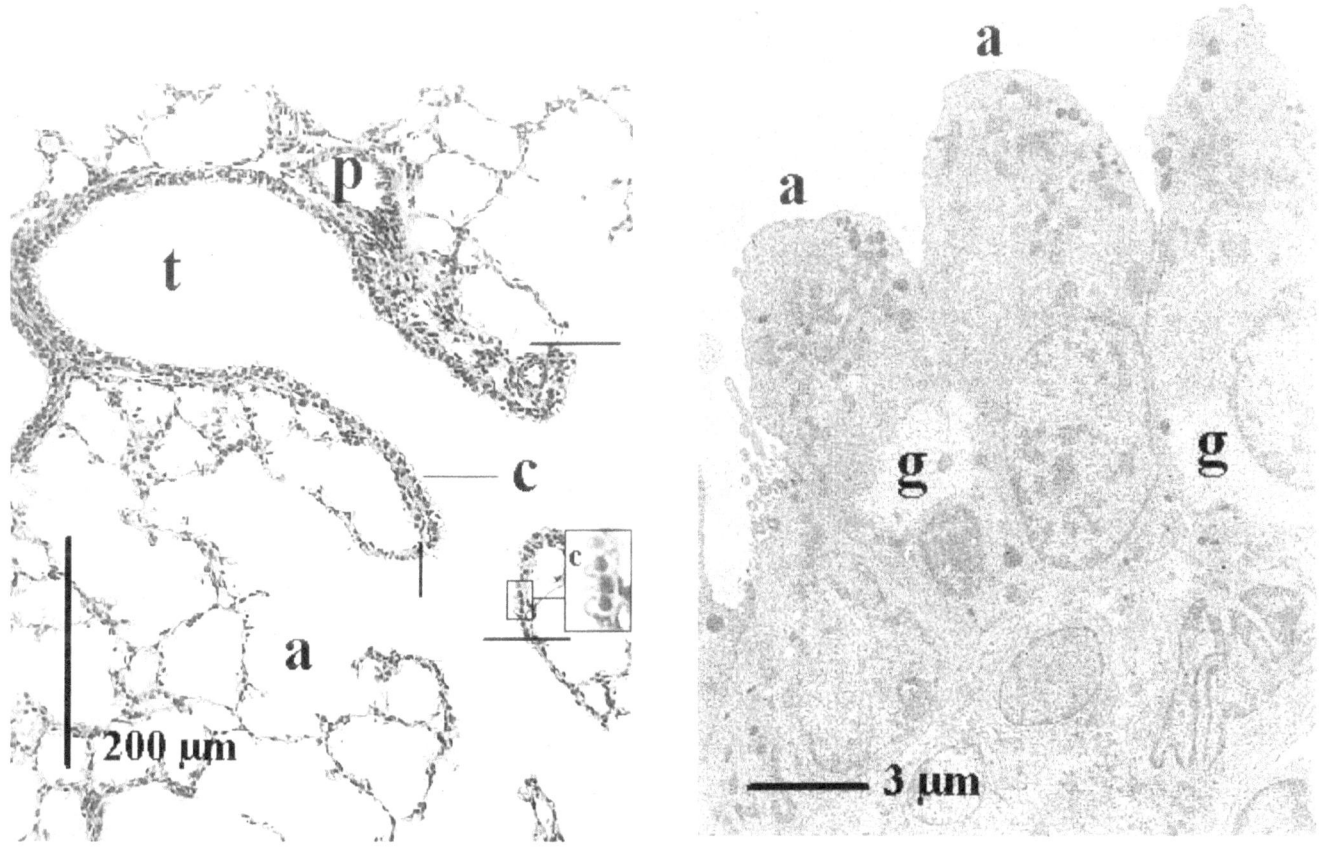

Fig. 4.14.8. (left) A terminal bronchiole (t) is lined with a simple cuboidal epithelium, composed of Clara cells (c). These cells have a clear cytoplasm and a bulging cell apex. At the bronchiolo-alveolar junction, it changes abruptly (lines) into the squamous epithelium of the alveoles (a). Next to the terminal bronchiole is a pulmonary arteriole (p). Lung, pig, HE. **Fig. 4.14.9.** (right) A few Clara cells, characterized by a bulging apex (a), which is loaded with mitochondria and lipid droplets. Glycogen (g) is dissolved in tissue preparations for light microscopy, explaining the clear aspect of these cells in Figure 4.14.8. See Figure 2.28. for a detailed view of the smooth endoplasmic reticulum. Lung, rabbit, TEM.

secretory mechanism is not well known, it may be merocrine.

The type II alveolar epithelial cells secrete a complex mixture of proteins and lipids, although the smooth endoplasmic reticulum is not as prominently present as it is in other lipid-secreting cells. This secretion is called **surfactant**, and is spread over the alveolar surface (Fig. 4.14.5.) as a lipid-rich layer with tensio-active properties: it regulates the alveolar surface tension.

In the alveolar parenchyma, air contacts fluid, e.g. cytoplasm, the surface of which behaves as an elastic membrane under tension, because the superficial fluid molecules are attracted by the deeper ones. This surface tension is a weak force, not usually apparent in the macroscopic world, but with important consequences on the microscopic scale of the alveoli. As a consequence of surface tension, a centripetal force develops, which tends to collapse the alveoles. This tendency is especially outspoken during exhalation, when the diameters of the alveoli decrease. In a sphere, surface tension is inversely proportional to the diameter. The smaller the alveole, the larger the surface tension and the larger its tendency to collapse. Badly working lungs can show numerous collapsed alveoli, a condition called emphysema. Since collapsed alveoli cannot be ventilated, this inhibits gas exchange. During inhalation, the alveoli tend to expand. In pathological circumstances, alveoli may even rupture: atelectasis. In normal lungs, the alveolar dimensions are relatively constant during successive inhalation and exhalation cycles, because surfactant stabilizes them by continuously adapting their surface tension. Surface tension in the surfactant film increases during inhalation, when the alveoles tend to expand, opposing their expansion. When, during exhalation, the alveoles tend to collapse, surface tension in the surfactant film decreases, limiting their tendency to collapse. This stabilization of alveolar diameters promotes the even distribution of air over the entire alveolar surface, and thus the efficiency of gas exchange.

In the alveolar lumen, **macrophages** may be observed (Fig. 2.27.). They remove foreign material and microorganisms, which were not intercepted in the airways. They do not stay in the alveolar spaces. Once they are loaded with undegradable residues, in which circumstances they may be called dust cells, they migrate to the airway lumen, from where they are carried off to the pharynx.

The septal fibrous tissue is loose and elastic, adapting the lungs to reversible deformation. This is especially important to diminish the lung's volume during exhalation, which is entirely passive. The fibrous tissue layer is extremely thin and may vanish completely. When this happens, the basement membranes of epithelium and endothelium merge. At the lung's periphery, the alveolar fibrous tissue is confluent with a serosa, rich in elastic fibrils, and lined with mesothelium, the **pleura** (Fig. 4.14.7.).

IV.14.1.2. Airways.

The airways are composed of concentric tissue layers. The lumen is lined with a **mucosa**, consisting of an epithelium that rests on a fibrous tissue lamina propria or corium. The mucosa is surrounded by a **musculosa** of visceral muscle tissue. The musculosa separates the mucosa from a deeper fibrous tissue layer, the **submucosa**. It is self evident that these layers are thickest and best developed in the larger, proximal airways, especially the bronchi. Here, the submucosa contains seromucous glands. External of the bronchial submucosa is an additional layer, which is composed of cartilage plates, the fibro-cartilaginous tunica. In the peribronchial fibrous tissue layer surrounding this, intramural ganglia and lymphoid tissue accumulations are found. The smaller, more distal airways, to begin with the bronchioles, have a much thinner wall, composed only of mucosa, musculosa, and submucosa. Individual layers are less well developed than those of the bronchi.

The airway epithelium is called **respiratory epithelium**, somewhat inappropriately, as airways only serve to conduct air and play no direct role in gas exchange.

In the smallest, peripheral airways, the terminal bronchioles (Fig. 4.14.8.), this epithelium is simple cuboidal. The transition from the squamous alveolar epithelium is brusque. This epithelium is almost entirely made up of **Clara cells** (Fig. 4.14.9.), typical representatives of the group of lipid-secreting gland cells (II.2.1.5.1.). Their apical cytoplasm contains mitochondria, lipid droplets and smooth endoplasmic reticulum, and bulges into the airway lumen. Basally, it also contains some rough endoplasmic reticulum. These cells contain fairly large amounts of glycogen, which is easily dissolved during tissue preparation for light microscopy, resulting in a translucent cytoplasm. The composition of the lipids is not exactly known, but it is supposed that they are analogous to the alveolar surfactant. Thus, Clara cells may contribute, by their exocrine secretory activity, to a tensio-active film in the peripheral airways. The secretory mechanism is

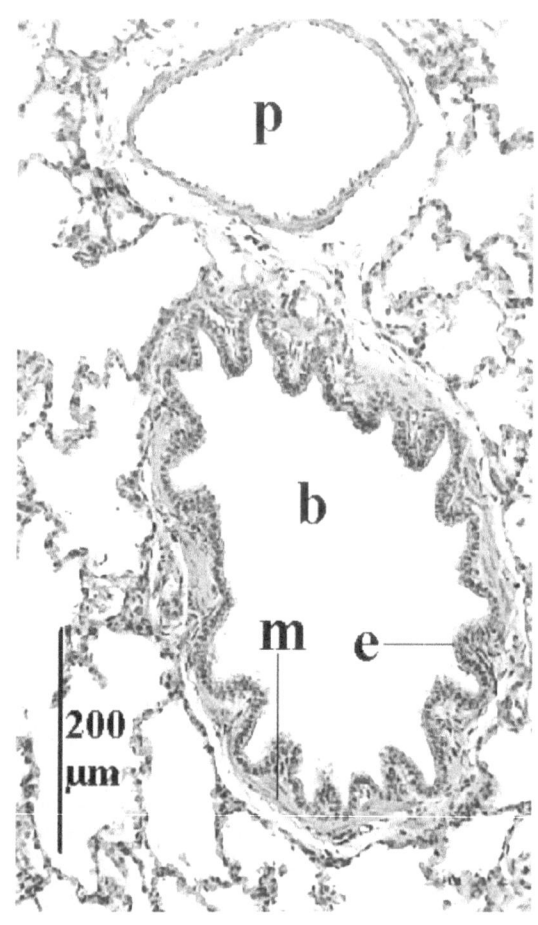

Fig. 4.14.10. A bronchiole (b) is lined with a simple to pseudostratified prismatic epithelium (e), containing ciliated cells. The bronchiolar wall also has a thin musculosa (m). Next to the bronchiole is a pulmonary arteriole (p). Its wall is much thinner than that of a corresponding arteriole of the systemic circulation (compare Figure 4.5.8.). Lung, cat, HE.

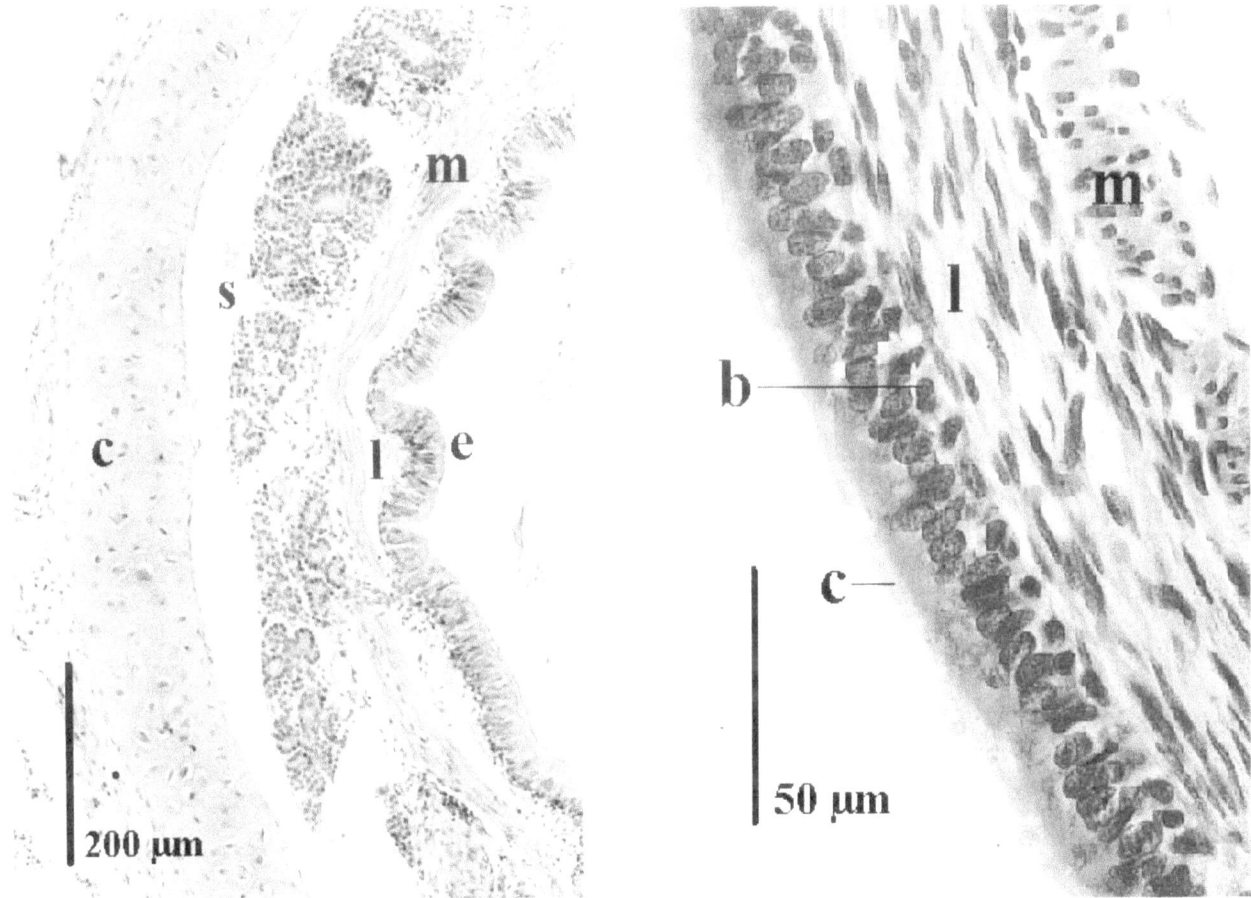

Fig. 4.14.11. (left) The bronchial wall is fairly complex. The mucosa is composed of respiratory epithelium (e) and a fibrous tissue lamina propria (l). A muscularis (m) separates it from the fibrous submucosa (s), which contains submucosal glands (g). The submucosa rests on a fibrocartilaginous tunica (c). Lung, guinea pig, HE. **Fig. 4.14.12.** (right) The bronchial mucosa consists of the respiratory epithelium, which is a pseudostratified epithelium, composed of prismatic ciliated cells (c: cilia) and cuboidal basal cells (b). It rests on a fibrous lamina propria (l). m = muscularis. Lung, pig, HE.

not well known either, and may be merocrine as well as apocrine.

In the smallest bronchioles, the respiratory epithelium contains numerous Clara cells. In the larger ones (Fig. 4.14.10.), more and more ciliated cells and goblet cells appear. In the largest bronchioles, basal cells appear, and the epithelium shows pseudostratification.

The respiratory epithelium is best developed in the bronchi (Fig. 4.14.11.), where it is distinctly pseudostratified and rich in **ciliated cells** and **goblet cells** (Figs. 4.14.12.-13.). Goblet cells produce mucus, which coats the airway wall, forming a mucus carpet in which foreign material and microorganisms are trapped. The mucus carpet rests on top of the cilia of the ciliated cells. The coordinated beating of the cilia transforms the mucus carpet into a conveyor belt, which moves, trapped particles and all, towards the pharynx. In normal circumstances, the amount of mucus produced is rather small, and most of it is swallowed imperceptibly.

In addition to goblet cells and ciliated cells, the respiratory epithelium contains a number of other functional cell types, which occur in small numbers. Among these are the widely dispersed **endocrine cells**, which are of the polarized, peptide or amine hormone-secreting type (Fig. 2.16.). They may occur as solitary cells or, predominantly at airway bifurcations and bronchiolo-alveolar junctions, as aggregates. These are contacted by sensory nerve fibers and are called neuroepithelial bodies. Neuroepithelial bodies are sensitive to low oxygen concentrations in the inhaled air, which may be a consequence of insufficient ventilation, i.e. ventilation hypoxia. They could be the pulmonary equivalent of the arterial chemoreceptors. They secrete a number of neurotransmitters and hormones, such as serotonin, calcitonin gene related peptide, and bombesin or gastrin releasing peptide. The first two are vasoactive agents, which may influence pulmonary perfusion. The third one is a growth factor. Neuroepithelial bodies are

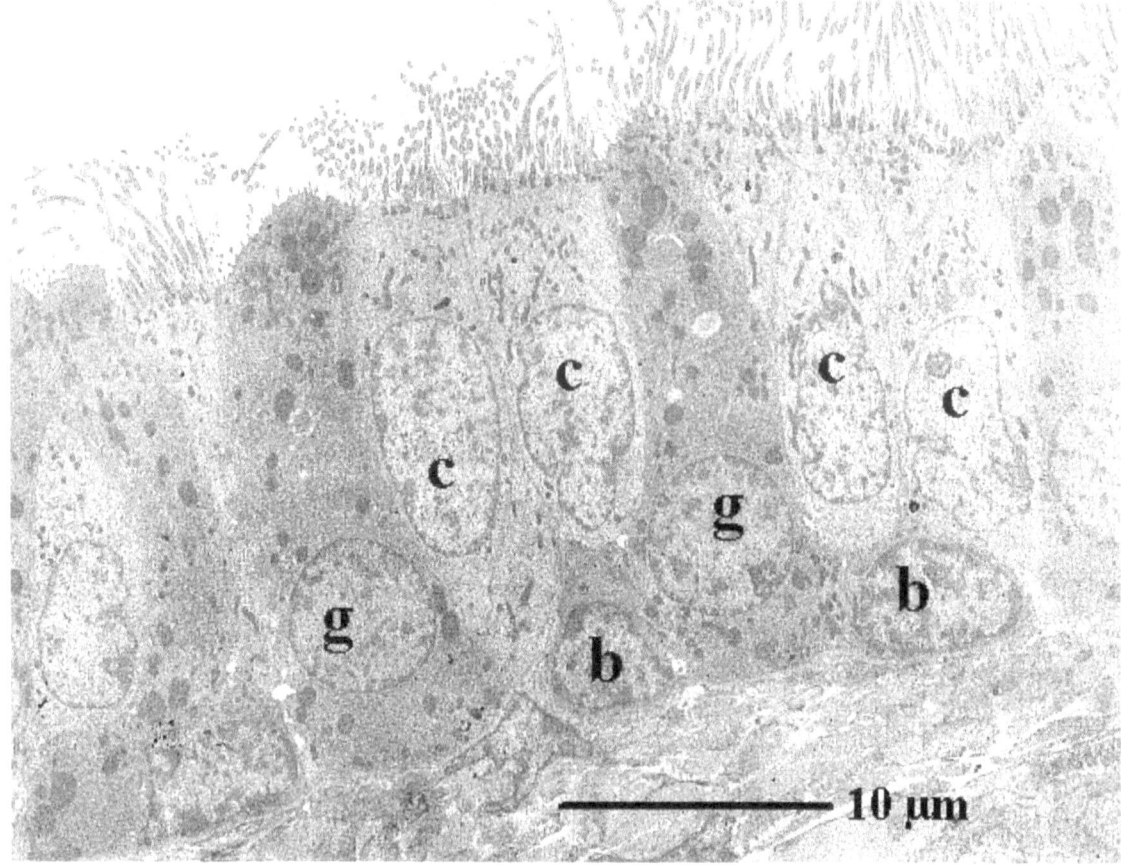

Fig. 4.14.13. Apart from non-functional, reserve basal cells (b), the bronchial pseudostratified epithelium contains 2 kinds of functional, prismatic cells: ciliated cells (c) and goblet cells (g). Lung, rabbit, TEM.

conspicuously present in the embryonic and fetal lungs and are regarded as regulators of lung growth and development.

The musculosa is thickest in the bronchi (Fig. 4.14.11.), progressively thinning out in the peripheral airways (Fig. 4.14.10.). Its smooth muscle fibers run more or less circularly. By contraction or relaxation, the musculosa influences the bronchial diameter. In the largest bronchi, sensory nerve terminals, rich in mitochondria, run between the smooth muscle fibers. These terminals are sensitive to deformation and constitute the pulmonary stretch receptor. During inhalation they are stretched, whereupon they inhibit, through a reflex mechanism, the respiratory muscles, initiating exhalation.

The submucosa is thickest in the bronchi and very thin to hardly present in the most peripheral airways. In the bronchi, it contains seromucous glands, the **submucosal glands** (Figs. 4.14.11., 4.14.14.). These are compound glands with serous and mucous acini, which produce mucus, contributing to the mucous conveyor belt operating in the bronchi. Capillaries occurring here and elsewhere in the airways (Fig.

4.14.14.) do not belong to the pulmonary circulation, which conducts deoxygenated blood to the alveolar parenchyma, but to the bronchial circulation, which supplies the walls of the larger airways with oxygenated blood.

In the bronchi, but not in the smaller airways, the submucosa rests on a **fibro-cartilaginous tunica** (Fig. 4.14.11.). This layer contains plates of hyaline cartilage, enveloped and interconnected by elastic tissue. This layer functions as a support, ensuring that the bronchial lumen is kept wide open. Air is a medium of low density, which has to be moved fast, continuously, and in large amounts. For this reason, the peristaltic mechanism of displacement, which operates in the intestine, is of no use. In stead, the bronchial wall is stiffened by a cartilaginous skeleton, creating a large lumen, through which air is pumped by the thoracic cage.

In the fibrous tissue layer enveloping the fibro-cartilaginous tunica, the **peribronchium**, nerve fibers are found, as well as **intramural ganglia** (Fig. 4.14.15.). These are motor ganglia, which contain the multipolar cell bodies of postsynaptic nerve cells.

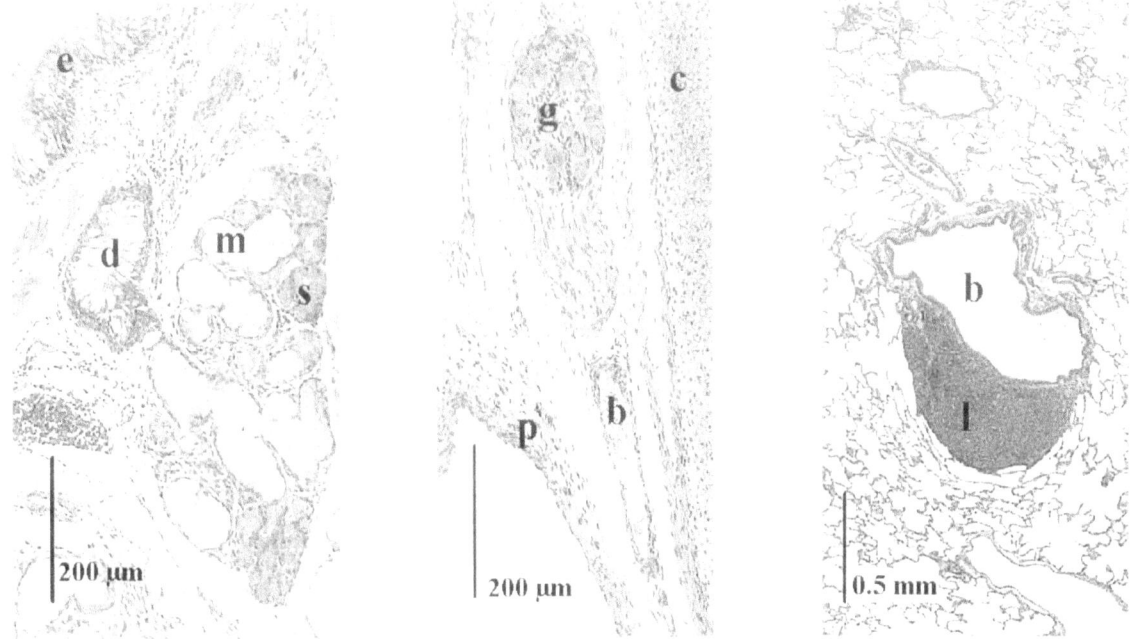

Left to right: **Fig. 4.14.14.** The submucosal glands of the bronchus are seromucous. The mucous acini (m) appear translucent. They secrete mucus. The serous acini (s) appear darker (= basophilic). They secrete a clear proteinaceous fluid. The duct (d) crosses the muscularis. e = epithelium. Lung, human, HE. **Fig. 4.14.15.** In the peribronchial fibrous tissue lie intramural ganglia (g) containing the perikarya of nerve cells of the autonomic nervous system, as well as bronchial blood vessels (b). The peribronchium is continuous with the adventitia of the large pulmonary vessels (p). c = bronchial hyaline cartilage. Lung, pig, HE. **Fig. 4.14.16.** The airway wall, such as in this bronchiole (b, no cartilage), may contain accumulations of lymphoid tissue (l): bronchus-associated lymphoid tissue. Lung, sheep, HE.

The fibrous tissue of the airways contains numerous lymphoid cells and other types of immune cells. This is to be expected since the lungs, as a consequence of continuous respiration, inhale large amounts of foreign material. This **bronchus-associated lymphoid tissue** may locally accumulate in impressive amounts (Fig. 4.14.16.), even forming true lymph nodes.

IV.14.2. Trachea and stem bronchi.

The trachea and stem bronchi are composed of the same tissues as the bronchi, but these are not always arranged concentrically. Over their entire length, they are reinforced by a cartilaginous skeleton, a **fibro-cartilaginous tunica**. This tunica does not consist of plates, but of rings, encircling the entire airway, except at the dorsal side, where they are open. In cross sections, they have the shape of a horseshoe. In the opening of the horseshoe is visceral muscle tissue, forming **Reisessen's muscle** (Fig. 4.14.17.). This muscle layer also contains stretch receptors. Since a typical musculosa is absent, there is no sharp

distinction between the lamina propria of the mucosa and the submucosa. In the deeper fibrous tissue, the secretory units of seromucous glands are observed, wherefore it is called submucosa. Trachea and stem bronchi lie free in the thoracic space, and the peribronchium is a serosa, lined with mesothelium.

IV.14.3. Larynx.

The larynx is the expanded cranial part of the trachea, which houses the **vocal cords**, and which opens in the throat or pharynx. During swallowing, it is closed by a valve, the **epiglottis**, so that saliva or food cannot enter the trachea.

The wall of the larynx is composed of hyaline and elastic cartilage (III.2.4.4.) plates, joined by fibro-elastic ligaments.
The vocal cords are two pairs of lateral folds of the mucosa. The cranial folds are the false vocal cords. The caudal ones, which can be voluntarily moved by skeletal muscle tissue, are the true vocal cords. The

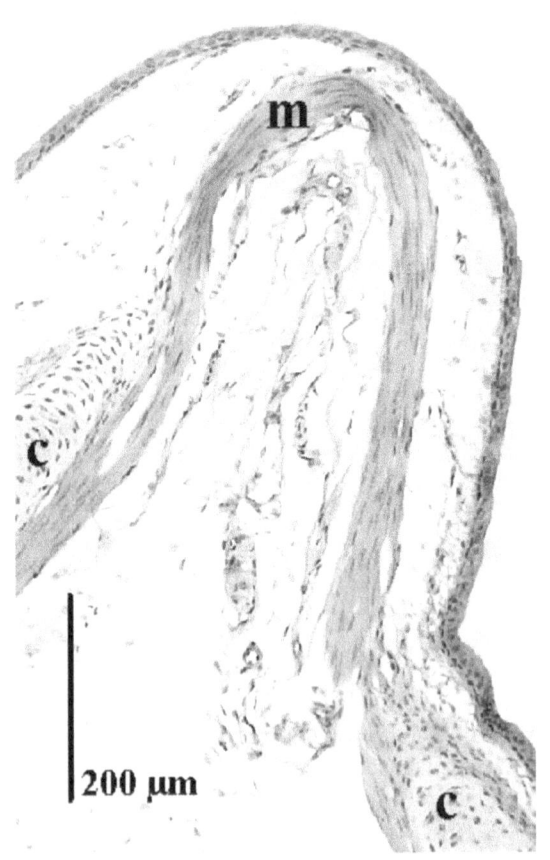

Fig. 4.14.17. The trachea is supported by cartilaginous plates (c), shaped like a horseshoe. The opening of the horseshoe is bridged by the tracheal muscle (m). Trachea, cat, HE.

true vocal cords have a core of elastic cartilage. Muscular contraction modifies the central opening, allowing sounds of different pitch to be produced when exhaled air is forced through it. The laryngeal epithelium is the usual respiratory epithelium, except in places where friction occurs, such as the vocal cords. These are lined with Malpighian epithelium.
The epiglottis contains a core of elastic cartilage, and its surface is lined, on both sides, with Malpighian epithelium.

IV.14.4. Nasal cavity.

The nasal cavity is subdivided in right and left halves by means of a septum of hyaline cartilage. They are connected with cavities in various skull bones, the sinuses. At the nasal openings, the epidermis forms large, stiff hairs, the vibrissae. Nasal cavity, sinuses, and the upper part of the pharynx are lined with respiratory epithelium, which rests on a richly vascularized lamina propria with seromucous glands. The goblet cells are frequently less high than the ciliated cells and occur in groups. The central ones are

the lowest and the peripheral ones incline towards them. Thus, characteristic intraepithelial glands, opening with a pore, are formed. The dense vascularization and the numerous glands are adaptations of the mucosa that enable it to moisten and warm inhaled air. This air conditioning effect is greatly promoted by surface expansion of the respiratory mucosa: it lines the turbinary bones or conches, which are convoluted, bony sheets, formed by the inside of the upper jawbones.

There are two small spots in the roof of the nasal cavity that are lined with **olfactory mucosa** (Fig. 4.14.18.), which is sensitive to chemical substances, or scents, in the inhaled air. The olfactory epithelium is pseudostratified, but distinctly higher than the ordinary respiratory epithelium. It contains receptor cells and the supportive cells.
The **supporting cells** (Fig. 4.14.19.) have a narrow basis and an expanded apex, which houses the nucleus. The apical membrane carries a well-developed brush border. The cytoplasm has a mixed character. It contains bundles of microtubules and microfilaments, but the apical cytoplasm also contains secretory vesicles with glycoproteins (mucus), which are secreted in merocrine fashion. These secretions help to dissolve scent substances, which cannot be detected otherwise. Golgi-complex and smooth endoplasmic reticulum are well developed, the rough endoplasmic reticulum somewhat less.
The **receptor cells** (Fig. 4.14.19.) are in fact bipolar nerve cells (II.2.3.), with a fusiform perikaryon, which is oriented at right angles to the plane of the epithelium. The perikarya and, consequently, the nuclei occupy the middle level of the epithelium, below the level occupied by the supportive cell nuclei. The central axon courses towards the olfactory bulbs of the cerebrum. The very short peripheral axon courses between the supportive cells towards the surface of the olfactory epithelium and forms junctional complexes with their apices. Its top extends above the epithelium and is dilated, forming an **olfactory knob**. The olfactory knob carries about ten fairly long (up to 5 micrometers) and abnormal, immotile, cilia or **olfactory hairs**. At their basis, these cilia have a normal structure, but towards their apex, they show eleven microtubular singlets in stead. At the top, they are very thin and devoid of microtubules. Starting at the olfactory knob, they follow a tortuous course between the microvilli of the supportive cells, but parallel to the epithelial surface. These olfactory hairs in all probability carry specific membrane receptors, which bind scent substances.
The underlying corium contains compound tubulo-acinar glands, **Bowman's glands** (Fig. 4.14.18.). They

272

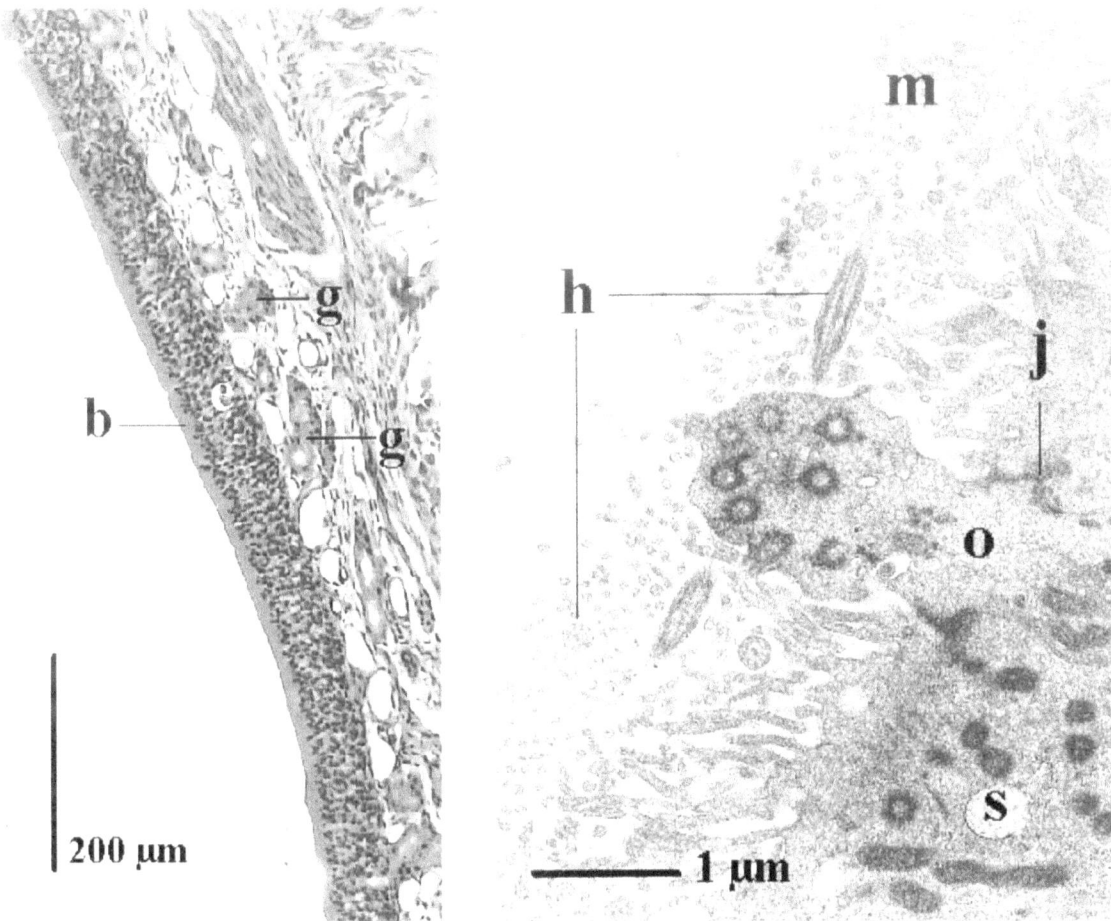

Fig. 4.14.18. (left) The olfactory mucosa is composed of olfactory epithelium (e), resting on a densely vascularized corium, which contains Bowman's glands (g). The clear brush border of this epithelium (b) is composed of the microvilli of its supporting cells (see Figure 4.14.19.). Compare the olfactory epithelium's thickness with the respiratory epithelium's (Fig. 4.14.12.). Olfactory mucosa, cat, HE. **Fig. 4.14.19.** (left) The olfactory epithelium contains chemoreceptive olfactory cells (o) and supporting cells (s), joined by junctional complexes (j). The supporting cells carry numerous microvilli (m), forming the brush border. The olfactory cells form an apical knob, the olfactory cone, which gives rise to several lengthy cilia, the olfactory hairs (h). These cilia are embedded in the brush border. Olfactory mucosa, cat, TEM.

secrete fluids that, in cooperation with those secreted by the supportive cells, dissolve scent substances, allowing these to interact with the receptor cells. Serous and mucous cells are encountered, which may intermingle, or may form their own secretory units. These cells secrete proteins and mucus, respectively.

The **vomeronasal organ** consists of two tubular cavities, which open in the upper part of the nasal cavity, on both sides of the septum. These tubules are lined with a sensory epithelium that strongly resembles the olfactory epithelium. It is probable that the vomeronasal organ is specifically sensitive to the body odors of other persons, which would have a subtle, imperceptible influence on our own behavior and physiology. In animals, the vomeronasal organ is well developed and its function in the detection of scents,

called pheromones, produced by other members of the same species, is indisputable.

References.

Breeze R.G., Wheeldon E.B.: The cells of the pulmonary airways. Am. Rev. Respir. Dis. 1977, 116: 705777.

Dormans J.A.M.A.: Morphology, function, and response of pulmonary type I cells: a review. Inhal. Toxicol. 1996, 8: 521-536.

Ferrari C.C., Carmanchahi P.D., Aldana Marcos H.J., Affani J.M.: Ultrastructural characterisation of the olfactory mucosa of the armadillo *Dasypus hybridus* (Dasypodidae, Xenarthra). J. Anat. 2000, 196: 269-278.

Krauhs J.M.: Morphology of presumptive slowly adapting receptors in dog trachea. Anat. Rec. 1984, 210: 73-85.

Penney D.P.: The ultrastructure of epithelial cells of the distal lung. Int. Rev. Cytol. 1988, 111: 231-269.

Van Lommel A.: Pulmonary neuroendocrine cells (PNEC) and neuroepithelial bodies (NEB): chemoreceptors and regulators of lung development. Paediatr. Resp. Rev. 2001, 2: 171-176.

IV.15. Digestive system.

The digestive system consists of an **oral cavity**, where food is prepared for swallowing by mastication and mixing with saliva, and an **intestine**, where food is digested and useful substances obtained from it are taken up by the body. The intestine is associated with two important glands: the **liver** and the **pancreas**.

IV.15.1. Oral cavity.

The oral cavity is lined with Malpighian **epithelium** (IV.1.3.4.). Food is chewed by means of **teeth**. Teeth and the structures that hold them in place are specialized forms of **supportive** and **connective**

tissue. Saliva is produced by the **glandular tissue** of the **salivary glands**. The tongue is not only an aid in speaking but also helps in swallowing. It is a mass of **muscle tissue**, lined with epithelium, which contains receptor organs, the **taste buds**. The oral cavity is a gateway through which foreign material enters the body. Therefore, it contains **lymphoid tissue**, which locally forms accumulations: the **tonsils**.

IV.15.1.1. Teeth.

During embryonic development, tooth formation starts in the primitive oral epithelium at the apex of the jaw arch (Fig. 4.15.1.), which is parallel to the occlusal plane of the later teeth. The epithelium grows, plate-

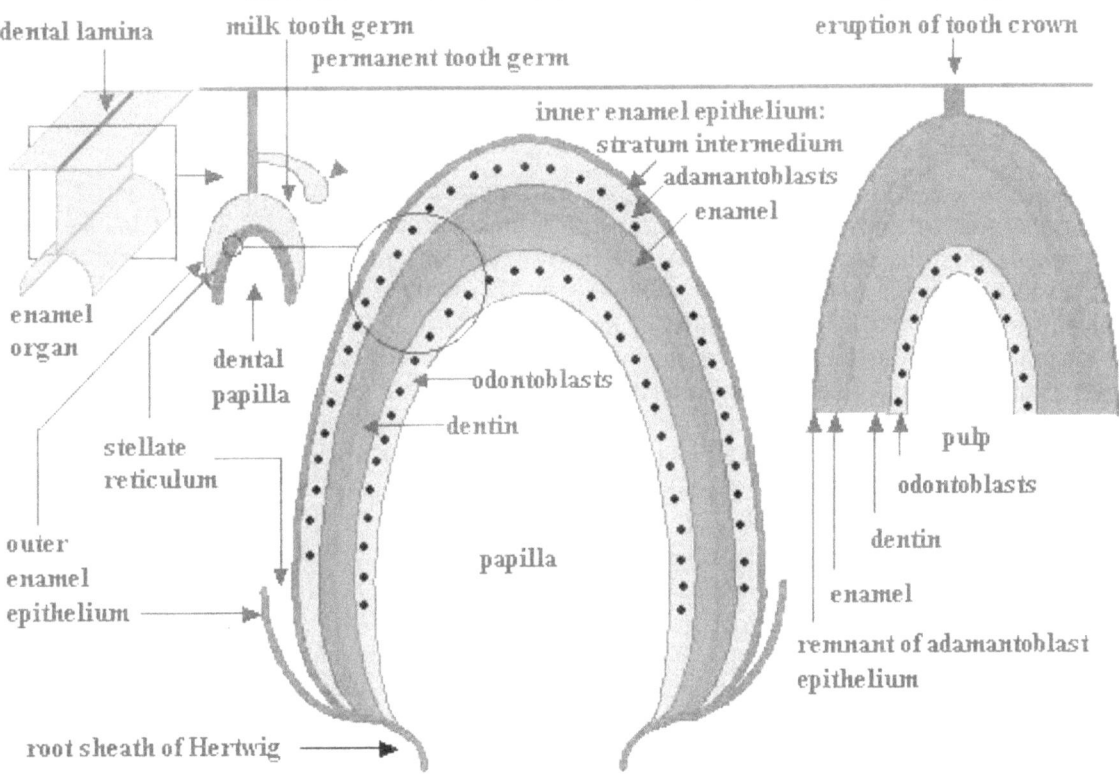

Fig. 4.15.1. Tooth germs arise from an infolding of the mouth's epithelium at the apex of the jaws: the dental lamina. The dental lamina is indented from below by fibrous tissue, the dental papillae, thus changing it into a series of bell-shaped enamel organs. The first germs to be formed thus are those of the milk teeth. Later, a permanent tooth germ develops as an outpocketing at the labial side of each milk tooth germ. Eventually, the enamel organ separates from the mouth's epithelium. The enamel organ is made of an outer and an inner epithelium, separated from each other by the stellate reticulum, a mesenchymal tissue. The inner epithelium consists of amelo- or adamantoblasts, which secrete enamel at their basal (!) pole. The dental papilla gives rise to an epithelium of mesodermal descent, composed of odontoblasts, which secrete dentin at their apical cell pole. The interior of the papilla develops into a pulp cavity. The tooth's crown erupts into the mouth upon formation and growth of a root. In this process, the outer epithelium of the enamel organ, which is strongly reduced by this time, merges with the mouth's Malpighian epithelium. During eruption, the last vestiges of the inner epithelium disappear.

like, into the underlying mesenchyme, giving rise to a **dental lamina**, which follows the curve of the jaw arch. The dental lamina fragments into separate pieces, each of which is indented by the mesenchyme, forming a **dental papilla** which points towards the occlusal plane and is capped with a bell shaped epithelium, the **enamel organ**. Thus, tooth germs are formed, which will give rise to milk teeth and to permanent molars. Each milk teeth germ forms a secondary germ at the labial side of the jaw, which will eventually form permanent incisors, canines, and premolars. Thus, teeth originate from both ectoderm and mesoderm. The bell-shaped enamel organ (Fig. 4.15.1.) consists of multiple layers of cells and is enveloped by a basement membrane. The outer cells, lying closest to the surface of the jaw arch, form a simple cuboidal epithelium, the outer enamel epithelium. The deeper cells secrete a viscous matrix and become star-shaped. They form the stellate reticulum. Near the dental papilla, the stellate reticulum changes into a few layers of cuboidal epithelial cells, the intermediate layer, and finally into a single layer of prismatic **ameloblasts**. The ameloblasts secrete enamel matrix on the occlusal top of the dental papilla, an activity that causes them to gradually recede from the papilla. This part of the tooth germ will later appear in the oral cavity, forming the tooth crown (Fig. 4.15.10.). The epithelium of the enamel organ initially covers deeper parts of the tooth germ, which will never appear in the oral cavity: the tooth root. Here, it does not form enamel. This part of the enamel organ, which disappears at an early stage, is the epithelial root sheath or Hertwig's sheath. The mesenchymal cells of the dental papilla, which border the enamel organ, develop into something which looks like an epithelium: a simple or pseudostratified layer of **odontoblasts** (Fig. 4.15.1.). The odontoblasts secrete the matrix of dentin, a tissue resembling bone, on the concave face of the enamel organ, receding from it as they do so. The odontoblasts will end up lining the tooth's pulp cavity and root canals (Fig. 4.15.10.). At the level of the later tooth root, **cementoblasts** develop out of mesenchymal cells, and secrete the matrix of cementum, another bone-like tissue (Fig. 4.15.10.). Tooth eruption, the appearance of the tooth crown in the oral cavity, is driven by the growth of the tooth root. At this time, the enamel organ is no longer functional. Its superficial epithelial layers merge with the oral epithelium lining the gingiva, and the tooth erupts. For a short while, the tooth crown may be covered with a rest of the enamel organ, Nasmyth's membrane. The interstitial tissue filling the pulp cavity and the root canals is a leftover from the original mesenchymal dental papilla. It is regarded as mucous tissue. Contrary to the mucous tissue of the umbilical

cord, it is vascularized and innervated. It contains a dense network of capillaries, which are formed by blood vessels entering through the root canals. There is also a dense sensory innervation, some fibers reaching into the dentinal tubules.

IV.15.1.1.1. Ameloblasts and enamel.

Ameloblasts are epithelial cells, derived from ectoderm. Initially, they rest on a basement membrane that borders the dental papilla, but degenerates at an early stage. In order to deposit enamel matrix in the right place, on top of the dental papilla, they have to secrete it at their basal pole. This means that the normal polarity of epithelial cells, which secrete at their apical pole, has to be reversed. Active ameloblasts are very tall, prismatic cells (Figs. 4.15.2.-3.) which have some characteristics in common with the matrix-secreting cells (II.2.1.1.3.) of connective and supportive tissues, especially so the osteoblasts, which show polarization and deposit matrix at one pole. Actually, they are epithelial cells that masquerade as matrix-secreting cells. In the ameloblasts, polarization is carried to much greater extremes still than in the osteoblasts, and they deposit matrix strictly at one pole, the basal one. The occlusal pole, which points away from the dental papilla, contains the nucleus and therefore looks like a basal cell pole, but it is in fact a camouflaged apical one. The give away is the presence of a terminal web, as well as occasional junctional complexes. Towards the dental papilla, an extensive rough endoplasmic reticulum and several Golgi-complexes develop (Fig. 4.15.4.). Both organelles line up at the cell's periphery, parallel to the cell membrane. In the center, along the cellular axis, secretory vesicles with an opaque content accumulate. Next to the dental papilla, the ameloblasts form a short, blunt process, **Tomes's process**, in which the secretory vesicles maintain their axial position (Fig. 4.15.5.). The vesicular content, the organic enamel matrix, is liberated, merocrine fashion, by exocytosis. The peripheral cytoplasm of Tomes's process is filled with filaments. Each ameloblast secretes a column of proteinaceous enamel matrix. When the enamel matrix has been deposited, the ameloblasts induce its calcification, which takes place by deposition of hydroxy-apatite. During calcification, the organic matrix is largely lost. Fully calcified enamel contains less than one percent of organic material and is the hardest substance of the body. The enamel layer consists of longitudinal prisms with a diameter of about 5 micrometers. Each is probably formed by a single ameloblast. These prisms run parallel to each other, from the dentin-enamel junction

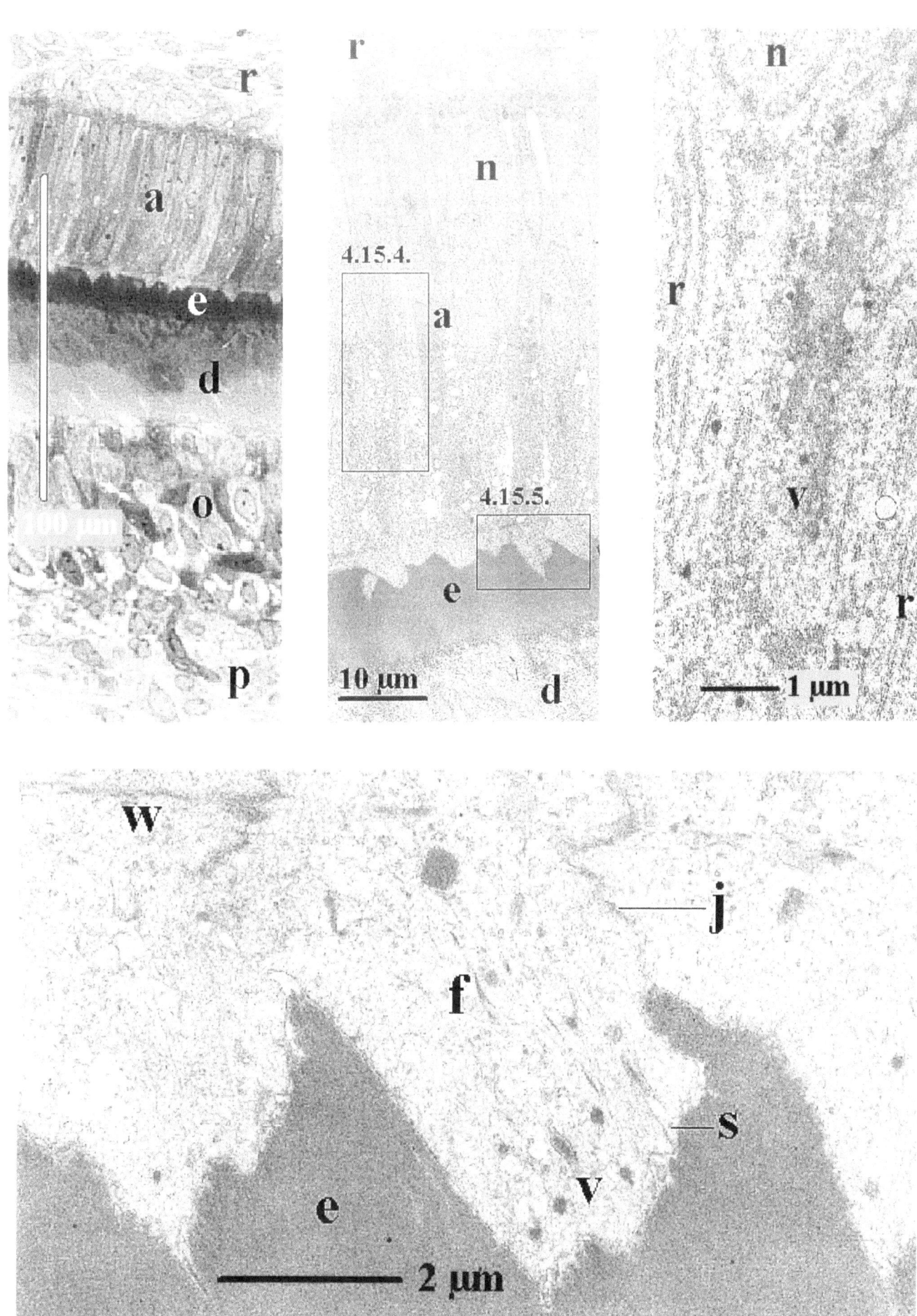

Fig. 4.15.2. (top left) The tooth germ's (or enamel epithelium's) wall is composed of a simple prismatic epithelium of ameloblasts (a) and a less regular "epithelium" of odontoblasts (o). Both have begun to secrete enamel (e) and dentin (d), respectively. The newly deposited dentin (clear layer) is as yet uncalcified. Nearer to the enamel lies older, calcified dentin (second darkest layer). r = stellate reticulum, p = pulp cavity. Tooth germ, rabbit, 1-micrometer plastic section, toluidin blue. **Fig. 4.15.3.** (top center) The enamel epithelium, composed of very slender and tall ameloblasts (a), rests on the stellate reticulum (r) (compare with Figure 4.15.2.). Ameloblasts are distinctly polarized cells, but the cell pole where the enamel matrix (e) is secreted is not the apical one, as it would be in typical polarized cells, but the basal one. The pole containing the nucleus (n) is in fact the apical pole. d = dentin. Tooth germ, rabbit, TEM. **Fig. 4.15.4.** (top right) In the middle part of the ameloblast, between the nucleus (n) and the enamel, lies a well-developed rough endoplasmic reticulum (r), its cisterns lined up along the cell membrane. In the cell's axis, secretory vesicles (v) accumulate. Tooth germ, rabbit, TEM. **Fig. 4.15.5.** (bottom) The basal ameloblast cytoplasm is rich in microfilaments (f). The axial region contains secretory vesicles (v) with a dense content that, after being liberated by exocytosis, or merocrine secretion (s) contributes to the deposition of enamel matrix (e). Typical components of an apical cell pole are seen, such as a junctional complex (j) and a terminal web (w). Notwithstanding, this is the basal pole. Tooth germ, rabbit, TEM.

to the crown's surface. When the enamel has been calcified, the ameloblasts die by apoptosis. Since the enamel organ thus degenerates prior to eruption, enamel cannot regenerate when it is damaged.

IV.15.1.1.2. Odontoblasts and dentin.

Odontoblasts have a mesodermal origin. Active odontoblasts form an "epithelium", the somewhat disordered initial organization of which indicates that it is not a true one (Fig. 4.15.2.). In contrast to ameloblasts, they are matrix-secreting cells that masquerade as epithelial cells. As odontoblasts grow older, the epithelium they form gradually acquires more order. The cells even develop junctional complexes of tight and intermediate junctions, associated with a terminal web. Contrary to true epithelia, however, these junctions do not appear to form complete, cell-encircling belts or fasciae. That part of the cell which is turned away from the enamel organ, and which may be called the basal cell pole, contains the nucleus, surrounded by a well-developed rough endoplasmic reticulum (Fig. 4.15.6.) and a few Golgi-complexes. As they deposit dentin matrix, the odontoblasts move away from the enamel-dentin interface. As they do so, each of them forms a thin, ever lengthening process, which trails behind them, as it were: **Tomes's fiber** (Figs. 4.15.7.-8.). Additional matrix may be deposited along the process. These processes lie in narrow, tubular canals, the **dentinal tubules** (Fig. 4.15.9.). Although dentinal tubules occupy the entire thickness of the dentin layer, Tomes's fibers only occupy the lower third of their length. Tomes's fibers are supported by axial microtubules and microfilaments. The matrix of dentin contains collagen and ground substance, and calcifies as it is deposited. Globally, dentin has the same composition as bone, but it is more strongly calcified and therefore harder. In addition to this, it is acellular, except for the odontoblastic processes.

IV.15.1.1.3. Periodontal ligament, tooth sockets, and gingiva.

Each tooth is implanted in its own socket (Fig. 4.5.10.), an opening at the apex of the jawbones. The tooth is held in place by a fibrous connective tissue, the **periodontal ligament**. The periodontal ligament is ordered fibrous tissue (III.2.4.2.), the bundles of collagen fibrils coursing in various directions (Fig. 4.15.10.). The gingival bundles are attached at the upper part of the tooth root and run toward the gingival fibrous tissue, where they end freely, while the interdental bundles connect the roots of several adjacent teeth (Fig. 4.15.11.). The alveolo-dental bundles connect the tooth root to the wall of the tooth socket. In this group, several subgroups with various orientations may be distinguished. Also in this group, but not in the others, at more or less equal distances from root and socket wall, the periodontal ligament shows a narrow band in which the collagen fibrils have an irregular course, the intermediary plexus (Fig. 4.15.12.). This area is rich in blood vessels and sensory nerve fibers. At one side of the periodontal ligament, collagen fibrils penetrate into the bone of the tooth socket wall, the lamina dura, and on the other side into the cementum of the tooth root, giving rise to Sharpey's fibers. Like tendons, the periodontal ligament is adapted to the accomodation of considerable tensile forces, which arise during biting and chewing. It transmits these forces to the jawbones. The various orientations of the fiber bundles enable the periodontal ligament to accommodate variously oriented tensile forces. The tooth socket wall is a specialized bony layer, the lamina dura. The lamina dura consists of a superficial layer of fibrous bone, in which the collagen Sharpey fibers of the periodontal ligament lie embedded, a middle layer of compact lamellar bone, and a deep layer of "circumferential" lamellae, which rest on the spongy bone core of the jaw. The tooth socket wall undergoes remodellation by local resorption of old bone and deposition of new

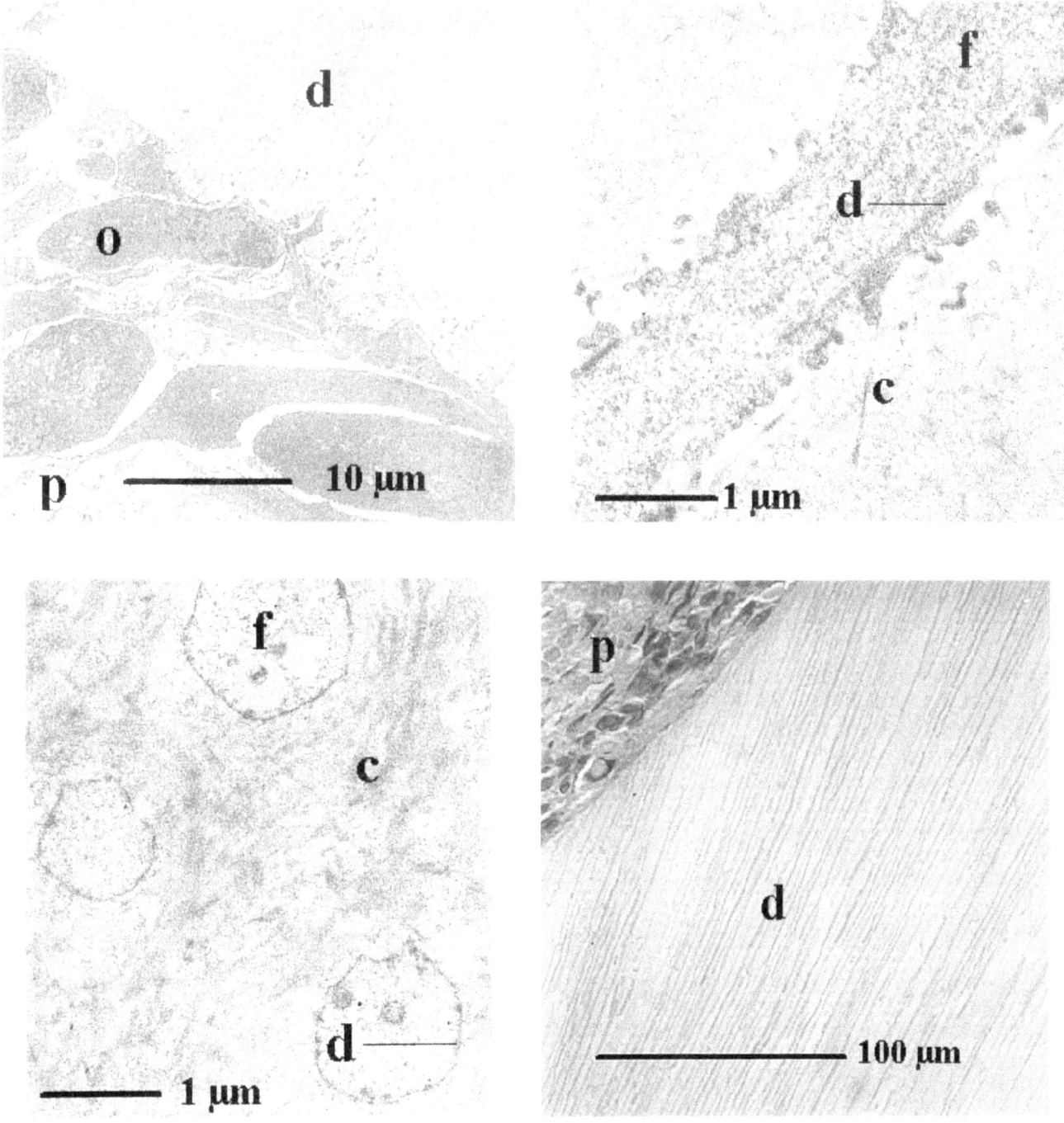

Fig. 4.15.6. (top left) The odontoblasts (o) border the tooth's pulp cavity (p). They secrete dentin matrix (d) in a way that is similar to that of osteoblasts, but contrary to these, they never get walled in by matrix: dentin is acellular bone. Tooth germ, rabbit, TEM. **Fig. 4.15.7.** (top right) As they deposit dentin matrix, the odontoblasts retreat from the dentin-enamel junction, forming an ever-lengthening process, Tomes's fiber. This fiber is supported by microfilaments (f). The cytoplasmic face of the cell membrane is coated with a dense layer (d). The dentin matrix contains collagen fibrils (c). Tooth germ, rabbit, TEM. **Fig. 4.15.8.** (bottom left) Tomes's fibers (t) in cross-section. Compare with Figure 4.15.7. Tooth germ, rabbit, TEM. **Fig. 4.15.9.** (bottom right) Under the light microscope, dentin (d) is characterized by numerous parallel dentin canals. Each of them contains an odontoblastic process, or Tomes's fiber. p = pulp cavity. Tooth, human, HE.

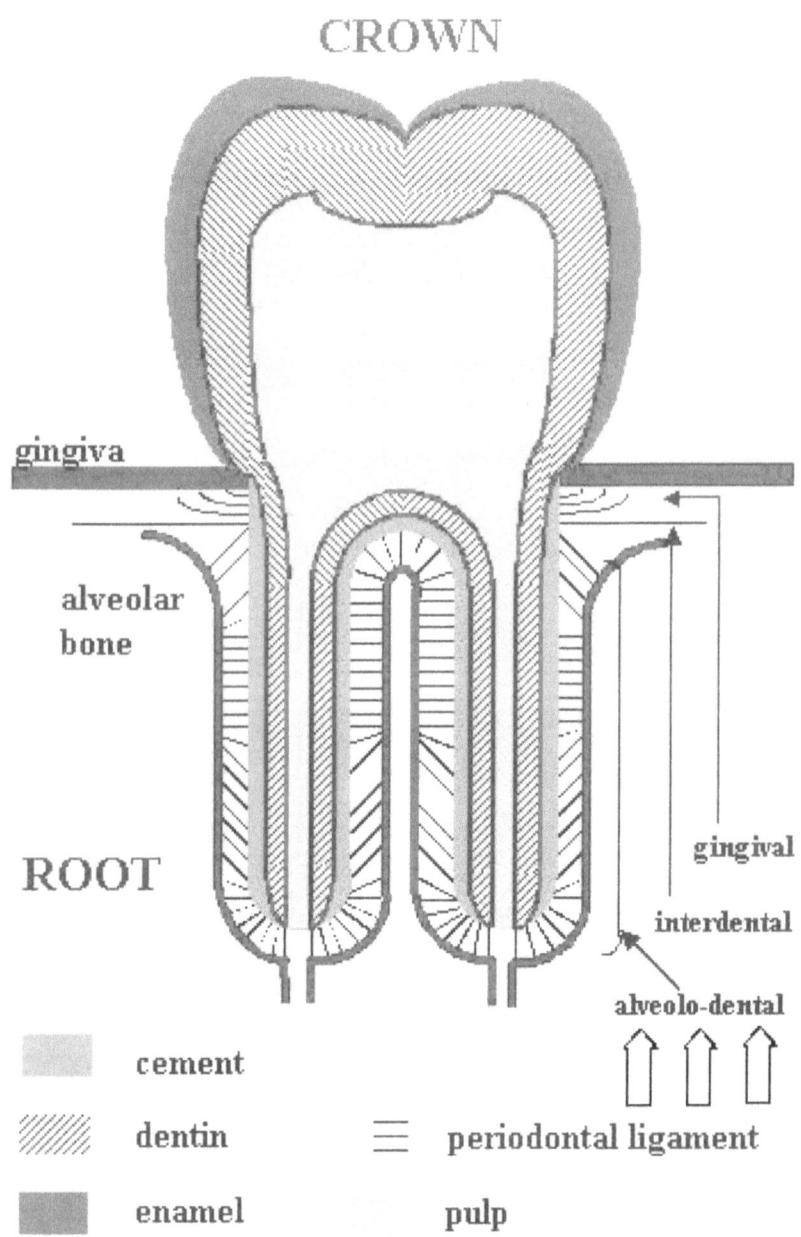

Fig. 4.15.10. The crown is that part of the tooth which is exposed in the mouth cavity, rising above the gum or gingiva. The pulp cavity extends into the crown. The crown's wall is made of dentin, coated with enamel. At the level of the root, the tooth is anchored into its socket by means of a periodontal ligament, composed of multiple fiber groups. The ligament's fibers are anchored into the root's cementum at one end. Cementum, like dentin, is acellular bone, but lacks canals. At the other end, the gingival ligament is anchored into the gum, the interdental ligament into the cementum of an adjoining tooth, and the alveolo-dental ligament into the bone of the tooth socket. In the alveolo-dental ligament, the orientation of the fiber groups varies according to their position, allowing them to withstand variously oriented tensile forces.

bone. Thus, the teeth can adapt themselves to changing load patterns, as they occur during growth of the jaws. This ability of remodellation is the basis of orthodontic corrections. The **gingiva** (Fig. 4.15.13.), or gum, is composed of the Malpighian epithelium of the oral cavity, which rests on a fibrous tissue corium.

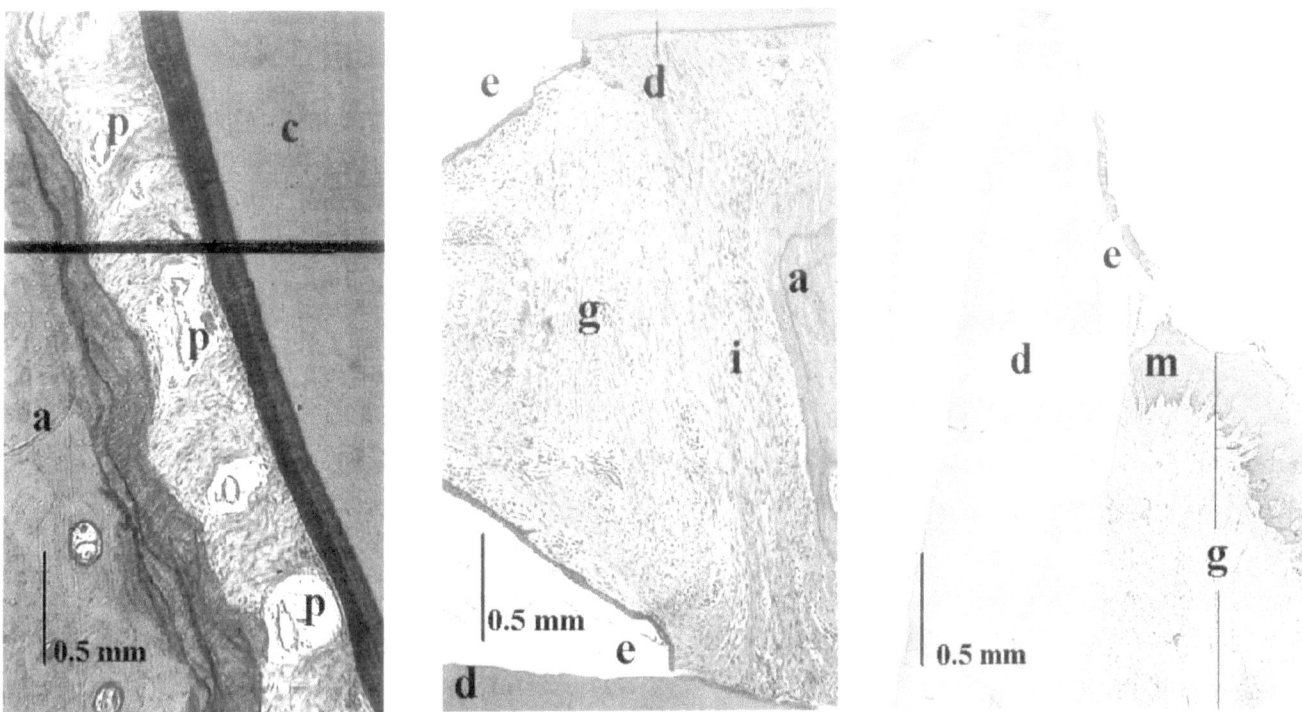

Left to right: **Fig. 4.15.11.** The gingival (g) and interdental (i) fiber groups of the periodontal ligaments. The wide spaces to the left and the right were occupied by the crown's enamel (e), which has disappeared upon decalcification of this tooth. d = dentin of two adjacent teeth, a = apex of the alveolar bone. Tooth socket, human, HE. **Fig. 4.15.12.** The alveolo-dental fiber group of the periodontal ligament contains a prominent intermediary plexus (p) with blood vessels. a = alveolar bone of the tooth socket, c = cementum of the tooth root. The dark ribbons at both sides of the periodontal ligament, especially next to the root, are artefactual folds of the tissue section. Tooth socket, human, HE. **Fig. 4.15.13.** The gingiva (g) is composed of Malpighian epithelium (m), which rests on a fibrous tissue corium. d = dentin, e = space previously occupied by enamel. Erupting tooth, human, HE.

The corium and the epithelium form papillae. The epithelium narrowly fits the base of the tooth crown, called the neck. The epithelial cells form hemidesmosomes, which join them to the enamel of the tooth's neck, which is covered with a fibrous layer resembling a basal lamina. This layer may grow fairly thick, forming a cuticle.

Fig. 4.15.14. (top left) Salivary glands are large, compound glands, enveloped in a fibrous tissue capsule (c) and subdivided into lobes (l) by means of fibrous tissue septa (s). The thickest septa carry excretory ducts (d) and blood vessels (v). Submandibular gland, human, HE. **Fig. 4.15.15.** (top right) The parotid gland is exclusively composed of serous acini (a). Intralobular, or striated, ducts (s) are found between the acini. The interlobular excretory ducts (e) course in the fibrous tissue septa. The epithelium forming their wall is stratified, consisting of a basal layer of cuboidal cells (c) and a superficial layer of prismatic cells (p). Parotid gland, human, HE. **Fig. 4.15.16.** (bottom left) The submandibular gland contains numerous serous acini (s), as well as relatively rare mucous acini (m). Saliva is evacuated via intralobular, or striated, ducts (d), lined with a simple prismatic epithelium. Submandibular gland, human, HE. **Fig. 4.15.17.** (bottom right) The sublingual gland contains numerous seromucous acini. These are mucous acini, the apex of which carries a cap of serous cells. In sections, this produces Gianuzzi's sickle (s). Between the acini, intralobular (striated) ducts are observed, which are lined with a simple prismatic epithelium (d). The interlobular excretory ducts (e) course in the fibrous tissue septa. The inset shows a detail of their stratified epithelium, consisting of basal cells (b) and prismatic cells (p). Sublingual gland, human, HE.

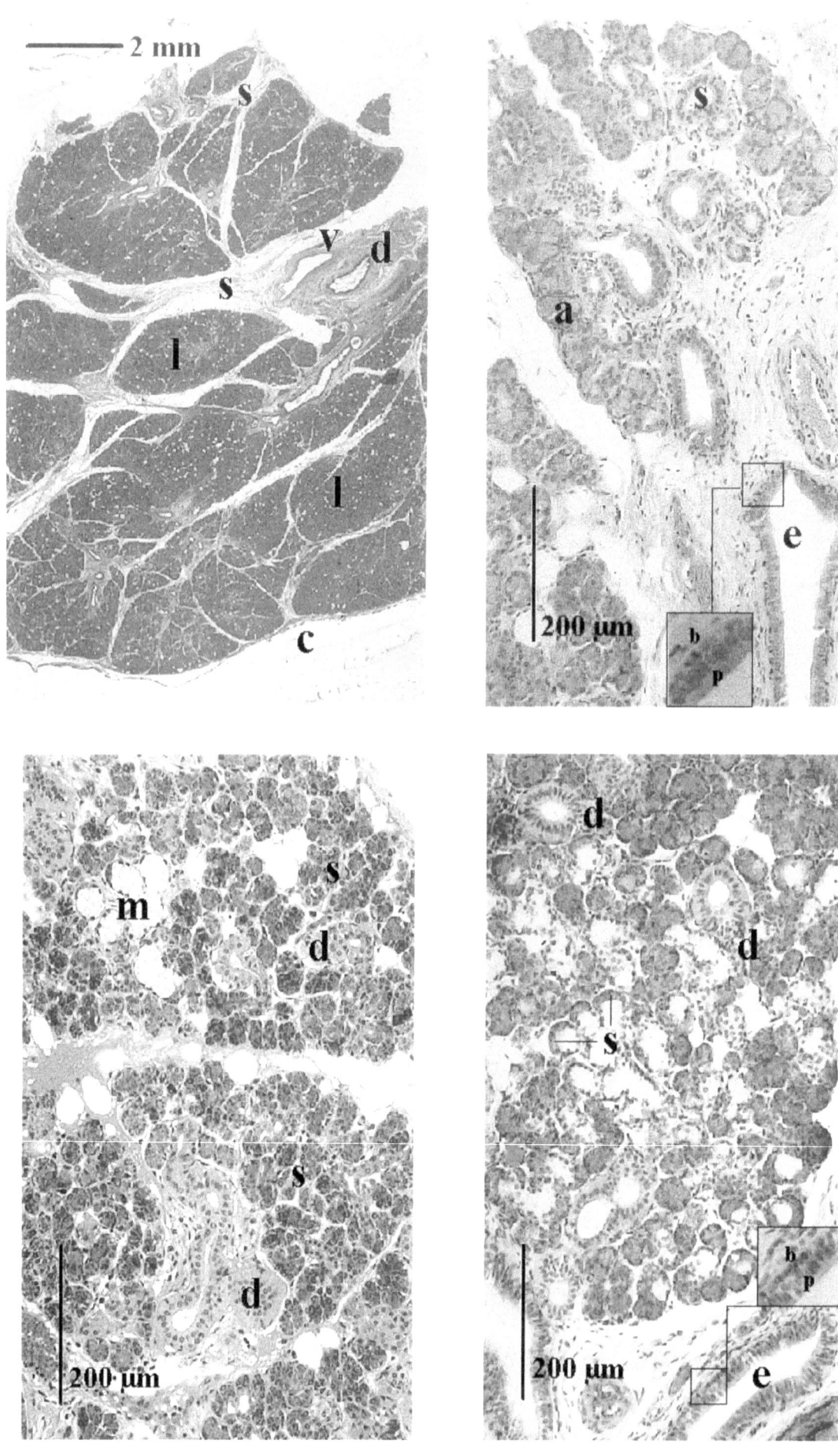

IV.15.1.2. Salivary glands.

Two kinds of salivary gland open into the oral cavity: the major salivary glands and the accessory salivary glands. There are three pairs of **major salivary glands**, named after their location. The lingual glands and the submandibular glands lie in the lower jaw, under the tongue, the first one at the front, the second one at the back. They open into the bottom of the oral cavity, on both sides of the tongue. The parotid glands lie in the hypodermis of the upper jaw, in front of the ears, and open into the oral cavity between the gums and the cheek, at the level of the second premolar. The major salivary glands are compound acinar or tubulo-acinar glands (III.5.1.). They consist of numerous lobes, separated from each other by fibrous tissue septa that carry nerve fibers, blood vessels, and ducts (Fig. 4.15.14.). The **parotid gland** is a purely acinar gland, containing exclusively **serous acini** (Fig. 4.15.15.). Serous acini consist of tall, pyramidal cells with basophilic cytoplasm and the cytological structure of exocrine, enzyme-secreting gland cells. Their secretory vesicles are spherical, have a moderately opaque content and reach diameters of about 1 micrometer. The serous cells are continuously active, although at a higher level during chewing, and produce a clear, copious, very fluid saliva, rich in enzymes like amylase and lysosyme. The **submandibular gland** is a tubulo-acinar gland, because it contains **mucous**

"acini" in addition to **serous** ones (Fig. 4.15.16.) that, strictly speaking, have to be regarded as tubules, since they are elongated instead of spherical. Mucous acini consist of cells with the cytological structure of exocrine, mucus-secreting gland cells. The secretory vesicles are fairly large, bigger than those of serous cells, but show little tendency to coalesce into a single bubble, as they would do in a goblet cell. The cells are much lower than serous cells, and this is largely explained by their secretory mechanism, which is apocrine, causing periodic loss of large portions of apical cytoplasm. Sometimes the nucleus lies flattened next to the basal cell membrane, which may be a consequence of excessive accumulation of secretory material. Mucous acini produce a thick, viscous saliva. A fair number of mucous acini carry a terminal cap of serous cells, forming a half moon shape in sections: **Gianuzzi's sickle**. Such acini are called **sero-mucous**. The **sublingual gland** is also a tubulo-acinar gland, but most of its acini are mucous or sero-mucous (Fig. 4.15.17.). The epithelium of the acini is associated with myoepithelial cells. A characteristic that the major salivary glands have in common is that their duct system consists of several segments. The distal branches of the duct system, in which the acini open, are Boll's intercalated ducts. These are very narrow ducts, the walls of which are an unspecialized, simple cuboidal epithelium, underneath of which myoepithelial cells are found. The intercalated ducts

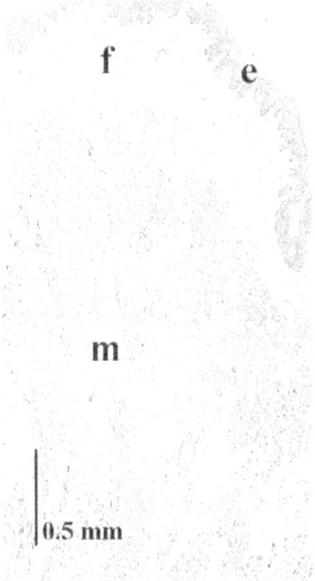 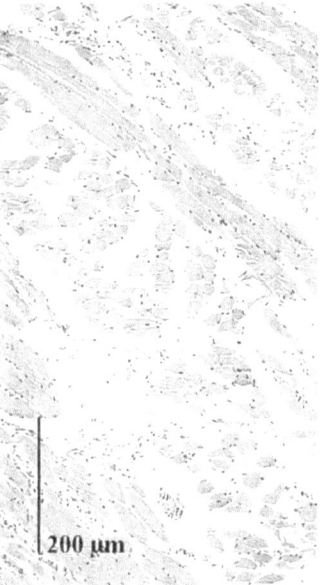

Fig. 4.15.18. (left) The tongue is a muscle (m), enveloped in a fibrous tissue layer (f), supporting a Malpighian, slightly keratinized, epithelium (e). Tongue, human, HE. **Fig. 4.15.19.** (right) The tongue's muscle fibers are typical skeletal muscle fibers, but they do not run strictly parallel (compare with Figure 3.3.3.). They lie in bundles, which course in various directions, accounting for the tongue's extreme mobility. Tongue, human, HE.

abruptly open into **Pflüger's ducts**. These ductal segments have a much larger diameter than acini or intercalated ducts and their wall is a simple prismatic epithelium with eosinophilic cytoplasm. The basal cell membrane forms deep, narrow, parallel folds, perpendicular to it. Between these folds lie rows of mitochondria. Light optically, this may produce a radial striation at the perimeter of the ducts. This is why these ductal segments are called **striated ducts**. The membrane folds increase the surface of the cell membrane, increasing the ability of these cells to resorb ions from the saliva, energy being supplied by the mitochondria. This way, the initially isotonic saliva becomes hypotonic. Thus, the major salivary glands function as osmoregulatory organs, as the kidneys and the sweat glands do. Beneath the epithelium, myoepithelial cells are found. The striated ducts have an exclusively intralobular course, amid the acini (Figs. 4.15.16.-17.). When Pflüger's ducts leave the lobes, they gradually change into branches of the **excretory duct**, which eventually opens into the oral cavity. Excretory ducts have an interlobular course, meaning that they run in the fibrous tissue septa between the lobes, and are much wider than Pflüger's ducts (Figs. 4.15.14.-15., 4.15.17.). The excretory duct is lined with a stratified epithelium. In the narrower, distal segments, it consists of a basal layer of cuboidal cells, and an upper layer of prismatic cells. This is an epithelium with a sealing function, blocking any exchanges between saliva and tissue fluids. The most proximal and widest segment, which opens in the oral cavity, is lined with Malpighian epithelium. The relative lengths of the three duct segments differ from gland to gland. Boll's intercalated ducts are longest in the parotid, Pflüger's ducts in the submandibular, and the excretory duct in the sublingual. The other segments are accordingly shorter. The **accessory salivary glands**, which are distributed over the mucosa of the oral cavity, except in the gums and the hard palate, are compound tubular or tubulo-acinar glands. The tubular glands are mucous, the tubulo-acinar glands are seromucous, with a predominance of mucous acini. The duct is lined with a simple, cuboidal to prismatic epithelium.

IV.15.1.3. Tongue and taste buds.

The tongue is a mass of skeletal muscle tissue, enveloped in a fibrous tissue layer, which is lined with Malpighian epithelium (Fig. 4.15.18.). The striated muscle fibers are grouped in bundles, which have various orientations (Fig. 4.15.19.). This explains the highly motile character of the tongue, which is essential for speech and for manipulation of food in the oral cavity. The striated muscle bundles are sheathed with a fibrous tissue perimysium. The subepithelial fibrous tissue is relatively dense, and can be regarded as an epimysium. In the peri- and epimysia, accessory salivary glands are found. The epithelium, though in principle Malpighian, shows a certain degree of keratinization, especially so at the dorsal side, giving the tongue surface a rough texture. The dorsal epithelium forms numerous outward bulges or papillae with a fibrous tissue core. The most common of these are the pointed and relatively strongly keratinized filiform papillae, which cover the anterior two thirds of the tongue. Distributed among these, but much more rare, are the knob-like fungiform papillae, which are less strongly keratinized. The rarest, biggest, and most complex type of papilla are the **circumvallate papillae**. There are only about ten of them, and they line up across the tongue, forming a demarcation line between the anterior two thirds and the posterior third of the tongue. They are knob shaped, a few millimeters in diameter, and surrounded by a deep epithelial fold. The walls of this fold contain taste buds. Specialized serous accessory salivary glands, Ebner's glands, open into the bottom of this fold. **Taste buds** are small chemoreceptive organs that are distributed in the epithelium of the oral cavity and the pharynx, and occur in larger concentrations in the epithelium lining the grooves surrounding the circumvallate papillae. A taste bud is spherical to fusiform, and occupies the entire epithelial thickness (Fig. 4.15.20.). It opens into the oral cavity through a taste pore (Fig. 4.15.21.). It is made up of a few tens of fusiform cells that stretch from the basement membrane to the taste pore. Distinction is made between taste cells and supporting cells. At the base of the bud, undifferentiated basal cells are found, which serve as replacements of the functional cells, which are continuously lost. This is a reminder that the taste cells and supporting cells are derived from a stratified epithelium, and are themselves modified epithelial cells. The **taste cells** carry apical microvilli (Fig. 4.15.21.) and the apical cytoplasm is rich in smooth endoplasmic reticulum. This is probably recycled cell membrane. The perinuclear cytoplasm is loaded with dense cored vesicles, so that the cells resemble endocrine, amine or peptide hormone-secreting cells (II.2.1.1.2.). Basolaterally, the taste cells are contacted by the terminals of sensory nerve fibers (Fig. 4.15.22.), and local synaptic junctions are formed. Here, the taste cell membrane is irregularly thickened, and dense cored vesicles accumulate in the cytoplasm, allowing the conclusion that the taste cells transmit stimuli to the nerve terminals. Cells which are contacted by sensory nerve fibers, but which do not themselves contain synaptic vesicles, have also been described.

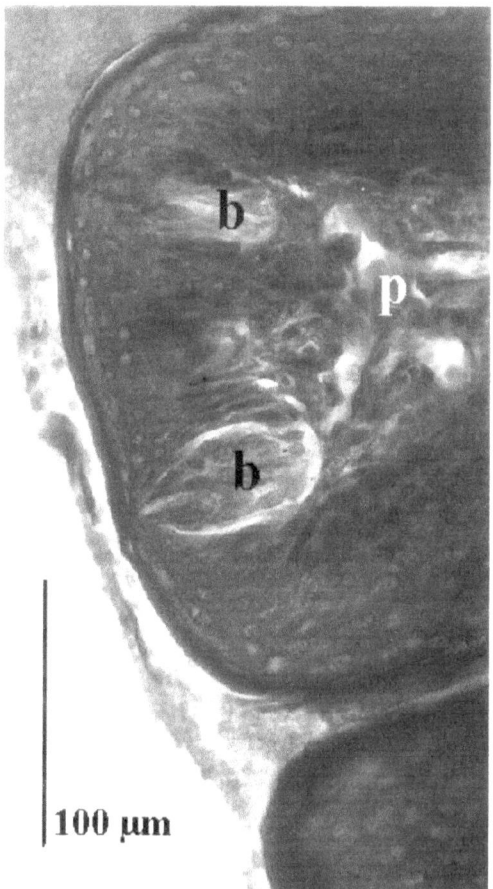

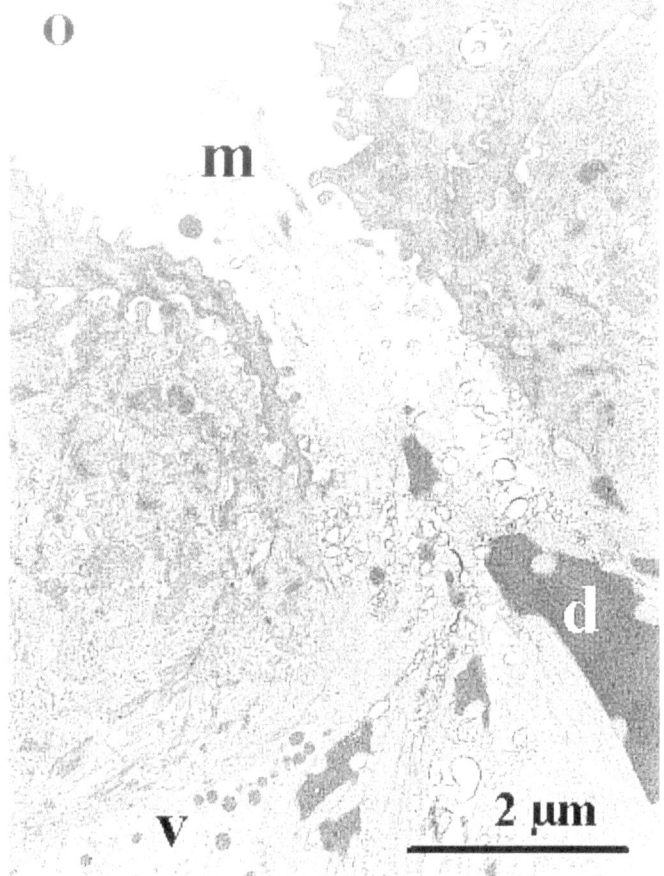

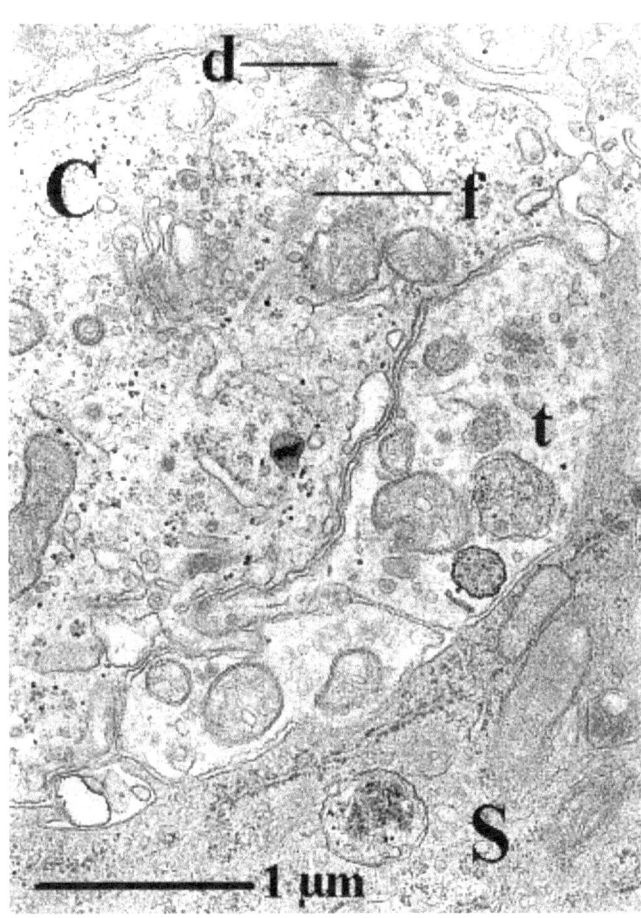

Fig. 4.15.20. (top left) The epithelium lining the tongue's papillae (p) contains taste buds (b). Tongue, cat, Masson stain. **Fig. 4.15.21.** (top right) The chemoreceptor cells of the taste bud carry microvilli (m) that project through a pore of the lingual epithelium into the oral cavity (o). Mark the secretory vesicles (v) of the supporting cells, the contents of which correspond to the dense intercellular material (d). This material is partly secreted into the oral cavity and may assist in trapping taste substances. Taste bud, rabbit, TEM. **Fig. 4.15.22.** (left) A taste bud is composed of chemoreceptor cells (c) and supporting cells (s). The chemoreceptor cells are contacted by the terminals (t) of sensory nerve fibers. Mark the presence of microfilaments (f) and desmosomes (d), which betray the epithelial nature of these cells. Taste bud, hamster, TEM.

They are also regarded as taste cells. Several types of supporting cell may be distinguished, which may represent different stages in the life cycle of a single cell type. Supporting cells also carry apical microvilli. The apical cytoplasm contains secretory vesicles. They contain variable amounts of rough endoplasmic reticulum, ribosomes, smooth endoplasmic reticulum, a Golgi-complex, mitochondria, and bundles of intermediary filaments. It is probable that these cells contribute to the accumulation of an opaque, mucous extracellular material in the taste pore, which would aid in dissolving taste substances, in which form they can interact with taste cells.

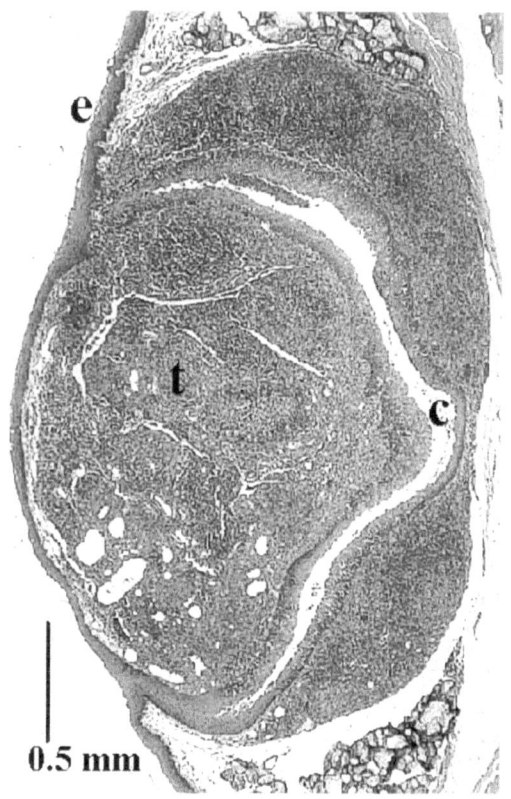

Fig. 4.15.23. In certain places, the Malpighian epithelium (e) lining the tongue, the palate, and the pharynx, forms deep crypts (c), wherein a tonsil (t) may develop. A tonsil is an accumulation of lymphoid tissue in the fibrous tissue corium, which partly disrupts the epithelial structure. Pharyngeal tonsil, rabbit, HE.

IV.15.1.4. Tonsils.

The tonsils are accumulations of lymphoid tissue, which are encountered in various places in the oral cavity and the pharynx, such as the posterior third of the tongue and the soft palate. The lymphoid tissue forms a globular or elongated mass, which bulges above the surrounding epithelium. The Malpighian epithelium overlying this mass is infolded, forming a number of deep, narrow crypts (Fig. 4.15.23.). It is often so heavily infiltrated with lymphocytes that its epithelial structure is hardly apparent.

The tonsillar lymphoid tissue forms follicles, the germinal centers of which contain large, proliferating B-lymphocytes, while the coronae contain smaller, immature B-lymphocytes. Frequently, the coronae are asymmetric: the side facing a crypt is wider than the opposite side. Between the follicles, T-lymphocytes accumulate and high endothelial venules are found.

The crypt epithelium is selectively permeable to antigens, which may be phagocytosed. The epithelial cells subsequently function as antigen presenting cells, activating lymphocytes and thus initiating immune responses. They are analogous to the M-cells that form the epithelium covering areas of lymphoid tissue concentration in the intestine.

IV.15.2. Intestine.

The intestine is a tubular organ, made up of concentric tissue layers (Fig. 4.15.24.). The innermost layer is **epithelium**. In combination with the underlying **connective tissue**, the corium or **lamina propria**, it forms the **mucosa**. In various places, the lamina propria supports outward folds of the epithelium, the intestinal villi, which carry specialized capillaries, made of endothelium. In other places, the epithelium folds in, and develops into **glandular tissue**: mucosal and submucosal glands. The continuous presence of foreign material inside the intestine explains the contribution of **lymphoid tissue** to the intestinal structure. The mucosa rests on a thin layer of **visceral muscle tissue**, the **muscularis mucosae**. Next is a relatively thick layer of connective tissue, the **submucosa**. The **musculosa** is a very thick layer of visceral muscle tissue below the submucosa. It is a compound layer, in principle composed of an inner circular layer and an outer longitudinal layer. The **serosa** is a thin connective tissue layer on the outside of the intestine, lined with mesothelium. The intestine contains massive amounts of **nerve tissue**. Most conspicuous are the ganglionic plexi in the submucosa and between the two layers of the musculosa.

The intestine is made up of a number of segments which differ in the details of their histological structure, which reflects their function: the **oesophagus**, the **stomach**, the **small intestine**, the large intestine or **colon**, and the **rectum**. The small intestine, which attains a length of five meters, is the longest segment of all. In its turn, it is composed of a cranial **duodenum**, an intermediate **jejunum**, and a

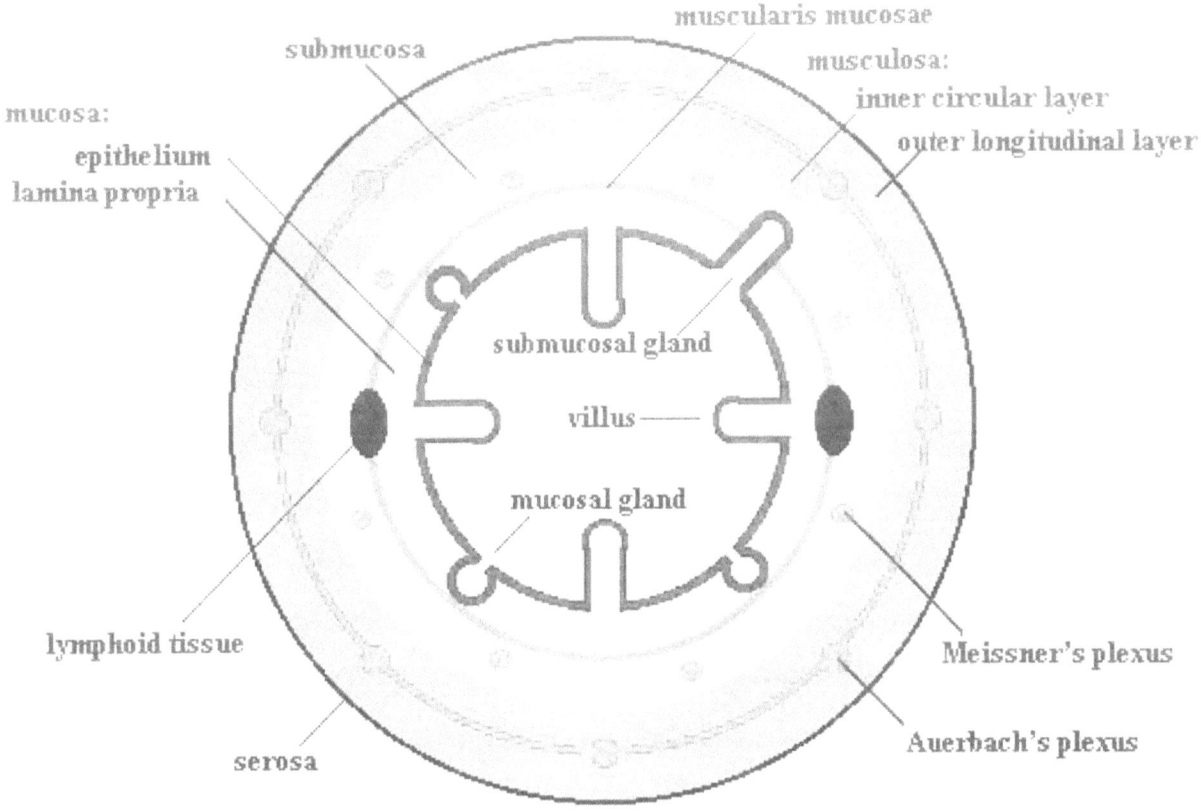

Fig. 4.15.24. The gut is made up of several concentric tissue layers. The lumen is bordered by a mucosa, which is a fibrous tissue lamina propria or corium, lined with epithelium. Locally, the mucosa forms villi. In various gut segments, the epithelium forms mucosal, as well as submucosal, glands. A thin layer of visceral muscle tissue, the muscularis mucosae, separates the mucosa from the fibrous tissue submucosa. The submucosa rests on a double layer of visceral muscle tissue, the musculosa. The inner layer of the musculosa consists of circularly running muscle fibers, the outer layer of longitudinally arranged fibers. The muscularis is sheathed with a fibrous tissue layer, lined with mesothelium, the serosa. At the junction of mucosa and submucosa, prominent accumulations of lymphoid tissue may form. The gut is densely innervated. The largest concentrations of nervous tissue are to be found in 2 ganglionic plexi: Meissner's plexus in the submucosa and Auerbach's plexus sandwiched between both muscle layers of the musculosa.

caudal **ileum**. At its origin, the colon forms a blind branch or caecum, which ends in the **appendix**.

The intestine is suspended from the roof of the abdominal cavity by means of the mesentery, a connective tissue membrane, lined with mesothelium, which is continuous dorsally with the peritoneum and which carries blood vessels and nerve fibers. At the level of the stomach, the mesentery forms specialized omenta. Omenta are perforated parts of the mesentery and show numerous milk spots, rare in other parts of the mesentery or the peritoneum. Milk spots are accumulations of immune cells, especially lymphocytes, and monocytes and macrophages.

IV.15.2.1. Mucosa and submucosa.

The **oesophagus** is lined with a **Malpighian epithelium** (Fig. 4.15.25.). The mucosa lies in longitudinal folds, which can flatten out when a food bolus passes by. This epithelium has a shielding function: in the oesophagus, no digestion or absorption as yet takes place.

Locally, the epithelium forms mucosal as well as submucosal glands, which secrete a lubrifying mucus. The **mucosal glands** are found predominantly at the beginning and at the end of the oesophagus. They are sessile, branched tubular glands, very like the cardiac glands of the stomach. The **submucosal glands** are found along the entire length of the oesophagus, with a slight preference for the cranial half. They are compound, branched tubular glands. The distal segments of their duct are lined with a simple prismatic epithelium, which changes into a Malpighian one at the mouth.

The **stomach** is lined with a **simple prismatic epithelium**, which forms mucosal glands. Depending on the microscopic structure and the cellular

287

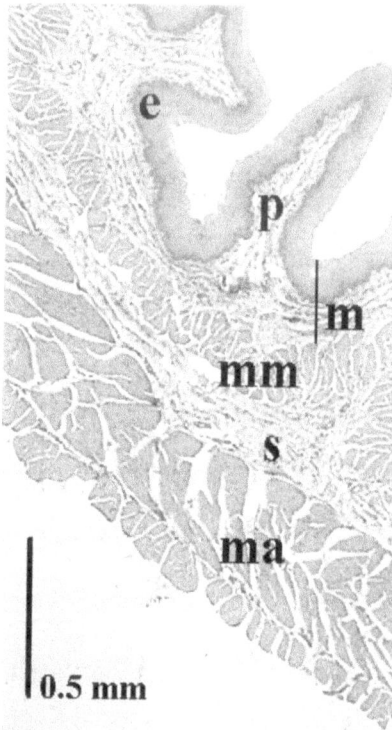

0.5 mm

Fig. 4.15.25. The most distinctive characteristic of the oesophagus is its Malpighian epithelium (e). With the underlying lamina propria (p) the epithelium forms the mucosa. The mucosa (m) is thrown into longitudinal folds. Also seen are the muscularis mucosae (mm), the submucosa (s), and the musculosa (ma). Oesophagus, cat, HE.

composition of the glands, three gastric regions can be distinguished. The **cardia** (Fig. 4.15.26.) is the stomach's connection with the oesophagus. The corpus with the **fundus** (Fig. 4.15.27.) is the stomach proper. The **pylorus** (Fig. 4.15.31.) opens into the duodenum. The mucosa is thrown into folds, which are irregular, branched, and run in various directions, the rugae (Fig. 4.15.27.).

The stomach's surface epithelium is made up of **superficial mucous cells** (Fig. 4.15.28.). They have the cytological structure of mucus-secreting gland cells, but their apical part, which bulges somewhat in the stomach lumen, is different from that of goblet cells. It does not contain a single mucus bubble, but looks spongy because of the presence of numerous mucus-containing vesicles. Many of these vesicles are electron opaque and their shape varies from spherical to discoid.

In numerous places, the stomach's superficial epithelium folds in, forming funnel-shaped infundibula or gastric pits (Fig. 4.15.28.). At the bottom of these open several sessile (III.5.1.) tubular **mucosal glands** (Fig. 4.15.27.), which touch the muscularis mucosae, occupying the entire thickness of the mucosa. There are about five glands per infundibulum. In the corpus and fundus, these glands are relatively long, up to 1 or 2 millimeters, unbranched, and straight. Their length

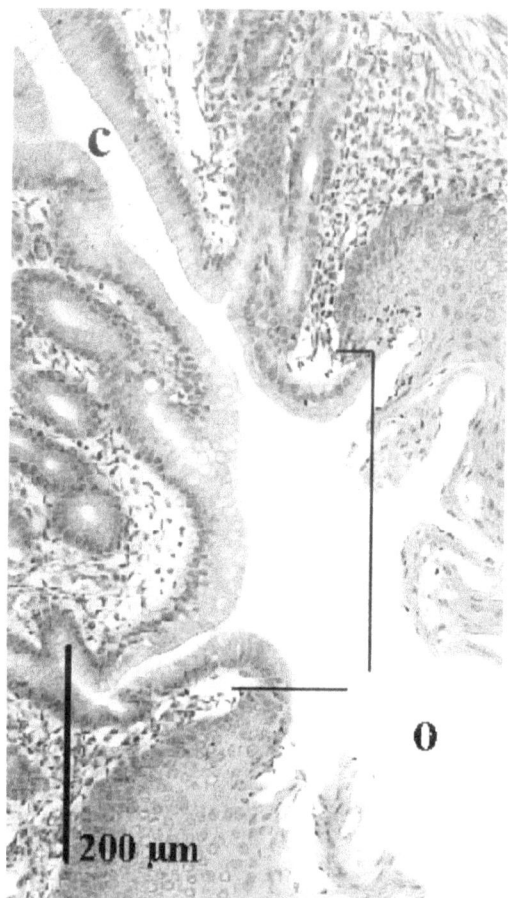

200 µm

Fig. 4.15.26. At the junction of oesophagus (o) and the stomach's cardia (c), there is an abrupt transition (lines) from Malpighian epithelium to simple prismatic epithelium, respectively. Oesophago-cardiac junction, cat, HE.

is at least three to four times that of the infundibula. They are so crowded that little fibrous tissue of the corium is visible (Fig. 4.15.29.). In the cardia, and especially so in the pylorus, mucosal glands are shorter, tend to branch, and are somewhat convoluted. The cardiac glands are at least twice as long, the pyloric glands at most twice as long, as the infundibula.

While the infundibula are lined with the same mucous cells as those of the surface epithelium, other cell types are found lining the glands. Just beneath the infundibula are found a second type of mucous cells: **mucous neck cells**. The cardiac and pyloric glands are almost exclusively made up of such cells. Contrary to goblet cells, and like superficial mucous cells, mucous neck cells have a spongy apical cytoplasm due to the accumulation of mucous vesicles. These vesicles are spherical and have and electron lucent interior. At the basis of the infundibula lie undifferentiated cells that multiply mitotically and differentiate into functional cells, most often superficial mucous cells. In this way, lost cells can be continuously replaced. In the fundic glands, other cells are found in addition to mucous neck cells. At the ends of the tubules, numerous

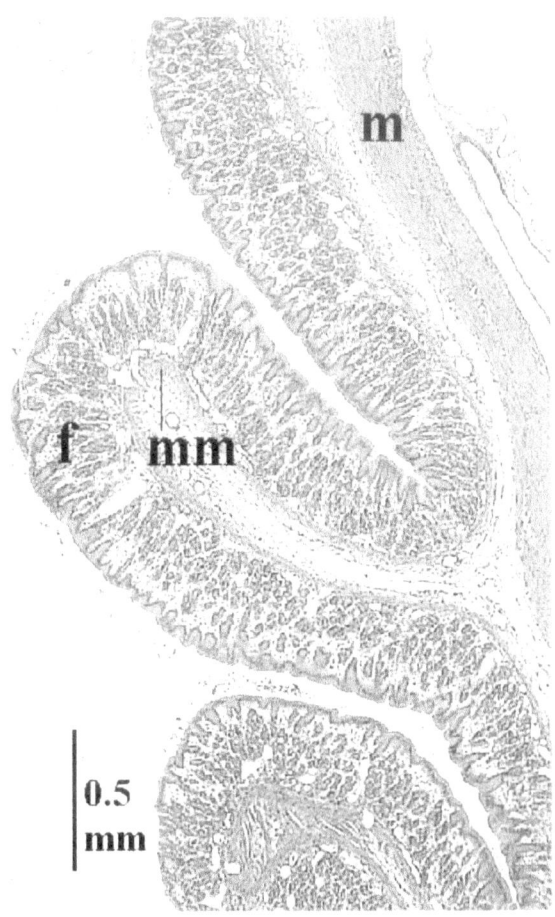

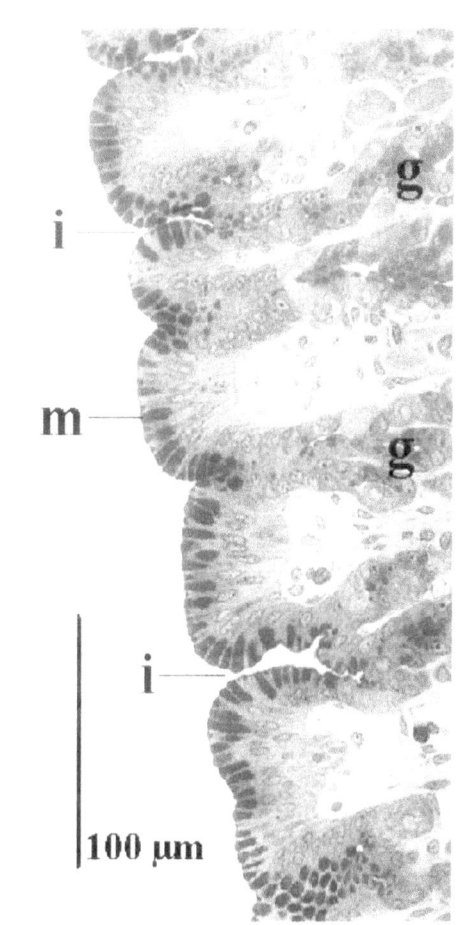

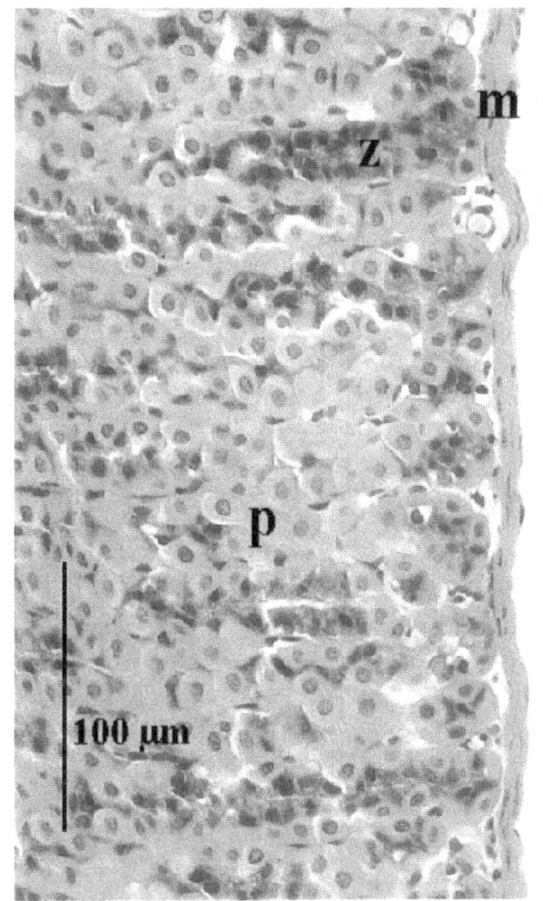

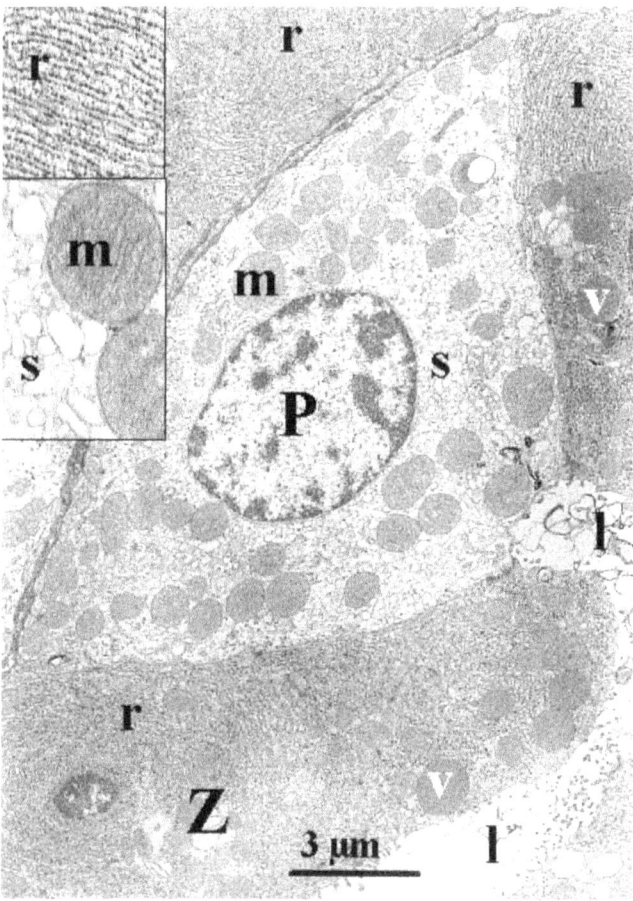

Fig. 4.15.27. (top left) The folded mucosa of the stomach's fundus is largely occupied by sessile, tubular, fundic glands (f). Also seen are the muscularis mucosae (mm) and the musculosa (m). Fundic stomach, cat, HE. **Fig. 4.15.28.** (bottom left) The fundic epithelium is composed of mucous cells (m). It folds in to form infundibula (i), at the bottom of which originate a number of fundic glands (g). Fundic stomach, cat, 1-micrometer plastic section, toluidin blue. **Fig. 4.15.29.** (top right) Fundic glands are unbranched, straight tubular glands that extend to the muscularis mucosae (m). The lamina propria fibrous tissue is almost completely crowded out. The glands contain 2 distinct types of gland cells: zymogen cells and parietal cells. Zymogen cells (z) are relatively small, conical, basophilic cells. Parietal cells (p) are large, globular cells with abundant eosinophilic cytoplasm. Fundic stomach, hamster, HE. **Fig. 4.15.30.** (bottom right) Zymogen cells (Z) are typical enzyme-secreting exocrine gland cells, with a strongly developed perinuclear rough endoplasmic reticulum (r) and apical secretory vesicles (v). Parietal cells (P) are not gland cells in the strict sense, but show the characteristics of ion transporting cells: a strongly developed perinuclear smooth endoplasmic reticulum (s) and numerous mitochondria (m). l = fundic gland lumen. Fundic stomach, rabbit, TEM.

zymogen cells are found. These are basophilic cells (Fig. 4.15.29.) with the typical cytological structure of enzyme-secreting gland cells (II.2.1.1.1., Fig. 4.15.30.). Their secretory vesicles are spherical, with a moderately opaque content, and have a diameter of about 1 micrometer. The more proximal stretches of the fundic glands are lined with **parietal cells**, which are very conspicuous, in the light microscope, because of their size and their eosinophilic cytoplasm (Fig. 4.15.29.). They are somewhat unusual cells with a central nucleus, numerous mitochondria, and a strongly developed smooth endoplasmic reticulum (Fig. 4.15.30.). Here and there, the cell membrane folds in, forming deep intracellular canals or canaliculi. The free cell membrane, as well as the one lining the canaliculi, carries numerous microvilli. Thus, these cells have some characteristics of brush border cells.

Distributed over the entire gastric epithelium, but distinctly concentrated in the pylorus, various types of **endocrine cells** are found, as they are elsewhere in the gut (Fig. 4.15.40.). These cells occur most often in the terminal stretches of the mucosal glands and have the cytological structure of polarized, amine or peptide hormone-secreting cells (II.2.1.1.2.). In the antral and pyloric mucosae, most are of the open type. Elsewhere, the endocrine cells usually are of the closed type. Most endocrine cell types specialize in the production of a single hormone substance, which may be an amine or a peptide.

Thus, the gastric epithelium, including the superficial one, is entirely glandular. The superficial mucous cells secrete a thick layer of neutral mucus with a lubricating function, and which protects the gastric lining against autodigestion. The mucus secreted by the neck cells is acid. The pyloric mucus is alcalic and protects the duodenum against the gastric acid. The zymogen cells secrete pepsinogen, the precursor of the digestive enzyme pepsin. The parietal cells pump chloride ions into the gastric lumen, which give rise to chloric acid. Chloric acid contributes to the transformation of pepsinogen to pepsin, allowing digestion of proteins. In addition to chloride, the parietal cells secrete intrinsic factor, a glycoprotein essential to the uptake of vitamin B12. The endocrine cells, especially so the open ones of the pyloric mucosa, are sensitive to chemical stimuli from the gastric lumen or the oesophagus, and their hormones act on the intestine itself or the glands associated with it. Amine hormones produced by these cells include serotonin, which influences gastric motility, and histamine, which stimulates the parietal cells. Peptide hormones secreted by these cells include gastrin and somatostatin. Gastrin stimulates the parietal cells and the smooth muscle fibers of the musculosa. It also stimulates Langerhans's islets in the pancreas to produce their own hormone, insulin. Somatostatin inhibits secretion of insulin, glucagons, gastrin, and somatotroph hormone.

The **small intestine** is lined with a **simple prismatic epithelium**, which is largely absorptive, but which also forms glands. The mucosa is thrown into transverse folds: Kerkring's plicae. In addition, the mucosa forms a large number of finger-like processes, the intestinal **villi**. These are most prominent in the middle part of the small intestine, the jejunum (Fig. 4.15.32.), where they may be up to a millimeter long. A square millimeter of mucosa numbers several tens of villi. At the basis of the villi, multiplication of undifferentiated cells, followed by differentiation, takes place. At their top, worn out cells are shed.

The villi are lined with absorptive epithelium, largely consisting of **enterocytes** (Figs. 2.40., 4.15.33.). The enterocytes digest polymeric substances, which they bind to their membrane, and absorb the simple molecules that are the digestive end products. Later they will pass these to the near capillaries. Enterocytes are absorbing brush border cells (II.2.2.2.1.), but when they are occupied with the absorption of lipids, they develop an extensive smooth endoplasmic reticulum.

When lipids, or triglycerides, are digested in the intestinal lumen, they give rise to monoglycerides and fatty acids, which diffuse through the enterocyte's cell membrane and into the smooth endoplasmic

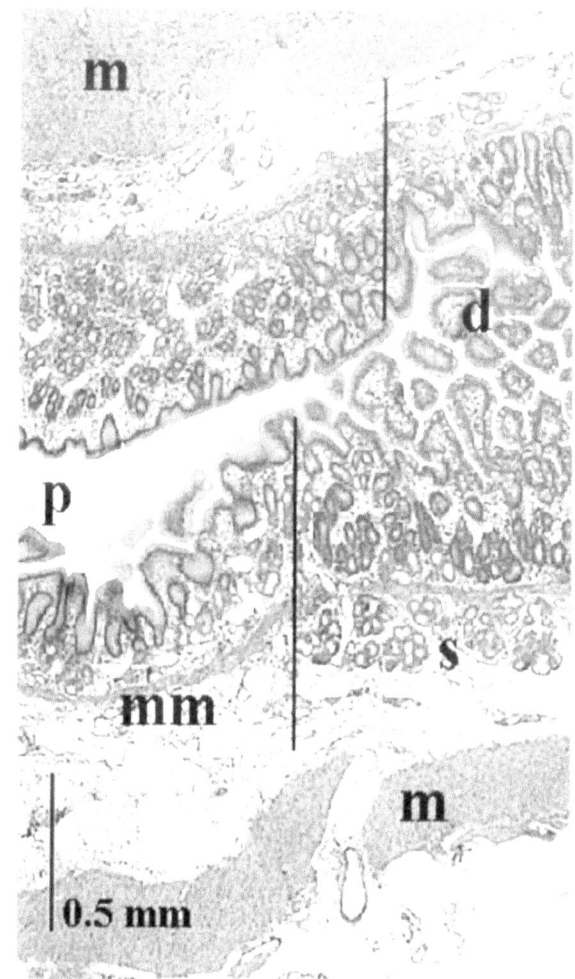

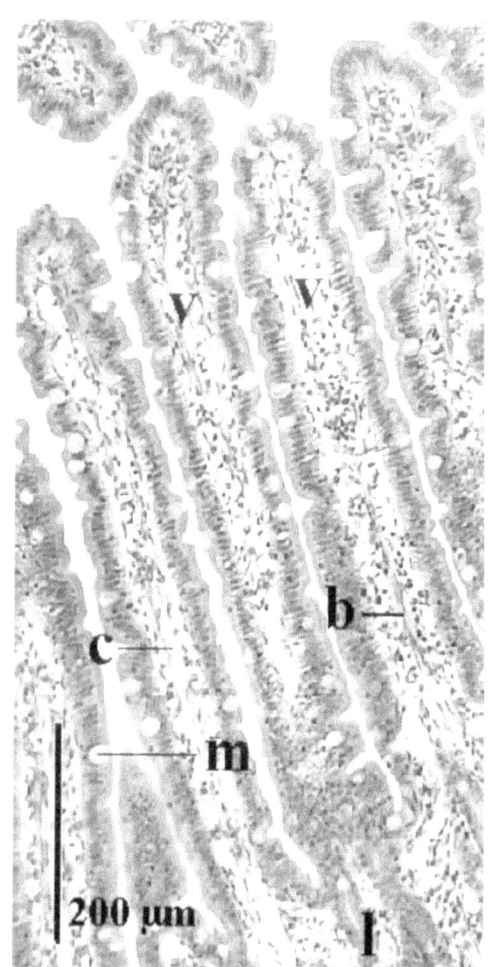

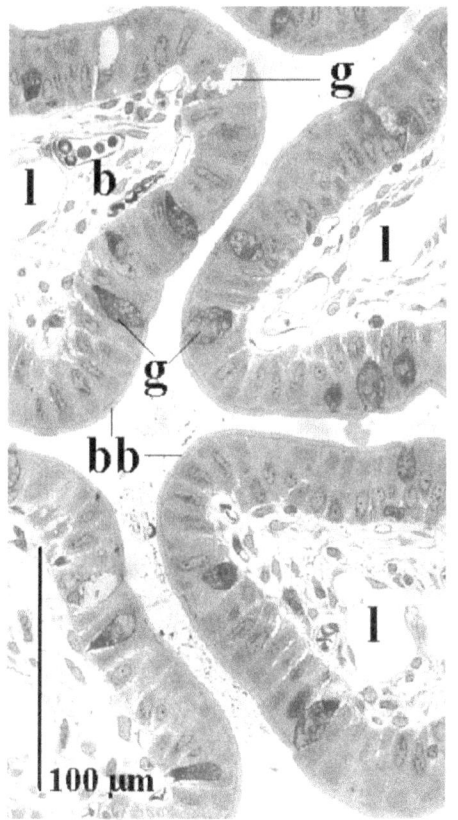

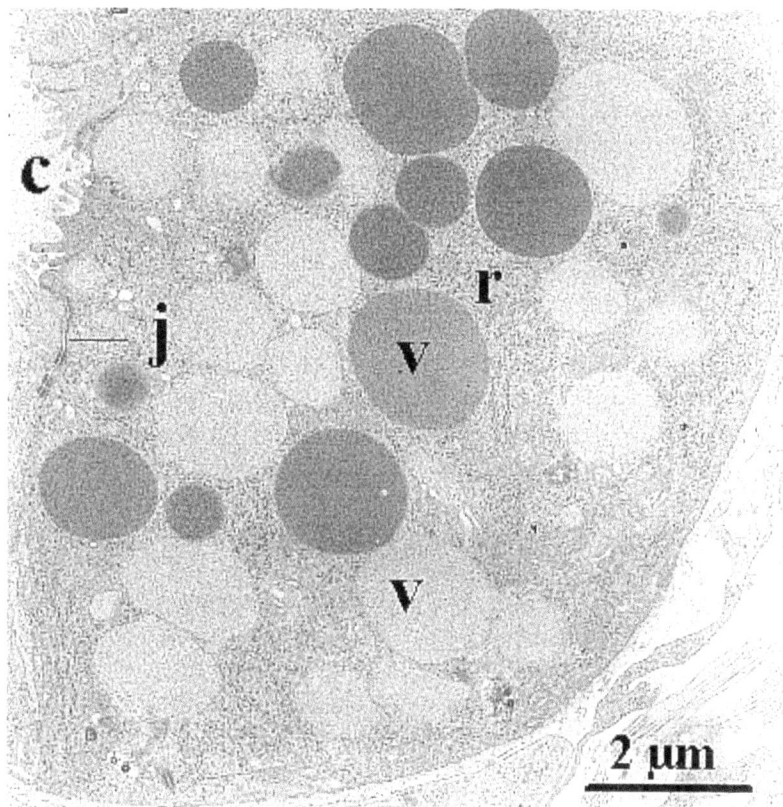

reticulum's interior. Here, they are reassembled into new triglycerides. These show up as electron opaque masses with variable dimensions in the interior of the reticulum's cisterns. Eventually, the reticulum gives rise to vesicles carrying lipid droplets with more or less standard sizes: chylomicrons. The droplets exit the cell by means of exocytosis at the basolateral cell membrane, entering the body proper.

In addition to enterocytes, the intestinal epithelium contains **goblet cells** (Fig. 4.15.32.). Their mucus lubrifies the intestinal wall and protects it against degradation by digestive enzymes.

Blood and lymph capillaries are very conspicuous in the intestinal villi. Many blood capillaries are fenestrated, and are places of uptake of the end products of digestion. The core of each villus contains one or more blind, relatively wide lymph capillaries, the **lacteals** (Fig. 4.15.33.). Lacteals are especially important in the uptake of lipids.

At the basis of the villi, the epithelium forms short, sessile glands: **Lieberkühn's crypts** (Fig. 4.15.32.). These contain cells with the cytological structure of enzyme-secreting gland cells: **Paneth's cells** (Fig. 4.15.34.). These secrete, among others, the bactericide enzyme lysozyme.

In the **duodenum**, the crypts lengthen into submucosal glands, **Brünner's glands** (Fig. 4.15.35.). These are sessile, branched tubular glands. Their prismatic gland cells show characteristics of both enzyme-secreting and mucus-secreting cells. The secretory vesicles are relatively small and have a fairly opaque content. Brünner's glands secrete mucus that, contrary to that produced by the goblet cells, is alcalic, helping to neutralize the gastric acid.

As in other gut segments (Fig. 4.15.40.), the small intestine's epithelium contains **endocrine cells** with the cytological structure of polarized, amine or peptide hormone-secreting cells (II.2.1.1.2.). The best known of these are **Kultschitzky's cells**, which are found in Lieberkühn's crypts. In the caudal duodenum and the cranial jejunum, the tips of the villi may carry endocrine cell clusters: Segi's caps. Depending on their type, the intestinal endocrine cells secrete, among others, secretin, cholecystokinin and serotonin. The first two are peptide hormones that promote the secretion of digestive enzymes by the exocrine pancreas. In addition, cholecystokinin stimulates contraction of the gall bladder, promoting the expulsion of bile into the duodenal lumen.

The lamina propria of the small intestine is very cellular because of the presence of large numbers of histiocytes, eosinophilic granulocytes, lymphocytes, plasma cells, and mast cells. Histiocytes and granulocytes phagocytose foreign material. The plasma cells secrete immunoglobin A, combined with a carbohydrate to make it resistant to digestive degradation, and which is liberated in the intestinal lumen. This allows elimination of pathogens even before they have entered the body proper. Immunoglobulin G and M are secreted in the mucosa. Many lymphocytes are T-lymphocytes, which can lodge themselves in the epithelium. Mast cells attract other immune cells, helping them to reach the intestinal mucosa.

The **large intestine** or colon (Fig. 4.15.36.), as well as the caecum and the appendix, are lined with a simple prismatic epithelium, consisting largely of **goblet cells**. No absorptive cells are found: the large intestine no longer contains digestible substances. Water is being absorbed, however, gradually solidifying the intestine's content. The secretions of the goblet cells lubrify the intestinal wall.

The **rectum** is initially lined with a typical colon epithelium. Its caudal stretch, the anal canal, is lined with Malpighian epithelium. The transition of one to the other is brusque, and forms the margo ani. The mucosa is thrown in longitudinal folds, which may flatten out during the passage of feces.

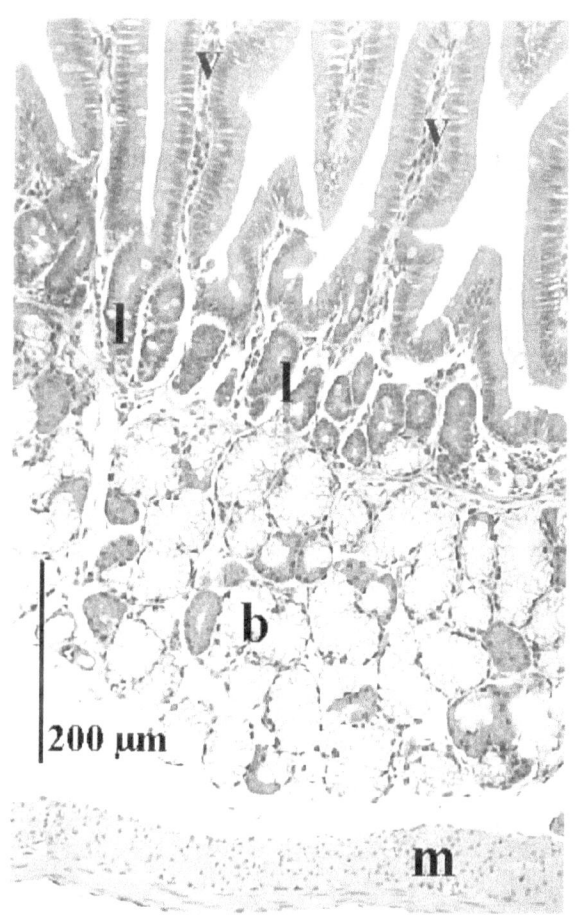

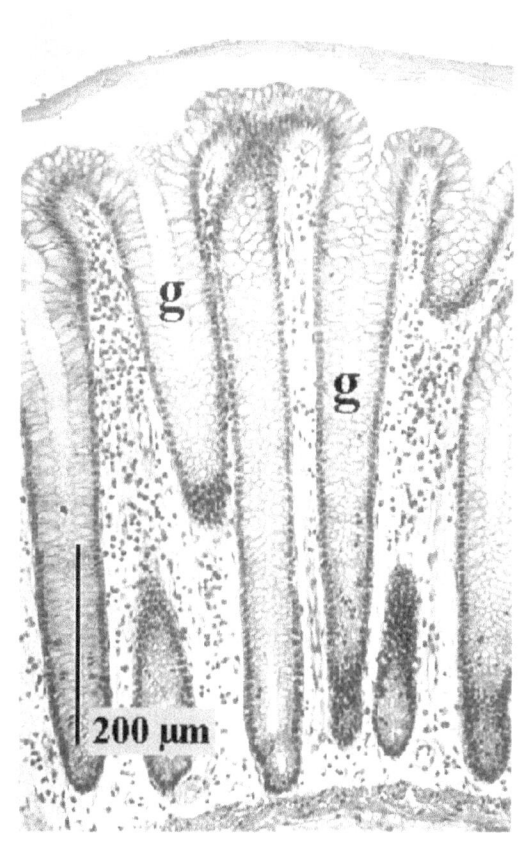

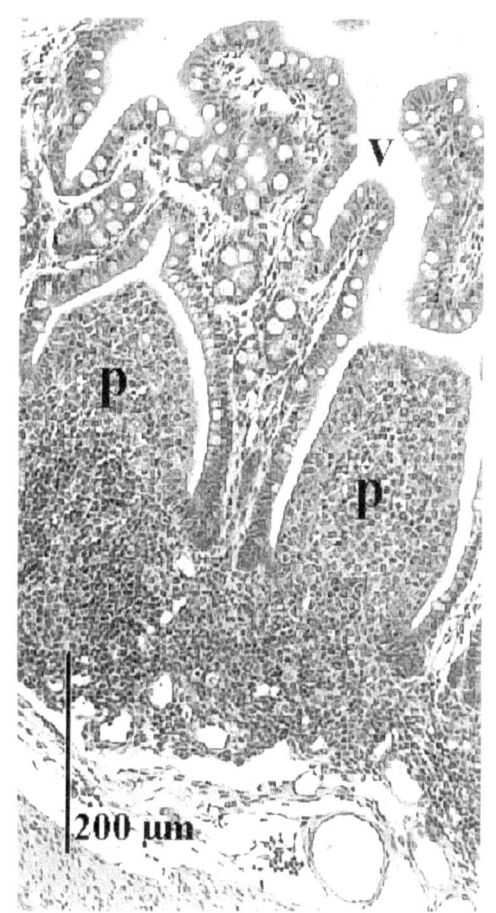

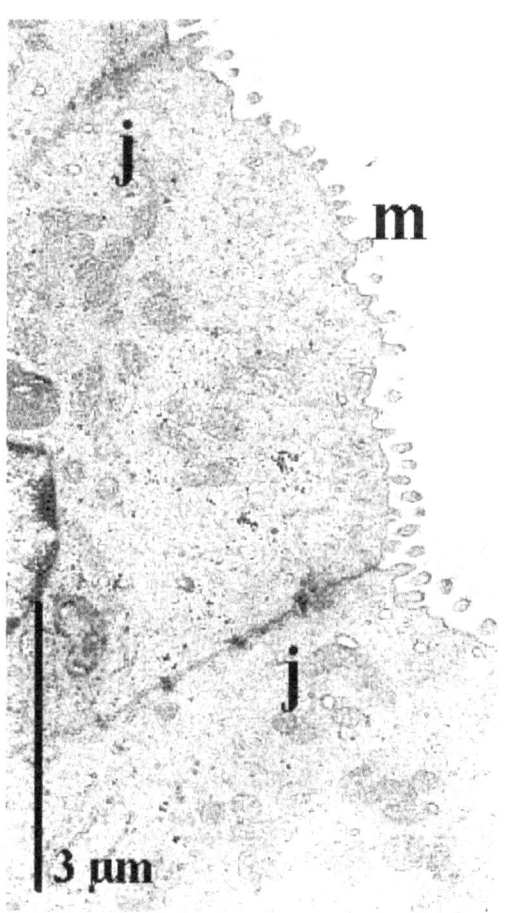

IV.15.2.2. Lymphoid tissue.

In addition to solitary immune cells, which can be regarded as diffuse lymphoid tissue, the intestinal mucosa locally contains organized lymphoid tissue. The mucosal structure is strongly disrupted by the accumulation of lymphoid tissue, and it may penetrate into the submucosa, disrupting the muscularis mucosae. Together, diffuse and compact lymphoid tissue form mucosa-associated lymphoid tissue (MALT).

One of the largest concentrations of lymphoid tissue is found in the caudal segment of the small intestine, the ileum, where it forms **Peyer's patches** (Fig. 4.15.37.). Peyer's patches are mounds, a few centimeters long, wherein lymph follicles develop. They bulge into the gut lumen and the overlying mucosa forms few and badly developed villi. The muscularis mucosa usually remains intact, limiting Peyer's patches to the mucosa. The germinal centers of these follicles contain numerous proliferating B-lymphocytes. Between the follicles are found concentrations of T-lymphocytes and high endothelial venules.

The overlying epithelium is specialized in the capture of antigens. It contains cells that lack a brush border, sharply contrasting them with neighbouring enterocytes: M-cells (Fig. 4.15.38.). The apical cell membrane carries short microvilli and microfolds (hence M-cells). It folds in, giving rise to endosomes, by means of which antigens from the gut lumen are internalized. The antigenic material is secreted at the basal cell pole, where it is taken up by macrophages, which will present it to lymphocytes, local ones or residents of lymph nodes. The basal cell pole of the M-cells may be thrown into complex folds to accommodate macrophages and lymphocytes.

Another distinct concentration of lymphoid tissue, with a follicular organization, is to be found in the **appendix** (Fig. 4.15.39.). M-cells cover the domes formed by this tissue. In contrast to Peyer's patches, it often penetrates into the submucosa.

IV.15.2.3. Muscle tissue.

The **muscularis mucosae** is a thin layer of visceral muscle tissue, separating the mucosa from the deeper submucosa. Its fibers have a circular course. **Brücke's muscles** are thin strands of muscle tissue which branch at right angles from the muscularis mucosae and extend into the cores of the villi (Fig. 4.15.32.). Contraction of these muscle fibers confers motility to the intestinal villi, promoting their contact with the intestinal content, and helps to expulse local secretory products and their mixing with the intestinal content. All this theoretically contributes to the efficiency of the digestive process.

In the cranial third of the oesophagus, the **musculosa** consists of skeletal muscle tissue. It is under voluntary control and contributes to swallowing. In caudal two thirds of the oesophagus, skeletal muscle tissue is progressively replaced with visceral muscle tissue, which continues in the rest of the intestine. Only in the rectum is the musculosa again made of skeletal muscle tissue.

The musculosa is double. In the inner layer, the muscle fibers run in a tight spiral. In the outer layer, their arrangement varies between a loose spiral and a longitudinal course. In the stomach, a third layer is added to the musculosa: it is an oblique layer at the inside of the inner circular layer. In the colon, the outer longitudinal layer is incomplete, consisting of three longitudinal ribbons, the **taenia coli**.

The musculosa contracts spontaneously at an inherent rhythm, which is modulated by the nervous system. Successive contractions run in a caudal direction, generating contraction waves. This mechanism of peristaltic contraction propels the intestine's content, like tooth paste in a tube. In the stomach, peristaltic contractions ensure mixing of its content.

At the junction of two intestinal segments, the inner layer of the musculosa may be thickened, forming a **sphincter** (Fig. 4.15.31.). The most important sphincter is the one separating the stomach from the

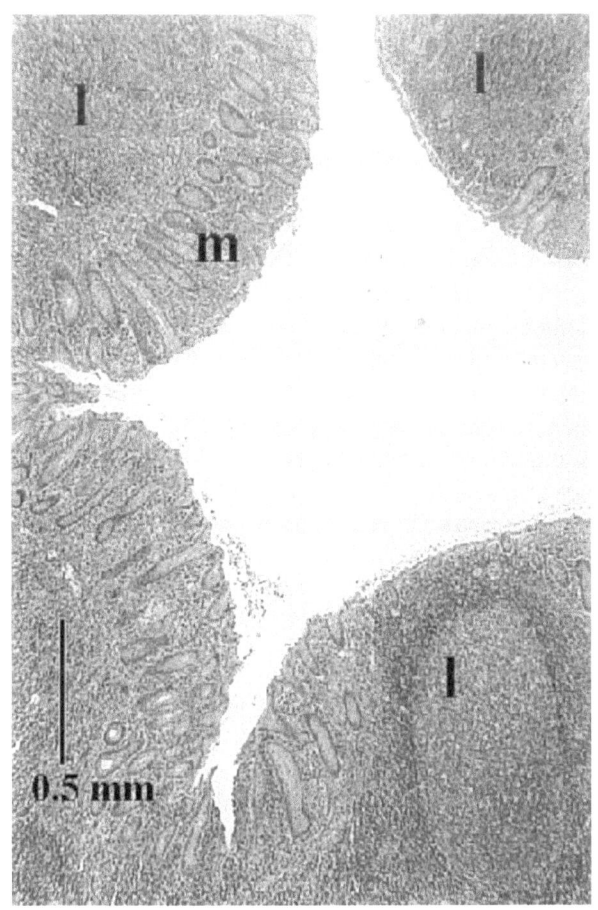

0.5 mm

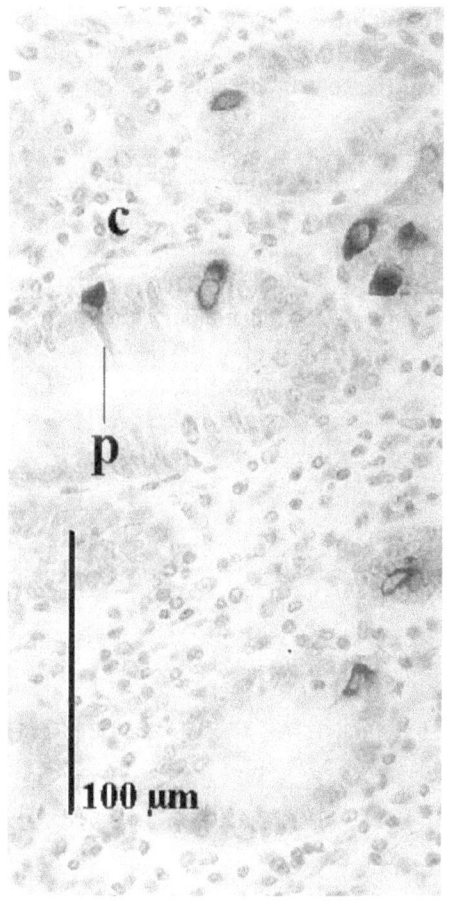

100 µm

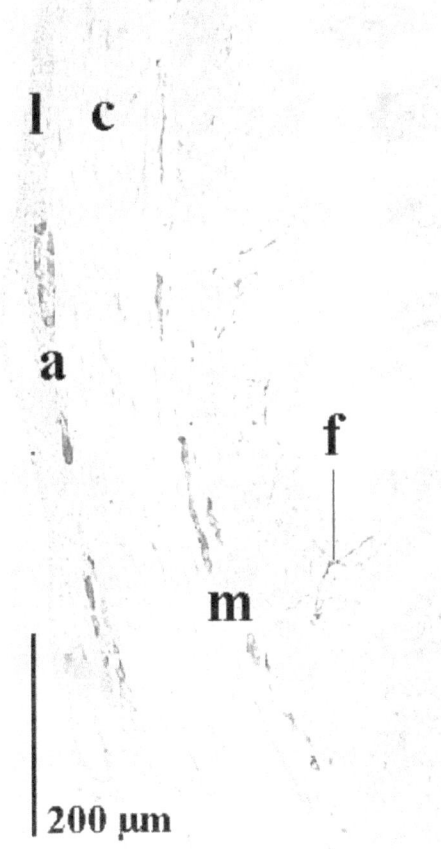

200 µm

Fig. 4.15.39. (top left) The appendix is characterized by massive accumulations of lymphoid tissue (l) in the mucosa and the submucosa. Locally, this may strongly disrupt the structure of the mucosa (m), which is otherwise identical to that of the colon. Appendix, human, HE. **Fig. 4.15.40.** (top right) The gut epithelium, such as here, in the appendix, contains endocrine gland cells. The wide basal cell part contains the unstained nucleus. The apical part thins into a slender process (p), which penetrates between the other cells and may reach (in open cells) the gut lumen. Hormones are secreted in the underlying corium (c). Appendix, human, immune reaction to chromogranin A, visualized with peroxidase. **Fig. 4.15.41.** (left) Sandwiched between the inner circular (c) and the outer longitudinal (l) muscle layers of the musculosa is a neural plexus containing relatively large ganglia: Auerbach's plexus (a). In the submucosa lie the smaller ganglia of Meissner's plexus (m). In the cores of the villi, bundles of nerve fibers are seen (f). Jejunum, cat, immune reaction to neuron-specific enolase, visualized with peroxidase.

295

duodenum, the gastro-duodenal sphincter. At the junction of the ileum and the colon, the ileo-caecal sphincter is found. The anal sphincter in the rectum contains a measure of skeletal muscle tissue. In addition to these, a pharyngo-oesophagal and an oesophageo-gastric sphincter are present. These sphincters, by closing or relaxation, control the cranio-caudal passage of the intestine's content. As long as they are closed, the content is withheld in the cranial segment. When its treatment is finished, the sphincter relaxes and the intestinal content moves into the next segment.

The intestinal visceral muscle tissue differs in one detail from visceral muscle tissue elsewhere: it contains a special type of cells: **interstitial cells of Cajal**. These cells are interposed between motor nerve endings and smooth muscle fibers. Cajal's cells are fusiform, with a central nucleus. They share a number of cytological characteristics with smooth muscle cells, such as longitudinal bundles of filaments, fusiform densities, and caveoli. The cytoplasm contains relatively abundant rough and smooth endoplasmic reticula, and mitochondria. Contrary to smooth muscle fibers, their basement membrane may be discontinuous. They are joined to smooth muscle fibers by means of gap junctions. They are contacted by the terminals of motor nerve fibers, although distinct synaptic junctions are not observed. It is assumed that Cajal's cells are pacemaker cells, analogous to cardiac Purkinje cells. They would generate spontaneous contraction stimuli, which would be transmitted through the gap junctions to the smooth muscle cells, thereby inducing peristaltic contractions in the musculosa, and be modulated by the nervous system.

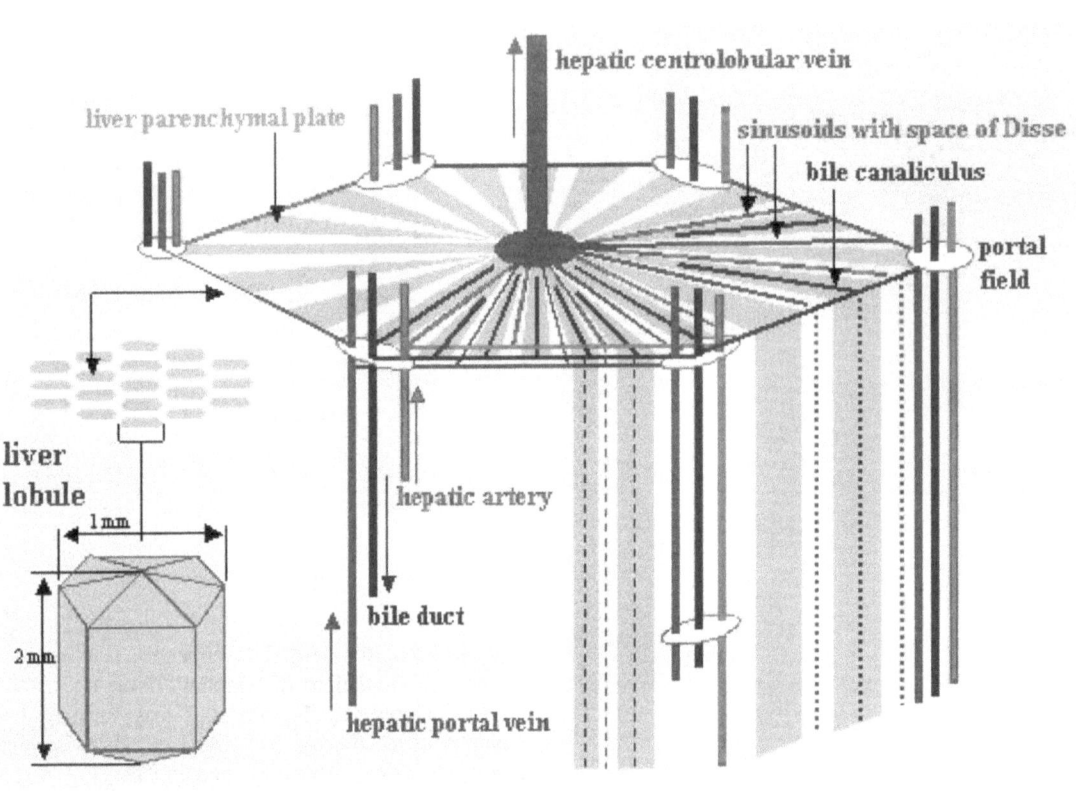

Fig. 4.15.42. The liver is a collection of hexagonal, closely joined lobules (left). A liver lobule is composed of radial plates of liver parenchyma. At the tips of these hexagons lie fibrous tissue portal fields. Each of these encloses a branch of the hepatic artery, which supplies the liver with oxygenated blood, a branch of the hepatic portal vein, which carries blood from the intestine, and a branch of the biliary duct system, via which bile is evacuated. The hepatic artery, as well as the portal vein, empty into sinusoids between the parenchymal plates. Beneath the sinusoidal endothelium is Disse's space. In the center of the lobule, the sinusoids merge into a centrolobular hepatic vein. The parenchymal plates are pervaded by a network of bile canaliculi, which conduct bile to the biliary ducts.

296

IV.15.2.4. Nerve tissue.

Nerve tissue pervades the intestine, but is concentrated in two plexi. **Meissner's plexus,** or the submucosal plexus, is located in the submucosa, **Auerbach's plexus**, also known as the myenteric plexus, between the two layers of the musculosa (Fig. 4.15.41.). The second one is more strongly developed than the first one. A third plexus, Schabadasch's, may be distinguished in the deeper layers of the submucosa.

Superficially, the intestinal nervous tissue resembles a collection of intramural, parasympathetic motor ganglia. It is, however, much more complex than this, to the extent that it deserves to be regarded as a subdivision of the peripheral nervous system in its own right, the enteric nervous system. To a considerable extent, it also functions independently from the rest of the nervous system. It regulates peristalsis, as well as secretion and absorption processes.

The neural plexi of the enteric nervous system consist

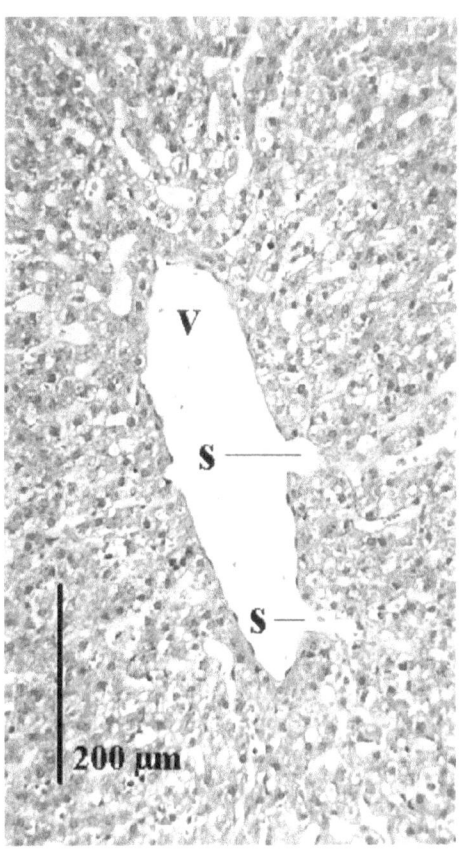 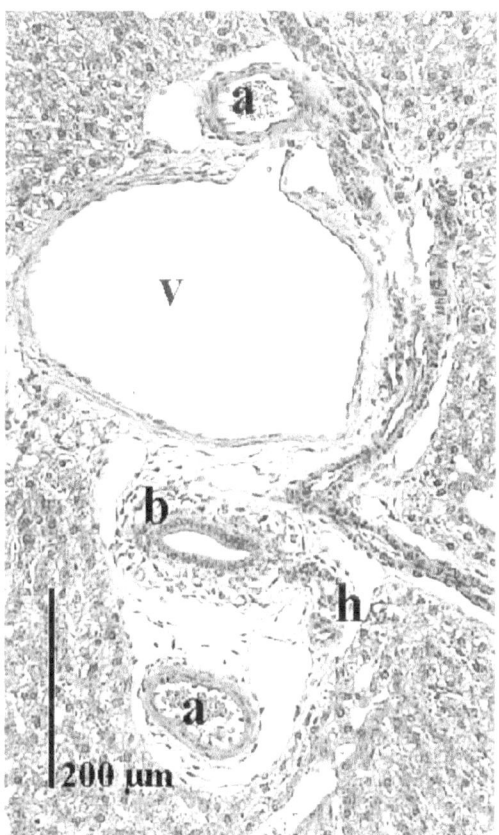

Fig. 4.15.43. (left) The wall of the centrolobular vein (v), surrounded by liver lobe parenchyma, is extremely thin and interrupted by sinusoids (s) that open into it. Liver, rabbit, HE. **Fig. 4.15.44.** (right) This portal field, surrounded by liver parenchyma, shows 2 sections of relatively thick walled blood vessels: liver arteries (a). The thin walled vessel is the portal vein (p). Another lumen is seen, lined with simple cuboidal epithelium: the biliary duct (b). A few narrower branches of the biliary tract, Hering's canals (h) emerge from the liver parenchyma. Liver, rabbit, HE.

of a dense network of nerve fibers and perikarya, and their associated glia cells. The nerve cells or ganglion cells are, in principle, multipolar motor nerve cells. There is a type of enteric nerve cell, however, which only has long unbranched processes with the ultrastructure of axons, similar to those of pseudounipolar nerve cells. This type is probably also a sensory nerve cell. In sharp contrast to motor ganglia elsewhere, the nerve cells are heterogeneous concerning the size and cytological structure of their

perikarya. They also differ in the structure of their dendritic trees. At least two categories of motor nerve cells can be distinguished: those with short, relatively simple dendrites and those with long, intensively branched dendrites. The nerve fibers are preganglionic (extrinsic) and postganglionic (intrinsic) motor nerve fibers, and sensory nerve fibers. The structure of the synaptic junctions, with their associated synaptic vesicles and membrane thickenings, is extremely variable. The glia cells have heterochromatic nuclei

297

and their cytoplasm is rich in intermediate filaments. They are analogous to Schwann's cells and satellite cells encountered elsewhere.

IV.15.3. Liver.

During embryonic development, the liver originates as an inpocketing of the primitive gut epithelium. In principle, the liver is an exocrine gland, but its functions are more complicated than this.

The liver is divided into four incompletely separated lobes, lined with a serosa. The liver lobes are composed of polyhedral **lobules** (Fig. 4.15.42.), about a million of them, which have a hexagonal cross section, and are separated from each other by thin to hardly present fibrous tissue septa. The lobules have a diameter of about 1 millimeter, and a length of a few millimeters. Their longitudinal axis is occupied by a branch of the liver vein, called a **centrolobular vein** (Figs. 4.15.42.-43.). Where the corners of three adjacent lobules touch, the septa widen into a **portal field** (Figs. 4.15.42., 4.15.44.). This area derives its name from the presence of a venule, a branch of the hepatic **portal vein**. The portal vein of the liver connects the capillary beds of the intestine, the pancreas and the spleen with those of the liver and supplies the liver directly (bypassing the heart) with products of digestion. The liver is supplied with oxygenated blood through the **hepatic artery**, branches of which also course in the portal fields. In addition to blood vessels, the portal fields also show sections of the liver's excretory duct system, the **bile ducts**. Both portal veins and hepatic arteries form a coalescing network of **sinusoids**, which pervade the liver lobules. Sinusoids differ from sinuses by the presence of phagocytosing cells in their endothelium. The sinusoids have a radial course and converge towards the centrolobular vein. Between the sinusoids lie the liver parenchyma cells or **hepatocytes**. They are arranged into sheets, one cell thick, which converge radially towards the lobular center. The cell sheets are branched and converge with neighbouring sheets. The length of a sheet, extending from the rim of the lobulus to the centrolobular vein, is about twenty cells. Between the cell sheets and the sinusoid endothelium is an extracellular space, **Disse's space**.

The portal bile ducts eventually converge towards a hepatic duct, which carries a branch, the cystic duct. Through the cystic duct, the gall bladder empties into the hepatic duct. Downstream from the cystic duct, the hepatic duct merges with the pancreatic duct, forming Vater's ampulla, which opens into the duodenum right beneath the stomach.

IV.15.3.1. Liver parenchyma.

Hepatocytes are relatively large, polyhedral cells with a central, spherical nucleus, which is rather euchromatic and contains a large nucleolus. The size of the nuclei varies, because many hepatocytes are tetraploid or even polyploid, which may also result in multinuclearity.

In principle, hepatocytes have two opposite vascular poles, which face Disse's space and a sinusoid. Here, the free cell membrane forms microvilli (Fig. 4.15.45.). The other cell membranes are joined, predominantly through tight junctions, to those of adjacent hepatocytes. At the center of the cell membranes facing each other, narrow intercellular **biliary canals**, with a minimal diameter of about 1 micrometer, can be made out (Figs. 4.15.45.-46.). Biliary canals arise by local, symmetric infolding of the membranes of two adjacent hepatocytes. On both sides of the canals, the extracellular space is sealed with tight junctions. Into these canals, the hepatocytes secrete bile. The hepatocyte poles facing adjacent hepatocytes are the biliary poles. The membranes making up the canals also carry microvilli. The pericanalicular cytoplasm contains microfilaments. Theoretically, therefore, it is possible that the canal's content is propelled actively. Eventually, the biliary canals will open into the portal bile ducts.

Besides the presence of microvilli and microfilaments, hepatocytes show characteristics of membrane-bearing cells (Fig. 4.15.46.): rough endoplasmic reticulum, lysosomes, and smooth endoplasmic reticulum. The cisterns of the rough endoplasmic reticulum form aggregates throughout the cell. Several Golgi-complexes are found, preferentially at the biliary pole. Lysosomes also have a preference for the biliary pole. The smooth endoplasmic reticulum is widespread and strongly developed. Between its cisterns lie large accumulations of glycogen granules. In addition to fibers and membranes, numerous primary organelles are present: mitochondria, ribosomes, and peroxisomes. Thus, hepatocytes are one of the most generalized cell types of the body, which indicates that they have many and varied functions.

Hepatocytes synthesize, secrete, excrete, and degrade a large number of substances.

Bile (or gall) is a complex mixture of substances, some secretory (synthesized by the hepatocytes), some excretory (taken up as such and subsequently liberated by the hepatocytes). Bile contains **bile salts**. These

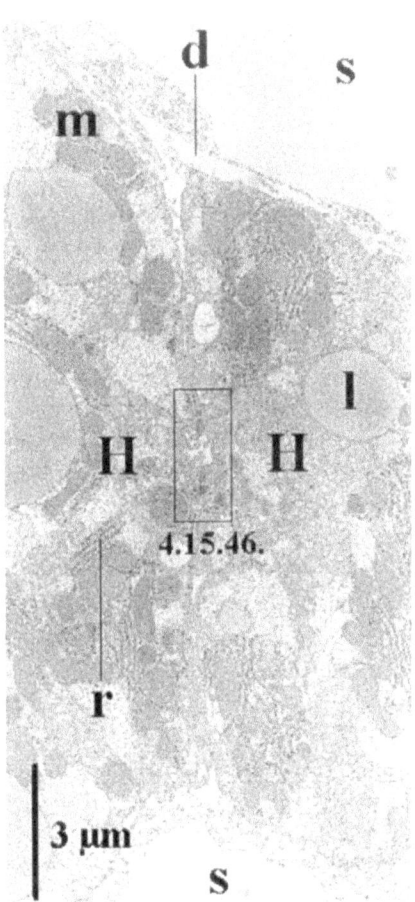

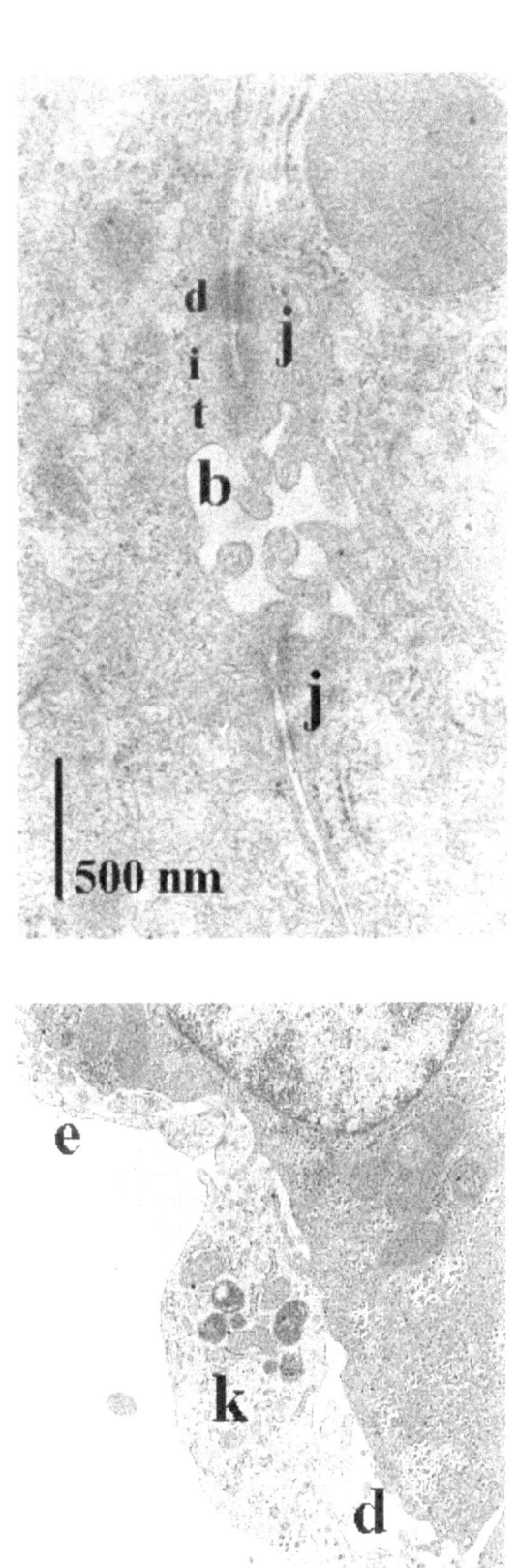

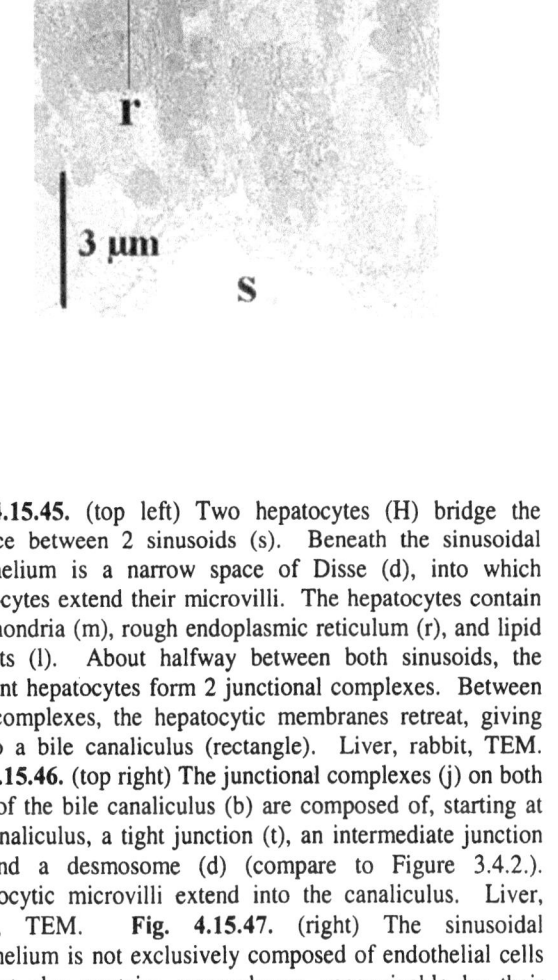

Fig. 4.15.45. (top left) Two hepatocytes (H) bridge the distance between 2 sinusoids (s). Beneath the sinusoidal endothelium is a narrow space of Disse (d), into which hepatocytes extend their microvilli. The hepatocytes contain mitochondria (m), rough endoplasmic reticulum (r), and lipid droplets (l). About halfway between both sinusoids, the adjacent hepatocytes form 2 junctional complexes. Between both complexes, the hepatocytic membranes retreat, giving rise to a bile canaliculus (rectangle). Liver, rabbit, TEM.
Fig. 4.15.46. (top right) The junctional complexes (j) on both sides of the bile canaliculus (b) are composed of, starting at the canaliculus, a tight junction (t), an intermediate junction (i), and a desmosome (d) (compare to Figure 3.4.2.). Hepatocytic microvilli extend into the canaliculus. Liver, rabbit, TEM. **Fig. 4.15.47.** (right) The sinusoidal endothelium is not exclusively composed of endothelial cells (e), but also contains macrophages, recognizable by their content of phagosomes and secondary lysosomes: Kupffer cells (k). Beneath the endothelium, in Disse's space (d) lie hepatocytic microvilli. Liver, rabbit, TEM.

are secretory products that emulsify lipids in the intestinal lumen, facilitating their uptake by enterocytes. Bile salts are synthesized by the smooth endoplasmic reticulum. Cholic acid, derived from cholesterol, is combined with the amino acids glycine or taurine (not found in proteins), forming glycocholic acid and taurocholic acid, respectively. These acids are secreted in ionic form and combine with sodium and potassium ions to form bile salts. The liver also recycles bile salts by reabsorbing them from the blood. Another bile component is bile pigment or **bilirubin**, a degradation product of hemoglobin. Senescent erythrocytes are degraded in various places of the body, including the spleen, the bone marrow, and the liver, and bilirubin eventually ends up in the hepatocytes. It is conjugated with glucuronic acid in the smooth endoplasmic reticulum, and secreted. The brown color of the stool is caused by this bile pigment. When the liver does not function properly, bilirubin may accumulate in the blood, causing jaundice.

Hepatocytes synthesize plasma proteins, such as albumin and fibrinogen, which they secrete into the blood.

Glycogen and lipids, such as cholesterol and triglycerids, are synthesized in the smooth endoplasmic reticulum. Glycogen is a polymerization product of glucose. In periods of enhanced energy requirements, it is degraded, liberating glucose and making it available to energy production. Fatty acids from the intestine are used to synthesize triglycerids, which are combined with cholesterol and proteins.

Hepatocytes have detoxifying abilities and degrade a large number of substances, such as amino acids, ethanol, and steroids. Amino acids are deaminated, producing urea, which is excreted by the kidneys. Most of the enzymes needed for this task reside in the smooth endoplasmic reticulum.

Disse's space is a wide extracellular space, loosely filled with reticulin (collagen type III) fibrils. Most of it may be occupied by hepatocyte microvilli.

Except for rare fibrocytes, Disse's space contains **hepatic stellate cells**. These have a cell body, which closely adheres to the abluminal sinusoidal endothelial surface, without forming junctions with it, and from where they extend processes, which encircle the sinusoids. Other processes contact hepatocytes. In addition to rough endoplasmic reticulum, the cell bodies contain multivesicular bodies and lipid droplets with diameters of 1 to 2 micrometers. Some of these "droplets" are vesicles, lined with a membrane. The lipid is predominantly vitamin A (esterified retinol), which is essential in vision and cellular differentiation, and of which the liver stores large amounts (It is an important component of cod-liver oil.). Apparently,

the enzymes that esterify retinol reside in the membrane of the multivesicular body, since it is in their interior that lipid accumulates. Sometimes, the vesicular membrane is lost, resulting in free lipid droplets. The processes contain bundles of microtubules and filaments. Stellate cells may function as pericytes, regulating sinusoidal blood flow by their contractile properties. They seem to synthesize, as well as to degrade, the matrix of the hepatic interstitial tissue. Finally, they secrete a number of mediators with profound influences on liver physiology.

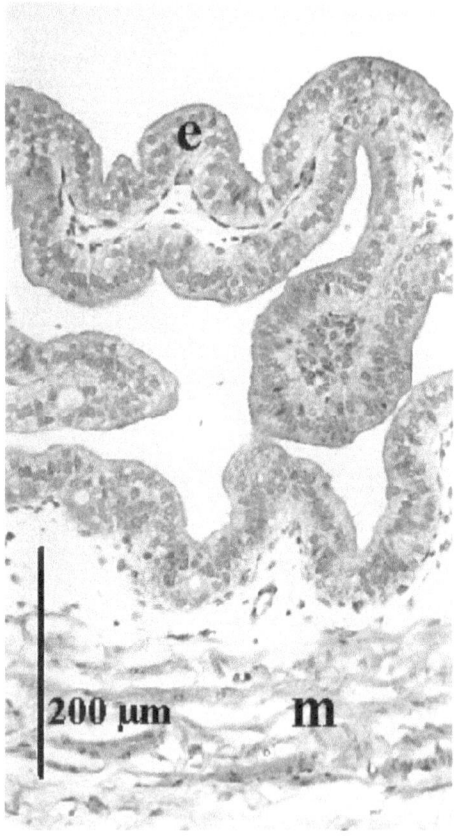

Fig. 4.15.48. The gall bladder mucosa is thrown into numerous, irregular folds, lined with a simple prismatic epithelium (e). m = musculosa. Gall bladder, rabbit, HE.

The endothelium separating Disse's space from the sinusoid lumen shows numerous fenestrations, many of which do not contain a diaphragm. In several places, there are openings between the endothelial cells and the basement membrane is frequently interrupted. All this explains why the sinusoid wall is highly permeable to blood plasma, carrying products of digestion. The sinus endothelial cells actively endocytose and contain numerous pinocytotic vesicles. Apart from the standard type of endothelial cells, the sinus wall

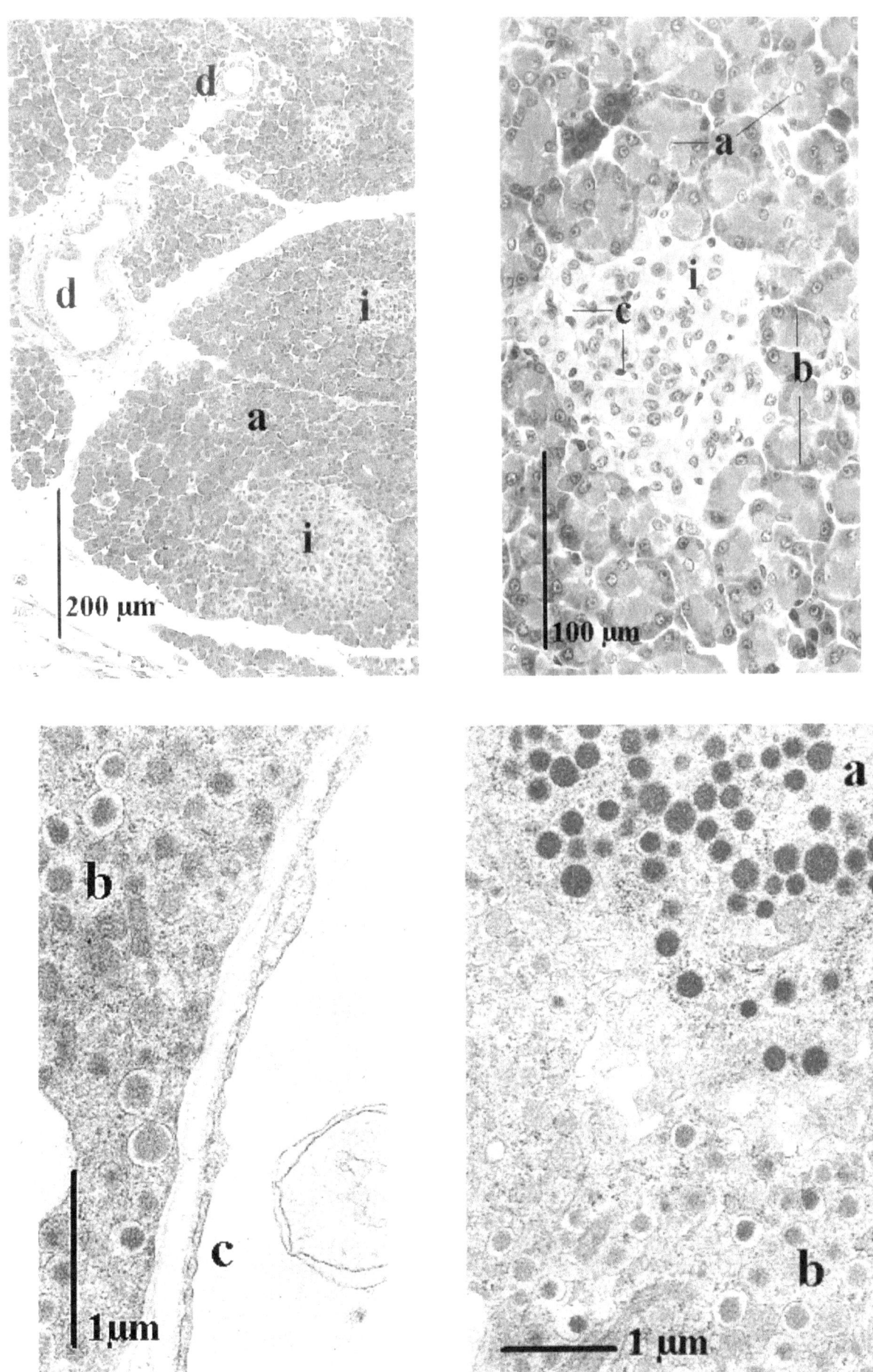

Fig. 4.15.49. (top left) The pancreas is made up of numerous lobules, separated from each other by fibrous tissue septa, which carry ducts (d). The ducts are lined with a simple, cuboidal to prismatic epithelium. The gland's lobules are collections of basophilic, serous acini (a). These constitute the exocrine pancreas, which produces digestive enzymes. Occasionally, groups of clearer cells are seen, Langerhans's islets (i). These represent the endocrine pancreas, which secretes hormones. The ducts naturally belong to the exocrine pancreas. Pancreas, human, HE. **Fig. 4.15.50.** (top right) The serous acini of the pancreas strongly resemble those of the salivary glands (compare Figures 4.15.15.-16.). Mark the basophilic stain (b), however, which is limited to the acinar rim, i.e. the basal part of the cells. Occasionally, a centroacinar cell shows (a). A Langerhans islet (i) is a massive (trabecular) group of cells, pervaded with capillaries (c). Pancreas, dog, HE. **Fig. 4.15.51.** (bottom left) The endocrine cells of Langerhans's islets, such as the B-cells (b) in this image, closely contact fenestrated, sinusoidal capillaries (c). Pancreas, rabbit, TEM. **Fig. 4.15.52.** (bottom right) The endocrine cells of Langerhans's islets are typical symmetrical peptide hormone-secreting cells. The 2 most common types are the A-cells (a), which secrete glucagon, and which contain very dense secretory vesicles, and the B-cells (b), which secrete insulin, and contain less dense vesicles. Pancreas, rabbit, TEM.

contains a specialized type: **Kupffer's cells** (Fig. 4.15.47.). These have the irregular shapes and cytological structure of macrophages (II.2.1.4.). It is evident that this endothelium contributes largely to the liver's degradative capacities.

IV.15.3.2. Bile ducts.

The biliary canals of the liver parenchyma open into the portal bile ducts through terminal ductules or Hering's canals. These have a diameter of about 10 micrometers and are lined with a simple epithelium, which is squamous at first and changes to cuboidal in the distal segments. The epithelial cells carry a few microvilli. They keep their structure when the terminal ductules open into the portal bile ducts, which have diameters of a few tens of micrometers. The largest portal ducts are enveloped with a thin layer of visceral muscle tissue. The extrahepatic bile ducts leave the liver lobes and merge into a single hepatic duct. They are lined with a simple prismatic epithelium, which forms a mucosa, a musculosa and, since they lie free in the abdominal cavity, a serosa.

The **gall bladder** (Fig. 4.15.48.) is lined with a simple prismatic epithelium. The apical membrane of the epithelial cells carries relatively short microvilli. They are absorbing brush border cells (II.2.2.2.1.), which absorb water from bile and thus concentrate it. The mucosa, which is lined by this epithelium, is thrown into complex folds. Some of these are temporary, caused by emptying of the gall bladder, others are permanent. Of these, rugae are formed when the mucosa bulges into the bladder lumen, while diverticula are infoldings of the epithelium into the lamina propria. Occasionally, mucous glands are present. Following the mucosa, a musculosa and a serosa are present. The connective tissue layers are rich in elastic fibers. The musculosa contracts under the influence of cholecystokinin, a hormone secreted by the duodenal endocrine cells, especially so after a lipid-rich meal.

The cystic duct has the same structure as the gall bladder. The mucosa forms a spiral fold, which may function as a kind of valve. Vater's ampulla, which also receives the pancreatic duct, functions as a sphincter and contains a well developed musculosa with longitudinal as well as circular layers of muscle tissue.

IV.15.4. Pancreas.

The pancreas is a large retroperitoneal gland, situated in the upper part of the abdominal cavity. Like the liver, it develops as an inpocketing of the primitive gut epithelium. It lacks a well-developed fibrous tissue capsule and looks like a diffuse mass. Anatomically, the gland has a cranial part, a corpus, and a caudal part. The cranial part lies close to the duodenum, the caudal part reaches the spleen. It is made up of both exocrine and endocrine glandular tissue.

The **exocrine pancreas** (Fig. 4.15.49.), as far as volume is concerned the most important of the two, is a compound acinar gland (III.5.1.). The **acini** are exclusively serous. The acinar cells (Fig. 2.14.) are a classic example of enzyme-secreting gland cells (II.2.1.1.1.). In contrast to parotid gland serous cells, the basophilic staining property is usually limited to the perinuclear part of the cell (Fig. 4.15.50.). The apical vesicles, or zymogen granules, confer eosinophilic properties to the cytoplasm. These are spherical vesicles with an electron opaque content, the largest of which may reach diameters of more than a micrometer. The proximal part of the **duct** has a tendency to bulge into the acinus, giving rise to a **centroacinar cell** in sections of the acini (Fig. 4.15.50.). Fibrous tissue septa divide the gland into lobes and lobules. The intralobular ducts (amid the acini) and the interlobular ducts (in the septa), are lined with a simple cuboidal to prismatic epithelium (Fig. 4.15.49.), respectively. The cells lining the intralobular ducts show little cytologic specialization. Those lining the interlobular ducts carry microvilli and may contain apical secretory vesicles. The final, widest section of the duct is the pancreatic duct.

The exocrine pancreas is the most important source of digestive enzymes. It secretes trypsin, chymotrypsin, carboxypeptidase, amylase, and lipase. The pancreatic fluid also contributes to the neutralization of the acid stomach contents when these are admitted into the duodenum.

The **endocrine pancreas** consists of isolated cell groups, which are distributed throughout the exocrine pancreatic tissue, with a slight preference for the caudal part: **Langerhans's islets** (Figs. 4.15.49.-50.). It is estimated that the human pancreas contains about a million of them. Each islet can be regarded as a trabecular gland and is made up of a few hundred polyhedral cells, interspersed with sinusoidal capillaries (Fig. 4.15.51.). With routine staining methods, these cells look paler than the exocrine cells, and are a little smaller. They have the cytological structure of peptide-hormone secreting gland cells (II.2.1.1.2.). The two most important hormones are insulin and glucagon, which regulate the blood's glucose level, and are synthesized by different cell types. Again we encounter the phenomenon of a multiple endocrine gland.

Insulin is synthesized and secreted by the **B-cells**, which represent about 75 percent of the total number of islet cells and predominate in the center of the islets. These cells have a relatively dispersed rough endoplasmic reticulum. The dense, crystalline core of the secretory vesicles has a rounded to angular shape and is relatively small, leaving a clear submembraneous halo. In the non-human pancreas, the vesicle core is usually homogeneous and moderately dense (Figs. 4.15.51.-52.). Insulin stimulates the uptake of glucose by the cells of the body and activates the polymerization of glucose to glycogen. Diabetes results from insufficient production of insulin.

Glucagon is synthesized and secreted by the **A-cells**, which represent about 20 percent of the total number of islet cells and predominate at the periphery of the islets. Their rough endoplasmic reticulum has a more compact distribution. The relatively large secretory vesicles have a uniformly dense, rounded core, which almost fills the entire vesicle, leaving only a narrow halo (Fig. 4.15.52.). Glucagon is insulin's antagonist. It stimulates glycogenolysis and the liberation of the resulting glucose.

The islets contain at least two rare cell types. The D-cells are squamous cells, predominating at the edges of the islets and their vesicles show a moderately dense, finely granular core. They secrete somatostatin, which inhibits the secretion of insulin, glucagon, and somatotroph hormone. The PP-cells are likewise squamous peripheral cells, but their secretory vesicles have a denser core. They secrete pancreatic polypeptide, which stimulates the secretion of gastric enzymes and inhibits the excretion of bile, as well as intestinal peristalsis.

References.

Bordi C., D'Adda T., Azzoni C., Ferraro G.: Classification of gastric endocrine cells at the light and electron microscopical levels. Microsc. Res. Tech. 2000, 48: 258-271.

Chen D., Zhao C.M., Andersson K., Meister B., Panula P., Hakanson R.: ECL cell morphology. Yale J. Biol. Med. 1998, 71: 217-231.

De Bleser P.J., Braet F., Lovisetti P., Vanderkerken K., Wisse E., Geerts A.: Cell biology of liver endothelial and Kupffer cells. Gut 1994, 35: 1509-1516.

Egerbacher M., Böck P.: Morphology of the pancreatic duct system in mammals. Microsc. Res. Tech. 1997, 37: 407-417.

Faussoni-Pellegrini M.S.: Histogenesis, structure and relationships of interstitial cells of Cajal (ICC): from morphology to functional interpretation. Eur. J. Morphol. 1992, 30: 137-148.

Gabella G.: Innervation of the gastrointestinal tract. Int. Rev. Cytol. 1979, 59: 130-193.

Gebert A., Rothkötter H.J., Pabst R.: M cells in Peyer's patches of the intestine. Int. Rev. Cytol. 1996, 167: 91-159.

Hand A.R., Pathmanathan D., Field R.B.: Morphological features of the minor salivary glands. Arch. Oral Biol. 1999, S3-S10.

Heel K.A., McCauley R.D., Papadimitriou J.M., Hall J.C.: Review: Peyer's patches. J. Gastroenterol. Hepatol. 1997, 12: 122-136.

Helander H.F.: The cells of the gastric mucosa. Int. Rev. Cytol. 1981, 70: 217-289.

Kanazawa H.: Fine structure of the canine taste bud with special reference to gustatory cell functions. Arch. Histol. Cytol. 1993, 56: 533-548.

Kawada N.: The hepatic perisinusoidal stellate cell. Histol. Histopathol. 1997, 12: 1069-1080.

Komuro T., Seki K., Horiguchi K.: Ultrastructural characterisation of the interstitial cells of Cajal. Arch. Histol. Cytol. 1999, 62: 295-316.

Kobayashi S., Iino S.: Segi's cap: group formation of gut endocrine cells at the tip of the villi in human embryonal intestine. Nagoya J. Med. Sci. 1993, 56: 43-52.

Kraehenbuhl J.P., Neutra M.R.: Epithelial M cells: differentiation and function. Annu. Rev. Cell Dev. Biol. 2000, 16: 301-332.

Mathew J., Geerts A., Burt A.D.: Pathobiology of hepatic stellate cells. Hepatogastroenterol. 1996, 43: 72-91.

Motta P.M., Macchiarelli G., Nottola S.A., Correr S.: Histology of the exocrine pancreas. Microsc. Res. Tech. 1997, 37: 384-398.

Ogata T.: Gastric oxyntic cell structure as related to secretory activity. Histol. Histopathol. 1997, 12: 739-754.

Orci, L., Vassalli J.D., Perrelet A.: The insulin factory. Sci. Am. 1988, september: 50-61.

Pinkstaff C.A.: The cytology of salivary glands. Int. Rev. Cytol. 63: 141-261.

Pinzani M.: Novel insights into the biology and physiology of the Ito cell. Pharmac. Ther. 1995, 66: 387-412.

Redman R.S.: Myoepithelium of salivary glands. Microsc. Res. Techn. 1994, 27: 25-45.

Robinson C., Kirkham J., Shore R.C.: Extracellular matrix of enamel and the ameloblast. Epith. Cell Biol. 1992, 1: 90-97.

Royer S., Kinnamon J.C.: Application of serial sectioning and three-dimensional reconstruction to the study of taste bud ultrastructure and organization. Microsc. Res. Tech. 1994, 29: 381-407.

Ruch J.V., Lesot H., Bègue-Kirn C.: Odontoblast differentiation. Int. J. Dev. Biol. 1995, 39: 51-68.

Rumessen J.J.: Identification of interstitial cells of Cajal. Significance for studies of human small intestine and colon. Dan. Med. Bull. 1994, 41: 275-293.

Sasaki T., Garant P.R.: Structure and organization of odontoblasts. Anat. Rec. 1996, 245: 235-249.

Tandler B.: Structure of mucous cells in salivary glands. Microsc. Res. Tech. 1993, 26: 49-56.

Tandler B.: Structure of the duct system in mammalian major salivary glands. Microsc. Res. Tech. 1993, 26: 57-74.

Tandler B., Phillips C.J.: Structure of serous cells in salivary glands. Microsc. Res. Tech. 1993, 26: 32-48.

Timmermans J.P., Scheuermann D.W., Stach W., Adriaensen D., De Groodt-Lasseel M.H.A.: Functional morphology of the enteric nervous system with special reference to large mammals. Eur. J. Morphol. 1992, 30: 113-122.

Wisse E., Braet F., Luo D., De Zanger R., Jans D., Crabbé E., Vermoesen A.: Structure and function of sinusoidal lining cells in the liver. Toxicol. Pathol. 1996, 24: 100-111.

GLOSSARY.

When the foundations of histology were laid, in the eighteenth and nineteenth centuries, English was not yet the universally accepted language of science it is today. In those days, scientists as a rule taught, published, and corresponded in Latin and classic Greek. Consequently, many terms which are used in histology are derived from these languages. Exceptions exist, but are few in number. This tradition has continued to the present day: several histologic terms exist which have been derived from the classic languages in comparatively recent times. The following list explains how histologic terms were derived, or may have been derived, from the classic languages. Hopefully, knowledge of a term's etymology will help to remember it.

acinus (-ni): Latin **acinus** (berry, many of which form a bunch, like a bunch of grapes). The three-dimensional structure of a compound gland indeed closely resembles a bunch of grapes, the acini being the grapes and the stems the ducts.

acrosome: Greek **acron** (top) and **sooma** (body). The acrosome is a body that lies at the top of the spermatozoon's head.

adamantoblast: Greek **adamas** (unbreakable, hard) and **blastè** (germ). The adamantoblast is a cell of the tooth germ, which produces the hard enamel substance.

adenohypophysis: Greek **adèn** (gland), **hupo** (beneath) en **phuoo** (to grow, or to make grow). The adenohypophysis is a gland that grows on the underside of the brain.

afferent: Latin **affere** (to conduct toward). Afferent (sensory) nerve fibers conduct signals toward the central nervous system. The afferent arterioles conduct blood toward the renal glomeruli.

alveolus (-li): Latin **alveus** (cavity), diminutive alveolus.

amnion: Greek **amnos** (lamb), the membrane which envelops a lamb (goats and sheep still appear to be the most common domestic animals in Greece) at birth.

ampulla (-lae): Latin **ampulla** (a small bottle or jug).

anaphase: Greek **ana** (several meanings: after, further, proper, ...) and **phainoo** (appear). The anaphase is a further stage of mitosis, it appears after the prophase and metaphase, it is the nuclear division proper.

apocrine: Latin **apex** (top) and Greek **krinoo** (to secrete). Secretion mechanism involving loss of the top cell half.

apoptosis: Greek **apo** (from) and **ptosis** (a fall). In cell death by apoptosis, cells never die in large numbers, all at the same time. They die one by one, in small numbers, one here, another one there. This is compared with the falling of leaves in the autumn.

arachnoidea: Greek **arachnion** (spider's web) and **eidos** (looking like something). The arachnoidea is so delicate as to resemble a spider's web.

artefact: Latin **ars** (work of art, handiwork) and **facere** (to make). Something that has not been made by nature, but by man.

arteria: Greek **artèria** (vein).

astrocyte: Greek **astèr** (star) and **kutos** (see cytoplasm).

atretic: Greek **a** (not, no, without) and **tresis** (opening, perforation). An atretic follicle does not show a central cavity.

atrium: Latin **atrium** (A front room, a room which had to be crossed before entering the living rooms proper. In this room, a fire was kept. Consequently, its walls were blackened with soot. The Latin word for black is ater.).

axon: Greek **axon** (axle). The shape of an axon is like a wheel axle.

basophilic: Greek **filein** (to love). Cell structures that are basophilic have a liking for basic stains.

blastocyst: Greek **blastè** (germ) and **kutos** (cavity, urn). The early embryo, or germ, is hollow.

bronchus: Greek **bronchos** (throat, windpipe).

cambium: Latin **cambire** (to exchange). A cambium is an immature tissue which is later replaced with, or exchanged for, a mature tissue.

capillary: Latin **capillus** (hair shaft).

caveola (-lae): Latin **cavus** (hollow).

cell: Latin **cella** (a small room, like a cloister cell).

centriole: Latin **centrum** (center, diminutive centriole).

chondrocyte: Greek **khondros** (granule) and **kutos** (see cytoplasm). When chewed, cartilage feels granular.

chorion: Greek **chorion** (membrane).

choroidea: Greek **chorion** (membrane) and **eidos** (to look like). A membrane that contains numerous blood vessels, and therefore resembles the chorion.

chromatolysis: Greek **chrooma** (color) and **luoo** (to detach, to dissolve). During chromatolysis, the nerve cell loses its staining properties, because the Nissl substance appears to dissolve.

chromosome: Greek **chrooma** (color) and **sooma** (body). Chromosomes may be visualized as distinctly colored cell bodies in the cell.

cilium: Latin **cilium** (eyelash).

cistern: Latin **cisterna** (an underground water tank).

cochlea: Greek **kokhlias** (snail). The cochlea is a spirally wound tube, resembling a snail's shell.

collagen: Greek **kolla** (glue) and **gennan** (to bring forth, to produce). Collagen of bones and hides can be broken down by boiling. The end product is a sticky mixture of amino acids and amino acid-derived molecules, gelatin, which can be used as glue. Therefore, collagen is a "glue maker".

conjunctiva: Latin **conjunctio** (bond, connection).

corium: Latin **corium** (hide, leather). The corium of a mucosa corresponds to the skin's dermis, from which leather can be made.

cornea: Latin **cornu** (horn).

corpora amylacea: Latin **corpus** (body) and Greek **amulon** (starch). The corpora amylacea resemble the starch granules of plant cells.

corpus albicans: see corpora amylacea, and Latin **albus** (white).

corpus ciliare: see corpora amylacea, and Latin **cilium** (eyelash).

corpus luteum: see corpora amylacea, and Latin **luteus** (yellow).

corpus rubrum: see corpora amylacea, and Latin **rubeus** (red).

cortex: Latin **cortex** (bark).

crista: Latin **crista** (crest, cock's comb).

crusta: Latin **crusta** (crust, nutshell).

crypt: Greek **cryptos** (hidden). Lieberkühn's crypts are inpocketings which would be hidden when viewed from the gut's lumen.

cuticula: Latin **cutis** (skin, diminutive cuticula).

cytogen: Greek **kutos** (see cytoplasm) and **gennan** (to bring forth). The cytogen stroma is an interstitial tissue that shows cell proliferation, bringing forth cells.

cytoplasm: Greek **kutos** (cavity, urn) and **plassoo** (to form).

cytotrophoblast: Greek **kutos** (cavity, urn), **trephoo** (to feed) and **blastè** (germ).

decidua: Latin **cadere** (to drop, to decay). The decidua is shed an decays when no embryo is implanted.

deferens: Latin **deferre** (to conduct downwards).

dendrite: Greek **dendron** (tree or bush).

derma: Greek **derma** (skin).

desmosome: Greek **dein** (to bind) and **sooma** (body). The desmosome is a body that binds cells.

diaphysis: Greek **dia** (asunder, through) and **phuoo** (to grow, or to make grow). The diaphysis, when it grows, causes the epiphyses to come asunder.

distal: Latin **dis** (asunder) and **stare** (to stand), to stand asunder. The kidney's distal corpuscles stand asunder from the glomeruli.

duct: Latin **ducere** (to carry, to convey).

duodenum: Latin **duodeni** (twelve). The human duodenum is about twelve finger lengths long.

dura mater: Latin **durus** (hard) and **mater** (mother), literally the "hard mother". This term is a (incorrect?) translation in Latin of an older Arabic term. "Mother" may have to be understood as "protectress" or "nurse".

ectoderm: Greek **ektos** (on the outside) and **derma** (skin).

efferent: Latin **effere** (to conduct away from). Efferent (motor) nerve fibers conduct signals away from the central nervous system. The efferent arterioles conduct blood away from the renal glomeruli.

enchondral: Greek **endon** (within, on the inside) and **khondros** (see chondrocyte).

endocard: see enchondral, and Greek **kardia** (heart).

endoneurium: see enchondral, and Greek **neuron** (see epineurium).

endothelium: see enchondral, and Greek **thèlè** (see epithelium).

endometrium: see enchondral, and Greek **metra** (womb).

endoplasmic: see enchondral, and Greek **plassoo** (see cytoplasm).

endocrine: see enchondral, and Greek **krinoo** (to secrete).

endocytosis: see enchondral, and Greek **kutos** (see cytoplasm).

endoderm: see enchondral, and Greek **derma** (skin).

enterocyt: Greek **enteron** (gut) and **kutos** (see cytoplasm).

ependyma: Greek **ependyma** (coat, tunic).

epicard: Grieks **epi** (on) and **kardia** (heart).

epididymis: see epicard, and Greek **didumis** (twin). An epididymis lies on or against both twins (i.e. the testes).

epineurium: see epicard, and Greek **neuron** (tendon, sinew). It may appear strange that the fibrous tissue that sheaths a nerve should derive its name from a word which means tendon or sinew. However, the perineurium is rich in collagen, and its white color gives nerves, macroscopically, a deceptive likeness to tendons. In classical times, people apparently were not that aware of the difference between the two.

epithelium: see epicard, and Greek **thèlè** (nipple). The epithelium lining the nipples stands out because of its darker pigmentation. Originally, the term "epithelium" exclusively signified the tissue lining the nipples. Later, the significance of this term was extended to include all lining tissues of ecto- and endodermal origin.

epiphysis: see epicard, and Greek **phuoo** (to grow, or to make grow). The epiphysis is a gland growing from the brain's upper side. The epiphysis is that part of a long bone which "grows" on top of the diaphysis.

epidermis: see epicard, and Greek **derma** (skin).

erythrocyte: Greek **eruthros** (red) and **kutos** (see cytoplasm).

erythroblast: Greek **eruthros** (red) en **blastè** (germ).

euchromatic: Greek **eu** (good, well, real, ...) and **chrooma** (color). This term designates the "real" chromatin (which does not stain!), actively involved in protein synthesis.

exocrine: Greek **exoo** (at the outside) and **krinoo** (to secrete). Exocrine glands liberate their secretory products in the outside world.

exocytosis: Greek **exoo** (at the outside) and **kutos** (see cytoplasm). Through exocytosis, substances end up at the cell's exterior.

fenestrated: Latin **fenestra** (window).

focus: Latin **focus** (hearth, fire place). Lenses allow concentration of the sun's rays in a single point, resulting in temperatures sufficiently high to ignite combustible materials, as in a fire place.

follicle: Latin **follis** (leather bag, air-filled pig bladder, diminutive folliculus).

fovea: Latin **fovea** (a pit or well).

fundus: Latin **fundus** (bottom).

fusiform: Latin **fusus** (spindle).

ganglion: Greek **gagglion** (swelling, tumor).

gingiva: Latin **gingiva** (gum).

gland: Latin **glans** (acorn). This term may signify the gland's shape or the smooth outer surface of its fibrous capsule.

glandula: Latin, diminutive of glans.

glia: Greek **glia** (glue). The glia cells "glue" the nerve cells to one another.

glomus: Latin **glomus** (a knot of wool).

glomerulus: Latin, diminutive of glomus.

glycocalyx: Greek **glukeros** (sweet) and **calux** (nutshell, rind). The glycocalyx is a layer of glycoproteins, containing a fraction with the chemical structure of carbohydrates, or sugars, coating the cell membrane.

glycogen: Greek **glukeros** (sweet) and **gennan** (to bring forth). Glycogen is a polymer of glucose, or sugar molecules, which can be liberated when the energy demands of the body require it. In this sense, glycogen brings forth sugar.

hemidesmosome: Greek **hemi** (half), and see desmosome.

heterochromatic: Greek **heteroo** (other, otherwise, other kind, different) and **chrooma** (color). The "other kind" of chromatin is the one that, in contrast to "true" chromatin or euchromatin, is not active in protein synthesis.

histiocyte: Greek **histos** (tissue) and **kutos** (see cytoplasm).

histology: Greek **histos** (tissue) and **logia** (doctrine), from **logos** (word) and **legoo** (to speak)

holocrine: Greek **holos** (wholly, complete) and **krinoo** (to secrete). In this secretion process, a cell's entire content is liberated.

hormone: Greek **hormaoo** (to drive, to incite). Hormones stimulate certain target cells and incite them to a specific action.

hyaline: Greek **hualos** (glass), **hualinos** (glassy).

hypertrophic: Greek **huper** (over, higher, more) and **trephoo** (to feed).

hypodermis: Greek **hypo** (under, beneath) and **derma** (skin).

incus: Latin **incus** (anvil)

infundibulum (-la): Latin **infundibulum** (funnel), from **infundere** (to pour in). The infundibula of the oviduct and the stomach glands are funnel-shaped.

interlobular: Latin **inter** (between)

interstitium: Latin **interstitium** (a space between).

intralobular: Latin **intera** (inside)

iris: Greek **Iris**, the goddess of the rainbow, because of the distinct color of the iris..

jejunum: Latin **jejunus** (an empty stomach). On autopsy or dissection, this gut segment is usually empty

juxtaglomerular: Latin **juxta** (next to one another), and see glomerulus.

keratinocyte: Greek **keras** (horn) and **kutos** (see cytoplasm).

kinetosome: Greek **kineoo** (to move) and **sooma** (body). The kinetosome is a body that forms the basis of the motile cilium.

lamina propria: Latin **lamina** (plate) and **propria** (self, own). The lamina propria is the mucosa's own fibrous tissue support. The other layers, e. g. submucosa, are not taken to belong to the mucosa.

ligament: Latin **ligare** (to bind).

limbus: Latin **limbus** (rim).

lumen: Latin **lumen** (the shining of light). The lumen of various organs is a place where, in theory, light may penetrate.

lysosome: Greek **luoo** (to loosen) and **sooma** (body). Lysosomes are bodies that engage in digestive processes.

macrophage: Greek **macros** (large) and **phagein** (to eat). The macrophage is a "big eater".

macula: Latin **macula** (spot, stain).

malleus: Latin **malleus** (hammer).

mast cell: German **mästen** (to feed, to fatten). Mast cells are filled with granules and look well fed.

matrix: Latin **matrix** (womb, or a female animal kept for breeding purposes). A medium wherein something can grow. The matrix of interstitial, connective, and supportive tissues looks as though it generates cells, or cells grow in it (actually, of course, the reverse is true: the matrix is a product of the cells).

mediastinum: Latin **mediastinus** (a servant of two masters). The mediastinum is an area which contacts several organs, e. g. the testis and the epididymis.

medulla: Latin **medulla** (marrow, as in bone and in plant stems).

megakaryocyte: Greek **megas** (large), **karuon** (nut, see nucleus) and **kutos** (see cytoplasm). The megakaryocyte is a large cell with a prominent nucleus.

melanocyte: Greek **melas** (black) and **kutos** (see cytoplasm).

meninges: Greek **meningx** (membrane).

merocrine: Greek **meros** (part) and **krinoo** (to secrete).

mesenchyme: Greek **mesos** (middle) and **enchuma** (what has been poured in). Mesenchyme fills the spaces between differentiated tissues, as thought it has been poured in.

mesothelium: see mesenchyme, and Greek **thèlè** (see epithelium).

mesoderm: see mesenchyme, and Greek **derma** (skin).

metaphase: Greek **meta** (next, after, behind) and **phainoo** (to appear).

metaphysis: Greek **meta** (see metaphase) and **phuoo** (to grow, or to make grow).

microscope: Greek **micros** (small) and **skopeoo** (to look).

microtome: see microscope, and Greek **temnoo** (to cut).

microtubule: see microscope, and Latin **tubus** (tube), diminutive tubulus.

microvilli: see microscope and villus.

mitochondrion: Greek **mitos** (thread) and **khondros** (granule). The resolving power of the light microscope is insufficient to make out individual mitochondria. They rather appear as beads that touch, forming a string of beads or a kind of "lumpy threads".

mitosis: Greek **mitos** (thread). During mitosis, thread-like chromosomes are formed.

mucosa: Latin **mucus** (slime).

muscle: Latin **mus** (mouse), diminutive musculus. Working muscles move under the skin, which evokes the image of mice scurrying about under a cloth.

myelin: Greek **myelos** (marrow).

myocard: Greek **mus** (muscle) and **kardia** (hart).

myometrium: Greek **mus** (muscle) and **metra** (womb).

nucleus: Latin **nux** (nut).

nucleolus: diminutive of nucleus.

odontoblast: Greek **odons** (tooth) and **blastè** (germ).

oligodendrocyte: Greek **oligos** (small, little), **dendros** (tree, bush) and **kutos** (see cytoplasm): a cell with a small number of branched processes.

organ: Greek **organon** (tool, instrument).

osteoblast: Greek **osteon** (bone) and **blastè** (germ).

osteocyte: see osteoblast, and **kutos** (see cytoplasm).

osteoclast: see osteoblast, and **klastos** (broken).

ovary: Latin **ovum** (egg).

oviduct: see ovary, and **ducere** (to carry, to convey).

papilla: Latin **papilla** (nipple).

pancreas : Greek **pan** (wholly) and **kreas** (flesh). This may refer to the curious fact that the pancreas almost completely lacks a connective tissue capsule.

parafollicular: Greek **para** (next, at, adjoining) and see follicle.

parathyroid: see parafollicular and see thyroid.

parietal: Latin **paries** (wall). The parietal cells of the stomach's fundic glands appear in the walls of the glands (not at the bottom, as the zymogen cells do).

perineurium: Greek **peri** (around) and **neuron** (tendon, sinew, see epineurium).

perimysium: see perineurium, and Greek **mus** (muscle).

pericard: see perineurium, and Greek **kardia** (hart).

perimetrium: see perineurium, and Greek **metra** (womb).

periosteum: see perineurium, and Greek **osteon** (bone).

periodontal: see perineurium, and Greek **odons** (tooth).

phagosome: Greek **phagein** (to eat) and **sooma** (body). The phagosome is an intracellular body that appears when the cell "eats".

pia mater: Latin **pia** (soft) and **mater** (mother), see dura mater.

pineal: Latin **pinea** (pine cone), the pineal gland is shaped like a pine cone.

pinocytosis: Greek **pinein** (to drink) and **kutos** (see cytoplasm). The cell appears to take in fluid droplets.

pituicyte: Latin **pitua** (nose slime) and Greek **kutos** (see cytoplasm). The glandula pituitaria, which is a close association of adenohypophysis and neurohypophysis, lies close to the nasal cavities. For this reason, this gland was once considered the source of nasal mucus.

placenta: Greek **plakous** (a flat cake)

pleura: Greek **pleura** (side, rib).

plexus choroideus: Latin **plectere** (to plaid, to braid) and **choroideus** (resembling the chorion, a membrane with blood vessels).

podocyte: Greek **pous** (foot) and **kutos** (see cytoplasm).

prophase: Greek **pro** (before, first) and **phainoo** (to appear):

prostate: Greek **prostates** (guard), from **proistanai** (to station in front). The prostate stands in front of the urine bladder.

proximal: Latin **proximus** (near, close). The proximal contorted tubules lie near a glomerulus.

pseudostratified: Greek **pseudos** (deceit, lie, and consequently false, untrue), and Latin **stratum** (a layer, what is spread out).

pseudounipolar: see pseudostratified, Latijn **unus** (one) and Greek **polas** (axis).

pseudopodia: see pseudostratified, and Greek **pous** (foot).

pycnotic: Greek **pucnos** (dense, thick)

pylorus: Greek **puloros** (gatekeeper) from **pulè** (gate). The pylorus is the gate or entrance to the small intestine.

rectum: Latin **rectus** (straight).

rete: Latin **rete** (net).

reticulum: diminutive of **rete**.

retina: from rete.

ribosome: from **ribo**nucleic acid and Greek **sooma** (body).

sacculus: Latin **saccus** (sack), diminutive sacculus.

scala tympani: Latin **scala** (ladder, gangway) and see tympanic.

scala vestibuli: see scala tympani and vestibulum.

scala media: see scala tympani, and Latin **medium** (middle).

sclera: Greek **sclèros** (dry, hard).

sebaceous: Latin **sebum** (fat, tallow).

secretion: Latin **secretio** (something that is given off).

septum: Latin **sepes** (hedge). A hedge separates adjoining area's of land, as a septum separates two lobes of an organ.

serosa: Latin **serum** (whey, watery fluid).

serous: see serosa.

sinus: Latin **sinus** (bay). Sinuses are wide, blood-filled spaces.

skeleton: Greek **skellein** (to dry), the "dry" part of the body, in contrast to the "fleshy" parts.

spermatocyte: Greek **sperma** (seed) and **kutos** (see cytoplasm).

spermatogonium: see spermatocyte, and Greek **gennan** (to bring forth).

spermatozoon: see spermatocyte, and Greek **zooön** (animal).

stapes: Latin **stapes** (stirrup).

stereocilia: Greek **stereos** (stiff, hard) and see cilium. A stiff, immotile cilium.

stratum corneum: Latin **stratum** (what is spread out, a layer) and **cornu** (horn).

stratum germinativum: see stratum corneum, and Latin **germinare** (to germinate).

stratum spinosum: see stratum corneum, and Latin **spina** (thorn, spine).

stroma: Greek **stroma** (bed, pillow). Something in or on which something else is resting. The stroma is an interstitial tissue on which other tissues rest, such as the fibrous stroma of lymphoid organs.

subperiostal: Latin **sub** (down, beneath, under) and see periost.

synapse: Greek **sunapsis** (link), from **sun** (together) and **haptein** (to bind, to connect).

syncytium: Greek **sun** (together) and **kutos** (see cytoplasm).

syncytiotrophoblast: see syncitium, and Greek **trephoo** (to feed) and **blastè** (germ).

synovium: Latin **ovum** (egg), synovial fluid resembles egg white.

tectorial: Latin **tectum** (roof). The tectorial membrane is a "roof" over Corti's organ.

telophase: Greek **tèle** (far, end) and **phainoo** (to appear).

tendinocyte: Greek **tenon** (tendon), from **teinein** (to stretch), and **kutos** (see cytoplasm).

testis (-es): Latin **testis** (witness). In Roman law, a man could legally testify only when he was in possession of these organs.

theca: Greek **thèkè** (case, chest).

thrombocyte: Greek **thrombos** (clot, lump) and **kutos** (see cytoplasm).

thymus: Greek **thumos** (hart, soul). The thymus lies near the hart.

thyroid: Greek **thura** (door). May be a reference to the thyroid's flattened aspect.

trabecular: Latin **trabecula** (a small beam).

trachea: Greek **artèria trakheia** (a "rough" blood vessel, rough from the presence of cartilage rings).

tubuli seminiferi: see microtubuli, Latin **semen** (seed) and Greek **pheroo** (to carry, to convey).

tunica adventitia: Latin **tunica** (upper garment, mantle), **ad** (on, at, to) and **venire** (to come). The adventitia is a coating which is added to the other two.

tunica albuginea: see tunica adventitia, Latin **albus** (white) and **gennan** (to bring forth).

tunica intima: see tunica adventitia, and Latin **intimus** (the innermost).

tunica media: see tunica adventitia, and Latin **medium** (middle).

tympanic: Greek **tumpanon** (drum).

uterus: Greek **hustera** (womb).

utriculus: Latin **uter** (leather flask), diminutive utriculus.

vagina: Latin **vagina** (sheath).

vasculosa: Latin **vas** (vessel).

vena: Latin **vena** (vein).

ventricle: Latin **venter** (belly), diminutive ventriculus. A ventricle is an expanded part, like a protruding belly.

vesicle: Latin **vesica** (bladder, blister), diminutive vesicula.

vestibulum: Latin **vestibulum** (fore-court, dedicated to the goddess Vesta).

villus: Latin **villus** (tousled hair).

visceral: Latin **visceris** (entrails).

zona fasciculata: Greek **zoanè** (belt) and Latin **fascis** (bundle), a belt-like zone with a fascicular structure.

zona glomerulosa: see zona fasciculata, and Latin **glomus** (a knot of wool).

zona pellucida: see zona fasciculata, and Latin **pellucidus** (translucent).

zona reticularis: see zona fasciculata, and Latin **rete** (net).

zymogen: Greek **zumè** (ferment, leaven) and **gennan** (to bring forth). Zymogen cells produce ferments, an alternative name for enzymes.

zygote: Greek **zugoo** (to connect two draft animals with a yoke).

The development of the science we call histology, as is the development of any science, has been the work of people. The majority of them are destined to live on as mere author names heading papers in scientific journals. A small number of these investigators have linked their names to the structure they discovered or described for the first time. Only a few are veritable scientific giants, whose work was of such fundamental nature, that it was important not only to histology, but to biological and medical science in general. Some of them earned the highest possible distinction for a scientist: the Nobel prize. Although they might not see themselves as histologists, here is my tribute to those I consider the greatest histologists of all times:

Cajal, Santiago Ramon Y. Petilla de Aragon 1852 - Madrid 1934. Professor of anatomy at Valencia, Barcelona, and Madrid. Here, his name is mentioned in connection with Cajal's cells of the visceral muscle tissue of the intestine. Cajal did not at all limit himself to this aspect of histology, however. His enormous merit for histology, and for biomedical science in general, lies in his fundamental research on the microscopic structure of the nervous system. He was one of the first and foremost proponents of the neuron theory, which states that nervous tissue is not a syncytium, but that it is composed of separate nerve cells. This may be obvious to us now, but it was not at all obvious in Cajal's days. His work was considered to be of such fundamental importance, and of such enormous consequence, that it earned him the 1906 Nobel prize in Medicine and Physiology, which he shared with another giant of histology, Camillo Golgi.

Golgi, Camillo. Corteno 1844 - Pavia 1926. Professor at the university of Pavia. He developed a staining method for nervous tissue, involving impregnation with silver salts, which carries his name. This technique only stains a fraction of the nerve cells present, but stains them in their entirety. With this method, the histological investigation of nervous tissue was greatly facilitated. It enabled him to demonstrate that nervous tissue was composed of separate cells, a decisive argument in favor of the neuron theory. In addition, his discoveries hinted at the way in which nerve cells were interconnected. This work earned him the 1906 Nobel prize in Medicine and Physiology, together with Cajal.

During his work on nervous tissue, he incidentally noticed a vesicular structure next to the nucleus of nerve cells, which he described as a "reticular apparatus". Decades later, electron microscopy demonstrated that this reticular apparatus is a membranous organelle, which we now know as the Golgi-complex. And so, Golgi became the only scientist after whom an organelle of first-rank importance is named.

Malpighi, Marcello. Bologna 1628 - Rome 1694. Professor at Bologna, Pisa and Messina, court physician to pope Innocent XII, honorary fellow of the Royal Society. Malpighi was one of the founders of modern biomedical science. He discovered the capillaries, linked his name to Malpighian epithelium and did fundamental research in entomology, embryology, physiology, and botany.

Purkinje, Jan Evangelista. Libochovice 1787 - Prague 1869. Professor of physiology at Prague and Breslau (Poland). Purkinje developed the microtome, as well as a number of additional devices and preparation techniques, essential to microscopic investigation. Purkinje cells of the hart and the cerebellum.

Schwann, Theodor. Neuss 1810 - Cologne 1882. Professor of anatomy at Leuven and Liège (Belgium). Schwann's great merit is his formulation, together with the botanist Schleiden, of the cell theory. This theory states that the cell is the fundamental building block of living beings. To us, this may be glaringly obvious, but it took years of precise observation, careful reasoning, and considerable argumentation to prove beyond doubt that this theory accurately described reality. He also worked on the microscopic structure of the nervous system. Schwann's cell of the nervous tissue.

A few additional names deserve mention.

Leeuwenhoek, Antonie van. Delft 1632 - 1723. Van Leeuwenhoek was a Dutch cloth merchant, without any formal training as a scientist. His hobby was the grinding of lenses. This led him to designing and building the first microscopes. His numerous observations and discoveries include the spermatozoa, the erythrocytes, and the microorganisms (bacteria and protozoa). He corresponded with the Royal Society of London and the Academie des Sciences of Paris.

Ruska, Ernst. Heidelberg 1906 - Berlin 1988. Ruska was an electrical engineer who, in 1933, developed the first working model of the electron microscope. The first commercial model he would built at the Siemens firm in 1939. But then the normal course of things was brutally interrupted for 5 years, and it would be more than a decade later, in the early fifties of the 20th century, before the electron microscope would come in widespread use. Contrary to the rocket engine and the nuclear bomb, the development of the electron microscope does not seem to have greatly benefited from the second world war. As a rather late recognition of his scientific merits, Ruska shared the 1986 Nobel prize in Physics with Rohrer and Binnig, the inventors of the scanning tunneling microscope, a device which makes use of some exotic quantum mechanical phenomena to detect single atoms.

INDEX.

Glycocalyx: 44
Glycogen: 35, 49, 167, 232
Glycolipids: 12
Glycolysis: 18
Glycosaminoglycans: 75
Goblet cells: 30, 269, 292
Goiter: 177
Golgi-complex: 28, 30
Gonadotroph cells: 176
Goormaghtig's cells: 192
Granular component of nucleolus: 17
Granular layer, keratinized epithelium: 98
Granular layer, cerebellar cortex: 155
Granulocytes: 65
Granulocytes, eosinophilic: 34, 66, 292
Granulocytes, neutrophilic: 34, 65
Granulocytes, basophilic: 66
Granulomere: 64
Granulosa cells: 226
Granulosa lutein cells: 37, 229
Gray matter: 153
Ground substance: 70, 75
Growth, appositional: 81
Growth, axial: 138
Growth, diametric: 138
Growth, epiphyseal: 139
Growth, interstitial: 80
Growth, longitudinal: 138
Growth plate: 138
Growth, subperiosteal: 135

Hair cells: 257, 260, 261
Hairs: 202
Hassal's bodies: 127
Havers's columns: 84, 138
H-band: 47
Heart: 165
Helper T-cells: 68
Hematoxylin: 7
Hemidesmosome: 98, 238, 281
Hemocytoblast: 60
Hemoglobin: 62
Henle's loops: 189
Hensen's disk: 47
Heparan sulfate: 75
Hepatocytes: 298
Herring bodies: 161
Heterochromatin: 17
High endothelial venules: 130
Histamine: 290
Histiocytes: 34, 74, 292
Histochemistry: 8
Histocompatibility antigens: 14
Holocrine: 35, 202
Horizontal cells: 247

Howship's lacuna: 83
Humoral immunity: 69
Hyaline cartilage: 80, 270
Hyalomere: 64
Hyaluronic acid: 75
Hybridochemistry: 8
Hypodermis: 205
Hypothalamic nuclei: 175
Hypothalamo-hypophyseal tractus: 175
Hypothalamus: 155

I-band: 46, 47
Ileum: 294
Immunity, cellular: 68
Immunity: humoral: 69
Immunochemistry: 8
Immunoglobulins: 68, 292
Incus: 254
Induction: 114
Infundibulum: 229
Inner plexiform layer: 246
Inner granular layer: 246
Insulin: 303
Intercalated disks: 88
Intercalated ducts: 283
Interdigitating cells: 132
Intermediary filaments: 44, 50, 52
Intermediary junction: 93
Internal root sheath, hair: 203
Interstitial cells of Cajal: 296
Interstitial cells, ovary: 37, 228
Interstitial tissue: 70, 79
Intervertebral disk: 141
Intestine: 286
Intima: 165
Intrafusal fibers: 145
Intraperiodic line: 112
Iodium: 177
Iris: 242
Isthmus: 229

Jejunum: 290
Joints: 142
Junctional complex: 93
Junctions: 87, 90
Juxtaglomerular apparatus: 191
Juxtaglomerular cells: 191

Karyoplasm: 17
Keratan sulfate: 75
Keratin: 51, 98
Keratinized layer: 99
Keratinocytes: 51, 98
Keratinosomes: 98

Respiratory chain: 19
Respiratory system: 263
Resting potential: 13
Rete testis: 217
Reticular tissue: 79
Reticulin fibers: 77
Reticuloblast: 71
Retina: 244
Retrograde transport: 53
Ribosomes: 18, 23
RNA: 15
Rod cells: 247
Rough endoplasmic reticulum: 23, 24, 26, 28, 53
Round window: 254
Ruffini's corpuscles: 206

Saccule: 254
Salivary glands: 283
Saltatory conduction: 114
Satellite cells of muscle tissue: 88
Satellite cells of sensory ganglia: 149
Scala media: 255
Scala tympani: 255
Scala vestibuli: 255
Schlemm's canal: 244
Schmidt-Lantermann clefts: 112
Schwann cell: 110
Sebum gland cells: 35
Sebum glands: 201
Secretin: 292
Secretory vesicles: 24, 25, 30, 66, 74, 176, 179, 182
Sections: 6
Segi's caps: 292
Semicircular canals: 254
Seminal vesicles: 219
Seminiferous tubules: 210
Serotonin: 64, 120, 290, 292
Serous: 25, 283
Sertoli's cells: 216
Sharpey's fibers: 144
SIF-cells: 152
Sinus: 103
Sinus, cortical: 130
Sinus, medullary: 130
Sinus, subcapsular: 130
Sinuses, splenic: 133
Sinusoids, hepatic: 298
Skeleton: 135
Skin: 195
Skin glands: 198
Slavjanski's membrane: 227
Small intestine: 290
Smooth endoplasmic reticulum: 35, 50, 182, 229
Sodium: 13, 182, 189, 198
Somatostatin: 290, 303

Somatotroph cells: 176
Spermatids: 214
Spermatocytes, primary: 212
Spermatocytes, secondary: 214
Spermatogenic cells: 212
Spermatogonia: 212
Spermatozoa: 214
Sphincter: 296
Spinal cord: 151,153
Spine, dendritic: 119
Spleen: 132
Spongious zone of endometrium: 232
Spongy bone: 84
Stains: 7
Stapes: 254
Stellate cells, hepatic: 300
Steroid droplets: 36
Stereocilia: 219, 257, 261
Stomach: 288
Stratum corneum: 99
Stratum germinativum: 98
Stratum granulosum: 98
Stratum spinosum: 98
Stretch receptor: 270
Striated ducts: 284
Stroma, of iris: 242
Stroma, of cornea: 238
Sublingual gland: 283
Submandibular gland: 283
Submucosal glands: 270, 292
Substance P: 121
Substantia nigra: 154
Summation: 117
Supporting cells: 51, 171, 258, 272, 286
Supportive tissue: 70
Suppressor T-cells: 68
Surfactant: 267
Sweat glands: 198
Sympathetic: 151
Synapse: 117
Synapses, afferent: 171
Synapses, axoaxonal: 119
Synapses, axodendritic: 119
Synapses, axosomatic: 118
Synapses, efferent: 171
Synaptic cleft: 118, 144
Synaptic rod: 249, 257, 258, 261
Synaptic vesicles: 118, 144, 156
Syncytiotrophoblast: 173
Syncytium: 46, 173
Synovium: 142

Taenia coli: 294
Taste buds: 284
Taste cells: 284